MEDICINE

A PRIMARY CARE

APPROACH

MEDICINE

A PRIMARY CARE

APPROACH

RICHARD H. RUBIN, M.D.
Assistant Professor, Division of General Medicine
University of New Mexico Health Sciences Center
Albuquerque, New Mexico

CAROLYN VOSS, M.D.
Assistant Professor and Associate Chief, Division of General Medicine
University of New Mexico Health Sciences Center
Albuquerque, New Mexico

DANIEL J. DERKSEN, M.D.
Associate Professor, Department of Family and Community Medicine
University of New Mexico Health Sciences Center
Albuquerque, New Mexico

ANN GATELEY, M.D.
Associate Professor and Residency Program Director, Department of Medicine
University of New Mexico Health Sciences Center
Albuquerque, New Mexico

RONALD W. QUENZER, M.D.
Professor of Medicine
Vice-Chair and Director of Clinical Affairs
Co-chief, Division of General Medicine
University of New Mexico Health Sciences Center
Albuquerque, New Mexico

W.B. SAUNDERS COMPANY
A Division of Harcourt Brace & Company
Philadelphia London Toronto Montreal Sydney Tokyo

W.B. SAUNDERS COMPANY
A Division of Harcourt Brace & Company

The Curtis Center
Independence Square West
Philadelphia, Pennsylvania 19106

Library of Congress Cataloging-in-Publication Data

Medicine: a primary care approach / [edited by] Richard H. Rubin . . .
[et al.].—1st ed.

p.   cm.

ISBN 0–7216–5200–X

1. Primary care (Medicine)   I. Rubin, Richard H.
[DNLM: 1. Primary Health Care.   W 84.6 M4891 1996]

RC46.M4752   1996   616—dc20
DNLM/DLC   95–21763

MEDICINE: A PRIMARY CARE APPROACH   ISBN 0–7216–5200–X

Printed in the United States of America

Last digit is the print number: 9   8   7   6   5   4   3   2   1

To

Joan, Greg, Daniel, and Ken

Dr. Virgil H. Voss

Krista, Shannon, and John

Dr. Harry L. Greene

Ginny, Barth, Branson, and Nick

Our teachers, colleagues, students, and patients

CONTRIBUTORS

SARAH E. ALLEN, M.D.
Assistant Professor of Medicine, Divisions of
General Medicine and Infectious Diseases,
University of New Mexico Health Sciences Center,
Albuquerque, New Mexico
Prevention of Infectious Diseases

SANJEEV ARORA, M.D.
Associate Professor of Medicine and Chief, Section
of Gastroenterology, University Hospital, University
of New Mexico Health Sciences Center,
Albuquerque, New Mexico
Inflammatory Bowel Disease

AMANDA A. BECK, M.D., Ph.D.
Assistant Professor of Medicine, Division of
Geriatrics and Sleep Disorder Center, University of
New Mexico Health Sciences Center, Albuquerque,
New Mexico
Insomnia

THOMAS M. BECKER, M.D., Ph.D.
Associate Professor of Medicine, Division of
Epidemiology and Preventive Medicine, University
of New Mexico Health Sciences Center,
Albuquerque, New Mexico
Prevention of Cancer

DAVID A. BENNAHUM, M.D.
Professor of Medicine and Family and Community
Medicine, University of New Mexico Health
Sciences Center, Albuquerque, New Mexico
Ethical Issues in Outpatient Medicine

CARL BETTINGER, M.D., J.D.
Clinical Assistant Professor of Medicine, University
of New Mexico Health Sciences Center,
Albuquerque; Shapiro and Bettinger, Albuquerque,
New Mexico
Legal Issues in Outpatient Medicine

CARL BIGLER, M.D.
Private practice, Flagstaff, Arizona
*Drug Rashes; Viral Infections of the Skin; Bacterial
Infections of the Skin; Fungal Infections of the Skin;
Melanoma*

ASKIEL BRUNO, M.D.
Associate Professor and Director, Indiana Stroke
Center, Department of Neurology, Indiana
University School of Medicine, Indianapolis,
Indiana
Unilateral Weakness or Numbness

IRENE J. BUÑO, M.D.
Resident in Dermatology, University of Colorado
Health Sciences Center, Denver, Colorado
Psoriasis

MARK R. BURGE, M.D.
Instructor in Medicine, Division of Endocrinology,
University of New Mexico Health Sciences Center,
Albuquerque, New Mexico
Hypercalcemia

JANETTE S. CARTER, M.D.
Assistant Professor of Medicine, Division of General
Medicine, University of New Mexico Health
Sciences Center; Attending Physician, Veterans
Administration Medical Center, Albuquerque, New
Mexico
Diabetes Mellitus; Team Approach to Chronic Care

KARA L. CATTON, R.D., C.D.E.
Ambulatory Care Dietician, Veterans Administration
Medical Center, Albuquerque, New Mexico
Team Approach to Chronic Care

DAVID B. COULTAS, M.D.
Associate Professor of Medicine and Chief, Division of Epidemiology and Preventive Medicine, University of New Mexico Health Sciences Center, Albuquerque, New Mexico
Prevention of Pulmonary Disease; Tobacco Use

MICHAEL H. CRAWFORD, M.D.
Robert S. Flinn Professor and Chief, Division of Cardiology, University of New Mexico Health Sciences Center, Albuquerque, New Mexico
Congestive Heart Failure

RICHARD E. CROWELL, M.D.
Associate Professor of Medicine, University of New Mexico Health Sciences Center; Chief, Pulmonary Section, Veterans Administration Medical Center, Albuquerque, New Mexico
Hemoptysis

BEN DAITZ, M.D.
Associate Professor of Family and Community Medicine, University of New Mexico Health Sciences Center, Albuquerque, New Mexico
Neck Pain; Leg Pain

LARRY E. DAVIS, M.D.
Professor of Neurology and Microbiology, University of New Mexico Health Sciences Center; Chief, Neurology Service, Veterans Administration Medical Center, Albuquerque, New Mexico
Dizziness and Vertigo

ROBERT D. DEFRANG, M.D.
Assistant Professor of Surgery, Division of Vascular Surgery, University of New Mexico Health Sciences Center, Albuquerque, New Mexico
Arterial Insufficiency of the Legs

DANIEL J. DERKSEN, M.D.
Associate Professor of Family and Community Medicine, University of New Mexico Health Sciences Center, Albuquerque, New Mexico
Diarrhea

MAXINE H. DORIN, M.D.
Associate Professor of Obstetrics and Gynecology, University of New Mexico Health Sciences Center, Albuquerque, New Mexico
Vaginal Bleeding; Amenorrhea and Other Menstrual Abnormalities

RICHARD I. DORIN, M.D.
Associate Professor of Medicine and Biochemistry, University of New Mexico Health Sciences Center; Chief, Endocrinology Section, Veterans Administration Medical Center, Albuquerque, New Mexico
Glucocorticoid Therapy

DOUGLAS EGLI, M.D.
Assistant Professor of Medicine, Division of General Medicine, University of New Mexico Health Sciences Center, Albuquerque, New Mexico
Effective Use of the Telephone in Outpatient Practice; Prostate Disorders

DENISE A. FARNATH, M.D.
Assistant Professor of Ophthalmology, University of New Mexico Health Sciences Center, Albuquerque, New Mexico
The Red Eye; Common Disorders of Vision

JERRY FELDMAN, M.D.
Assistant Professor of Dermatology, University of New Mexico Health Sciences Center, Albuquerque, New Mexico
Acne; Psoriasis; Contact Dermatitis; Urticaria; Nonmelanoma Skin Cancer

LAURA M. FERRIES, M.D.
Private practice, Sheridan, Wyoming
Glucocorticoid Therapy

WALTER B. FORMAN, M.D.
Professor of Medicine, University of New Mexico Health Sciences Center; Associate Chief of Staff, Geriatrics/Extended Care, Veterans Administration Medical Center, Albuquerque, New Mexico
Approach to the Cancer Patient in the Primary Care Setting

DANA FOTIEO, M.D.
Assistant Professor of Medicine, Division of General Medicine, University of New Mexico Health Sciences Center, Albuquerque, New Mexico
Jaundice and Liver Function Abnormalities

GREGORY G. FOTIEO, M.D.
Assistant Professor of Medicine, Division of General Medicine, University of New Mexico Health Sciences Center; Attending Physician, Veterans Administration Medical Center, Albuquerque, New Mexico
Involuntary Weight Loss

LUCY FOX, M.D.
Clinical Assistant Professor of Medicine, University of New Mexico Health Sciences Center; Chief, Division of Nephrology, Lovelace Health Systems, Albuquerque, New Mexico
Dysuria and Urinary Tract Infections

ANN GATELEY, M.D.

Associate Professor of Medicine, Division of
General Medicine, and Residency Program Director,
Department of Medicine, University of New Mexico
Health Sciences Center; Attending Physician,
Veterans Administration Medical Center,
Albuquerque, New Mexico
Obesity

MICHAEL W. GAVIN, M.D.

Hanover Medical Specialists, Wilmington, North
Carolina
Acute Pancreatitis; Chronic Pancreatitis; Gallstones

FRANK D. GILLILAND, M.D., Ph.D.

Assistant Professor of Medicine, Division of
Epidemiology and Preventive Medicine, University
of New Mexico Health Sciences Center,
Albuquerque, New Mexico
Occupational and Environmental Disorders

NONA M. GIRARDI, M.D.

Clinical Instructor, Department of Family and
Community Medicine, University of New Mexico
Health Sciences Center; Attending Physician,
Albuquerque Family Health Center, Albuquerque,
New Mexico
Nausea and Vomiting

HOWARD K. GOGEL, M.D.

Adjunct Professor of Medicine, University of
New Mexico Health Sciences Center; Southwest
Gastroenterology Associates, Albuquerque, New
Mexico
*Dysphagia and Odynophagia; Upper Gastrointestinal
Bleeding*

DAVID V. GONZALES, M.D.

Assistant Professor of Medicine, Division of General
Medicine, University of New Mexico Health
Sciences Center, Albuquerque, New Mexico
Lower Gastrointestinal Bleeding

GARY M. GREENBERG, M.D.

Assistant Professor of Medicine, Division of
Cardiology, and Director, Arrhythmia and
Pacemaker Service, University of New Mexico
Health Sciences Center, Albuquerque, New Mexico
Palpitations and Arrhythmias

ALAN K. HALPERIN, M.D.

Professor of Medicine, Division of General
Medicine, Case Western Reserve School of
Medicine; Research Director, Division of General
Medicine, Cleveland Clinic Foundation, Cleveland,
Ohio
Clinical Reasoning; Hypertension

WILLIAM R. HARDY, M.D.

Professor of Medicine, Division of General
Medicine, Associate Professor of Pathology,
University of New Mexico Health Sciences Center,
Albuquerque, New Mexico
Anemia; Bleeding Disorders

FRED HASHIMOTO, M.D.

Professor of Medicine, Division of General
Medicine, University of New Mexico Health
Sciences Center, Albuquerque, New Mexico
The Use and Misuse of Medical Tests

FRED S. HERZON, M.D.

Professor and Chief, Division of Otolaryngology,
University of New Mexico Health Sciences Center,
Albuquerque, New Mexico
*Ear Pain; Hearing Loss and Tinnitus; Rhinorrhea and
Nasal Stuffiness; Epistaxis*

MARTIN E. HICKEY, M.D.

Adjunct Associate Professor of Medicine, University
of New Mexico Health Sciences Center; Senior Vice
President and Chief Medical Officer, Lovelace
Health Systems, Albuquerque, New Mexico
Cost-Effective Approach to Primary Care Practice

MICHAEL HOLLIFIELD, M.D.

Assistant Professor of Psychiatry, University of
New Mexico Health Sciences Center, Albuquerque,
New Mexico
The Somatizing Patient

ANDREW C. HSI, M.D., M.P.H.

Assistant Professor of Pediatrics, Director of
Newborn Nursery and Director of Los Pasos
Program, University Hospital, University of
New Mexico Health Sciences Center, Albuquerque,
New Mexico
Developmental-Behavioral Issues in Pediatrics

LOURDES M. IRIZARRY, M.D.

Assistant Professor of Medicine, Division of
Infectious Diseases, University of New Mexico
Health Sciences Center; Attending Physician,
Veterans Administration Medical Center,
Albuquerque, New Mexico
Fever

M. MAZEN JAMAL, M.D.

Assistant Professor of Medicine, Division of
Gastroenterology, University of New Mexico Health
Sciences Center, Albuquerque, New Mexico
Diverticular Disease

DAVID S. JAMES, M.D.
Assistant Professor of Medicine, Division of Pulmonary Medicine, University of New Mexico Health Sciences Center; Attending Physician, Veterans Administration Medical Center, Albuquerque, New Mexico
Asthma and Chronic Obstructive Pulmonary Disease

LESLEY W. JANIS, M.D.
Assistant Professor of Medicine, Division of General Medicine, University of New Mexico Health Sciences Center; Director, Women's Health Clinic, Veterans Administration Medical Center, Albuquerque, New Mexico
Prevention of Osteoporosis; Vaginitis; Menopause and Postmenopausal Symptoms

DOUGLAS R. JEFFERY, M.D., Ph.D.
Assistant Professor of Neurology, Bowman Gray School of Medicine, Winston-Salem, North Carolina
Seizure Disorders

CURTIS O. KAPSNER, M.D.
Associate Professor of Medicine, Division of General Medicine, and Vice-Chair for Education, Department of Medicine, University of New Mexico Health Sciences Center; Attending Physician, Veterans Administration Medical Center, Albuquerque, New Mexico
Hematuria; Kidney Stones

PATRICIA KAPSNER, M.D.
Associate Professor of Medicine, Division of General Medicine, University of New Mexico Health Sciences Center, Albuquerque, New Mexico
Thyroid Disorders

SUSANNA J. KEARNY, B.A.
Program Specialist, University of New Mexico Health Sciences Center, Albuquerque, New Mexico
Cultural Considerations in Primary Care

MOLLY K. KING, M.D.
Assistant Professor of Neurology, University of New Mexico Health Sciences Center; Director, Neurophysiology Laboratory, Veterans Administration Medical Center, Albuquerque, New Mexico
Unilateral Weakness or Numbness

MARK LANGSFELD, M.D.
Assistant Professor of Surgery, Division of Vascular Surgery, University of New Mexico Health Sciences Center, Albuquerque, New Mexico
Arterial Insufficiency of the Legs

CAROL M.J. LARROQUE, M.D.
Assistant Professor of Psychiatry, University of New Mexico Health Sciences Center, Albuquerque, New Mexico
Depression

CHI CHI LAU, M.D.
Assistant Professor of Medicine, Division of Rheumatology, University of New Mexico Health Sciences Center, Albuquerque, New Mexico
Generalized Achiness

LYDIA LAWSON, M.D.
Lovelace Health Systems, Albuquerque, New Mexico
Contraception

JOHN LEGGOTT, M.D.
Assistant Professor of Family and Community Medicine, University of New Mexico Health Sciences Center, Albuquerque, New Mexico
Screening for Disease

MARK D. LEHMAN, M.D.
Chief Resident, Division of Dermatology, University of New Mexico Health Sciences Center, Albuquerque, New Mexico
Bacterial Infections of the Skin

EDWARD N. LIBBY, M.D.
Assistant Professor of Medicine, Division of General Medicine, University of New Mexico Health Sciences Center, Albuquerque, New Mexico
Knee Pain

JONATHAN LISANSKY, M.D.
Associate Professor of Psychiatry, University of New Mexico Health Sciences Center; Associate Chief, Psychiatry Consultation and Liaison Service, Veterans Administration Medical Center, Albuquerque, New Mexico
Anxiety

BARBARA LUDWIG, Q.M.R.P., L.P.C.
Director, Transdisciplinary Evaluation and Support Clinic, Department of Family and Community Medicine, University of New Mexico Health Sciences Center, Albuquerque, New Mexico
Patients With Chronic Disability

F. CLAUDE MANNING, M.D.
Private practice, Everett, Washington
Dementia; Special Problems in the Elderly

ELAINE MARCUS, M.D.
Assistant Professor of Family and Community Medicine, University of New Mexico Health Sciences Center, Albuquerque, New Mexico
Hemorrhoids and Other Common Anorectal Disorders

MELISSA MARTINEZ, M.D.
Clinical Assistant Professor of Family and
Community Medicine, University of New Mexico
Health Sciences Center; Clinical Supervisor,
Albuquerque Family Health Center, Albuquerque,
New Mexico
Abdominal Pain

MARC MASOTTI, M.D.
Chief Resident, Department of Medicine, University
of New Mexico Health Sciences Center; Veterans
Administration Medical Center, Albuquerque, New
Mexico
Jaundice and Liver Function Abnormalities

MELVINA McCABE, M.D.
Assistant Professor of Family and Community
Medicine, University of New Mexico Health
Sciences Center, Albuquerque, New Mexico
Cultural Considerations in Primary Care

DENIS M. McCARTHY, M.D. M.Sc.
Professor of Medicine and Chief, Division of
Gastroenterology, University of New Mexico Health
Sciences Center; Chief, Gastroenterology Service,
Veterans Administration Medical Center,
Albuquerque, New Mexico
Peptic Ulcer Disease; Gastroesophageal Reflux

TERESITA McCARTY, M.D.
Assistant Professor of Psychiatry and Chief,
Psychiatry Consultation Service, University
Hospital, University of New Mexico Health Sciences
Center, Albuquerque, New Mexico
The Difficult Patient

CHRISTOPHER A. McGREW, M.D.
Assistant Professor of Family and Community
Medicine, Assistant Professor of Orthopedics and
Rehabilitation, University of New Mexico Health
Sciences Center, Albuquerque, New Mexico
Shoulder Pain

MARTHA COLE McGREW, M.D.
Assistant Professor of Family and Community
Medicine, University of New Mexico Health
Sciences Center, Albuquerque, New Mexico
Prenatal Care

CARYN McHARNEY-BROWN, M.D.
Assistant Professor of Family and Community
Medicine, University of New Mexico Health
Sciences Center; Medical Director, Southeast
Heights Center for Family Health, Albuquerque,
New Mexico
The Abnormal Pap Test

CELIA A. MICHAEL, Ph.D.
Adjunct Assistant Professor of Psychiatry,
University of New Mexico Health Sciences Center;
Director of Behavioral Medicine, Veterans
Administration Medical Center, Albuquerque, New
Mexico
Alcohol and Substance Abuse

GLEN H. MURATA, M.D.
Professor of Medicine, University of New Mexico
Health Sciences Center; Chief, Division of General
Medicine, Veterans Administration Medical Center,
Albuquerque, New Mexico
Chest Pain; Headache

BETTY NEWVILLE, M.D.
Private practice, Albuquerque, New Mexico
Dyspnea

CAROL Y. NISHIKUBO, M.D.
Chief Resident, Department of Medicine, University
of New Mexico Health Sciences Center; Veterans
Administration Medical Center, Albuquerque,
New Mexico
Irritable Bowel Syndrome

LARRY A. OSBORN, M.D.
Associate Professor of Medicine, Division of
Cardiology, University of New Mexico Health
Sciences Center, Albuquerque, New Mexico
Syncope

TOBY B. PALLEY, M.D.
Assistant Professor of Family and Community
Medicine, University of New Mexico Health
Sciences Center, Albuquerque, New Mexico
Constipation

JAMES R. PHELPS, M.D.
Staff Psychiatrist, Samaritan Mental Health, Good
Samaritan Hospital, Corvallis, Oregon
Facilitating Patient Adherence

RONALD W. QUENZER, M.D.
Professor and Vice-Chair for Clinical Affairs,
Department of Medicine, and Co-chief, Division of
General Medicine, University Hospital, University of
New Mexico Health Sciences Center, Albuquerque,
New Mexico
Bronchitis and Pneumonia

VEENA RAIZADA, M.D.
Professor of Medicine, Division of Cardiology,
University of New Mexico Health Sciences Center,
Albuquerque, New Mexico
Murmurs and Valvular Heart Disease

MICHAEL T. REED, Pharm.D.
Associate Professor of Clinical Pharmacy, Arnold and Marie Schwartz College of Pharmacy and Health Sciences, Long Island University, Brooklyn, New York; Drug Therapy Consultant, Medical Intensive Care Unit, Mt. Sinai Hospital and Medical Center, New York, New York
Prevention of Adverse Drug Reactions

ESTHER P. REINHARDT, R.N., C.D.E.
Diabetes Educator, Veterans Administration Medical Center, Albuquerque, New Mexico
Team Approach to Chronic Care

LAURA WEISS ROBERTS, M.D.
Assistant Professor of Psychiatry, University of New Mexico Health Sciences Center, Albuquerque, New Mexico
The Difficult Patient

GLENN C. ROBINSON, M.D.
Private practice, Coeur d'Alene, Idaho
Hepatitis

RICHARD J. ROCHE, M.D.
Assistant Professor of Medicine, Division of Geriatrics, Director, Geriatric Evaluation and Management Unit, University of New Mexico Health Sciences Center, Albuquerque, New Mexico
Special Problems in the Elderly

RICHARD H. RUBIN, M.D.
Assistant Professor of Medicine, Division of General Medicine, University of New Mexico Health Sciences Center, Albuquerque, New Mexico
Differences Between Inpatient and Outpatient Medicine; Chronic Cough

MARK C. SADDLER, M.D.
Private practice, Farmington, New Mexico
Proteinuria; Chronic Renal Failure

JOHN H. SAIKI, M.D.
Professor of Medicine, Division of Hematology and Oncology, University of New Mexico Health Sciences Center, Albuquerque, New Mexico
Breast Disorders; Lymphadenopathy and Splenomegaly

KERRIE R. SEEGER, M.D.
Assistant Professor of Family and Community Medicine, University of New Mexico Health Sciences Center, Albuquerque, New Mexico
Patients With Chronic Disability

BRUCE K. SHIVELY, M.D.
Associate Professor of Medicine, University of New Mexico Health Sciences Center; Chief, Cardiology

Section, Veterans Administration Medical Center, Albuquerque, New Mexico
Leg Edema

WILMER L. SIBBITT, JR., M.D.
Professor of Medicine, Division of Rheumatology, University of New Mexico Health Sciences Center, Albuquerque, New Mexico
Approach to the Patient With Arthritis

BARBARA E. SMALL, M.D.
Assistant Professor of Pediatrics and Director, General Ambulatory Services, Department of Pediatrics, University of New Mexico Health Sciences Center, Albuquerque, New Mexico
Common Pediatric Infections

DONALD E. STEHR, M.D.
Associate Professor of Medicine, Division of General Medicine, University of New Mexico Health Sciences Center; Attending Physician, Veterans Administration Medical Center, Albuquerque, New Mexico
Chronic Pain

PETER G. STEIN, M.D.
Assistant Professor of Family and Community Medicine, University of New Mexico Health Sciences Center, Albuquerque, New Mexico
Sore Throat

VICTOR C. STRASBURGER, M.D.
Associate Professor of Pediatrics, Chief, Division of Adolescent Medicine, University of New Mexico Health Sciences Center, Albuquerque, New Mexico
Special Problems in Adolescents

CRAIG TIMM, M.D.
Assistant Professor of Medicine, Division of Cardiology, and Director, Cardiac Catheterization Laboratory, University of New Mexico Health Sciences Center, Albuquerque, New Mexico
Prevention of Coronary Artery Disease; Coronary Artery Disease

BERTHOLD E. UMLAND, M.D.
Associate Professor and Residency Program Director, Department of Family and Community Medicine, University of New Mexico Health Sciences Center, Albuquerque, New Mexico
The Patient in the Context of the Family, the Community, and Society

CHRISTOPHER E. URBINA, M.D., M.P.H.
Assistant Professor of Family and Community Medicine, University of New Mexico Health Sciences Center, Albuquerque, New Mexico
Cultural Considerations in Primary Care; Prevention of Injuries

B. SYLVIA VELA, M.D.
Assistant Professor of Medicine, Division of Endocrinology, University of New Mexico Health Sciences Center; Attending Physician, Veterans Administration Medical Center, Albuquerque, New Mexico
Hyperlipidemia; Male Sexual Dysfunction

ALBERT V. VOGEL, M.D.
Associate Professor of Psychiatry, University of New Mexico Health Sciences Center, Albuquerque, New Mexico
The Somatizing Patient

CAROLYN VOSS, M.D.
Assistant Professor of Medicine and Associate Chief, Division of General Medicine, University Hospital, University of New Mexico Health Sciences Center, Albuquerque, New Mexico
Diagnostic and Therapeutic Aspects of the Medical Interview; Breast Disorders

DANIEL C. WASCHER, M.D.
Assistant Professor of Orthopedics and Chief, Division of Sports Medicine, University of New Mexico Health Sciences Center, Albuquerque, New Mexico
Wrist and Arm Pain

ERIC S. WEINSTEIN, M.D.
Associate Professor of Surgery and Chief, Division of Vascular Surgery, University of New Mexico Health Sciences Center, Albuquerque, New Mexico
Arterial Insufficiency of the Legs

ROBERT E. WHITE, M.D., M.P.H.
Associate Professor of Medicine, Division of General Medicine, University of New Mexico Health Sciences Center; Attending Physician, Veterans Administration Medical Center, Albuquerque, New Mexico
The Role of Primary Care; Low Back Pain

WILLIAM H. WIESE, M.D., M.P.H.
Professor of Family and Community Medicine and Director, Center for Population Health, University of New Mexico Health Sciences Center, Albuquerque, New Mexico
Screening for Disease

JOSEPHINE WILLIAMS, M.D.
South Denver Infectious Disease Specialists, Englewood, Colorado
Sexually Transmitted Diseases

BRUCE WILLIAMS, M.D., M.P.H.
Assistant Professor of Medicine, Division of Infectious Diseases, University of New Mexico Health Sciences Center, Albuquerque, New Mexico
Approach to the HIV-Positive Patient in the Outpatient Setting

BRONWYN E. WILSON, M.D.
Assistant Professor of Medicine, Division of General Medicine, University of New Mexico Health Sciences Center, Albuquerque, New Mexico
Chronic Tiredness

PREFACE

Since the mid-1970s, much has been written about the growing need for primary care physicians in the United States. Why most U.S. medical school graduates opt to become specialists rather than generalists has been commented on extensively, and a number of proposals aimed at reversing this trend have been set forth in both the popular and the medical press.

Although a multitude of factors undoubtedly influence each medical student's career choice, our concern is that many students may be rejecting primary care out-of-hand because of two commonly held misconceptions. The first is that the content of primary care is so vast, so *unwieldy,* that trying to gain a handle on it is inherently impossible. The second is that primary care lacks the ferment and dazzling breakthroughs so evident in the specialties—that, in effect, everything worth knowing in primary care is already known.

This book is meant to dispel both misconceptions. We believe that the content of primary care, though undeniably broad, is eminently definable; furthermore, we believe that the fundamentals of primary care can be mastered by medical students even during a 4- to 6-week clinical rotation.

In addition, we contend that primary care offers not only intellectual challenges that are truly extraordinary, but also a treasure trove of research opportunities that we are just beginning to explore; we believe that by encouraging our students to ask the right questions, now and in the future, we are advancing the care of tomorrow's patients as well as today's.

This book is designed primarily for medical students for use during their ambulatory care experience. We suspect, however, that many residents—and many physicians caring for patients in the community—will find it useful as a practical (and affordable) guide and as an up-to-date review.

We have intentionally begun each chapter with a case history, followed by a brief list of questions raised by the case history. Our aim is straightforward: we hope the reader will use these questions as a framework to which subsequently presented information can be attached. The emphasis throughout is on problem-solving—a method of learning that seems particularly valuable for students who also happen to be adults. After reasoning their way through the commonly encountered problems posed by the case histories, readers should soon feel much more at ease when faced with analogous problems in their "real-life" outpatients. Although we have included a resolution of the case history at the end of each chapter, our goal is most assuredly not to promote a "one right answer" mentality; on the contrary, our hope is that the opening case history will pique the student's intellectual curiosity and that a rational approach to the problem at hand will quickly become evident as each brief chapter unfolds.

This book allows the student to meld new clinical information with knowledge already acquired during the first 2 years of medical school. All too often, an unfortunate gap seems to exist between our students' preclinical and clinical experiences, and we hope to bridge that gap as much as possible in the pathophysiology section of each chapter. We believe that by emphasizing the connection between the basic sciences and clinical medicine, we will be able to promote better understanding and retention of the new material as well as relatively painless reinforcement of the old.

At the conclusion of each chapter is a series of questions that spotlights pieces of the puzzle still glaringly missing from our current knowledge base. We hope that readers of this book, in the course of their careers, will provide answers to many of these; in fact, nothing would give us, as teachers of medicine, greater pleasure.

Although most of the material presented deals with commonly faced outpatient problems, we have also included chapters on other topics pertinent to primary care, such as prevention, doctor-patient communication, health economics, and medical ethics in the ambulatory arena. In our view, students are well served when they begin to explore these highly relevant issues as early in their training as possible.

Finally, we cannot refrain from pointing out the large percentage of our authors who are practicing primary care physicians in addition to being medical educators. We also note with pride that this book is a joint effort involving both a department of internal medicine and a department of family medicine. At many institutions, such a collaboration would have been difficult, if not impossible; for the faculty at the University of New Mexico Health Sciences Center, however, this book represents a true labor of love.

We hope this book will make clear why all of us continue to find primary care so satisfying and so challenging—and yes, such great fun so much of the time.

RICHARD H. RUBIN, M.D.
CAROLYN VOSS, M.D.
DANIEL J. DERKSEN, M.D.
ANN GATELEY, M.D.
RONALD W. QUENZER, M.D.

ACKNOWLEDGMENTS

The authors would like to thank Bill Schmitt, Anne-Marie Shaw, and Carol Vartanian, our intrepid editors at W.B. Saunders, without whose patience and nurturing this book would not have been possible. In addition, we would like to express our appreciation to Yolanda Viramontes, Tanya Morga, Shelli Doyle, Jan Frank, and Shirley Rey Lovato, whose tirelessness in the preparation of this manuscript deserves special applause and commendation.

CONTENTS

SECTION III

Physician-Patient Communication

SECTION IV

Prevention in Primary Care

SECTION V

COMMON CONSTITUTIONAL SYMPTOMS

SECTION VI

COMMON EYE, EAR, NOSE, AND THROAT PROBLEMS

SECTION VII

COMMON PULMONARY PROBLEMS

S E C T I O N   V I I I

COMMON CARDIOVASCULAR PROBLEMS

S E C T I O N   I X

COMMON GASTROINTESTINAL PROBLEMS

SECTION X

COMMON GENITOURINARY PROBLEMS

SECTION XI

COMMON SEXUALLY TRANSMITTED DISEASES

SECTION XII

COMMON ISSUES IN WOMEN'S HEALTH

S E C T I O N   X I I I

Common Endocrine Problems

S E C T I O N   X I V

Common Hematologic-Oncologic Problems

S E C T I O N   X V

Common Musculoskeletal Problems

SECTION XVI

COMMON NEUROLOGIC PROBLEMS

SECTION XVII

COMMON PSYCHIATRIC PROBLEMS

SECTION XVIII

COMMON BEHAVIORAL ISSUES IN PRIMARY CARE

SECTION XIX

COMMON DERMATOLOGIC PROBLEMS

SECTION I

THE ROLE OF PRIMARY CARE

CHAPTER 1

THE ROLE OF PRIMARY CARE

Robert E. White, M.D., M.P.H.

H$_x$ Two medical students are considering their career choices.

"When I started medical school, I wanted to be a general type of doctor, and I think that's still what I want, but it's hard to decide."

"You won't see me in primary care. It's orthopedics all the way!"

"Why are you so sure?"

"Have you forgotten those long hours on your medicine rotation? After all that hard training, those generalists don't know enough, they see the same incurable problems over and over, they don't get to do anything exciting like surgery, and they don't earn as much money. I rest my case!"

"Our hospital rotation didn't show us what primary care is really like. Besides, in a few years you might have a hard time finding a job, while primary care physicians will have lots of choices."

Questions

1. What is primary care, who provides it, and why is there a primary care doctor shortage?
2. What will my future be like if I choose to become a primary care physician?

WHAT IS PRIMARY CARE?

The glossary in Box 1–1 defines primary care, which involves first contact with a patient, predominantly outpatient care, knowing patients thoroughly (problems and personal issues), and integrating many different aspects of medical knowledge and services. The primary care, or generalist, physician sees basic problems (Table 1–1). However, since even the 20 most common problems account for only 38% of all visits, primary care doctors also see a wide variety of problems. Conversely, the more a physician specializes in the care of one organ, the more that person is likely to become expert in a small number of diseases (Table 1–2).

Over the past 10 years, as more activities move out of the expensive hospital environment, the time clinicians spend in outpatient practice has been increasing. On average, practicing physicians provide 50 hours of direct patient care per week, 50%–75% of those 50 hours in outpatient settings and the remainder in hospitals or nursing homes. The average family practitioner spends 75% of his or her time seeing 100 patients per week in the office. He or she also makes 14 inpatient visits and discharges three hospital patients per week. Internists and pediatricians perform 60 to 100 outpatient visits and 20 to 30 inpatient visits per week and discharge 3 to 5 patients from the hospital each week. They spend on average 60% of their time in clinics or offices; subspecialized pediatricians and internists spend less than 60% and their primary care colleagues spend more than 60%.

BOX 1-1. Definition of Primary Care

Accessible	Is patient's first medical contact, is available when patient has urgent or chronic complaints, is financially affordable and geographically accessible. Is usually delivered in an office or clinic in either urban or rural setting.
Comprehensive	Provides broad range of services, including acute and chronic disease management, prevention and psychosocial management, care in clinic, hospital, nursing home, or via telephone.
Coordinated	Is aware of patient's entire list of problems and is central source of information about patient's care. Controls patient referrals to specialists, manages care delivered by team of health care workers, and translates specialty advice for patient.
Continuous	Develops long-term relationships with patient, maintains longitudinal record of patient problems, and promotes health over the long term.
Accountable	Is responsible for broad range of health issues and outcomes and is patient advocate in health care system. Educates patient about treatment outcomes and prognosis and understands patient preferences.

TABLE 1–1. The Top 20 Reasons Patients Visit Their Doctor*

Diagnosis	Percentage of All Visits
1. General medical examination	4.4
2. Cough	3.6
3. Routine prenatal examination	2.9
4. Symptoms referable to throat	2.7
5. Postoperative visit	2.4
6. Earache or ear infection	2.0
7. Well-baby examination	2.0
8. Back symptoms	1.9
9. Skin rash	1.8
10. Stomach pain/cramps/spasm	1.7
11. Fever	1.5
12. Headache, pain in head	1.5
13. Vision dysfunction	1.5
14. Knee symptoms	1.4
15. Nasal congestion	1.3
16. Blood pressure test	1.1
17. Head cold/upper respiratory infection	1.1
18. Neck symptoms	1.1
19. Depression	1.1
20. Low back symptoms	1.1
All other reasons	61.8

*690 million patient visits made in the offices of 1400 randomly selected, nonfederal physicians. Source: S. M. Schapert. National Ambulatory Medical Care Survey: 1991 Summary. Advance Data from Vital and Health Statistics. No. 230. Hyattsville, Maryland, National Center for Health Statistics, 1993.

Thinking about the Future

Maintaining competence in primary care is no more difficult than in specialty disciplines. A satisfying and challenging career in medicine depends on learning and using the knowledge base appropriate for the patient, whether as a specialist or generalist. Primary care physicians rely on history and physical examination skills and on human interaction more heavily than on technology, and they learn how to tolerate uncertainty while making decisions. They are stimulated by variety and take professional pride in appropriately using

TABLE 1–2. Variety of Patient Care Problems Seen by Different Physicians

	Number of Presenting Problems Accounting for 50% of Visits	Percentage of All Visits Accounted for by the 50 Most Frequent Presenting Problems
Family medicine	27	65.3
Internal medicine	21	69.3
Pediatrics	6	84.9
Cardiovascular medicine	7	90.5
Dermatology	5	87.0
General surgery	22	71.0
Obstetrics/gynecology	3	91.7
Ophthalmology	3	91.7
Orthopedic surgery	8	92.9
Otolaryngology	7	93.2
Urology	10	92.0
Psychiatry	4	97.0
Neurology	9	90.0

Reprinted, with permission, from B. Starfield. *Primary Care: Concept Evaluation and Policy.* New York, Oxford University Press, 1992, p. 99.

consultants and in pragmatically focusing their self-education. Primary care physicians report great satisfaction with personally knowing their individual patients and bringing the great variety of medical services to bear on patients' diverse problems.

WHO DELIVERS PRIMARY CARE?

Many different generalists are trained to provide the care described in Box 1–1. Family practice residency is specifically designed for primary care; internal medicine and pediatrics residencies provide both primary and specialty care training. In the United States, many internal medicine and pediatric subspecialists deliver part-time primary care, usually because their patients require more than subspecialty expertise or because there are more specialists in the community than needed. (By contrast, specialists in Canada and some European countries cannot practice primary care because they can treat only patients referred to them by generalists.)

Some general surgeons and obstetrician/gynecologists provide primary care but usually only for patients who are generally healthy and do not have multiple or chronic problems.

Nonphysicians (nurses, nurse practitioners, and physician assistants) also provide primary care.

Thinking about the Future

There are 20,000 first-year residency positions available each year in the United States for 16,000 graduating medical students. Half those positions can lead to generalist careers: family practice (2800), internal medicine (5300), pediatrics (2000), and medicine/pediatrics (300). Because many of these programs are hospital based and allied with highly specialized teaching centers, the primary care educational content will vary.

WHY IS THERE A SHORTAGE OF PRIMARY CARE PHYSICIANS?

Today, everyone hears about the primary care physician shortage. This shortage, unique to the United States, evolved over many years. A substantial growth in medical student numbers started around 1970. It was followed by two decades of specialized training and research program expansion, along with proliferation of community services based on specialization and technologic innovation. These changes were fostered by several factors, including governmental policies, methods of paying for health care, physicians' desire to develop the full potential of medical knowledge and technology, and the public's faith in this approach.

The success and growth of specialty medicine has been enormous (Fig. 1–1), but it has also encouraged physicians to seek the prestige, life-style, and monetary awards of specialty medicine over primary care. As a result, only 35% of all U. S. physicians today consider themselves primary care doctors, whereas in Canada the number is 52%, in Germany 45%, in Great Britain 70%, and in Australia 73%.

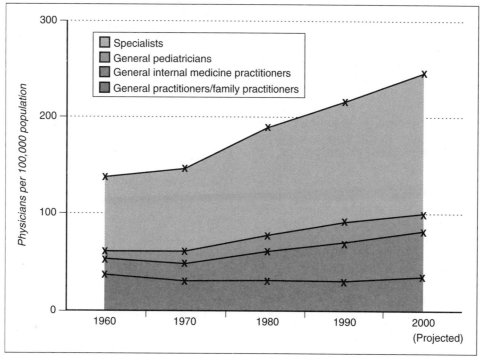

FIGURE 1–1. *Growth in physician numbers per 100,000 people in the United States.*

Thinking about the Future

The mismatch between ordinary patient needs (Table 1–1) and the kind of physicians available (Fig. 1–1) is generating governmental pressure on medical schools and residency programs to train more generalists. However, if the 35% of students who now enter primary care increases to 50% after 1994, it will take 25 years before half of all practicing physicians in the United States are generalists. If 100% of all medical students pursue primary care training, the 50/50 balance would still not be reached until 2004. Therefore, specialty physicians may experience escalating monetary, regulatory, and organizational pressures to abandon specialty practice and become generalists. On the other hand, primary care physicians can be sure their skills will be needed and that multiple career paths will be open to them.

WHERE IS PRIMARY CARE DELIVERED?

The principal sites of primary care delivery (office, clinic, hospital, and nursing homes) need little description, but their organization is rapidly changing. The range of organizational possibilities is displayed in order of increasing complexity in Table 1–3. **Solo practice** is the simplest and oldest type but is becoming less common. Only 9% of newly trained physicians expect to enter solo practice, usually in small communities or special niches in the medical marketplace. In those locations, the generalist usually has broad autonomy and responsibility and is paid fees for each service given to individual patients.

The environment for urban or suburban generalists is changing rapidly. Traditionally, they have practiced in **single** or **multispecialty groups** and have been paid

TABLE 1–3.   Where Primary Care Physicians Practice

	Physician Number			Physician Organizational Role	Generalist Autonomy	Physician Payment*	Means of Providing Care	
	Generalist	Total	Place				In Hospital	By Specialists
1. Solo practice	1	1	Rural > urban	Owner	Highest	FFS	Individual	Referral
2. Single specialty group	2–6	2–6	Rural = urban	Partner	High	FFS/CAP	Individual	Referral
3. Multispecialty group	0–20	10–75	Urban > rural	Partner or member	Medium	FFS/CAP	Individual	Within group
4. Generalist organization	30–100	30–100	Urban	Partner or employee	Medium	Salary	Contract	Capitation contract
5. Multispecialty organization	25–50	50–150	Urban	Employee	Low	Salary	Within group	Within group
6. Integrated physician-hospital organization	> 100	> 100	Multiple urban sites	Employee	Medium	Salary	Within group	Within group

*FFS = fee for service; CAP = capitation.

on a fee-for-service basis. Now most young doctors enter salaried or capitation-based practices in organizations. With capitation, the organization providing care receives a monthly lump sum for each patient for whom that organization is responsible, whether or not that patient requires any medical services. Capitation is fueling the growth of larger and more complex physician groups and organizations.

Multispecialty organizations have been present for many years but are becoming more primary care oriented. **Generalist** and **integrated organizations** are newer. The former employ only generalists and subcontract their expensive specialty and hospital care. Integrated organizations employ many different health care workers in many different facets of medical care across community and state boundaries, thereby benefiting from economies of scale. As larger organizations proliferate and absorb smaller, independent groups, doctors lose autonomy and experience different financial incentives. Increasingly, doctors must be concerned with organizational, as well as personal, goals. As physician income shifts from fee-for-service to salary or capitation, the doctor must seek to offer the fewest possible services that provide appropriate care.

Thinking about the Future

Many health experts expect and hope that "managed care" will evolve in the late 1990s to control costs while improving efficiency and quality of patient care. Managed care is not a specific insurance plan or type of group practice but rather a set of principles intended to bind patients and doctors together and encourage them to conserve resources. Patients enter these plans because their employers increasingly choose them (more than half of American workers were covered by such plans in 1992) and because they promise set benefits. In exchange, patients accept a reduced choice of doctors and hospitals, are encouraged to be cost conscious in seeking medical attention, and are sometimes encouraged to adopt healthy habits. Doctors enter these plans because they provide patients. In exchange, they accept scrutiny of their practice habits as well as financial incentives to be cost efficient.

Managed care relies heavily on "gatekeeper" generalists who try to solve their patients' problems before obtaining specialty consultation or expensive services and who efficiently coordinate patient care. Because managed care plans are rapidly expanding and are competing for a dwindling supply of primary care doctors, generalists will experience increased stature, income, and influence within organizations. Conversely, fewer of the abundant, urban specialists and hospital-based specialists will be needed, so their influence, autonomy, and income will decrease as they compete for pools of managed care patients.

Generalist physicians face two challenges. One is the acquisition of managed care skills (Table 1–4). The second is to avoid losing the patient's trust while changing from providers of service to case managers.

TABLE 1–4. Physician Skills and Knowledge Needed in the Managed Care Environment

Medical Decision Making
Biostatistics
Clinical epidemiology
Probabilistic reasoning
Dealing with uncertainty
Using decision algorithms and guidelines

Quality of Patient Care Outcomes
Assessing functional status and patient preferences
Communicating risks, benefits, alternatives, and outcomes
Gauging benefit versus cost of treatments
Understanding computer databases
Being aware of legal aspects of outcomes

Medical Economics
Health care economy and policy
Insurance and risk-sharing concepts
Health delivery organizations
Physician payment incentives
Computer database profiling of physician performance

Managing Patient Access to Care
Management of consultative care
Team participation and leadership
Prevention strategies
Home care assessment and support services
Interpersonal communication
Medical ethics, liability, and responsibility

Research Questions

1. How can generalists, specialists, and other health care workers in integrated organizations work together to deliver care that is "personal"?
2. How will patients, doctors, and society at large learn to conserve medical care resources?

Case Resolution

The student who completed primary care training received multiple job offers with a confusing array of contract arrangements, but she was able to select a practice arrangement that suited her personality and needs. The student who completed orthopedic training was not immediately successful in finding a position. When he did, he received a salary that was lower than what he was expecting. In addition, he was not able to perform selected specialized procedures until he achieved partnership status in the group that hired him.

Selected Readings

Gonzales, M. (ed.). *Socioeconomic Characteristics of Medical Practice 1994.* Chicago, Center for Health Policy Research, American Medical Association, 1994, p. 49.
Nash, D. *Future Practice Alternatives in Medicine,* 2nd ed. New York, Igaku-Shoin, 1993.
Starfield, B. *Primary Care: Concept, Evaluation, and Policy.* New York, Oxford University Press, 1992.

Differences Between Inpatient and Outpatient Medicine

Richard H. Rubin, M.D.

H$_x$ After completing two rigorous back-to-back clerkships on the medicine and surgery wards, a third-year medical student views his upcoming rotation in the outpatient clinic as something of a vacation. The first patient he sees in clinic, however, is a 55-year-old, overweight female interior decorator with diabetes who, when asked the reason for her visit, removes a legal-sized sheet of paper from her handbag and proceeds to relate what seems to be an interminable list of complaints, including inability to lose weight, chronic headaches, episodic abdominal bloating, right shoulder pain, left knee pain, bilateral foot pain, extreme tiredness, and "funny spots" on her tongue. The medical student spends an hour and a half with the patient, dutifully exploring every symptom. By the time he leaves the examining room, *he* is experiencing extreme tiredness, wondering how to make any sense out of this bewildering morass of information.

Questions

1. Why is the delivery of health care increasingly being shifted from the inpatient to the outpatient arena?
2. How does the approach to the patient in the outpatient setting differ from that in the inpatient setting?

Third- and fourth-year medical students typically receive most of their clinical training in the inpatient setting—interviewing, examining, and learning how to manage hospitalized patients. This traditional inpatient focus has been shaped by a number of factors, including (1) the long-standing, close relationship between medical schools and large teaching hospitals; (2) what seemed, in the past at least, to be a never-ending supply of hospitalized patients presenting interesting diagnostic and therapeutic challenges; and (3) the apparent belief that students (and residents) could readily acquire the skills relevant to outpatient care once they had mastered the presumably more difficult problems posed by inpatients.

For more than a decade, however, the delivery of health care in the United States has been shifting from the inpatient to the outpatient setting. This change has been spurred, in large measure, by the harsh realities of medical economics. Since outpatient care is much less costly for most disorders than is inpatient care, third-party payers have grown increasingly insistent that each day a patient spends in the hospital be absolutely necessary and fully justifiable.

Forces other than cost containment also have contributed to the inpatient-to-outpatient shift in health care delivery (Table 2–1). The result of these various forces acting in concert is that outpatient care is assuming greater prominence.

DIFFERENCES IN EDUCATIONAL MODEL

The change in health care delivery has far-reaching implications for American medical education. In the past, for example, a particularly perplexing patient might easily have been admitted to a teaching hospital for a lengthy diagnostic workup, allowing students and residents ample opportunity to expand their base of clinical experience as well as sharpen their reasoning skills. Today, however, if such a patient were to be admitted at all, it would most likely be for one of the decreasing number of procedures that can be performed only on an inpatient basis; the patient would arrive at the hospital having been exhaustively "worked up" as an outpatient and would probably be hospitalized only briefly. In short, the educational value of this patient to the residents and students on the inpatient team would be greatly diminished, since most of the key decision making about care would have already taken place in the outpatient setting.

Because the real (i.e., postresidency) world of medicine is placing increasing emphasis on outpatient care, it would seem logical for medical education to follow suit, and this is already occurring at many institutions. Students need to be aware of the ways in which practicing in the outpatient setting differs from practicing in the inpatient setting (Table 2–2). Several of these differences, particularly those relating to patient care and physician-patient interactions, are discussed below.

DIFFERENCES IN DISORDERS

Anyone who works in an outpatient setting soon recognizes the truth behind the dictum that "common

---

TABLE 2–1. Reasons for the Increasing Shift of Health Care from the Inpatient to the Outpatient Setting

Expense (outpatient care tends to be much less costly)
Technologic advances (which allow sophisticated diagnostic and therapeutic measures to be performed without hospitalization)
Patient preference

TABLE 2–2.   Differences Between Outpatient and Inpatient Medicine

Differences in Disorders
Different spectrum of ailments (common, often chronic)
Symptoms often nonspecific
Frequent psychosocial component
Differences in Approach to Evaluation and Management
More stepwise approach, using time as ally
In addition to cure, goals include prevention and maintenance of highest possible level of functioning
Differences in Physician-Patient Relationship
Physician less paternalistic, more of a health advisor and counselor
Differences in Physician Rewards
Medical "successes" often less dramatic but still immensely gratifying over time

things occur commonly." Unfortunately, many common disorders receive little attention in medical school. The inpatient model of education frequently paints an extremely skewed picture of mankind's afflictions: scleroderma and lupus are fascinating diseases, but low back pain and such "periarticular" problems as tendinitis and bursitis are vastly more common. Such disorders may not be life threatening, but their impact on patients' lives makes them anything but trivial.

Many patients, in fact, present with no well-defined illness at all but instead are plagued by nonspecific symptoms such as tiredness or dizziness. Often, the cause of such symptoms remains unclear even after a thorough evaluation. Learning how to approach (and subsequently help) the patient with such nonspecific complaints is a skill unique to outpatient practitioners.

Psychosocial problems, although highly relevant to inpatient care, assume even greater importance in the outpatient setting. It is estimated that approximately half of all outpatient visits have a significant psychosocial component. The outpatient physician thus has the unparalleled opportunity to intervene (and provide benefit) in both the psychological and physical realms—a distinction that is, of course, arbitrary in many patients.

DIFFERENCES IN APPROACH TO EVALUATION AND MANAGEMENT

Patients are usually admitted to the hospital because of an acute illness (or sudden exacerbation of a preexisting illness) that requires rapid evaluation and management. Most problems encountered in the nonemergency outpatient setting, however, are subacute or chronic in nature, and such problems can often be prioritized and evaluated over time in a more stepwise fashion. Time, in fact, is frequently a valuable ally in outpatient practice, unlike the situation in inpatient practice where the more frenetic pace often causes time to be an adversary. The mere passage of time may help sort out problems that are initially unclear and frustrating and may even allow some symptoms to disappear entirely.

The goals of outpatient care also differ in several important respects from the goals of inpatient care. Cure—or at least reversing an acute process—is what drives much of inpatient management. Although selected conditions (especially infectious diseases) can be cured in the outpatient setting, major emphasis is also placed on the prevention of disease and the maintenance of the highest possible level of functioning, both of which are rightfully considered important long-term goals. In short, the focus is not simply on disease or even symptoms, but on the patient's well-being and all that it entails.

DIFFERENCES IN PHYSICIAN-PATIENT RELATIONSHIP

For most patients, being hospitalized is an unnatural and extremely artificial experience; people who are used to making decisions for themselves are placed in a highly dependent position in which they have relatively little choice about what they eat, wear, and do. In this setting, the physician-patient relationship tends to be paternalistic. Physicians write "orders" about their patients, and these orders are carried out by nurses and other hospital personnel. Medical care often seems to be directed anonymously by "teams" of house staff, attending physicians, and consultants, and it is a sad commentary that many hospitalized patients are unable to name the person who is actually in charge of their care.

In contrast, patients seen in the outpatient clinic have lives of their own, with personal matters to attend to and often jobs to perform. Their personal health may be quite important to them, but in reality, it is just one of many things on their minds. A paternalistic physician-patient relationship, in which an authoritarian physician tells the patient what to do (or what is going to be done), is usually inappropriate in the outpatient setting. Here, the physician is more accurately regarded as a health advisor whose ability to educate, persuade, and negotiate will likely determine whether that advice is followed or not.

DIFFERENCES IN PHYSICIAN REWARDS

The aims of outpatient practice are simple: to cure (and even better, to *prevent*) disease whenever possible and to offer comfort and support to all who seek help. Medical successes are sometimes less dramatic in outpatient practice than they are in the high-tech inpatient setting, but they are no less personally satisfying. Caring for patients over time—keeping them out of the hospital and as healthy and functional as possible—is both the challenge and the joy of outpatient primary care. This sentiment was poignantly expressed by the celebrated poet William Carlos Williams, himself a family practitioner, in his autobiography:

It's the . . . day-in, day-out everyday work that is the real satisfaction of the practice of medicine; the million and a half patients a man has seen on his daily visits over a 40-year period of weekdays and Sundays . . . [It is] the actual calling on people, at all times and under all conditions, the coming to grips with the intimate conditions of their lives, when they were being born, when they were dying . . . watching them get well when they were ill, [that] has always absorbed me.

Research Questions

1. How can the education of medical students and residents be changed to more closely mirror the primarily outpatient focus of most practicing physicians?
2. What should be the role of community physicians in this educational process?

Case Resolution

The medical student and his clinic attending discussed various strategies for prioritizing the patient's complaints. The patient was included in this discussion, and she expressed the wish that her tiredness and right shoulder pain be addressed during this initial visit. A 40-minute follow-up visit was scheduled in 2 weeks' time, and the

student—at the suggestion of his attending physician—made a note to question the patient further about her life situation at the next visit.

Selected Readings

Federman, D. D. Relation of the internal medicine residency and the medical school curriculum. Ann Intern Med 116(12 part 2):1061–4, 1992.

Feltovich, J., T. A. Mast, and N. G. Soler. Teaching medical students in ambulatory settings in departments of internal medicine. Acad Med 64:36-41, 1989.

Howell, J. D., N. Lurie, and J. O. Woolliscroft. Worlds apart: Some thoughts to be delivered to house officers on the first day of clinic. JAMA 258:502–3, 1987.

Starr, P. *The Social Transformation of American Medicine.* New York, Basic Books, 1982.

MEDICAL TESTING AND CLINICAL REASONING

| C H A P T E R   3 |

THE USE AND MISUSE OF MEDICAL TESTS

Fred Hashimoto, M.D.

H$_x$ A 26-year-old female medical student telephones and says that she has pancreatitis. During the previous 2 weeks, she has experienced several episodes of intermittent epigastric discomfort lasting for several hours. It was worsened by eating. The patient, who occasionally takes 200 mg of ibuprofen for headaches, denies nausea, vomiting, or blood in her stools. Yesterday she ordered a screening panel on herself from a local laboratory that publicly offers test screening panels. She says that her amylase result was abnormally high at 150 U/L (normal, 0–130 U/L).

Questions

1. What is the significance of the abnormal amylase result? How sensitive and specific is it for pancreatitis?
2. Are large screening panels helpful for general diagnostics?
3. What tests, if any, should you order next?
4. What are the most probable diseases this woman might have? Is it important to know exactly how probable they might be?
5. What test characteristic is important when a test is used to confirm a disease? To exclude a disease?
6. What is Bayes' theorem?

Testing is immensely important to busy practitioners. Magnetic resonance imaging (MRI) of the head reveals more about intracranial masses than physical examinations can, and echocardiograms provide more information about the heart than stethoscopes do. Ordering large screening panels can be a time-effective way of investigating vague complaints such as fatigue. Because testing is easy to obtain and requires less effort than traditional history taking and physical examinations do, more tests might be performed as physicians feel pressure to see more patients quickly or make a diagnosis immediately.

Testing constitutes a large part of physicians' interactions with their patients and their medical problems.

In the primary care setting, frequently ordered tests include blood chemistries, hematology profiles, urinalyses, cultures, x-rays, diagnostic imaging, electrocardiograms (ECGs), and gastrointestinal endoscopies. Test results change doctors' *probabilistic assessment of the existence of possible disease states*. In a sense, questions to patients, physical examinations, and even referrals to consultants can also be considered "tests." Often a verbal question yields more information than a serum assay. Testing in medicine is basically a question and then an answer.

However, many tests—some of which are very costly—are being done that are not needed for patient care decisions. In addition to their expense, these unnecessary tests contribute to the problem of **false-positive results.** The more tests that are ordered, the greater the number of false-positive results that occur; these results must be approached properly to avoid unnecessarily increasing costs by further inappropriate testing. Tests should be ordered with discretion.

Testing opportunities occur at strategic junction points in decision trees. The test result, which changes the **pretest probability** for the disease in question, influences the way in which the problem will be managed. The cost and possible adverse effects of a test should be included in the expected value or cost of the management alternatives.

The major purposes of testing are to confirm, or rule in, a diagnosis; exclude, or rule out, a diagnosis; screen a population for a disease; and monitor a clinical situation. Other possible purposes are to give a prognosis, identify risk, reassure the patient (or doctor), generate income, shift efforts and costs in the diagnostic effort, save time, make time (i.e., have the patient wait a certain interval), and reduce litigation risks (many times at great cost and without changing the probability estimate significantly).

The relationship between a disease and a test for that disease can be summarized by the 2 × 2 matrix in Figure 3–1.

Disease

		Present	Absent	
Test Result	+	a	b	(a + b)
	−	c	d	(c + d)
		(a + c)	(b + d)	(a + b + c + d)

Where

a = persons with disease who test positive
c = persons with disease who test negative
d = persons without disease who test negative
b = persons without disease who test positive
(a + c) = persons with disease
(b + d) = persons without disease
(a + b) = persons who test positive
(c + d) = persons who test negative
(a + b + c + d) = total persons
(a + c)/(a + b + c + d) = prevalence of disease

Sensitivity = true positive rate = a/(a + c)
false negative rate = c/(a + c)
(true positive rate) + (false negative rate) = 1

Specificity = true negative rate = d/(b + d)
false positive rate = b/(b + d)
(true negative rate) + (false positive rate) = 1

Predictive value positive = a/(a + b)
Predictive value negative = d/(c + d)

FIGURE 3–1. *Test characteristics.*

TEST CHARACTERISTICS

A test has defined characteristics relative to the disease it tests for. **Sensitivity** is the proportion of people with the disease who test positive for the disease. This proportion is also known as the **true positive rate.** **Specificity** is the proportion of people without the disease who test negative for the disease. This is also called the **true negative rate.** For example, if a serum amylase level is abnormally high in 75 of 100 persons who have acute pancreatitis, the test sensitivity is 75%. If it is high in the absence of pancreatitis 30% of the time (i.e., the false-positive rate is 30%), the test specificity is 70%.

The **posttest probability** of disease is the probability of a patient having the disease after the test results for it are known. This posttest probability can be calculated from the 2×2 matrix or by **Bayes' theorem,** which uses the pretest probability of the disease and the test's characteristics (Fig. 3–2). The posttest probability of a disease for which the test is positive is synonymous with the predictive value positive in the 2×2 matrix. For example, if the physician feels that the probability of the patient profiled in the case history above having pancreatitis is 25% and if a serum amylase is abnormally high, then the posttest probability of pancreatitis can be calculated from Bayes' theorem as follows:

$$(0.25 \times 0.75)/[(0.25 \times 0.75) + (1 - 0.25)(1 - 0.70)] = 45\%$$

If the pretest probability of pancreatitis is very high or very low, a positive or negative test result will usually change it relatively little. For example, if the pretest probability for pancreatitis is 0.90, then the posttest disease probability, obtained from Bayes' theorem or the 2×2 matrix, is 96% after a positive result. If the pretest probability is a more intermediate 0.65, the posttest probability after a positive test increases by 17% to 82%. Testing is most likely to affect patient care decisions when the pretest probability for the disease is intermediate.

Although diagnostic test results are often described as being either positive or negative—or abnormal or normal—they are not necessarily categorical but often relative. A serum sodium level of 134 mEq/L is hardly abnormal when one of 135 mEq/L is normal. Test results usually lie on a continuum and a statistical consideration—two standard deviations from the mean—often defines the cutoff point between normal and abnormal results. An abnormal state statistically can be normal physiologically for a given individual.

Choosing a cutoff point to include test values of more persons with disease increases the sensitivity of the test but decreases the specificity; therefore, more false-

Bayes' theorem is usually written

$$P(D+/T+) = \frac{P(D+)\ P(T+/D+)}{P(D+)\ P(T+/D+) + P(D-)\ P(T+/D-)}$$

Where
   P(D+/T+) = the posttest probability of having the disease given a positive test result
   P(T+/D+) = the probability of a positive test in one having the disease
   P(T+/D-) = the probability of a positive test in one not having the disease
   P(D+)   = the pretest probability of having the disease; this can be the disease
              prevalence in a population of such patients

When the conditional probabilities are translated into test characteristics, Bayes' theorem can be restated

$$P(D+/T+) = \frac{prevalence \times sensitivity}{(prevalence \times sensitivity) + (1 - prevalence)\ (1 - specificity)}$$

Thus, the posttest probability of having the disease after testing positive for it depends on both the test characteristics and the pretest disease probability.

For those who prefer odds to probabilities [odds = probability/(1 – probability)], this relationship can be restated. Dividing P(D+/T+) by P(D-/T+) yields

$$\frac{P(D+/T+)}{P(D-/T+)} = \frac{P(D+)}{P(D-)} \times \frac{P(T+/D+)}{P(T+/D-)}$$

which, for a positive test, is

$$\begin{array}{ll} posterior\ odds \\ of\ disease \end{array} = \begin{array}{ll} prior\ odds \\ of\ disease \end{array} \times \begin{array}{ll} sensitivity/(1 - specificity) \\ ("likelihood\ ratio") \end{array}$$

The increase in probability or odds that the disease is present after a positive test for it can be computed by the above formulas. The decrease in probability or odds after a negative test can be similarly computed.

FIGURE 3–2. *Bayes' theorem.*

positive results will occur. Conversely, moving the cutoff point to be more restrictive increases the test's specificity but decreases its sensitivity. For example, changing the cutoff point of the prostate-specific antigen (PSA) test from 4.0 ng/mL to 2.0 ng/mL will result in picking up more cases of prostatic cancer but will also generate more false-positive results. Often, test results should not be considered as either positive or negative, but rather the magnitude of the result's abnormality should be taken into account. A PSA of 25 ng/mL is more likely to be indicative of prostate cancer than is one of 10 ng/mL.

Currently, it is not possible to have precise test characteristics, prevalence data, and pretest probabilities readily available. The populations in which testing has been done to determine the test's characteristics may not be representative of the specific patient to be tested. Prevalences can vary depending upon the designated "gold standard" for the disease. Advances in sensitive techniques such as imaging technology have resulted in an increase in the diagnosis and reported prevalence of diseases. As extensive databases are compiled, more exact information will become available.

TESTING IN OUTPATIENT CLINICS

Testing is an important activity in outpatient clinics. Between planned screening and monitoring tests and unplanned diagnostic tests, testing often determines, at least in part, the frequency at which many patients return to a clinic.

In the outpatient setting, testing has a different complexion than in inpatient services. Periodic screening tests (e.g., Pap smears and mammograms) and surveillance tests (e.g., serum levels of glycosylated hemoglobin, potassium, phenytoin, and thyroglobulin) are routinely ordered. Testing is often contemplated when new medical problems arise. These new problems are usually less health-threatening than inpatient problems are, and tests are therefore less urgently needed. Many of these problems resolve of their own accord after a short time; for this reason, appropriate restraint can save money and other resources.

Time is an important factor to understand and use well. The need to quickly resolve uncertainty by establishing an immediate diagnosis should be tempered. Clinical follow-up often is more important than testing; in a way, watchful waiting with clinical follow-up is also a "test" that yields results. For example, a 40-year-old woman presents with a vague right upper quadrant (RUQ) abdominal pain. An RUQ ultrasound and an upper GI x-ray series should not be reflexively ordered. Watchful waiting might be the best course. Obviously, urgent and emergent problems do present in outpatient clinics, and in those cases, testing and treatment must be done as expeditiously as possible.

BASIC GUIDELINES FOR TEST ORDERING

The following guidelines incorporate considerations from Bayes' theorem, concepts of formal decision making, and common sense.

Reasons for Tests

There should be a good reason to order a test. Studies have shown that physicians frequently order excessive, hard-to-justify admission chemistry panels, sedimentation rates, hematology profiles, and coagulation screens.

An old maxim is that if a test will not affect patient management, it should not be done. For example, if a diabetic's daily blood glucose levels have been averaging around 260 mg/dL, then a glycosylated hemoglobin level need not be ordered, since the result will undoubtedly be high and will not change what the patient should do. The maxim doesn't imply that a change in patient plan *must* follow a test because no change is often deemed, after testing, to be the best alternative.

However, just because the test result *might* change management options is not reason enough to test. Other issues might include the cost of testing and the probability of obtaining a result that will cause a change. Ordering an expensive test in an attempt to diagnose a non-dangerous disease that is very unlikely usually is not indicated.

Test Consequences

The physician should know the big picture of the patient's health and where the test—and its possible results—fit in. The following must be considered: (1) alternative management courses, including not testing or treating; (2) the importance of the diagnosis being entertained—if it is a significant diagnosis that should not be missed, testing for it should be contemplated even if the pretest probability is rather low; (3) patient values regarding the different interventions and outcomes; (4) the test costs, risks, and degree of invasiveness (e.g, ordering an expensive imaging test to work up what is probably a tension headache usually is not indicated); and (5) concurrent problems, especially those that might be end-stage or terminal (e.g., aggressive workup of possible gallstones might not be indicated in a patient with metastatic adeno-carcinoma of the colon).

If several tests are available, the choice of which to use will depend on the disease being tested for and on the tests' characteristics, possible invasiveness, and cost.

Pretest Disease Probability

Estimate the pretest disease probability. The pretest probability depends on findings from the history, physical examination, and previous test results. Although probabilistic thinking is often not rigorously applied and precise probabilities might be hard to come

by, rational decision making requires pretest probability estimates. The following conditions reflect the considerations that should be taken into account when contemplating pretest probabilities and testing.

When the pretest probability is very high or very low, testing should be done cautiously. For example, screening the general public for the HIV antibody is not worthwhile, since the prevalence of HIV infection in the general population is very low and the predictive value of a positive result is very low. Most of the positive results generated will be falsely positive, and additional tests will be required to substantiate that. However, screening prison populations for HIV might make more sense because disease prevalence is higher in that setting and there will be a larger proportion of true positives. Another example is obtaining exercise ECGs when the pretest disease probability is very high or very low. Such testing is usually not worthwhile because a positive or negative test is unlikely to change the pretest disease probability.

When a test will be used to exclude a disease, that disease should not have a high pretest probability.

When a test will be used to confirm a disease, that disease should not have a low pretest probability.

The prevalence of serious disease for outpatients is generally less than that for inpatients.

Screening Tests

Tests for screening serve the specific purpose of finding asymptomatic disease. Therefore, a screening test needs high sensitivity for the screened disease.

Groups such as the U. S. Preventive Services Task Force and the Canadian Task Force have considered test characteristics when recommending specific screening guidelines. Local experts or a review of the literature can provide guidelines on how often nonscreening surveillance tests—such as mammograms following up abnormal mammograms or Pap tests following up mildly dysplastic smears—should be ordered.

A mammogram in a young woman with relatively dense breast parenchyma is a poor screening test for cancer because of low sensitivity. Tests that have only moderate sensitivity can be used for screening if they are repeated at given intervals. An example is the Pap smear for cervical cancer.

When a screening test is used in a population with relatively low disease prevalence, the test should also have high specificity; otherwise many false-positive results will occur. Working up many false-positive tests can significantly increase the costs of screening.

Confirmatory Tests

A confirmatory test should have relatively high specificity to minimize false-positive results. Examples of confirmatory tests are the Western blot test for HIV disease and biopsy of a mass during flexible sigmoidoscopy. Many confirmatory tests—such as coronary angiography and specific tissue biopsies—lie within the domain of the subspecialists and the inpatient service.

Excluding Tests

An excluding test should have relatively high sensitivity to minimize false-negative results. This type of test is often used in the outpatient setting. Examples are chest x-rays (CXR) to rule out significant pneumonia and serum transaminase levels to exclude acute hepatitis.

Examples of tests that have low sensitivity for the disease in question and therefore should not be used as excluding tests are CXRs to rule out lung cancer, electrocardiograms for coronary artery disease or arrhythmias, stool guaiac tests for colon cancer, bone x-rays for osteomyelitis, one set of pulmonary function tests (PFTs) for asthma, or serum creatinine for kidney disease.

Sensitivity in a testing situation can be enhanced by repeating the test (e.g., multiple stool guaiacs), lengthening the testing interval (e.g., a 24-hour Holter monitor instead of a 15-second ECG), enhancing the test (e.g., methacholine-stimulation PFTs), or adding other tests (e.g., serum creatinine plus urinalysis).

Parenthetically, just because a disease is not ruled out does not mean that it is ruled in, and conversely, just because it is not confirmed does not mean that it is excluded.

Test Panels

Tests should be ordered selectively. The physician should beware of general panels and should approach an incidental abnormal test result with caution. The more tests that are ordered, the greater the number of abnormal results that will occur. In most clinics, it is as easy to order a whole battery of tests, called a "panel" (e.g., "admission panel," "hepatitis panel," "thyroid panel," "liver panel"), as it is to order just one test; many clinicians order the battery, thinking that more information is better (even though the "more" may be unrelated to the problem at hand). The battery usually costs more than the one or two indicated tests. In addition, the problems introduced by any incidental abnormal test values must be addressed. For instance, a standard 20-test "admission panel" will yield all normal results for only 64% of well persons.

When an incidental abnormal test result occurs, the physician should consider the following before ordering more tests: What was the pretest probability—and the posttest probability—that the disease indicated by the abnormal result is present? The test should be repeated; often the repeat result will be normal.

Case Resolution

The patient's mildly abnormal amylase level was not impressive. The test's sensitivity and specificity for acute pancreatitis are not high—about 70%–75%. The physician asked to examine the patient in the office within the next few days. That examination showed mild epigastric tenderness without rebound or guarding. The physician learned that the patient's mother and sister had had cholecystectomies. Two weeks later after the patient ate a greasy hamburger, her pain recurred. Her amylase was 155 U/L. The physician obtained a right upper quadrant ultrasound, which showed gallstones. After her gallbladder was removed, the patient had no similar pains. A year later, her amylase was still 160 U/L. This mildly "abnormal" elevation was normal for her and not related to her symptoms.

Selected Readings

Black, W. C., and H. G. Welch. Advances in diagnostic imaging and overestimation of disease prevalence and the benefits of therapy. N Engl J Med 328:1237–43, 1993.

Griner, P. F., R. J. Mayewski, A. I. Mushlin, et al. Selection and interpretation of diagnostic tests and procedures: Principles and applications. Ann Intern Med 94(4 part 2): 557–600, 1981.

Kassirer, J. P. Our stubborn quest for diagnostic certainty. N Engl J Med 320:1489–91, 1989.

McNeil, B. J., E. Keeler, and S. J. Adelstein. Primer on certain elements of medical decision making. N Engl J Med 293:211–5, 1975.

Panzer, R. J., E. R. Black, and P. F. Griner. *Diagnostic Strategies for Common Medical Problems.* Philadelphia, American College of Physicians, 1991.

Pauker, S. G., and R. I. Kopelman. Trapped by an incidental finding. N Engl J Med 326:40–3, 1992.

Ransohoff, D. R., and A. R. Feinstein. Problems of spectrum and bias in evaluating the efficacy of diagnostic tests. N Engl J Med 299:926–30, 1978.

Reuben, D. B. Learning diagnostic restraint. N Engl J Med 310:591–3, 1984.

Sox, H. C. Probability theory in the use of diagnostic tests. Ann Intern Med 104:60–6, 1986.

Woolf, S. H., and D. B. Kamerow. Testing for uncommon conditions. Arch Intern Med 150:2451–8, 1990.

CLINICAL REASONING

Alan K. Halperin, M.D.

H$_x$ A 58-year-old male lawyer makes an urgent appointment. His chief complaint is "I have been having chest pain." The patient is overweight, has a cigarette pack in his front pocket, and appears anxious.

Questions

1. What diagnostic possibilities should you consider and why?
2. How can these hypotheses be further refined to ascertain the most probable diagnosis?

Medical educators have a long history of teaching medical students both the factual knowledge and the clinical skills necessary to evaluate patients. However, the teaching of clinical reasoning has received little attention in the medical curriculum. Despite this omission, clinical reasoning is critical to ensure the best outcome for patients by maximizing the benefits and reducing the risks of the physician's decisions. It is also a process by which costs can be controlled.

Patients frequently consult physicians because they have complaints. It is the prime function of the physician to accurately gather data from the history and physical examination, formulate a diagnostic hypothesis, select and interpret the results of appropriate tests, and recommend a course of action. This chapter will explain the components of the diagnostic process. This process, termed **iterative hypothesis testing,** utilizes the principles of medical decision making and includes the following components: **hypothesis formation, hypothesis refinement** (including diagnostic testing and causal reasoning), and **hypothesis confirmation.** The purpose of the diagnostic process is to reduce uncertainty so that the practitioner can make the best decisions about evaluation and management. Iterative hypothesis testing contrasts with the method of exhaustion that is commonly used by medical students. Students using this technique do an exhaustive history and physical examination lasting hours, write up their findings on numerous pages, and still have no idea what is wrong with the patient.

HYPOTHESIS FORMATION

In the case history presented, hypotheses can be formulated about the cause of the client pain soon after the chief complaint is established. Experienced clinicians start to form diagnostic hypotheses within seconds. There are numerous causes of chest pain, and the role of the physician is to discover the most likely diagnosis from a long list of possible causes. Establishing the diagnosis in this patient is important because some causes of chest pain are life threatening and require emergency intervention (e.g., myocardial infarction or pulmonary embolus), others have considerable risks of morbidity or mortality and require further testing (e.g., cancer, coronary heart disease), and still others cause morbidity but are not life threatening (e.g., musculoskeletal pain).

Although it is impossible to be certain of the diagnosis from such little information, there are clues that can help generate and prioritize different diagnostic hypotheses. One possible diagnosis is coronary heart disease (CHD). CHD is common in this patient's age group, and the patient has several risk factors that might predispose him to coronary heart disease (smoking, obesity). However, there are many other possible diagnoses. Some of the more common include gastroesophageal reflux disease, musculoskeletal chest pain, pneumonia, cancer of the lung, and pulmonary embolus or infarction. This list of diagnostic possibilities is termed the differential diagnosis. The initial diagnostic impression is important because it provides the framework for further questioning. A different differential diagnosis would be obtained if the patient had been a 20-year-old woman taking birth control pills. In that case, CHD would be extremely unlikely and other causes (e.g., pulmonary embolus) more likely.

HYPOTHESIS REFINEMENT

As new information is gathered from the history and physical examination, the initial diagnosis may be revised, refined, or made more specific. Several strategies for eliciting information can be used. The "confirmation" strategy is used to enhance the probability of a hypothesis, while the "rule-out" strategy is used to reduce the probability of a hypothesis.

Upon further questioning of the patient with chest pain, the following additional information is gleaned. The patient first experienced chest pain 1 month ago when he developed severe sharp, substernal chest pain with radiation to his left arm while walking quickly. The pain was associated with diaphoresis but not shortness of breath and was relieved by rest within 5 minutes. It has occurred five times in the last month: four times with exertion and once at rest. He was otherwise healthy except for a remote history of peptic ulcer disease.

From the further description of the pain, it is now possible to rank-order the diagnoses in our differential diagnosis and choose a working diagnosis. From the available data, CHD is now the most likely diagnosis. The chest pain fits the pattern of CHD pain, and the patient has several risk factors for CHD. Further questioning should be directed at ruling out or confirming the other common causes of chest pain listed above such as trauma, connective tissue disease, infection, neoplasm, etc. The physical examination can often yield information that affects the probability of the working diagnosis (e.g., a heart murmur consistent with aortic stenosis or a vesicular rash suggestive of herpes zoster). Even after a thorough history and physical examination, however, there is often uncertainty about the diagnosis. This is not the fault of the physician but is inherent in the diagnostic process.

Physicians frequently use words such as probably, unlikely, or certain to describe their assessment of the likelihood of the diagnosis. Such words, however, are imprecise and may convey different meanings. Using probabilistic statements avoids this ambiguity. **Probability** is a number between 0 and 1 that expresses the likelihood of an event. For example, one might estimate the probability of CHD in this patient as 0.70 given the results of the history and physical examination.

Physicians frequently use cognitive processes or **heuristics** (rules of thumb) to help estimate probability. It is possible to form probabilistic statements by using personal experience, published data, and specific attributes of the patient. **Personal experience** is the most important factor in formulating a probability assessment. One heuristic is called the **representativeness** heuristic, in which the probability is estimated based on how closely the patient resembles others known to have the condition. This patient has many characteristics of those who have CHD. The **availability** heuristic is used when the probability of an event is judged by the ease with which it is remembered. Frequent events are more easily remembered. The **anchoring and adjustment** heuristic allows for the special characteristics of the patient. Physicians often make an initial probability assessment (the anchor) and adjust it based on additional characteristics of the patient. In this patient, the probability of CHD would increase if it was known that he had a strong family history of coronary disease.

Clinical experience and knowledge can affect the quality of the diagnostic process. If a student does not recognize the classic pain pattern of patients with coronary heart disease or appreciate atypical presentations or special attributes of patients, mistakes in clinical diagnosis can be made.

In addition to personal experience, physicians also use **published data** to estimate probability. For example, one can look up the expected **prevalence** of CHD in patients of different ages presenting with various types of chest pain. This method of assigning patients is imprecise, however, because the process is not standardized. Another method to estimate probability is a clinical **prediction rule,** which has the following attributes. It is based on clinical studies in which historical data are obtained from many patients with chest pain. The diagnosis is established by a "gold standard" (cardiac catheterization) independently of these data. The independent predictors are identified by statistical techniques, and a method is developed to use these predictors, usually a mathematical formula. The prevalence of disease in various groups can then be determined by cardiac catheterization. Finally, the rule can be tested on new patients. When using prediction rules, it is important to know the population from which it was derived and how similar your patient is to that population. For example, if the rule was developed in a population of middle-aged men and the patient is a young woman, the rule may not be applicable.

Another approach to diagnosis using the published literature is to use **algorithms,** which are step-by-step instructions to facilitate problem solving. The diagnostic process is represented by a series of yes/no decision points. The goal is to place the patient in a group in which the prevalence of disease is high or low. Algorithms exist for common problems such as coronary heart disease and pharyngitis secondary to B-hemolytic streptococcus. Unfortunately, patients don't always fit into yes-or-no decision points. The process using iterative hypothesis testing is the strategy used by most physicians.

HYPOTHESIS CONFIRMATION

After gathering the appropriate information from the history and physical examination, the next step is to select the most likely diagnosis (working diagnosis) from the differential diagnosis. In the patient profiled above, CHD is the most probable diagnosis. Based on the history, the physical examination, published reports, and personal experience, the probability of CHD can be estimated as 0.70. This is called the **prior probability.** In this range of probability, there is still diagnostic uncertainty. Further tests are necessary. Should the "gold standard" test (cardiac catheterization), which is costly and invasive, be performed, or should an exercise tolerance test, which is less costly and noninvasive but not as good a test, be performed instead? If the prior probability is very high (e.g., 0.95), then it might be reasonable to proceed directly to the coronary arteriogram. If the probability is very low (e.g., 0.10), then no further testing may be necessary. When the results are in between, then further noninvasive testing is warranted. Proceeding directly to the coronary arteriogram when there is diagnostic uncertainty would subject patients to an unnecessary invasive and potentially dangerous procedure, waste resources, and increase costs. Such limits are called treatment thresholds. Knowing the prior probability and the sensitivity and specificity of a test, it is possible using Bayes' theorem to calculate the **posterior (posttest) probability** given a positive or negative test result (Chapter 3). The better the test (i.e., the higher the sensitivity and specificity), the closer the posterior probability approaches 1.

SUMMARY

Clinical reasoning is a critical cognitive process for physicians to master. It includes the following steps: hypothesis generation, which occurs early in the patient interview, hypothesis refinement, and hypothesis confirmation. The physician commonly uses several heuristics (rules of thumb) to aid in the diagnostic process. Understanding the basic principles of medical decision making will help the physician pinpoint the most likely diagnosis.

Research Questions

1. Do physicians who understand the principles of medical decision making interpret diagnostic tests more accurately than those who do not?
2. What is the best method of teaching clinical reasoning?

Case Resolution

The physician obtained the additional history that the patient's chest pain occurred only with exertion. A stress-test was performed, and after 4 minutes, the patient developed chest pain and 2 mm of ST segment depression. Subsequently, cardiac catheterization demonstrated severe three-vessel disease, and the patient was referred for coronary bypass surgery.

Selected Readings

Kassirer, J. P., and R. I. Kopelman. *Learning Clinical Reasoning.* Baltimore, Williams & Wilkins, 1991.
Sox, H. C., M. A. Blatt, M. C. Higgins, and K. I. Marton. *Medical Decision Making.* Stoneham, Massachusetts, Butterworth-Heineman, 1988.

CHAPTER 5

COST-EFFECTIVE APPROACH TO PRIMARY CARE PRACTICE

Martin E. Hickey, M.D.

Hx A 50-year-old female travel agent diagnosed with non–insulin-dependent diabetes mellitus (NIDDM) 5 years ago now presents with 2 days of progressively worsening urinary frequency, dysuria, and fever. Until the present illness she had been doing relatively well on 70/30 NPH/regular insulin, 50 units in the morning, and a sliding scale of up to 20 units in the afternoon based on home glucose monitoring (which she often skips). She has gained 4.5 kg (10 lb) over the past year, and her home monitoring glucose level, when she measures it, ranges from 150 to 250 mg/dL. Her mother died at age 60 of a myocardial infarction and had a 20-year history of NIDDM. The physical examination is remarkable for obesity (weight, 88 kg [194 lb], height, 163 cm [5 ft, 4 in.]), blood pressure of 150/100, temperature of 38.7° C (101.6° F), and questionable right costovertebral angle tenderness. She appears mildly ill but in no significant distress. Urinalysis reveals white blood cells and bacteria, and a dipstick test is positive for leukocytes, nitrites, and 1+ ketones. Blood chemistry is notable for glucose of 358 mg/dL, bicarbonate of 16 mEq/L, and HbA$_{1c}$ of 12.3%. The patient is a member of a health maintenance organization (HMO) that has contracted with the physician group to which the primary care practioner belongs. This organization no longer uses a fee-for-service payment method but pays the physician group through capitation.

Questions

1. Should this patient be managed as an inpatient or an outpatient?
2. What is the cost difference between inpatient and outpatient management?
3. Should the patient be referred to an endocrinologist for consultation and management of her diabetes?
4. Should you be concerned about the cost of her care?
5. What is meant by capitation?

Over the last three decades, health care costs in the United States have been rising at a rate of two to three times general inflation. In 1993, over 900 billion dollars were spent on health care, which is three times the defense budget and four times the cost for all education. The percentage of gross national product (GNP) spent on health care in 1963 was 6.5%, 15% in 1993, and may surpass 20% by the turn of the century. Premiums for health insurance have been increasing at a rate of 10%–20% per year. This high cost has led many employers to drop health insurance as an employee benefit, causing more people to become uninsured each year (with approximately 37 million people uninsured in 1993). Although the physician is not solely responsible for these increases, 70%–80% of health care expenditures pass through the physician's pen. As such, the decision to admit or not admit a patient takes on significant economic importance.

THE PHYSICIAN'S ROLE IN HEALTH CARE COSTS

A major way to reduce health care costs is to shift patient care out of the hospital and into the outpatient setting. A measure of inpatient utilization is the number of hospital days used per year per 1000 people. For patients under age 65 years, this figure had been as high as 1200/1000 in the 1980s. The national average is now about 600/1000, and in health care markets with high managed care penetration (e.g., California) it is approaching 150/1000. Many West Coast health plans intend to reduce this number to about 50/1000 by the year 2000. By treating more people in the ambulatory setting (e.g., outpatient surgery), letting patients convalesce at home with the support of home health nursing (e.g., home IV therapy), and employing principles of case management for chronic diseases, inpatient days can be significantly reduced.

Most health care costs pass through physicians. Although physicians play a role in reducing hospital use, they have had little direct incentive to keep costs down. Under "fee-for-service" reimbursement, providers are paid to treat illness by each episode of care, which encourages higher utilization of resources and a subsequent increase in costs. To turn this incentive around and to contain costs, a new payment methodology, called "capitation," is being utilized by payers. A monthly payment is made from the health plan to the physician for each patient regardless of whether that patient is ill or not. Thus, the physician has an incentive to keep the patient well. Further, since utilization of hospital services, specialists, tests, and various therapies may also come out of this monthly payment, the physician is motivated to utilize resources more appropriately. Because the usual primary care physician will care for about 2000 patients, most of whom will not suffer major illness, capitation provides a large pool of funds to cover the risk of illness within this group. The risk for illness and high expenditures is thus being passed from the payer or insurer to the physician. This is particularly true for primary care physicians, who are becoming the entry point for most patients into the health care system.

In a capitated system, the primary care clinician must think carefully about the intensity of resources brought to bear in dealing with a patient problem. If too many resources are used, especially ones that may not be needed to effectively diagnose and treat the problem, then the physician and his peer group, who pool their capitation risk, may overexpend the funds available to treat their patients. Careful consideration must be given to (1) hospitalizing patients versus treating them as outpatients with careful follow-up; (2) referring patients to consultants, especially when long-term follow-up can be done by the primary care physician; (3) using appropriate diagnostic tests; and (4) prescribing cost-effective drugs and other therapies. Under capitation, prevention takes on a highly significant role.

Whatever the system, the primary concern must continue to be the best result or outcome for the patient. Physicians cannot lose sight of this goal, especially in a system with potential rewards for doing less. Capitation seeks to motivate the clinician to appropriately utilize resources so that efficient as well as effective care can be provided. Thus, the primary care physician not only manages clinical care but also the clinical resources necessary to deliver high-quality care.

APPROACHES TO CLINICAL RESOURCE MANAGEMENT IN PATIENT CARE

Reduction in Hospital Utilization

Hospital expenditures account for over 40% of all health care costs. Reducing the number of hospital days will have the single largest impact of any cost reduction activity. Thus, before hospitalizing any patient, one should always ask, "Can this problem be handled on an outpatient basis?" Will the use of family members, home health nursing, home IV therapy, careful patient instructions, and close telephone and office follow-up suffice in caring for the problem? Can the workup and management be done on an ambulatory basis? Is the procedure, such as tubal ligation, amenable to day surgery? If a patient does need to be hospitalized, then discharge planning should become part of the admitting process. Many patients can convalesce at home or in an intermediate care facility with daily follow-up by telephone or home health nursing. Such approaches have allowed many primary care physician groups to reduce their hospital days per year per 1000 patients to less than 200 and in the process greatly reduce hospital expenditures.

Appropriate Specialty Consultation and Referral

The first question to ask is whether or not consultation is truly needed. Does the medical problem exceed the limits of one's training and experience, or is there an unfamiliar or complex procedure involved? By the same token, a good ambulatory care clinician should not go on a differential "fishing expedition" with multiple, random, and expensive tests, when a specialist might make the diagnosis clinically or with fewer tests.

If a referral is indicated, then the goals of the referral should be clearly spelled out. If possible, the consultation should be limited to one or a few visits. The specialist should then provide instructions to the referring doctor regarding care for the patient after the diagnosis has been made. Documentation of all test results and pertinent past medical records should be sent so that these expenditures do not have to be repeated.

If the patient has a complex chronic disease, such as end-stage renal disease, the specialist could well become the "primary care" provider, and the patient should be transferred to the specialist's care. If a physician has a large number of patients with the same problem in his practice, then focused medical education about the specific problem can reduce the number of referrals.

Case Management

For patients with chronic disease, case managers can reduce costs. This person is usually a nurse who can take the time to work closely with patients who are difficult to manage or have high hospitalization risk. Case managers provide patient education, coordinate support services, arrange ambulatory follow-up, discuss prevention, and in the process save expenditures well beyond their own costs. This close attention may also result in better outcomes and improve the patient's quality of life, since case managers also pay close attention to socioeconomic and home support factors.

Appropriate Use of Diagnostic Modalities

Before any test is undertaken, a clear purpose for it should be established. Another question to ask is whether the information gained will have a true impact on the management of the patient problem. Finally, the test should be efficacious; i.e., it should have good sensitivity and specificity and produce significant change in the positive predictive value if used (Chapter 3).

Therapeutic Cost Control

First, the clinician should be sure that the intervention is likely to be successful in treating the problem at hand. If not, the alternatives (including no intervention) should be thoroughly discussed with the patient. The well-informed patient may choose not to have an intervention of uncertain benefit. Second, if several different approaches or drugs achieve the same outcome, then the less expensive approach or drug should be utilized.

COST EFFECTIVENESS IN THE FUTURE

"Effectiveness" is the key word. In addition to containing costs through reducing hospital days, obtaining only appropriate consultation, and utilizing the services of case managers, the next focus should be on assuring successful outcomes; i.e., assessing whether a particular diagnostic and therapeutic approach to a problem achieves the positive benefit desired. Despite the science that provides the foundation of modern medical care, few studies objectively evaluate whether current diagnostic and therapeutic interventions for common medical problems are effective. From the common

upper respiratory tract infection to the management of angina, the comparative outcomes of different approaches are often unknown. This "outcomes" research will serve as the basis for primary care in the future. Once a specific approach is found that produces a better or more cost-effective outcome, it is likely to become a guideline, a management strategy that should ideally decrease morbidity and reduce costs.

Such work will require the compilation and analysis of extensive data and the utilization of sophisticated medical information systems. By the turn of the century, a primary care practitioner may well be able to enter a patient's problem, demographics, and comorbid conditions into a computer and be given an approach that will lead to the best predicted outcome at the least cost.

Society is demanding high-quality, affordable health care with universal access. These features can only be achieved if the provider is conscious of costs and can assure quality of outcome at the same time. The most effective locus of control for these two goals is in the mind of the clinician. This is the only place where all the parameters having impact on the patient and the interests of society can be measured and balanced appropriately. Thus, today's medical student and trainee will need to learn several new skills and knowledge bases. Included in these are medical economics, medical decision analysis, fiduciary—as well as biomedical—ethics, medical informatics, quality improvement, epidemiology and the health of populations, prevention, outcomes assessment, and group leadership and participation skills.

Research Questions

1. How can information on outcomes and the costs of different approaches to a medical problem be made easily accessible to the busy primary care practitioner?
2. Is either quality or outcome of care compromised by delivering and coordinating care through the primary care practitioner?

Case Resolution

The patient profiled above has an acute urinary tract infection (UTI). Her poorly controlled NIDDM puts her at risk for frequent UTIs. Her serum glucose is elevated above normal, and she has 1+ ketones and a low normal serum bicarbonate level. Her questionable costovertebral angle tenderness suggests possible pyelonephritis, but the finding is not a definitive sign. She does not appear to be in significant distress and is able to take oral fluids and medications. Since she is not in ketoacidosis, appears to have a UTI, is able to take to take fluids and medications, and has family at home to care for her, she can be treated as an outpatient.

She should be instructed to call if she starts to vomit, develops a fever over 40° C (104° F), develops significant flank pain, or symptomatically feels worse. A home health nurse will check on her the next day (to take vital signs, check a urine sample for ketones, and take a finger-stick glucose reading), and she will be seen in the office again in

3 days. This approach assures immediate intervention if the patient worsens, and greatly reduces the cost of this acute illness.

In addition to the cost savings, which are extremely important in prepaid capitated health plans, it is important to note that careful outpatient management should lead to a successful outcome. Some clinicians might argue that treating her as an inpatient would protect them against malpractice claims should the patient take a turn for the worse. Careful documentation of the reasoning for outpatient management, plus written patient instructions (with a copy in the chart), should protect the physician from litigation. The law requires that the care and approach be reasonable and in accordance with community standards, not that a perfect outcome be achieved all the time.

This patient should have more aggressive management of her poorly controlled NIDDM to prevent complications. A single consultation with an endocrinologist for suggestions on daily glucose control and a long-term management regimen might be helpful. However, this chronic disease does not require ongoing, expensive management by a specialist. A nurse case manager might be of major benefit to the patient. Working closely with the patient, the case manager could develop a weight reduction program (the treatment of choice in obesity-induced NIDDM), provide intensive blood pressure monitoring (to reduce the risk of future end-stage renal disease and coronary artery disease), and teach better home control of the NIDDM. A nurse case manager would be significantly less expensive than an endocrinologist and might be able to prevent expensive future complications and hospitalizations.

Selected Readings

Boland, P. (ed.). *Making Managed Healthcare Work: A Practical Guide to Strategies and Solutions.* Rockville, Maryland, Aspen Publishers, 1993.

Drumond, M. F., G. L. Stoddard, and G. W. Torrance. *Economic Evaluation of Health Care Programmes.* New York, Oxford University Press, 1987.

Kongstevdt, P. R. (ed.). *The Managed Care Handbook.* Rockville, Maryland, Aspen Publishers, 1993.

Shulkin, D. J., and A. H. Rosenstein. Toward cost effective health care. *In* D. B. Nash (ed.). *The Physician's Guide to Managed Care.* Gaithersburg, Maryland, Aspen Publishers, 1994, pp. 119–57.

Vogel, D. *The Physician and Managed Care.* Chicago, American Medical Association, 1993.

PHYSICIAN-PATIENT COMMUNICATION

CHAPTER 6

DIAGNOSTIC AND THERAPEUTIC ASPECTS OF THE MEDICAL INTERVIEW

Carolyn Voss, M.D.

H$_x$ A 28-year-old female sales clerk comes in because she has been experiencing left-sided chest pain daily for the past 2 months. During the interview, she also reveals that she has had "almost constant" abdominal pain and bloating since her teenage years, but quickly states that she has "just learned to live with it." She has pain in multiple joints, especially in the evening, and frequent headaches. On further questioning, she reveals that she has been to the emergency room at least a dozen times in the past month for the above symptoms, as well as for a motor vehicle accident that occurred in her words, "because my husband was drunk and wouldn't give me the keys." In taking her sexual history, she reveals that she has not had intercourse in over a year, because of "pelvic pain." The patient seems pleasant but aloof and somewhat distracted. The physical examination is normal. By the end of the interview, she seems more concerned with her frequent headaches than with her chest pain. As the examiner leaves the room, feeling exhausted and somewhat anxious, the patient expresses hope that the examiner can "get to the bottom of this."

Questions

1. How can the medical interview aid in making a diagnosis?
2. How might the interview hinder making a diagnosis?
3. In what ways might the interview be therapeutic?

Of all the activities physicians perform, perhaps the most important is the medical interview. This interaction ranges from a superficial exchange between two strangers to an intimate, emotional experience between two people who know each other well. With the time pressures that are present in the current health care milieu, time available for the interview is often quite limited. Consequently, conducting an effective medical interview requires considerable skill in adjusting the form and content according to the situation at hand.

The interview is the foundation of the science of medicine. It is from the interview that the physician obtains the "raw material" from which to formulate diagnoses, workup plans, and research questions. A 1975 study showed that 82% of diagnoses were made on the basis of the medical interview alone. But the medical interview is also the cornerstone of the art of medicine. It is in this interaction that trust, understanding, and empathy can be fostered; indeed, it is essential that these qualities be actively sought in every medical interaction in order to optimize patient outcomes.

To function effectively as a physician, it is not enough to know just the structure of the medical interview. Almost anyone can be trained in a very short period of time to ask a structured set of questions. This is a task most students master in the first or second year of medical school; as daunting as it may seem at the time, learning the basic format of the interview is relatively straightforward. The real challenge is to master the *art* of the medical interview, and it is in the mastery of this art that a true physician is born.

THE DOCTOR-PATIENT DYNAMIC

Most encounters between physicians and patients have three major goals. First, the physician must come to understand, by talking with and observing the patient, what is actually troubling the patient. What is troubling the patient may or may not be a clearly definable "medical" problem, and failure to recognize this will not only impede the physician's ability to get needed information but may also impair the physician's ability to appropriately treat the patient. For example, a woman who complains of insomnia since she lost her job may benefit far more from a supportive discussion of the stress she is under than from a prescription for a sleeping pill.

Sometimes understanding what the patient really means is not as easy as it sounds. For example, patients may use medical terminology inappropriately or even name body parts incorrectly (e.g., complaining that "my stomach hurts" when experiencing pelvic pain). More often, patients may complain of things that they feel are "all right" to complain about ("I have a headache") to legitimize a visit to the physician for problems that they feel are not "all right" to talk about ("My son was sent to jail"). The need to find out "what's really wrong" is especially important in cases where symptoms cannot be explained by a definable medical problem. However, discovering what the patient is most concerned about is *always* important, since one of the key steps in building rapport is making sure the patient feels that he or she has been heard. Without this feeling, patients are much less likely to experience trust or to follow medical advice.

Second, the physician must be able to restructure the information received from the patient so that the patient's concerns make sense within a medical framework. The facts or "raw material" elicited from the patient need to be organized and interpreted to create the "history." For example, the symptoms of crushing chest pain, sweating, and shortness of breath are rephrased in the physician's mind to "possible heart attack."

Finally, the physician must "retranslate" medical knowledge into an answer or explanation that makes sense to the individual patient. This can be especially difficult in situations where the cultural background, life experiences, or education of the physician differ markedly from those of the patient.

DIAGNOSTIC ASPECTS OF MEDICAL INTERVIEWING

Fact Gathering

As natural as having a conversation with a patient may seem, the use of selected techniques will make the interview an even more effective tool. The time-honored concept of beginning the interview by letting the patient tell his or her story, in his or her own words, is useful because it makes it less likely that important clinical data will be missed. Asking leading questions or interjecting one's own ideas into the interview too soon effectively closes the door on any information the patient might have that is contrary to expectations, thus decreasing the diagnostic sensitivity of the interview. Most patients are eager to find an answer to their problems and therefore are very willing to agree when one is suggested, no matter how erroneous it may be. If patients perceive that they are expected to have certain symptoms, they will tend to agree (or believe) that they have them. The physician should try to remain quiet for a moment after the patient finishes speaking (this is often not easy to do) in order to help the patient share difficult aspects of his history. Not interrupting can be as helpful as asking the right questions.

Nonverbal Communication

The interview should ideally be performed in a setting where privacy is maximized and the patient can feel that the physician's attention is undivided. This not only makes it easier to conduct the interview but also sends the patient a wealth of nonverbal information—that the physician is interested, cares about confidentiality, and believes that the patient's description of the problem is of utmost importance. Maintaining eye contact, sitting at eye level with the patient, and touching the patient appropriately during the interview all increase the likelihood of finding out what is needed to help the patient. Both parties send nonverbal cues to each other. Eyes tearing up is an obvious example, but these cues are often more subtle—breaking eye contact, changing the tone of voice, or turning away slightly. Paying attention to these cues can help determine which lines of questioning will be fruitful and which represent uncomfortable territory for the patient. Acknowledging this can help the interview move forward, whereas charging forward unaware is likely to impede the development of a good patient-physician relationship.

Despite the best intentions, physicians can decrease the diagnostic value of the medical interview by impairing the patient's ability to supply the needed "raw material." Failure to constantly be aware of one's own interviewing style and nonverbal messages—as well as the patient's verbal and nonverbal responses—will result in less reliable information and a less satisfying physician-patient relationship. Some common pitfalls to avoid are listed in Table 6–1.

The Symptoms in Context

Along with providing the information necessary to formulate diagnostic hypotheses, the interview is also useful for obtaining important experiential data from the patient. A patient's previous responses to illness or other adverse life events will help the physician understand how the patient will react to and experience the situation at hand. For example, a patient who prides himself on always keeping a "stiff upper lip" will be much less likely to report certain symptoms. Additionally, the patient's family and cultural milieu will determine not only what information the patient feels he or she can give, but also how he or she will respond to and interpret the diagnosis or medical advice. Taking into account the patient's world view, no matter how different from one's own, can greatly help in establishing a therapeutic alliance.

TABLE 6–1. Common Pitfalls to Avoid in the Medical Interview

Failing to introduce yourself
Failing to say the patient's name
Allowing distractions to remain (TV, radio, etc.)
Standing throughout the interview
Asking too few open-ended questions
Interrupting the patient's answers
Using medical jargon or other terms the patient doesn't understand
Asking "double questions"
Failing to make eye contact
Frowning, looking at your watch, or turning away from the patient while the patient is speaking

---

THERAPEUTIC ASPECTS OF MEDICAL INTERVIEWING

The process of obtaining information from the patient and getting to know the patient is, in and of itself, a form of treatment. The pleasure, trust, and relief that a patient may feel after an encounter with a physician are powerful therapies and sometimes may be *all* the physician has to offer.

The Patient-Centered Interview.

As described above, the patient-centered interview (using open-ended questions, etc.) is a technique by which the most useful information can be obtained. In addition, the act of talking with patients in this manner is therapeutic. Patients who feel they have been heard are also more likely to comply with advice and return for follow-up visits.

Empathy

Empathy has been defined by Zinn as "a process for understanding an individual's subjective experience by vicariously sharing that experience while maintaining an observant stance." Using a combination of memories, personal experiences, and fantasy (as well as an ardent attempt to understand the patient's own experience), an empathic physician can more fully share the subjective *experience* of illness with patients while maintaining an objective stance. This can be therapeutic in several ways. Physicians who are perceived by their patients as being more empathic are generally more effective in relieving their patients' concerns. In addition, empathic physicians are usually viewed by their patients as being more competent overall, thus improving patient motivation for following the physician's advice. Empathy on the part of the physician validates the patient as a person and enhances the patient's ability to express "hidden agendas" as well as express (and thereby relieve to a certain extent) the anxiety experienced because of illness.

Trust

Fostering trust is another therapeutic benefit that results from an effective medical encounter. By exhibiting patience, consistency, and unconditional positive regard, the physician can win and maintain patients' trust, even in the event of mistaken diagnoses or therapeutic mishaps. Trust in the physician allows the patient with an acute illness to agree to undergo otherwise unthinkable procedures.

In the case of the patient with chronic illness, trust in the physician helps the patient maintain hope and experience less anxiety as he or she learns to live with long-term problems. By fostering and maintaining the patient's trust, the physician can improve the quality of the patient's illness experience and also lessen the patient's suffering—therapeutic effects that are often difficult to achieve with medications alone.

INTROSPECTION

Another aspect of medical interviewing is being aware of one's own particular personality traits and reactions. These reactions can be either beneficial or harmful, depending on the reaction itself and the physician's degree of insight into it.

For example, what Sapira terms "autodiagnosis" is often quite helpful if it is understood and appreciated by the interviewer. This is the phenomenon whereby the physician can make a diagnosis, or have an insight, on the basis of the feelings a patient generates *within* the physician (e.g., a depressed patient who leaves the physician feeling depressed). Autodiagnosis can be very useful in evaluating a patient with multiple, seemingly unconnected complaints, to help uncover "what's really wrong."

A related concept is the role of physician anxiety in the interview process. If the physician feels anxiety during an interview, that may be a hint that the patient feels it too. Physician performance anxiety can interfere with the patient-centered approach, especially if the interviewer's focus is on "getting it right" instead of on the patient. For a student learning interviewing skills, it is helpful to be aware of and to acknowledge anxiety. Doing so will not only help ease one's own anxiety but will also help develop empathy with anxious patients.

A final physician factor to be aware of is bias. A human being does not exist who is not biased in some way. What is important in the process of medical interviewing is to be thoroughly aware of one's biases and to work at keeping them from coloring interpretations, reactions, and expectations. For example, many in the medical profession quickly develop biases regarding the "type" of patient who abuses intravenous drugs. Not recognizing this bias will result in failure to identify intravenous drug users who are counter to the type. Other biases are more subtle, and it is worth the effort and introspection required to find those that are within oneself.

SUMMARY

The medical interview is the source from which the rest of medicine springs. Learning the skills to perform an interview that is useful diagnostically and therapeutically—and that sets the stage for a satisfying patient-physician relationship—is a lifelong process. Without these skills, not only the art and science of medicine, but also the pleasure of medicine surely suffers.

Research Questions

1. How can the process of medical education be improved to foster empathy and good communication skills on the part of physicians?
2. How might more effective physician-patient communication save health care dollars?

Case Resolution

During subsequent interviews, the physician allowed sufficient time for the patient to describe how her life has been affected by her multiple symptoms. By making appropriately placed empathic statements ("It sounds like all this has been very hard on you"), the physician eventually established a trusting and therapeutic relationship with the patient. At the time of her fourth visit, the patient revealed information that she has never discussed with anyone: at age 9 years, she was sexually abused by a friend of her parents. The patient asked whether any of her current symptoms might be related to that event.

Selected Readings

Matthews, D. A., et al. Making "connexions": Enhancing the therapeutic potential of patient-clinician relationships. Ann Intern Med 118:973–7, 1993.

Sapira, J. D. The interview. In J. D. Sapira and J. D. Orient. *The Art and Science of Bedside Diagnosis.* Baltimore, Urban & Schwarzenberg, 1990.

Siegler, M. Falling off the pedestal: What is happening to the traditional doctor-patient relationship? Mayo Clin Proc 68:461–7, 1993.

Zinn, W. The empathic physician. Arch Intern Med 153:306–12, 1993.

CHAPTER 7

THE PATIENT IN THE CONTEXT OF THE FAMILY, THE COMMUNITY, AND SOCIETY

Berthold E. Umland, M.D.

H_x A 68-year-old female retired domestic worker who has wintered in Arizona for the past 2 years returned to her long-time primary care physician complaining of almost constant abdominal pain. A gastroenterologist in Arizona had evaluated the pain with barium contrast studies, upper and lower gastrointestinal endoscopy, and a CT scan of the abdomen, all with negative (i.e., normal) results. A variety of medications have not helped the pain. A detailed history obtained from the patient and her husband revealed no obvious pattern to her symptoms. During the physical examination—with her husband absent—the patient burst into tears, saying, "This move to Arizona has been terrible. Johnny has been drinking a lot, and then he screams at me and calls me the most horrible names. My first husband never treated me this way." Additional questioning revealed a connection between the abdominal pain and episodes of verbal abuse.

Questions

1. Why did it take 2 years for the patient to describe her stress to her physician?
2. How does psychosocial stress cause abdominal pain?
3. Is it always necessary to understand the biomedical "cause" to help the patient?

People who become patients spend only a small fraction of their lives in medical settings. Physicians are taught to focus almost exclusively on the signs, symptoms, and biomedical issues patients present with at the time of the medical encounter. However, patients bring with them their own socioeconomic and educational context, cultural belief systems about illness and health, and individual habits and behaviors, all of which may have a profound impact on the outcome of the doctor-patient interaction. While physicians have an acquired biomedical perspective, they also have their own biases, attitudes, and belief systems. Even the most sophisticated and scientifically inclined physicians have been known to resort to their grandmother's advice when counseling patients about problems that do not fit a strict biomedical model. Physicians give advice freely, but they are often guilty of "noncompliance" in their own life-style—often for the same reasons as their patients.

To better understand the patient's perspective, one needs to recognize the difference between illness and disease. The patient experiences an *illness,* whereas the clinician diagnoses and manages a *disease*. The experience of illness is much broader than the disease itself because it includes everything in the patient's life that is affected by the disease. The patient's theories of causation are often related to the illness, not the disease. Physicians usually think in terms of pathophysiology, but patients might view illness as punishment for a sin or transgression. They may believe an enemy has cast an evil eye or put a hex on them. If a clinician ignores that broader context, communication between physician and patient is likely to be incomplete and unsatisfactory.

In 1977, George Engel described a biopsychosocial model of health and illness that takes into account the complex interplay between the patient's body, the social situation, and the person's psychological state. Engel's model thus attempts to reconcile the mind-body dualism that has separated psychiatry and medicine throughout most of the 20th century.

PATHOPHYSIOLOGY

Some medical problems seem straightforward: a broken arm, at first glance, appears to be a biomedical event. Casting the broken arm in plaster for 3 to 6 weeks usually allows it to heal. However, the fracture occurred in the context of the patient's social setting. The injury may have been secondary to a drunken fall or physical abuse by another person. Ignoring the social setting puts the patient at risk for similar episodes.

Recent research shows an association between environmental tobacco smoke and respiratory disease in children and adults. Side-stream smoke contains the same toxic substances as inhaled smoke. Our society is beginning to recognize the rights of nonsmokers, and many cities and states have enacted laws that ban smoking in certain designated areas. However, children cannot prevent their parents from smoking in the home or car and thus may be susceptible to illness brought on by parental behavior.

Although some people feel that exposing children to secondhand smoke is a form of child abuse, a more flagrant example of abuse was first described approximately 25 years ago in the medical literature and termed the "battered baby syndrome." More recently, it has been recognized that adolescents as well as young children can be victims of family violence and abuse and that this abuse can be physical, sexual, or mental. Such abuse may present as an unexplained injury or a more subtle change such as poor performance in school or withdrawal from social activities. Unless domestic violence and abuse are considered in the differential diagnosis, the symptoms are likely to progress. An accurate diagnosis is critical to appropriate intervention.

Although abuse can be seen in families at all socioeconomic levels, socioeconomic status can have a profound effect on the pathophysiology of specific diseases. Infectious diseases have historically been more prevalent among impoverished people living in crowded conditions with poor sanitation. A classic example is rheumatic fever. Other diseases are more likely to occur amidst the relative affluence of more highly industrialized societies. There appear to be clear links, for example, between coronary artery disease and a high-fat diet. In China, where coronary disease had previously been uncommon, increasing affluence appears to be increasing the incidence of diabetes and hypertension, leading to a recent epidemic of coronary disease.

An elderly demented person repeating the same question time after time will likely try the patience of an otherwise loving caretaker. The caretaker reaches a limit and strikes out in frustration. Injury occurs, not from deliberate or malicious action, but from frustration. If the caretaker does not receive respite, another injury may occur. When the elderly person is seen in the emergency room, more than the injury needs to be dealt with. The social situation must be addressed to prevent recurrence.

EVALUATION

Medical students are taught to collect information regarding the present illness, review of systems, past medical history, family history, and—in what often seems to be an afterthought—social history. Extensive teaching is done to perfect physical examination maneuvers. Expensive laboratory tests and other investigations are discussed at great length during the training years. However, there never seems to be enough time to *listen* to the patient describe the context in which the illness occurs and is experienced. Diagnosis in the absence of a management plan is not helpful other than for self-limited disease or disease so serious that intervention will not change the outcome. Neglecting the context in which the illness arises—and the patient's capacity to deal with the illness—usually precludes successful management.

MANAGEMENT

"Noncompliance" means that the patient is not doing what the physician has advised. It is often used as an epithet depicting the patient as somehow stubborn and deliberately disobedient. However, the patient may not (1) be able to afford the medication prescribed, (2) know how to read instructions on a prescription label (a large percentage of the U.S. population is functionally illiterate), or (3) have the resources to carry out the special treatment recommended. Most companies provide sick leave for employees, but do not allow compensated time off when a parent needs to care for an ill child. An injunction to spend hours in bed will be ignored when there are child care or other family responsibilities that no one else can handle. Facilitating patient adherence requires recognition of the many factors that interfere with a patient's best intentions.

An incomplete understanding of community resources can also lead physicians astray. Medical training occurs mainly in tertiary care institutions. Practicing in a rural area is perceived as difficult because resources that a physician is accustomed to using may not be available. A "context specialist" can provide help to physicians in all settings. Nurses, social workers, and home health care providers are often aware of the importance of "context" and can mobilize resources to overcome the barriers that might otherwise inhibit patient compliance.

PATIENT AND FAMILY EDUCATION

Patients are usually more aware of the interdependence of biopsychosocial factors than are physicians. They have not been through the scientific socialization process that minimizes causality not fitting the biomedical model. Physicians should listen carefully to the patient's explanatory model of illness even when the linkages are to a social or cultural situation rather than a biomedical event. Conversely, patients have been heavily influenced by the media and the health care establishment to always expect a biomedical cause. They have learned to discount their own observations and intuition about psychosocial etiologies of illness. They have also learned that a psychosocial cause may be misinterpreted as malingering. They fear that their physician will say "it's all in your head" and that they will be humiliated and accused of faking illness.

As physicians become trained in the biopsychosocial model of illness, they can in turn educate their patients and their patients' families. Viewing the patient in context allows a broader interpretation of events. As a clinician collects data and translates this information back to the patient and the family, the meaning of disease in the patient's life will be better understood. In addition, compliance usually improves when the patient and family understand the rationale of the physician's recommendation.

Research Questions

1. How can we educate physicians and other health care providers to use the biopsychosocial model routinely?
2. Aside from the epinephrine response, what physiologic mechanisms are responsible for the somatic manifestations of "stress"?

Case Resolution

When the patient's husband returned to the examination room, he was persuaded by the circumstantial evidence that his drinking was responsible for his wife's symptoms and he expressed a willingness to discontinue alcohol use entirely. He left the office with a prescription for disulfiram (Antabuse). With continued counseling and support, the patient's abdominal pain disappeared.

Selected Readings

AMA Council on Scientific Affairs. Adolescents as victims of family violence. JAMA 270:1850–6, 1993.

Boyle, P. The hazards of passive and active smoking. N Engl J Med 328:1708–9, 1993.

Chilmonczyk, B. A., et al. Association between exposure to environmental tobacco smoke and exacerbation of asthma in children. N Engl J Med 328:1665–9, 1993.

Engel, G. L. The need for a new medical model: A challenge for biomedicine. Science 196:129–36, 1977.

CHAPTER 8

CULTURAL CONSIDERATIONS IN PRIMARY CARE

Melvina McCabe, M.D., Susanna J. Kearny, B.A., and Christopher E. Urbina, M.D., M.P.H.

Hx   A 55-year-old Native American male presents with the chief complaint of pain in his chest that began upon awakening and has continued intermittently throughout the day. He reports that "somewhat similar" pains in the past were partially relieved by antacid use. The current pain is described as "very mild," radiates to the left arm, and is associated with shortness of breath and nausea. The patient is a member of the governing body of his community and chairs several subcommittees. He is accompanied by his wife, children, parents, and sister, who report that he has recently been unable to fully perform job-related activities because of fatigue. He came to the clinic today at their insistence. His medical history is significant for adult-onset diabetes mellitus and hypertension, and his current medications are glyburide and lisinopril. The patient had a cholecystectomy 10 years ago and was involved in a motor vehicle accident 5 years ago. He denies the use of alcohol or tobacco and has no history of allergy to medications. He is afebrile and has a pulse of 110/min and blood pressure of 100/50 mm Hg. His respiratory rate is 24/min. The remainder of the physical examination is unremarkable except for dark smudges noted on the skin over various parts of his body.

Questions

1. What might have caused the dark smudges on the patient's body?
2. What impact do cultural considerations have on the delivery of health care?

The phenomenon of cultural diversity and the importance of its impact on health care delivery are being increasingly recognized. The experiences of many Native American, Hispanic, African American, and Asian American patients related to health, disease, and wellness differ greatly from models presented in traditional Western medical education.

Cultural diversity exists *within* groups as well as *between* ethnic populations. Although tremendous cultural diversity exists among non-Hispanic whites, this patient population generally accepts the prevailing Western notions of health and illness and therefore is not included in this discussion. It is important to note, however, that no single ethnic group is considered the norm, and culture does not fully determine an individual's behavior. Key issues for each ethnic group include (1) cultural attitudes and beliefs about health and illness, (2) patient use of dual (i.e., Western as well as culturally specific) health systems, (3) the nature of patient interactions with health professionals, (4) disease prevalence, and (5) provider expectations.

NATIVE AMERICAN PERSPECTIVE

The top five leading causes of death in the Native American population are coronary artery disease, accidents, neoplastic disease, cerebrovascular disease, and liver disease including cirrhosis (Table 8–1). Life expectancy at birth is 75.1 years for Native American females, compared to 78.1 years for white females, and 67.1 years for Native American males, compared to 70.7 years for white males.

The population of Native Americans in the United States is estimated at approximately 2 million. There are 500 federally recognized American Indian tribes and Alaskan Native groups. The Native American tribes are distributed throughout the United States with the greatest concentration in the Western states. The cultural complexity is enormous given the number of distinct tribal groups.

Approximately 51% of Native Americans reside in urban settings, with the remainder residing in rural or reservation sites. American Indians living on a reservation can receive their medical care at Indian Health Service (IHS) facilities. Because many reservation-dwelling Native Americans live in outlying areas with unpaved roads, access to IHS facilities may sometimes be difficult. American Indians living in urban areas may not always have IHS facilities available to them and must therefore find other health care options.

Cultural beliefs vary greatly among the members of different tribes. Beliefs can also vary among members of the *same* tribe, and such intratribal heterogeneity must be taken into account when interacting with Native American patients. The degree of acculturation and the influence of Christianity are but two of the many factors accounting for these intratribal differences.

Beliefs concerning health and disease also vary significantly among Native American individuals. A Western physician, to become a truly effective healer, must demonstrate respect for these cultural beliefs by acknowledging them and incorporating them whenever possible into the Western medical paradigm. In addition, patients need to be accepted for who they are. The Western health professional must assess Native American patients in the context of their environment, society, and ethnic values and beliefs.

Many Native American patients will have been treated by traditional healers before they seek Western medical intervention. It is important to ask whether traditional healers have been involved in the patient's care, and it is key that this question be asked in a nonjudgmental manner. Such a discussion often reveals to the Western healer the patient's beliefs about the cause of the illness and the most effective intervention. A specific example of disease causation from the Navajo perspective is the concept of disharmony with nature. Harmony with nature is evidenced by wellness; disease is a symptom of disharmony.

Native Americans maintain strong family ties. The Western healer must, at the very least, acknowledge the presence of each family member and include them, when appropriate, in the discussion. To find out what is culturally appropriate in a given situation, one must not be ashamed to ask.

Native American patients may minimize the degree of pain or discomfort they are experiencing. Reported pain levels may thus not be an accurate indicator of the severity of the patient's problem.

TABLE 8–1.   Leading Causes of Death among Different Ethnic Groups

	Cause of Death				
	1	2	3	4	5
Native Americans	Heart disease	Accidents	Neoplastic disease	Stroke	Liver disease, including cirrhosis
Asian Americans	Heart disease	Neoplastic disease	Stroke	Accidents	Respiratory infections
African Americans	Heart disease	Neoplastic disease	Stroke	Homicide	Accidents
Hispanic Americans	Heart disease	Neoplastic disease	Accidents	Stroke	Diabetes mellitus

Data from U. S. Department of Health and Human Services, National Center for Health Statistics. *IHS Trends in Indian Health 1991.* Hyattsville, Maryland, Public Health Service, 1992.

AFRICAN AMERICAN PERSPECTIVE

African Americans often do not receive adequate primary care, and access to health care in general is lacking. In 1989, the infant mortality rate for African Americans was more than twice that for whites, and African American infants were almost three times as likely as white infants to have very low birth weights. According to the National Center for Health Statistics, African Americans are disproportionately affected by the nation's leading causes of death. In 1989, the death rate for cancer was higher in African American males than in any other race/sex subgroup—230.6 deaths per 100,000 persons compared with 157.2 deaths per 100,000 persons for white males. In 1989, the mortality rate due to heart disease for African American males was 272.6 per 100,000 persons compared with 205.9 for white males. For African American females, the corresponding death rate due to heart disease was 172.9 per 100,000 persons compared with 106.6 for white females.

Additional data from the National Center for Health Statistics indicate that hypertension and diabetes are among the leading causes of death for African American females and homicide is currently the leading cause of death among African American males aged 15–34 years. African Americans are almost twice as likely as whites to experience severe hypertension, and obesity is twice as prevalent among African American women as in white women. In a health survey conducted in 1990, 15.1% of African Americans rated their health as poor, compared to 8.1% of whites.

U. S. census figures for 1990 reveal that of a total African American population of approximately 30 million, 5 million people live outside metropolitan areas, 8 million people live in non-central city metropolitan areas, and 17 million live in central cities. The fragmented social conditions associated with inner-city life mean that an African American patient is less likely to have the support of an extended family. The 1991 Census Bureau Population Survey revealed that 40% of African Americans were without health insurance. Problems with transportation, inability to leave work, and past experiences with racism are all barriers to effective treatment.

Sociocultural and organizational problems in health care delivery are compounded by communication barriers. A frequent source of misunderstanding between African American patients and their often non–African American physicians relates to the prevention and treatment of hypertension. While a physician may know that African Americans are at risk for hypertension and prescribe antihypertensive medication for this chronic health problem, African American patients often believe that hypertension is related to a particular stressful situation and may stop taking their medication once that stressful situation has passed.

Although African American patients are likely to be acculturated to traditional Western medicine, their problems and cultural beliefs related to health are extremely diverse. African Americans often seek health-related support and advice from individuals outside the formal health care system. In addition, they not uncommonly maintain cultural perceptions and beliefs outside the mainstream of Western medicine, including the benefits of herbs and other home remedies. Physicians thus need to determine their patients' belief systems and incorporate these beliefs into clinical decision-making.

HISPANIC PERSPECTIVE

Although the Hispanic population of the United States may share a common language and certain cultural traditions, differences among the various Hispanic groups (e.g., Puerto Rican Americans, Mexican Americans, Cuban Americans, etc.) can be as dramatic as differences between Hispanics and the non-Hispanic white majority. A Mexican American may be culturally closer to citizens of Mexico than to citizens of Puerto Rico. Another key issue is the degree of acculturation and assimilation into the majority culture. A fifth generation New Mexican Hispanic, for example, may not speak Spanish, may have been educated at private schools, and will likely earn a considerably higher income than a recently arrived Mexican immigrant working in the chile fields of the Rio Grande Valley.

The U. S. Hispanic population is thus quite heterogeneous with many geographic, historical and cultural differences. Since the late 15th and 16th centuries, Hispanics have lived in the Americas. The arrival of the Spanish in the Americas simultaneously led to the destruction of native populations and the proliferation of several "new" populations united by language, religion, and a number of cultural traditions. Today, Hispanics in the United States are generally categorized by their nation of origin: Mexican Americans, Cuban Americans, Puerto Rican Americans, and South or Central Americans. In 1990, United States Hispanics numbered over 22 million and are projected to be the largest ethnic minority by the beginning of the 21st century.

Hispanics suffer disproportionately from several major illnesses. Although Hispanics die of heart disease and cancer at lower rates than do non-Hispanic whites, Hispanics suffer from an excess incidence of cancer of the stomach, esophagus, and pancreas. Hispanic women develop cervical cancer twice as often as non-Hispanic white women. In addition, Hispanics have more undiagnosed hypertension and are three times more likely to develop diabetes mellitus than non-Hispanic whites. Unintentional injuries, homicide, chronic liver disease (including cirrhosis), and AIDS are also growing problems among Hispanics. Violent deaths account for an increasingly high mortality rate among Hispanic adolescents. In general, family, language, and religion play a major role in day-to-day decisions about health, life, and death.

ASIAN AMERICAN PERSPECTIVE

The five leading causes of death in Americans of Asian or Pacific Islander descent are heart disease, malignant neoplasms, cerebrovascular disease, accidents, and respiratory infections (especially pneumonia and influenza). According to the National Center for Health Statistics, diabetes mellitus is the sixth leading cause of death in Asian or Pacific Islander females and chronic obstructive pulmonary disease the sixth leading cause of death in Asian or Pacific Islander males. Additional statistics, however, show that these disease prevalence figures can obscure the considerable cultural variability among Asian Americans. Asian cultures are heterogeneous; language, customs, religion, and even food are distinct for each ethnic group. It is particularly important to gain an understanding of Asian-American patients' attitudes toward health and illness and their expectations and apprehensions regarding Western medicine.

Many of the most recent Asian American immigrants came to the United States from Southeast Asia during two periods, the first in 1975 and the second in 1979. The majority of the first group of refugees were (1) educated Vietnamese, (2) under 45 years of age, (3) in good physical health, and (4) accompanied by family members. The second wave of Southeast Asian refugees were more heterogeneous—generally not as well educated, not as healthy, and less familiar with Western institutions and the English language. Physicians whose Southeast Asian patients arrived after 1979 may find that these patients speak very little English, know little about the U. S. health care system, and continue traditional health care practices including the use of herbal remedies.

A strong belief in the curative power of nature, a mistrust of invasive procedures, and the use of explanatory models for health and illness that include concepts of "cold," "hot," "wet," and "dry" are all common in the more recent Southeast Asian immigrants and may prove frustrating to a practitioner of Western medicine. Misunderstanding the patient's concepts of health and sickness may also cause the physician to misinterpret the patient's behavior. Noncompliance, for example, may really represent noncommunication between patient and physician, especially if the patient decreases or discontinues medication because of the commonly held Southeast Asian perception that Western drugs are excessively potent. A patient's physical complaints may mask psychiatric or psychosomatic problems, particularly if there is no easily identifiable medical cause. Refugee trauma increases the likelihood of anxiety, depression, delayed grief, and posttraumatic stress disorder. A bilingual interpreter can be extremely helpful in communicating with an Asian American patient, but attention to, and respect for, the patient's point of view is the most important element in successful management.

SUMMARY

The many cultures within our society, with their attendant values and beliefs, make for a rich and fascinating mosaic. This great variety of attitudes and experiences makes it impossible to apply only one health care model to every patient and every clinical situation.

Cultural beliefs exert a strong influence on how readily a patient accepts Western medicine's explanations of health and disease. Western medical views are but one path to wellness and health. The existence of many other paths must be acknowledged to truly understand and help patients from non-Western backgrounds.

Research Questions

1. What is the impact of traditional Native American healing practices on the most prevalent diseases in this population?
2. In your community, what are the expectations of the health care system by the Hispanic, African American, Asian American, and other minority populations?

Case Resolution

The patient's ECG was normal, but the physician believed that the chest pains might have been due to unstable angina and recommended hospitalization. After consulting with his family, the patient agreed. The patient requested—and received—the inclusion of a traditional healer in his care. The admitting physician was initially unaware of the significance of the dark smudges on the patient's skin but later learned from the family that these were incurred during a ceremony performed by a tribal healer.

Selected Readings

Council on Scientific Affairs. Hispanic health in the United States. JAMA 265:248–52, 1991.

Muecke, M. A. In search of healers: Southeast Asian refugees in the American health care system. West J Med 139(6):31–6, 1983.

National Center for Health Statistics. *Health United States, 1991.* Hyattsville, Maryland, Public Health Service, 1992.

U.S. Bureau of the Census. *The Hispanic Population in the United States: March 1991.* Current Population Reports Series P-20, No. 455. Washington, D.C., U.S. Department of Commerce, 1991.

U.S. Department of Health and Human Services, National Center for Health Statistics. *IHS Trends in Indian Health 1991.* Hyattsville, Maryland, Public Health Service, 1992.

FACILITATING PATIENT ADHERENCE

James R. Phelps, M.D.

H$_x$ A 45-year-old male insurance agent has a history of reflux esophagitis, peptic ulcer disease, and hypertension. Despite his continued use of cimetidine, which he takes religiously, he is now experiencing epigastric pain on exertion. The patient has a prominent family history of heart disease and has not responded to his physician's repeated admonitions to stop smoking. His physician, concerned about new ST-T segment changes on the patient's electrocardiogram, schedules a treadmill test, and changes the patient's medication from an ACE inhibitor to a β-blocker. The patient does not understand the doctor's concern; he is sure that his pain represents "just another problem with his stomach." He stops taking the β-blocker after a few doses because he feels "too slowed down." He plans to discuss this further with his physician after his treadmill test. Two days later, he suffers a myocardial infarction.

Questions

1. Why didn't the patient adhere to the physician's treatment recommendations?
2. What could the physician have done differently to increase the likelihood that the patient would follow the advice given?

BOX 9-1. Four Steps to Facilitate Patient Efforts

1. **Suspect** low adherence rates; if necessary, focus your facilitating efforts on those whose perceptions of cost and benefit predict highest risk.
2. **Detect** the factors that will influence adherence by inquiring about patients' perceptions (severity, susceptibility, treatment efficacy, and self-efficacy).
3. **Facilitate** patients' adherence by minimizing the complexity of their treatment, inquiring about potential barriers, and writing a summary of plans for the patient to take home.
4. **Respect** patients' autonomy and the fact that they, not you, control outcomes.

The rate-limiting step in improving patients' health frequently is not under physicians' control. In most outpatient situations, patients exercise ultimate control, since even the most accurate diagnoses and the most efficacious therapies will not be of benefit unless patients are willing and able to carry out the designated treatment plan. As primary care providers, physicians must recognize that they are dependent upon their patients' adherence to treatment plans if the desired results are to be achieved.

The following is a four-step guide to help physicians facilitate their patients' efforts; it also provides a structure for students' continued learning (Box 9–1).

STEP 1: SUSPECT

Not all patients are at risk for low adherence rates. Patients who perceive their treatment regimens to be highly effective and of minimal bother are at far less risk than are those who perceive their regimens to be of little benefit and are concerned about potential side effects.

By considering the patient's view of treatment benefits and costs (the latter including treatment risks and side effects), physicians can identify those patients most in need of a systematic approach to increasing adherence. In which of the squares shown in Figure 9–1 does the patient in the introductory case history fall?

STEP 2: DETECT

Surprisingly, not many patient characteristics have a strong effect on adherence: intelligence, age, and socio-

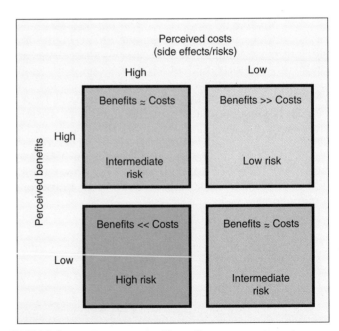

FIGURE 9–1. *Stratifying the risk of low adherence rates by patient perception of cost and benefit of treatment.*

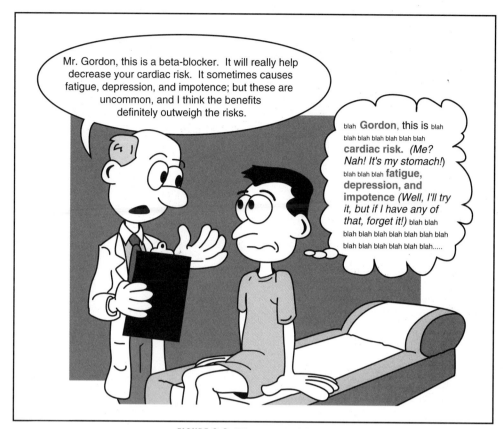

FIGURE 9–2. *What a patient hears.*

economic status have only weak influence. Not even the severity of disease is predictive. Instead of the *actual* risk of morbidity or mortality, it is the patient's *perceived* risk of debility or death that more powerfully affects adherence.

Often there is little resemblance between actual risk and perception of risk. When perceived risk exceeds actual risk (e.g., in a hypochondriacal patient), the physician is very likely to be aware of the disparity. But when a patient's actual risk exceeds the perceived risk (e.g., in the case profiled above), the disparity can easily be missed by the physician.

When doctors do not directly inquire about their patients' beliefs, a circumstance such as that shown in Figure 9–2 can arise. Research suggests that patients' information retention rate is about 50% at best, declining linearly in proportion to the volume of information transmitted. Even when patients actually hear physicians' words, they edit the physicians' statements and recommendations on the basis of their own health beliefs.

How can this scenario be avoided? The answer is simple, though not always easy to implement in practice: the physician must weave patient education into the patient's preexisting knowledge and beliefs. Thus, in the same way that the diagnostic process begins with a detailed history of the present illness, effective patient education begins with inquiries into the patient's health belief system.

What specifically should the physician inquire about?

To answer that question, the way in which physicians generally approach "patient education" needs to be examined. Most physicians follow the format in which they themselves were educated: usually they deliver mini-lectures to patients on the risks and benefits of the various treatments under consideration. They believe that if the benefits outweigh the risks, patients will opt in favor of treatment and adhere to the advised regime (Fig. 9–3).

However, even when patients hear the description exactly as physicians intend, they may not arrive at the same conclusion. It is their *perception* of their illness that makes the difference. They must believe that (1) they are at risk ("perceived susceptibility"), (2) the risk is serious ("perceived severity"), (3) the treatment will work ("treatment efficacy"), and (4) they can carry out the treatment ("self-efficacy").

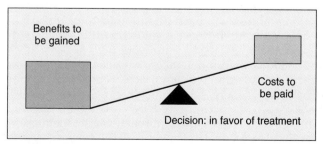

FIGURE 9–3. *Physician's model of patient's decision making.*

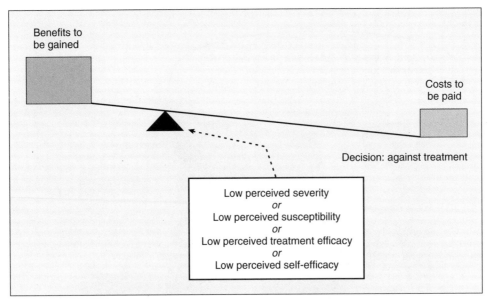

FIGURE 9–4. *Effect of health beliefs on patient's decision making.*

The model in Figure 9–4 shows how the patient can understand and even agree completely with the physician's exposition of risks and benefits, yet still arrive at a different decision regarding treatment, or even worse, simply not "comply."

The Interview

Just as the chief complaint routinely prompts physicians to ask questions about location, duration, and so on, adherence-facilitating patient education should prompt physicians to routinely include questions about the following four health beliefs:

1. What does the patient know about *severity?* e.g., "What is your understanding of a heart attack?"
2. What does the patient know about *susceptibility?* e.g., "How likely is this to happen to you, do you think?"
3. What does the patient know about treatment *effectiveness?* e.g., "What have you heard about ways to prevent heart attacks?" "Do you think this could work for you?"
4. Does the patient believe he or she could *carry out* the treatment? e.g., "What might get in the way of sticking with this treatment?"

After conducting such an inquiry, physicians can address the specific needs of individual patients: some will simply need more information about the treatment options, others will need attention to their underlying beliefs about their disease, and still others will need a systematic approach to improving their self-efficacy.

The inquiry approach takes only seconds longer than the physician-directed approach. Moreover, this approach is usually more effective because patients' beliefs can be incorporated into treatment planning. Patients who require this approach can be identified in Step 1. A key axiom to remember is this: *when preparing to educate patients about a treatment plan, ask—don't tell.*

STEP 3: FACILITATE

Three basic measures will help most patients maintain high adherence rates:

Minimize the complexity of the treatment by keeping the **total number of medications** to an absolute minimum and the **number of administration times** to an absolute minimum as well. For patients whose medications are many and must be administered at different times, a pill-minder box—prepared with the patient by a nurse in the clinic and refilled by a visiting nurse—is an effective, albeit resource-intensive, approach.

Ask patients to identify potential barriers to full adherence. A patient frequently knows what is likely to interfere with adherence. Simply asking patients, "What is likely to get in the way of your taking this medication?" will usually reveal one or several specific barriers, e.g., financial concerns, fear of side effects, lack of access to a pharmacy, or the more subtle issues discussed in Step 2.

Extend your presence beyond your office door. A simple, hand-written summary outlining the treatment plan, prepared by the physician, can significantly improve adherence rates. Patients often remark that carrying a prn medicine in their purse or pocket is like having their doctor accompany them wherever they go. Likewise, a list of instructions or recommendations taped to their bathroom mirror—or carried along with the pills themselves—helps extend the physician's reach. A supply of auto-carbon paper in the examination room allows doctors to put a copy of their summary in the chart, thus documenting their adherence-promoting efforts.

STEP 4: RESPECT

When physicians control the data-gathering process, the decision-making process, and the communication process during encounters with patients, they should be neither surprised nor angry when patients do not assume responsibility for carrying out the treatment.

For most patients, especially those at high risk (see Fig. 9–1), physicians should promote a sense of responsibility by encouraging a *collaborative* relationship. This means deliberately and consistently (1) *asking questions,* not making statements; (2) *suggesting options,* not making decisions; and (3) *facilitating patients' efforts,* not making plans. Sharing power in this manner should lead to better results.

Research Questions

1. What factors affect physicians' adherence to guidelines aimed at improving patient adherence?
2. What other measures can be taken in outpatient settings to promote a stronger sense of responsibility on the part of patients for their own health outcomes?

Case Resolution

The patient was hospitalized following his myocardial infarction. The shock of this event led him and his physician to engage in a more collaborative relationship in which his concerns could be aired completely. The physician recognized the patient's desire to return to a physically active life-style and arranged a meeting with the cardiac rehabilitation team early in the hospitalization. Following the patient's discharge, the physician worked with him to find an antihypertensive agent that would not affect his sexual functioning. In addition, the two are working together to plan a stepped approach to smoking cessation.

Selected Readings

Becker, M. H. Theoretical models of adherence and strategies for improving adherence. *In* S. A. Schumaker, S. B. Shron, and J. K. Ockene (eds.). *The Handbook of Health Behavior Change.* New York, Springer Publishing Company, 1990.

Beckman, H., and R. Frankel. Can I really improve my listening skills with only 15 minutes to see my patients? HMO Practice 5(4):114–20, 1991.

Ley, P. *Communicating With Patients: Improving Communication, Satisfaction and Compliance.* New York, Croom Helm, 1988.

Meichenbaum, D., and D. Turk. *Facilitating Treatment Adherence: A Practitioner's Guidebook.* New York, Plenum Press, 1987.

Miller, W. R., and S. Rollnick. *Motivational Interviewing: Preparing People to Change Addictive Behaviors.* New York, Guilford Press, 1991.

O'Brien, M. K., K. Petrie, and J. Raeburn. Adherence to medication regimens: Updating a complex medical issue. Med Care Rev 49:435–54, 1992.

CHAPTER 10

EFFECTIVE USE OF THE TELEPHONE IN OUTPATIENT PRACTICE

Douglas Egli, M.D.

H$_x$ A physician is on call over the weekend for a group practice of six family practitioners. A 46-year-old male house painter who is followed by one of the other partners telephones. The patient states that he has a history of chronic low back pain, dating to a work-related injury 10 years ago. For no explicable reason, his pain is much worse this evening, and he is requesting narcotics. He claims that acetaminophen, aspirin, and nonsteroidal anti-inflammatory drugs (NSAIDs) have recently been ineffective in controlling his pain. He denies radiation of pain to his legs, bowel or bladder incontinence, or saddle anesthesia.

H$_x$ Later that day, a 57-year-old female advertising executive calls complaining of severe midepigastric discomfort associated with nausea and light-headedness. The pain was acute in onset, is currently moderately severe, and has been unrelieved by multiple doses of antacids. She has no previous history of gastrointestinal disorders. Her past medical history is significant for a 60 pack-year smoking history and hypertension. She is scheduled to leave town in the morning and would like some medication to relieve the discomfort.

Questions

1. In general, how should after-hour medical calls be handled?
2. How should calls related to narcotics be handled?
3. What are possible causes of the second caller's pain, and how should this situation be dealt with?
4. On average, what percentage of medical care provided by primary care physicians is delivered over the telephone?

A significant amount of medical care is delivered over the telephone. Although research in this area is limited, an estimated 15% (or greater) of primary care physicians' time is spent on patient-related telephone calls. Phone calls occur for a variety of reasons and can be to or from patients, pharmacists, hospital staff, home health personnel, and other physicians.

These calls last a variable amount of time. Calls to pharmacies are usually quick; many calls to patients will also be brief. However, calls from or to patients with complex medical or psychosocial problems have the potential of lasting much longer. It is often best to have these patients come in for a formal appointment.

Patients call doctors for a number of reasons. A call may be the means by which they first enter the health care system. More often, patients seek guidance regarding symptoms. Some patients call to request specific treatments; others call simply to make sure that their particular problem is not life-threatening or serious. A small subgroup of patients abuses the health care system. These patients tend to have psychiatric or chronic medical problems. Their primary complaints may seem like medical issues when, in fact, their repeated calls and requests for drug therapy (including pain medication) may mask a "hidden agenda" related to psychosocial problems or drug addiction.

Doctors usually try to return calls at specific times during the workday (e.g., during a lunch break or before or after clinic sessions). It is generally not practical for physicians to be interrupted each time a call comes in. Most patients realize this and don't expect immediate responses to nonemergency calls. Some physicians instruct their office personnel to interrupt them for calls from other physicians; however, this is not a universal practice.

In general, physicians do not charge for phone calls, especially since it is currently difficult to receive third-party (insurance) reimbursement for this activity. Most patients regard phone conversations as part of the total service physicians provide for them.

TYPES OF CALLS

Calls that physicians receive fall into two general categories: those which occur during regular working hours and those which occur after hours. Office calls can be further separated into those requiring a physician's attention and those that support staff can handle. Most offices depend heavily on receptionists or nurses to triage phone calls.

Nonmedical Calls

Most office calls are related to appointments, cancellations, and billing-related matters; they do not require physician involvement and are more appropriately handled by office personnel. Telephone courtesy on the part of office staff is important, since it is often nonmedical issues that frustrate patients the most and sometimes lead to hostility or even litigation.

Overworked receptionists may consider phone calls an inconvenience rather than an essential part of medical practice. They may treat the callers as adversaries rather than as customers. Patients' impressions of physicians are often shaped by their impressions of the office staff and, in particular, the reception staff. In order for doctors to recruit and retain patients, their reception staffs must treat callers courteously and efficiently.

Prescription Refills

Prescription refill requests are typically handled by a nurse under physician supervision. Most pharmacies will accept a prescription for an uncontrolled medication called in by a nurse. Documentation of medication refills is essential and should be the responsibility of either the nurse or the supervising physician.

Medical Problems

Offices vary in the way they treat calls related to medical problems. Some offices develop specific protocols for common problems such as upper respiratory tract infections or urinary tract infections. Such protocols can greatly decrease the amount of time physicians spend on the phone. Medical advice, however, should be dispensed only by trained medical personnel such as a nurse or doctor. Some offices train nurses to screen all medically related calls, extracting key bits of information so that when the physician calls the patient, the conversation will be more focused and time-efficient. Some physicians take all medically related phone calls themselves, without prior screening by a nurse. Protocols for emergency calls should be established in all offices. These calls should be thoroughly documented, and it is good practice to ask patients to call back later if their symptoms do not improve or if they worsen.

After-Hours Medical Calls

After office hours, the telephone is the principal means by which patients can reach their physicians. Physicians may receive an occasional call after hours for medication refills, but the majority of these calls are symptom-related. Physicians typically respond to these calls by providing advice or possibly by prescribing medication and arranging for appropriate follow-up.

Common problems such as upper respiratory tract infections or urinary tract infections can be handled quickly, whereas unusual or complex complaints are much more difficult to attend to over the telephone. It is important to recognize that there is no legal imperative to prescribe medication on the basis of a phone call. In fact, when a prescription is issued as a result of a phone conversation, the episode moves toward a true patient encounter with all its medicolegal ramifications. All calls that occur after hours should be documented and placed in patients' medical records. If the problem is complex or unusual, it is often best for the physician to arrange for some type of immediate evaluation in an emergency room or urgent care center, perhaps agreeing to meet the patient there or at least alerting the appropriate personnel of the patient's imminent arrival.

After-Hours Prescription Refills

Refilling narcotics after hours can be a difficult issue. Some physicians simply refuse to prescribe controlled substances to anyone other than their own patients. Others may give a small prescription calculated to last only until patients can reach their primary physician during regular working hours. Some physicians will even ask patients to meet them at a specific location (e.g., an emergency room) in order to discourage drug-seeking behavior.

THE TELEPHONE ENCOUNTER

The key ingredient in any phone encounter is open communication. Important nonverbal cues that physicians rely on during an office visit are missing. Therefore, physicians must actively listen to patients to ensure that the encounter is as thorough as necessary for appropriate decision making. Historical information should be accurately obtained, and physicians should be alert for the emotional underpinning of patients' complaints. Keeping an open mind is essential. It is tempting to come up with an immediate diagnosis and treatment plan during a brief phone encounter. If the approach is too superficial, however, crucial information will not be elicited, possibly resulting in erroneous diagnoses and inappropriate treatment or advice. Whether to treat patients over the phone (or make arrangements for further evaluation) has to be decided on an individual basis. Decisions are based on the severity and urgency of the problem, the physician's confidence in the diagnosis, the physician's prior knowledge of the patient, and the setting in which the call occurs. For example, are there medical facilities close by the patient where further evaluation could be carried out, or is the patient miles away from the nearest emergency room or health center?

MEDICOLEGAL ASPECTS

Improperly used, the telephone can be the means by which patient confidentiality is breached or test results miscommunicated. In addition, poor communication over the phone can easily lead to hostile or even litigious patients.

Written authorization from patients is mandatory before information is released to anyone other than themselves. If verbal authorization for release must be accepted (i.e., in an emergency), it is best to follow up with written authorization. For information that is potentially stigmatizing (e.g., problems related to drug abuse or HIV status), a specific release should always be obtained. For legal as well as medical reasons, it is good

practice to adequately document all calls to pharmacies, other physicians, etc.

As the push for cost-effective health care increases, the practice of medicine over the telephone undoubtedly will escalate because it is an efficient and cost-effective means of providing care. No one has yet examined the quality of care delivered over the telephone; however, as insurance regulators, government agencies, and professional societies increase their scrutiny of the quality of care delivered in a variety of venues, this issue surely will become a focus of future investigation.

Research Questions

1. To what extent is medical care delivered over the telephone in different primary care settings?
2. Is the outcome of patients treated over the telephone different from that of patients treated during an office or emergency room visit?
3. What factors are most important in the decision-making process when physicians deliver medical care over the phone?

Case Resolutions

The physician on call prescribed a small amount of a codeine-containing analgesic, calling in the prescription to the pharmacy. The physician instructed the patient to call again that evening if the pain worsened or neurologic symptoms developed and to contact his usual physician in the morning.

The physician, who was suspicious that the second patient's pain might be due to cardiac ischemia, instructed her to call for an ambulance and arranged to meet her in the emergency room of a nearby hospital. Arriving 20 minutes later, the physician learned that the patient went into ventricular fibrillation in the ambulance but was successfully defibrillated by the paramedics. Her ECG showed an acute inferior wall myocardial infarction.

Selected Readings

Curtis, P. Improving the use of the telephone. Practitioner 235:514–20, 1991.

Curtis, P., and A. Talbot. The telephone in primary care. J Community Health 6:194–203,1981.

Fischer, P. M., and S. R. Smith. The nature and management of telephone utilization in a family practice setting. J Fam Pract 8:321–7, 1979.

Johnson, B., and C. Johnson. Telephone medicine: A general internal medicine experience. J Gen Intern Med 5:234–9, 1990.

Spencer, D., and A. Davgird. The nature and content of physician telephone calls in a private practice. J Fam Pract 27:201–5, 1986.

Walter, L. Why plaintiffs' lawyers love your phone. Med Economics 70:33–9, 1993.

PREVENTION IN PRIMARY CARE

CHAPTER 11

SCREENING FOR DISEASE

William H. Wiese, M.D., M.P.H., and John Leggott, M.D.

H$_x$ A 49-year-old male meteorologist presents for a routine checkup. He has not seen a doctor since his physical examination upon joining the Marine Corps 27 years ago. The patient is mildly obese, but the physical examination is otherwise unremarkable.

Questions

1. Which history questions screen for health behaviors that put this patient at risk?
2. What are the leading causes of morbidity and mortality in this age group?
3. What screening laboratory tests are recommended for this patient?

BACKGROUND

In 1922, the American Medical Association first proposed the annual physical examination in an attempt to encourage preventive medicine. It has become increasingly clear, however, that age, genetics, and personal health behaviors strongly influence an individual's risk for the development of disease. In a policy statement in 1983, the AMA withdrew endorsement of the annual physical examination and supported the periodic visit tailored to the unique health risks of the individual patient. This recommendation coincided with those developed in the late '70s and '80s by the Canadian Task Force on the Periodic Health Examination, the U. S. Preventive Services Task Force, and the American College of Physicians. Each task force consisted of a panel of experts collaborating to systematically review evidence regarding the clinical effectiveness of preventive interventions. Guidelines were then developed for implementing these services in clinical practice.

The U. S. Preventive Services Task Force further suggested that clinicians obtain histories to identify behaviors associated with known health risks. Smoking, not wearing seat belts, physical inactivity, poor nutrition, and excessive use of alcohol are examples of behaviors that increase morbidity and mortality. Mod-

ification of such behaviors prior to the development of disease is an example of primary prevention. The clinician should identify health risks while providing information and support to help the patient change such life-style behaviors.

Screening for disease is another major component of the primary care provider's overall preventive responsibility. The periodic health assessment is the prototype of secondary prevention. It allows the physician to make age- and gender-specific recommendations modified by the patient's individual risk profile as determined by family history, previous health history, health-related behaviors, and environmental and occupational exposures.

SCREENING CRITERIA

Screening for disease is to be distinguished from diagnostic evaluation and hypothesis testing. Screening presumes that the patient has no symptoms related to the target condition and that there is no reason to suspect the condition other than the patient's general risk profile. In general, the likelihood of the condition being present in the asymptomatic individual is low. For example, the likelihood of an asymptomatic woman having breast cancer detectable by mammography and confirmed by tissue diagnosis might be 1:300. In contrast, the odds of a woman with a new breast nodule having cancer may be 1:5. These are contrasting examples of prior probabilities, which are the estimated statistical likelihoods that testing in a given patient will yield a true-positive result. The former is an example of screening, the latter of diagnostic assessment.

A screening maneuver, whether assessed by specific questions, physical examination, or a test or procedure, yields a result that is generally either "positive" or "negative." Positive results trigger further testing to determine whether the condition actually exists. For example, a positive screening mammogram may be followed by a biopsy. Negative screening usually results in no further action until subsequent screening is performed or symptoms or signs emerge. Some screening result, neither positive or negative. A repeat test may be indicated unless the provider decides to pursue further diagnostic or therapeutic interventions.

It is important that screening maneuvers be sensitive (i.e., show a positive result when the asymptomatic condition is truly present) and specific (i.e., not show a positive result when the condition is truly absent) (see Fig. 3–1). Specificity is of particular concern in screening because the prevalence or prior probability of a positive result is apt to be low. In screening, therefore, a non-specific test will likely produce too many false positives for every true positive. In a population that is mostly without the condition, even a test with high specificity can yield an overwhelming number of false-positive results. An example is the testing of serum for prostate-specific antigen (PSA) as a screen for preclinical cancer of the prostate. Using test criteria that give adequate sensitivity, there may be four false-positive results for every true positive. All positive tests require further assessment, which is usually costly and may be invasive. In this example, one true positive test out of five total positive tests yields a positive predictive value of only 20%. Positive predictive value is the proportion of all positive tests that are true positives. The positive predictive value of initial screening mammography for cancer of the breast in women aged 40 to 49 was 4% in one U. S. study. The positive predictive value of CA-125 for cancer of the ovary in unselected postmenopausal women is less than 1%.

Screening is an inherently imperfect process. Most screening tests are less than completely sensitive, and some persons with the targeted condition will have false-negative test results. As discussed above, most screening maneuvers will yield a certain percentage of false-positive results requiring follow-up testing that can be costly or dangerous.

For screening to be justified, the following criteria should be met:

1. The targeted condition should be serious and sufficiently prevalent in the group being screened to justify the costs and risks of the screening procedure and the subsequent evaluation of all positive results.

Example: Breast cancer, the targeted condition screened for by mammography, is prevalent and usually has tragic consequences unless diagnosed early. Mammography is safe and, though uncomfortable, generally well tolerated. The fear of cancer and severity of the diagnosis typically outweigh the anxiety, inconvenience, and cost of working up false-positive examinations. However, this is a highly personal decision that should be discussed by the clinician and patient prior to ordering the test. As with all screening tests, the possible consequences of the test result—positive or negative—should be understood by the patient and clinician prior to ordering the test.

2. The patient's risk of future morbidity or mortality must be reduced as a result of early (i.e., presymptomatic) detection of the condition.

Example: The early detection and treatment of hypertension is partially responsible for the decrease in age-adjusted mortality from strokes. Stroke mortality has decreased by more than 50% since 1972.

3. The screening maneuver itself must be acceptable to the patient.

Example: Many Americans can quote their cholesterol level or last blood pressure reading. These screening maneuvers are accomplished easily and without significant patient objection. On the other hand, flexible sigmoidoscopy as a screening tool has failed to gain widespread patient acceptance. Patients are required to only drink liquids for several days or take laxatives and enemas in preparation for the examination. The examination is uncomfortable, invasive, and time consuming and requires skill and expensive equipment on the part of the provider. Despite these objections, the procedure can be lifesaving and is recommended as a screening tool in selected populations.

APPROPRIATE SCREENING VERSUS OVERSCREENING

There are pitfalls and hazards from omitting screening and from overscreening. Obviously, failure to screen for serious conditions that can benefit from early intervention will result in missed opportunities for early management. Overscreening occurs when a screening maneuver is performed too frequently or when it is unlikely to yield information that will benefit the patient. Overscreening can lead to costly workup of "abnormal" results owing to statistical variation in normal results, trivial abnormalities, and abnormalities unlikely to benefit from early detection. Indiscriminate use of chemistry panels, electrocardiography, or chest radiography on unselected asymptomatic individuals is an example of overscreening.

Patients with known disease are generally treated and then monitored for disease progression or the development of complications. Such tertiary prevention dominates much of the current practice of medicine. Patients frequently do not seek medical attention prior to the development of symptoms. The opportunity for primary or secondary prevention may have passed once a patient is symptomatic. Barriers to early preventive care exist in part because of the clinician's traditional role of diagnostician rather than counselor and educator. Reimbursement favors procedure-oriented tertiary patient care rather than the often time-consuming processes of (1) helping patients change behavior (primary prevention) and (2) eliciting sufficient information to effectively screen for disease (secondary prevention).

GUIDELINES FOR SCREENING

Recommendations for screening are available from many authorities, notably the U. S. Preventive Services Task Force (USPSTF), the Canadian Task Force on the Periodic Health Examination, the American College of Physicians, and the American Cancer Society. Not all of these authorities agree on every issue. A major

TABLE 11–1. Screening Guidelines for Patients Aged 40–64 years.*

Leading causes of death

Heart disease	Breast cancer
Lung cancer	Colorectal cancer
Cerebrovascular disease	Obstructive lung disease

Screening	Counseling	Immunizations
History	*Diet and Exercise*	Tetanus-diphtheria (Td) booster¶
Dietary intake	Fat (especially saturated fat), cholesterol, complex carbohydrates, fiber, sodium, calcium‖	*High-Risk Groups*
Physical activity		Hepatitis B vaccine
Tobacco/alcohol/drug use		Pneumococcal vaccine
Sexual practices	Caloric balance	Influenza vaccine
Physical Examination	Selection of exercise program	
Height and weight		This list of preventive services is not exhaustive. It reflects only those topics reviewed by the U. S. Preventive Services Task Force. Clinicians may wish to add other preventive services on a routine basis, and after considering the patient's medical history and other individual circumstances. Examples of target conditions not specifically examined by the Task Force include:
Blood pressure	*Substance Use*	
Clinical breast examination†	Tobacco cessation	
High-Risk Groups	Alcohol and other drugs:	
Complete skin examination	Limiting alcohol consumption	
Complete oral cavity examination	Driving/other dangerous activities while under the influence	
Palpation for thyroid nodules	Treatment for abuse	
Auscultation for carotid bruits	*High-Risk Groups*	
	Sharing/using unsterilized needles and syringes	
Laboratory/Diagnostic Procedures		Chronic obstructive pulmonary disease
Nonfasting total blood cholesterol	*Sexual Practices*	Hepatobiliary disease
Papanicolaou smear‡	Sexually transmitted diseases; partner selection, condoms, anal intercourse	Bladder cancer
Mammogram§		Endometrial disease
High-Risk Groups		Travel-related illness
Fasting plasma glucose	Unintended pregnancy and contraceptive options	Prescription drug abuse
VDRL/RPR		Occupational illness and injuries
Urinalysis for bacteriuria	*Injury Prevention*	
Chlamydial testing	Safety belts	
Gonorrhea culture	Safety helmets	Remain alert for
Counseling and testing for HIV	Smoke detector	Depressive symptoms
Tuberculin skin test (PPD)	Smoking near bedding or upholstery	Suicide risk factors
Hearing	*High-Risk Groups*	Abnormal bereavement
Electrocardiogram	Back-conditioning exercises	Signs of physical abuse or neglect
Fecal occult blood/sigmoidoscopy	Prevention of childhood injuries	Malignant skin lesions
Fecal occult blood/colonoscopy	Falls in the elderly	Peripheral arterial disease
Bone mineral content	*Dental Health*	Tooth decay, gingivitis, loose teeth
	Regular tooth brushing, flossing, and dental visits	
	Other Primary Preventive Measures	
	High-Risk Groups	
	Skin protection from ultraviolet light	
	Discussion of aspirin therapy	
	Discussion of estrogen replacement therapy	

*For screening, counseling, and immunization guidelines listed for high-risk groups, the reader should consult the U. S. Preventive Services Task Force (USPSTF) *Guide to Clinical Preventive Services* for identifiers of persons at high risk.

†Annually for women.
‡Every 1–3 years for women.
§Every 1–2 years for women beginning at age 50 (age 35 for those at increased risk).
‖For women.
¶Every 10 years.
#Annually.

reason for disagreement is that scientific evidence for the effectiveness of many maneuvers is often weak or lacking. Only a few preventive interventions have been subjected to carefully executed, prospective, randomized, controlled trials using mortality or clear-cut measures of morbidity as outcomes. Lesser levels of scientific assessment are subject to error or otherwise limited by biases, confounders, or other variables. Even a well-executed prospective trial must be judged by whether the results can be generalized to other specific populations.

For every condition there are anecdotes of how periodic screening led to early diagnosis and presumably beneficial or lifesaving intervention. The physician should guard against the temptation of using anecdotal evidence alone as the basis for general screening behaviors. The USPSTF and Canadian Task Force take into account the strength of the available scientific evidence in making screening recommendations.

The guidelines emphasize determining whether a patient has a higher than usual risk for a specified condition. This practice increases the prior probability of a patient having the condition and the likelihood that screening will yield a true positive result. An age- and gender-specific screening protocol augments or modifies the patient's overall risk profile and the likelihood that the screening maneuvers will benefit the individual. Individual risk profiles are influenced by genetics, behaviors, environmental and occupational exposures, and prior and current medical history.

When the various expert guidelines are in agreement, standards for preventive practice emerge. Such standards will have increasing relevance for the financing of primary care practice and also will have medicolegal implications. Primary care providers have longitudinal patient care responsibility, including primary and secondary prevention. Providers have become increasingly accountable for whether and how screening is done. It would be inappropriate, however, to utilize guidelines as rigid requirements. The provider should always apply judgment in using any guideline, including when it may not be appropriate or when it may be insufficient.

SCREENING OF ADULTS

A periodic health assessment should be scheduled annually or every 2 years for each well adult. A mechanism such as a flow sheet in the medical record can improve provider adherence. It should include patient-specific modifications based on identified risks. Availability of tests and how the results will affect the individual should also be considered. Positive results should be entered or highlighted on the flow sheet. Automated systems are becoming available to assist the provider with these tasks.

Research Questions

1. Are the USPSTF and similar guidelines applicable to all patients in a nation as culturally diverse as the United States?
2. What should be the clinician's role in screening versus advocating for health risk behavior change?

Case Resolution

Screening guidelines for the patient profiled in the introductory case history are summarized by the USPSTF guidelines presented in Table 11–1. Clinician effectiveness in implementing these recommendations largely depends on the patient's willingness to comply. The rapport established between provider and patient is key in the provision of lifelong health care (including screening for disease).

The patient presented at the beginning of the chapter was mildly obese. Obesity is a risk factor for heart disease, which is the leading cause of death in the 40- to 64-year-old age group. The physician counseled the patient about life-style changes that promote weight loss, including exercise and dietary habits.

Selected Readings

American Cancer Society. *Summary of American Cancer Society Recommendations for the Early Detection of Cancer in Asymptomatic People.* Atlanta, American Cancer Society, 1992.

American Medical Association, Council on Scientific Affairs. Medical evaluation of healthy persons. JAMA 249:1626–33, 1983.

Canadian Task Force on the Periodic Health Examination. The periodic health examination. Can Med Assoc J 121:1194–254, 1979.

Eddy, D. M. (ed.). Common screening tests. Philadelphia, American College of Physicians, 1991.

U.S. Preventive Services Task Force. *Guide to Clinical Preventive Services: An Assessment of the Effectiveness of 169 Interventions.* Baltimore, Williams & Wilkins, 1989.

CHAPTER 12

PREVENTION OF INFECTIOUS DISEASES

Sarah E. Allen, M.D.

Hx A 28-year-old male requests a physical examination before entering nursing school.

Questions

1. What information pertaining to life-style, home life, and employment is needed to determine which vaccinations the patient requires?
2. What should be done if the patient is unsure whether he has received immunization against measles, mumps, and rubella (MMR), or does not remember which type of "measles" he had as a child?

With the exception of clean water, the development and widespread use of immunizations have had the most significant positive impact on the health of humankind, far beyond the treatment of established infections with antibiotics. Immunization programs are responsible for the global elimination of smallpox and the near elimination from the Americas of such highly fatal and morbid diseases as diphtheria and polio. In countries with inadequate vaccine programs, tetanus, rabies, and measles continue to kill millions each year. Even in developed countries, several vaccine-preventable diseases are poised to make a comeback: over 60,000 polio-virus infections have occurred in the Netherlands in recent years, and the incidence of diphtheria is reported to be increasing in the former Soviet Union. These disease outbreaks may have an impact on the United States through travel and immigration.

Immunizations are highly cost effective. The cost-benefit ratio of the MMR vaccine, for example, was estimated to be 1:14.4 when it was introduced. Many physicians, however, fail to immunize their patients against preventable disease. During their training, generalist physicians are repeatedly advised to obtain mammograms, check blood pressures and serum cholesterol levels, and discuss smoking. Without immunization programs, however, measles and tetanus would be seen far more often than breast cancer or heart disease. Routine health maintenance must include a vaccination history and adequate social and sexual histories to determine which immunizations are indicated for each patient.

PHYSIOLOGY OF ACTIVE AND PASSIVE IMMUNIZATION

Immunization may be either active or passive. **Active immunization** is the administration of an antigenic substance in the form of a vaccine that results in two general immune responses. Through **humoral immunity,** antibodies (IgM, IgG, or IgA) are produced; through **cellular immunity,** a T-lymphocyte response occurs. This combination of humoral and cellular immunity provides the individual with protection against the index pathogen. An Arthus-type (antigen-antibody complex) reaction may occur following immunization, resulting in soreness, occasionally erythema, and rarely necrosis at the site of injection.

Vaccines are composed of one of four types of antigens: (1) toxoids; (2) nonviable components of viruses or bacteria; (3) killed but whole viruses or bacteria; or (4) attenuated, but live, viruses or bacteria. Toxoid vaccines are derived from pathogenic bacterial toxins that have been altered chemically to be nonpathogenic but remain antigenic. Vaccines prepared from viruses or bacteria may contain the entire pathogen or just an antigenic portion. If the whole pathogen is used, it may be live-attenuated or killed. Use of a live-attenuated pathogen may evoke the best immune response but is usually associated with more risk to the host, since some of the organism's pathogenicity can remain. Killed pathogens, particularly whole bacteria such as in the whole cell pertussis vaccine, are often highly immunogenic but may also be associated with adverse reactions. The safest vaccines are usually produced when just an antigenic portion of the pathogen is used in vaccine preparation, but some immunogenicity may be lost in the process. Recently, some vaccine components such as *Haemophilus influenzae* capsular proteins have been conjugated to immunogenic substances such as diphtheria toxoid to form highly immunogenic and effective "conjugate" vaccines.

Passive immunization is the administration of preformed immunoglobulins after, or in anticipation of, disease exposure. Passive immunization does not stimulate a host immunologic response. Immunoglobulin used in passive immunization may be **specific** (e.g., hyperimmune globulin) to an index pathogen such as hepatitis B, or **nonspecific** (e.g., gamma globulin) and include not only antibodies to the index pathogen but other antibodies as well. Gamma globulin, for example, is used after exposure to hepatitis A as well as after exposure to measles. Passive immunization may protect an individual from overt disease but not necessarily from infection. For specific indications for immunoglobulin, see Table 12–1.

TABLE 12–2. Vaccination Schedules for Adults*

Born after 1957
  dT, 0.5 mL intramuscularly every 10 years†
  MMR-2‡, 0.5 mL subcutaneously
Born before 1957 but less than 65 years of age
  dT, 0.5 mL intramuscularly every 10 years†
65 years of age or older
  dT, 0.5 mL intramuscularly every 10 years†
  Pneumococcal vaccine, 0.5 mL intramuscularly every 5–6 years
  Influenza A/B vaccine, 0.5 mL intramuscularly every autumn

*dT, adult-dose diphtheria and tetanus; MMR, measles, mumps, rubella.
†With serious tetanus-prone wounds, patients with no history of tetanus immunization should receive a primary vaccination series as well as tetanus immunoglobulin; some experts advise giving tetanus toxoid to patients if none has been given in the preceding 5 years.
‡The recommendation for two lifetime doses of MMR was made in 1989. Most patients receive a first dose of MMR at 15 months of age; many adults have not received a second dose.

VACCINATIONS FOR ROUTINE HEALTH MAINTENANCE

Tables 12–2 and 12–3 summarize vaccine schedules for adults and children. This section contains a brief natural history of and immunization recommendations for each index disease.

Diphtheria

Diphtheria is caused by *Corynebacterium diphtheriae* and its highly potent toxin. This often fatal disease, which was widespread in the early 1900s, is marked by inflammation and fibrinous exudate in the throat, nose, and tracheobronchial tree. The toxin causes degeneration in peripheral nerves, heart muscle, and skin. The diphtheria vaccine is made of nonpathogenic toxoid derived from diphtheria toxin. After a primary vaccination series (see Table 12–3), diphtheria toxoid is given every 10 years, usually with tetanus toxoid, designated "DT" in children and "dT" in adults. The lowercase "d" indicates the lower dose of diphtheria toxoid given to adults, who experience increased adverse reactions with the higher dose of the toxoid. Adverse reactions include soreness at the sight of injection and very rarely anaphylaxis.

Tetanus

Tetanus is caused by the toxin tetanospasmin produced by *Clostridium tetani*. Painful muscular contrac-

TABLE 12–1. Indications for Immunoglobulin Use*†

Gamma Globulin (Nonspecific)
Anticipated or recent exposure to hepatitis A
Exposure to measles >72 hours or unable to receive vaccination

Hyperimmune Globulin (Specific to Pathogen)
Exposure to hepatitis B without demonstrable immunity
Exposure of immunocompromised, susceptible host to varicella
Highly tetanus-prone wound in unimmunized host
Rabies exposure without preexposure vaccine

*Immunoglobulin also comes in an IV preparation for use in specific immunodeficiency disorders.
†If given with vaccine, immunoglobulin should be given at a separate site.

TABLE 12–3. Vaccine Schedule for Infants and Children*

Birth	Hep B-1
2 months	DTP-1, OPV-1, Hlb-1, Hep B-2
4 months	DTP-2, OPV-2, Hlb-2
6 months	DTP-3, Hlb-3, Hep B-3
15 months	MMR-1, DTaP-4, OPV-3, Hlb-4
4–6 yrs	DTaP-5, OPV-4, MMR-2
14–16 yrs	dT

*OPV, oral polio vaccine; DTP, pediatric-dose diphtheria, tetanus, pertussis; aP, acellular pertussis; MMR, measles, mumps, rubella; dT, adult-dose diphtheria and tetanus; Hlb, *Haemophilus influenzae* type *b* conjugate vaccine; Hep B, hepatitis B.

tions result from the toxin's action on the central nervous system. The highly effective tetanus vaccine is made up of nonpathogenic toxoid. After a primary vaccination series (see Table 12–3), tetanus toxoid is given every 10 years, usually with diphtheria toxoid. In the case of a highly tetanus-prone wound such as a puncture, tetanus toxoid should be given to individuals whose last vaccination was more than 5 years earlier. Tetanus immunoglobulin and tetanus toxoid are recommended for patients with tetanus-prone wounds with no history of immunization or whose immunization status is unknown. Adverse reactions to tetanus toxoid include soreness at the site of injection and rarely anaphylaxis.

Measles

Measles is marked by catarrhal inflammation of the respiratory tract, a generalized maculopapular eruption, fever, and other constitutional disturbances. Complications that may result in death include dehydration from severe odynophagia, pneumonia, encephalopathy, and subacute sclerosing panencephalitis. Measles can be severe in malnourished individuals and is a major killer worldwide. The vaccine is a live-attenuated virus usually given with mumps and rubella vaccines as MMR. In 1989 after a dramatic increase in measles cases in the United States, it was recommended that two lifetime vaccine doses be given to individuals born after 1957. Individuals born before 1957 have usually had natural measles. The first dose is usually given at 15 months and the second dose at grade school entry. An older child or adult who has not received a second MMR dose may receive it at any time unless contraindicated. Pregnant women and immunosuppressed individuals other than patients with HIV should not receive MMR because of the live virus.

Individuals exposed to measles may be protected by administration of vaccine within 72 hours. Pregnant patients, immunocompromised patients, and individuals exposed more than 72 hours earlier may be given gamma globulin up to 6 days following exposure.

Many individuals are unsure whether they have had natural measles or have been previously immunized. Neither additional doses of MMR nor administration of MMR following natural measles has been associated with increased adverse reactions. The physician may either give MMR or check antibody titer (IgG) to rubeola virus to determine the need for immunization.

Adverse reactions to the measles vaccine include fever up to 12 days following the vaccine. Transient rashes have been reported. Encephalitis following measles vaccine occurs at a lower frequency than encephalitis of unknown cause in the general population and is less frequent than encephalitis following natural measles.

Mumps

Mumps, or epidemic parotitis, is usually mild in children but may cause severe orchitis in adults. Over 4000 cases occurred in 1988 in the United States, and an estimated 16% of young adults lack immunity. Mumps immunization is usually given as MMR. Adverse reactions are rare.

Varicella (Chickenpox)

Varicella is a herpesvirus infection with primary, latent, and reactivation disease states. Primary infection results in a pruritic vesicular rash, fever, and usually mild systemic symptoms. Most children have a mild illness. However, immunocompromised children and normal adults can suffer severe complications including bacterial superinfection, encephalitis or meningitis, pneumonia, hepatitis, thrombocytopenia, and glomerulonephritis. The virus persists in a latent stage after primary infection and may reactivate in the form of a painful neuritis as herpes zoster (shingles). A recently released vaccine is available although at the time of this writing, appropriate indications are still being determined. Primary infections may be prevented with varicella zoster hyperimmune globulin (VZIG). VZIG is given within 96 hours of exposure (earlier, if possible) to persons both likely to be susceptible to varicella and likely to develop complications.

Rubella

Rubella is an acute but mild exanthematous disease resulting in marked enlargement of lymph nodes but usually little fever or constitutional reaction in children or adults. Infection during the first several months of fetal life, however, may result in severe congenital deformities. The goal of vaccination programs is to prevent infection in pregnant women. Infants are vaccinated with live-virus vaccine at 15 months with MMR and again at school entry. Women planning to become pregnant should have a rubella IgG titer checked to ensure immunity prior to becoming pregnant. Vaccine should be given to women who lack immunity, but pregnancy should be delayed for 3 months following immunization because of the theoretical effects of the live-virus vaccine on the fetus.

Influenza

Influenza is an acute infectious respiratory disease caused by orthomyxoviruses that produce catarrhal inflammation and may result in secondary pneumonia. Influenza commonly occurs in epidemics or pandemics, when it is responsible for 10–40 thousand deaths per year, mostly in the elderly population. The clinically most important types of influenza are A and B. The vaccine is composed of nonviable components of the influenza A and B strains that are most likely to occur in a given year. The vaccine is associated with a 70%–80% reduction in clinical illness but not necessarily a reduction in infection. The vaccine does not cause the "flu"; the rate of side effects of the vaccine is equal to that of placebo. Vaccine is given to patients 65 years of age and older and patients with chronic illnesses, such as diabetes mellitus (DM), congestive heart failure (CHF), chronic obstructive pulmonary disease (COPD), human immunodeficiency virus (HIV) infection, and end-stage renal disease (ESRD), situations in which influenza would not be well tolerated. In addition, influenza vaccination should be given to health care workers and family members of chronically ill patients and offered to people who are essential in their place of employment.

Streptococcus pneumoniae

Pneumococcal disease in the form of pneumonia, bacteremia, or meningitis is responsible for 40,000 deaths each year in the United States. The 23-valent vaccine decreases the rate of bacteremia in immunocompetent patients but not the rate of infection. Immunization is recommended every 5–6 years to patients 65 years of age and older and to patients with chronic illnesses such as COPD, CHF, DM, HIV, and ESRD who are either susceptible to or would not tolerate serious infection due to pneumococcus. The vaccine should also be given to patients prior to undergoing splenectomy (or as soon after as possible) and to patients with defective spleens (as seen in sickle cell anemia). Studies have challenged the vaccine's effectiveness in immunocompromised and chronically ill patients. In the future, the vaccine may be produced as a conjugate vaccine with anticipated increased immunogenicity.

Hepatitis B

Hepatitis B causes an annual 300,000 infections and 5000 deaths in the United States. Worldwide, an estimated 200 million are chronically infected. The U. S. incidence has increased since vaccine introduction despite its effectiveness. This rising infection incidence led to the recommendation for universal vaccination at birth. Infants born to mothers with detectable hepatitis B surface antigen should also receive hepatitis B immunoglobulin.

In adults, vaccination is recommended to individuals at increased risk for acquiring hepatitis B: men whose sexual partners are other men, health care workers, intravenous drug users, commercial sex workers, sexual partners of infectious (acute or chronic) patients, and other individuals such as police officers, fire fighters, and morticians who are exposed to blood and other body fluids. Some experts suggest that individuals with a history of sexually transmitted disease are at increased risk for hepatitis B and should also be immunized. Because of the expense of the vaccination series, it is usually cost effective to rule out previous exposure and chronic infection by checking hepatitis B core IgG and surface antigen prior to initiating the vaccination series. The vaccine is composed of surface antigen prepared by recombinant DNA technique and is administered at 0, 1, and 6 months.

Although the vaccine is generally highly effective, some individuals do not develop protective antibody following inoculation. It is therefore advisable to check a surface antibody titer following the vaccination series

to ensure immunity. Lack of response to vaccination is associated with obesity, age over 40, and immunosuppression. Recent studies suggest that in patients who do not respond to the intramuscular primary vaccine series, two 0.25-mL booster doses of vaccine given intradermally (in the same fashion as a tuberculin skin test) stimulate adequate antibody production in 90% of subjects.

PEDIATRIC IMMUNIZATIONS

In addition to MMR, diphtheria, tetanus, and hepatitis B, infants should be vaccinated against the following diseases.

Haemophilus influenzae Type B

Haemophilus influenzae type B in infants may result in highly morbid and fatal illnesses such as meningitis, sepsis, or epiglottiditis. Before the development of the conjugate vaccine, infection with *H. influenzae* was common in the pediatric population. Prepared from capsular antigen conjugated to diphtheria toxoid, the vaccine is highly immunogenic. Immunization is given in infancy at 2, 4, 6, and 15 months.

Pertussis

Pertussis, or whooping cough, is an upper respiratory infection caused by *Bordetella pertussis*. Cough may progress to severe paroxysms followed by a characteristic inspiratory whoop and vomiting. Pertussis is particularly severe in the first year of life. Complications include apnea, seizures, pneumonia, encephalophy, and death. Older children and adults may present atypically with a persistent cough without a whoop. Duration of illness, even in uncomplicated cases, is 6 to 10 weeks. There are two preparations of pertussis vaccine: a standard whole cell preparation and a newer purified acellular vaccine. Infants may receive the acellular preparation in lieu of the whole cell vaccine for the fourth and fifth doses (see Table 12–3). Both whole cell and acellular preparations are given with diphtheria and tetanus toxoids, designated DPT and DaPT.

Adults are often carriers of pertussis. An estimated 25% of adults with a recent cough of at least a week's duration have been documented to have pertussis. Because of adverse reactions to the whole cell vaccine, adults are not immunized at present. The acellular preparation may be used for adults in the future.

Poliomyelitis

Polio, an enteric viral infection, may progress to inflammation of the central nervous system (CNS) gray matter and lead to paralysis. Polio has been eradicated from the United States and the Americas but occurs commonly in other parts of the globe and remains a threat to the Western Hemisphere.

There are two types of poliovirus vaccines: oral, live-attenuated (OPV) and parenteral, killed (IPV). Each preparation has advantages and disadvantages. The oral, live vaccine is more immunogenic, protecting both the gastrointestinal (GI) tract and CNS from infection. Oral vaccine virus is excreted through the GI tract. Through fecal-oral contamination, the vaccine is spread to recipient contacts and in this way extends immunization beyond the initial vaccine recipient. If the contact is immunosuppressed, however, live vaccine virus may infect the CNS, resulting in vaccine-associated encephalopathy. Parenteral, killed polio vaccine is a safer vaccine, causing no vaccine-related CNS infections in recipients or contacts. However, the parenteral preparation provides only CNS immunity and induces no GI tract protection. Because no vaccine virus is excreted, no extension of immunity is provided to contacts.

The decision whether to use OPV or IPV depends on the age, immune status, and vaccination history of the recipient. The present recommended schedule is four OPV doses in infancy as outlined in Table 12-3. Immunocompetent adults anticipating exposure through travel may receive a single booster dose of OPV if they were immunized with OPV in childhood and all household contacts are immunocompetent. Adults who did not receive oral vaccine in childhood, who are immunocompromised, or who have immunocompromised household contacts should receive IPV. Revisions to the use of OPV in the United States are being considered because the risk of vaccine-associated encephalopathy, while small, now outweighs the risk of wild-type poliovirus infection.

SPECIAL SITUATIONS

Rabies

Rabies is a highly fatal viral infection usually transmitted by carnivorous animal bites. The virus infects the central nervous system and salivary glands. Patients manifest excitement, aggressiveness, and madness followed by paralysis and death. Human rabies is rare in the United States but common in developing countries. Individuals likely to be exposed to rabid animals such as veterinarians or travelers to endemic areas should receive a preexposure vaccine series. Should exposure occur, a limited postexposure vaccine series is still required. Individuals exposed to rabies who have not received a preexposure vaccine series should receive a complete vaccination series as well as rabies immunoglobulin.

Pregnancy

Vaccination, especially with live-virus vaccines, is usually contraindicated in pregnancy because of unknown or speculated adverse effects on the fetus. In the situation where there has been or will be a high likelihood of disease exposure, the use of killed or even live-virus vaccine may be indicated. More commonly, when a pregnant patient is exposed to a vaccine-preventable disease such as measles, passive immunization with immunoglobulin is used. Tetanus toxoid is safe in pregnancy, and immunization should be current

to prevent neonatal tetanus in infants delivered in unsanitary conditions.

HIV Infection

While HIV-infected patients may have inadequate responses to immunizations because of depressed cellular immunity, they should receive all standard vaccinations as well as influenza and pneumococcus. The use of MMR has not been associated with adverse reactions in HIV-infected children or adults, and it is recommended in infected children and in adults born after 1957 if measles exposure is likely. HIV-infected patients should otherwise not receive live-virus vaccines. Acquisition of natural hepatitis B after becoming infected with HIV is associated with a high likelihood of chronic hepatitis B infection. Therefore, HIV patients should receive hepatitis B vaccine unless prior exposure, evidenced by surface antigen, core antibody, or surface antibody, has occurred.

Splenectomy

Functionally asplenic patients (as a result of surgery, sickle cell disease, or lymphoma) should receive pneumococcal vaccine. It should be given prior to surgical splenectomy whenever possible.

Other Immunocompromised Patients

Although their response may be inadequate, most immunocompromised individuals should receive killed, toxoid, and subunit vaccinations including influenza and pneumococcal vaccines, preferably prior to becoming immunocompromised if this can be anticipated. In general, immunocompromised patients should not receive live-virus vaccinations, and passive immunization should be considered if exposure is likely. Individuals living with immunocompromised patients should not receive enterally spread live-virus vaccines such as OPV because of the danger of oral-fecal spread to the immunocompromised person.

Anecdotal reports have suggested that tetanus toxoid may result in allograft rejection, and some transplant centers recommend the use of tetanus immune globulin for the management of tetanus-prone wounds.

PATIENT EDUCATION

Patients are often concerned about possible side effects of immunization, and subsequent but unrelated illness is often incorrectly attributed to immunization.

TABLE 12–4. Maximizing Opportunities to Vaccinate*

1. Every patient visit is an opportunity to vaccinate. Take advantage of it.
2. Patients may receive multiple vaccinations in a single clinic visit.
3. Mild febrile illnesses (e.g., upper respiratory tract infections or otitis media) are not contraindications to vaccination.

---

*Few absolute contraindications exist to killed or toxoid vaccines (see Table 12–5).

TABLE 12–5. General Contraindications to Vaccination*

1. Prior anaphylactic reaction to the specific vaccine
2. Prior anaphylactic reaction to a vaccine component (e.g., egg protein or specific antibiotic used in the preparation)
3. Concurrent moderate or severe illness
4. Pregnancy and immunodeficiency are usually contraindications to live virus vaccination (e.g, MMR and polio); exceptions to this guideline exist

*See text for specific vaccine contraindications.

Risks and benefits of each vaccine should be explained (Tables 12–4 and 12–5). The National Childhood Vaccine Injury Act of 1986 has required the development of vaccine information statements for commonly used vaccines including MMR, DPT, and polio vaccines. Once available, these statements must be given to all persons, regardless of age, who receive any of these vaccines. Adverse reactions to MMR, DTP, and polio vaccines must be reported.

Research Questions

1. How can vaccines with limited immunity be made more immunogenic?
2. How can the acceptance of immunizations by physicians and the general public be increased?

Case Resolution

The student in this case is a heterosexual male. His wife is a kidney transplant patient. He should receive hepatitis B vaccine if he is seronegative. He should receive the flu vaccine to protect both himself and his wife. He should not receive a live polio vaccine because of the possibility of transmitting the live vaccine virus to his wife. He can be given the killed polio booster if needed for travel. The student should be immune to measles, mumps, and rubella. He can receive MMR even if he has had prior vaccinations or illnesses.

Selected Readings

Centers for Disease Control and Prevention. Recommendations of the Advisory Committee on Immunization Practices (ACIP). MMWR 43(RR-1):1-38, January 28, 1994.

Guide For Adult Immunization, 3rd ed. Philadelphia, American College of Physicians, 1994.

Peter, G. Childhood immunizations. N Engl J Med 327:1794-1800, 1992.

CHAPTER 13

PREVENTION OF CORONARY ARTERY DISEASE

Craig Timm, M.D.

H$_x$ A 50-year-old male electrical engineer is concerned about his risk of developing heart disease. He denies any cardiovascular symptoms but desires evaluation because "heart attacks run in his family": his father and several aunts and uncles had documented myocardial infarctions in their 50s. The patient has a 25 pack-year history of cigarette smoking. His blood pressure has been noted to be as high as 160/100 mm Hg. He also recalls that his cholesterol level was elevated several years ago. He is not active physically, taking only occasional short walks. He denies a history of diabetes. He has gained 14 kg (25 lb) over the last 5 years. The physical examination is normal except for mild to moderate obesity.

Questions

1. What are the major risk factors for atherosclerosis and coronary artery disease (CAD)?

2. How can the risk for development of CAD be diminished in a patient who does not yet have CAD (i.e., primary prevention)?
3. How can the risk for progression of CAD—and adverse events such as myocardial infarction—be reduced in a patient known to have CAD (i.e., secondary prevention)?

Despite reduction in the mortality rate for CAD over recent decades, it remains the leading cause of death in the United States. Approximately 1.5 million Americans have a myocardial infarction (MI) each year, more than 500,000 die of CAD-related causes, and over 500,000 undergo percutaneous transluminal coronary angioplasty (PTCA) or coronary artery bypass graft surgery (CABG).

Extensive research has identified risk factors for CAD. Generally accepted modifiable risk factors include diabetes, hypercholesterolemia, hypertension, and tobacco smoking. Other innate, nonmodifiable factors predisposing to CAD include older age, male sex, and a family history of premature CAD.

PATHOPHYSIOLOGY

The atherosclerotic lesions that cause coronary artery disease develop over a period of years to decades. The most widely held theory of atherogenesis is the response-to-injury hypothesis, which postulates that atheromatous lesions begin with damage to the endothelial lining of the blood vessel. Subsequently, circulating monocytes adhere to the damaged endothelium and migrate to the media of the vessel. There they convert into macrophages and act in a variety of ways to facilitate plaque formation. They ingest large amounts of cholesterol in the form of low-density lipoprotein (LDL) and ultimately become the foam cells that are responsible for the earliest lesion of atherosclerosis—the fatty streak. Macrophages also release chemotactic factors that (1) stimulate proliferation of smooth muscle cells and fibroblasts and (2) promote their migration into the damaged intima. This proliferation of a cellular and extracellular connective tissue matrix results in steady growth of the atherosclerotic plaque. As the lesion begins to encroach on the vessel lumen, symptoms of myocardial ischemia develop owing to the imbalance between oxygen supply and demand. A stable coronary lesion that produces symptoms only in situations of increased demand (e.g., exercise) may become "unstable" if the plaque ruptures and causes total or subtotal occlusion of the vessel. Plaque rupture can lead to unstable angina, myocardial infarction, or sudden death.

Numerous risk factors for CAD have been identified. These include acquired (and potentially modifiable) factors as well as factors that are fixed or unchangeable (Table 13–1).

Hypertension (see Chapter 38) is an acquired condition associated with increased risk of atherosclerosis. There is no absolutely defined "normal" blood pressure; the risk of CAD rises steadily as either the systolic or diastolic blood pressure increases. Elevated blood pressure is generally defined as > 140/90 mm Hg.

Hypercholesterolemia (see Chapter 79) may be characterized as elevation of total cholesterol or of LDL cholesterol. A decreased level of high-density lipoprotein (HDL; the so-called good cholesterol) is also a risk factor for CAD. As is the case with hypertension, there is a con-

tinuum of risk: higher levels of LDL or total cholesterol are associated with increased risk of atherosclerosis as are lower levels of HDL. The National Cholesterol Education Program (NCEP) guidelines recommend (1) LDL < 160 mg/dL in patients with no or one risk factor for CAD, (2) LDL < 130 in patients with two or more risk factors for CAD, and (3) LDL < 100 in patients with known CAD.

Any amount of tobacco **smoking** leads to increased risk of atherosclerosis, and again there is a continuum of risk related to the number of cigarettes smoked. The risk of developing a myocardial infarction is nearly three times as high in current smokers as in nonsmokers. With smoking cessation, the excess risk decreases substantially over time but may not reach the baseline level of risk. Heavy cigarette smoking has an adverse effect on the lipid profile, resulting in lowered HDL and increased LDL.

Diabetes and impaired glucose tolerance are well-established risk factors for CAD and vascular disease. Together, diabetes and impaired glucose tolerance occur in 20%–25% of the adult population of the United States. The evidence that strict control of diabetes leads to lower complication rates is controversial. However, the recently reported Diabetes Complications and Control Trial (DCCT) demonstrated a lower incidence of eye complications with tighter control of blood sugar and by inference suggested that other vascular complications may also be reduced by tighter control.

Other potentially modifiable risk factors for CAD include exercise, psychosocial factors (stress level, personality type), obesity, and alcohol intake. The evidence that they independently alter CAD risk is not conclusive.

The fixed or nonmodifiable risk factors of **age, male sex,** and **family history** are also important in determining the likelihood of CAD in a given patient. As a risk factor, male sex is more important in young and middle-aged populations. As women pass menopause, they develop more atherogenic lipid profiles and their risk for CAD converges with that of men.

EVALUATION

History

The history should identify CAD risk factors as well as any symptoms suggestive of myocardial ischemia. Eliciting the details of a chest pain history is described in Chapter 35. It is important to recognize that a patient may answer "no" to the question "Do you have chest pain?" even when symptomatic ischemia is present. Questions related to chest discomfort or tightness (as opposed to pain), breathing difficulties, abdominal pain, or arm or jaw pain may identify symptoms suggestive of ischemia.

Physical Examination

The physical examination should focus on the cardiovascular system, the eyes (looking for signs of long-standing diabetes or hypertension), the chest and lungs

TABLE 13–1. Risk Factors for Cardiovascular Disease

Fixed	Acquired
Male sex	Cigarette smoking
Family history of coronary artery disease	Hypercholesterolemia
Older age	Diabetes mellitus
	Hypertension

(looking for evidence of tobacco use), and the skin (looking for evidence of xanthomas or xanthelasmas).

Measurement of blood pressure, especially on several occasions over a period of days to weeks, will identify the hypertensive patient. Many people may have a single, mildly elevated reading in a stressful circumstance, but repeated or significant elevations help document the presence of hypertension.

Examination of the retina may reveal evidence of diabetic vascular complications, including microaneurysms, hemorrhages, and exudates. People with long-standing hypertension will commonly have arteriolar narrowing and arteriovenous nicking. Older men with elevated lipids may have a corneal arcus.

Xanthelasmas are lipid deposits in the skin that appear as small yellowish growths, commonly seen on or adjacent to the eyelids. Xanthomas are lipid-laden nodules of varying size. Another skin finding related to CAD risk factors is the presence of yellow-brown "nicotine" stains on the fingers of cigarette smokers.

An increased anteroposterior diameter or other evidence of chronic lung disease may be present in long-time smokers.

The cardiovascular examination is usually normal in patents with risk factors for CAD. However, a previous (perhaps silent) myocardial infarction is suggested by finding evidence of an enlarged heart, including a displaced or abnormal point of maximal impulse or the presence of an S_3. An S_4 is commonly present in patients with hypertension.

Additional Evaluation

If the patient is asymptomatic, only minimal additional evaluation is recommended.

An ECG should be obtained to look for evidence of left ventricular hypertrophy, especially in patients with hypertension.

Blood testing for glucose, glycosylated hemoglobin, and blood urea nitrogen (BUN) or creatinine levels is indicated in patients with diabetes to assess glycemic control and evidence of end-organ complications. BUN and creatinine may also be elevated in patients with hypertension, suggesting long-standing disease.

A lipid profile is beneficial in all adult patients as a screening test. Some authors would argue that only a total cholesterol is necessary in the younger, asymptomatic patient without risk factors. The pattern of lipid abnormality is helpful in planning the type of treatment, if needed. In those with a normal lipid profile, the NCEP recommends repeat measurement of total and HDL cholesterol every 5 years.

MANAGEMENT

While the strength of evidence varies for each risk factor, available data suggest that control of any CAD risk factor leads to a decreased risk of cardiovascular disease.

Many therapeutic agents are available for the treatment of hypertension. The physician should observe the patient carefully for efficacy and side effects, as well as for possible adverse effects on other CAD risk factors (e.g., both β-blockers and thiazide diuretics may cause elevations in serum lipids).

Strict control of glucose appears to decrease vascular complications of diabetes. Diabetes should be managed by a dedicated team (see Chapter 124).

The initial management of hypercholesterolemia should focus on dietary modification (to decrease both saturated and total fat intake) along with encouraging other interventions that might improve the patient's lipid status, such as regular physical activity and good diabetes control. Patients needing pharmacologic therapy should have therapy tailored to their specific lipid abnormality.

While the benefits of smoking cessation are substantial and unequivocal, this is one of the hardest risk factors to modify because of the addictive nature of nicotine. A variety of methods are available to help patients quit smoking, including behavior modification and the use of nicotine patches. Although success rates vary, it is clear that physicians who play a supportive, nonjudgmental, and educational role can have a significant impact on their patients' smoking behavior.

The relationship between physical activity and the risk of developing coronary disease is controversial, although evidence suggests a beneficial effect. Exercise (1) favorably alters lipid profiles, (2) reduces blood pressure, and (3) improves glucose tolerance, independently of any benefit on the risk of CAD. Exercise programs should be tailored to the patient's abilities and interests, and there are very few people for whom a regular exercise program is not advisable. Patients over age 40 who have been sedentary are generally advised to undergo a medical evaluation and an exercise tolerance test before beginning rigorous exercise training.

PATIENT AND FAMILY EDUCATION

The CAD-related information available to the general public from mass media and various industry sources is staggering, both in terms of volume as well as its frequently inaccurate or confusing nature. The patient and family thus often rely on the primary care physician for clarification and elaboration.

Important aspects of education include information about (1) the harmful effects of tobacco and the benefits of smoking cessation, (2) the importance of following a low-fat diet, and (3) the health-promoting benefits of physical activity. Patients who are taking medication should be counseled about possible adverse effects, the importance of compliance, and the need to speak with their provider before stopping or changing medications.

Because risk factor reduction is beneficial for everyone, family members should be encouraged to (1) know their own risk factor profiles; (2) work with the patient on having everyone in the household stop smoking; (3) engage in regular exercise, perhaps as a family activity; and (4) adjust eating habits toward a heart-healthy diet.

NATURAL HISTORY/PROGNOSIS

Coronary artery disease develops and progresses over a period of years to decades. The fatty streak, present in young adults, may not progress to a lesion causing angina or infarction until the person is 50, 60, or 70 years old. Substantial evidence supports the hypothesis that risk factor modification is helpful in both primary and secondary prevention. Regarding secondary prevention, several large prospective studies using serial coronary angiography have shown a modest degree of coronary disease regression in some patients—and lack of progression in others—following aggressive risk factor modification. The more striking finding is that risk factor modification (e.g., cholesterol reduction) is associated with a substantial and significant reduction in coronary events that is out of proportion to the angiographic differences noted. These findings suggest that risk factor modification may stabilize the atherosclerotic plaque, making it less susceptible to rupture and the ensuing unstable coronary syndromes.

Research Questions

1. What are the roles of other postulated risk factors for CAD (e.g., a hypercoagulable state, the presence of an oxidizing environment, or a possible infectious agent initiating atherosclerosis)?
2. What are the most effective large-scale public education methods of informing people about the risk factors for CAD?
3. What are the most effective ways to teach physicians and medical students about CAD risk factors, so that they will incorporate risk factor modification into their clinical practice?

Case Resolution

Together, the patient and his physician formulated a plan for risk factor reduction. The plan included (1) screening for diabetes mellitus and hyperlipidemia, (2) entering a smoking cessation program and using a nicotine patch (for a tapering course over 2 months), (3) switching to a low-fat diet with the aim of gradual weight loss, and (4) engaging in a gradually increasing exercise regimen to which the patient thinks he can adhere over the long term.

Selected Readings

Criqui, M. H. Cholesterol, primary and secondary prevention, and all-cause mortality. Ann Intern Med 115:973–6, 1991.

Farmer, J. A., and A. M. Gotto. Risk factors for coronary artery disease. *In* E. Braunwald (ed.). *Heart Disease,* 4th ed. Philadelphia, W. B. Saunders Company, 1992.

Kottke, T. E., et al. The systematic practice of preventive cardiology. Am J Cardiol 59:690–4, 1987.

Summary of the second report of the National Cholesterol Education Program (NCEP) Expert Panel on Detection, Evaluation, and Treatment of High Blood Cholesterol in Adults. JAMA 269:3015–23, 1993.

CHAPTER 14

PREVENTION OF PULMONARY DISEASE*

David B. Coultas, M.D.

H$_x$ A 25-year-old white male auto mechanic presents for a second opinion about medications he has been prescribed for asthma. About 2 years ago he began to experience episodic coughing, wheezing, and shortness of breath. At that time, he was given a β-agonist metered-dose inhaler, which he uses as needed, and an oral theophylline preparation, which he takes every 12 hours. Although these medications provide symptomatic relief and his symptoms have become less frequent, he is unhappy about taking them because he feels they make him "shaky and nervous." He wants to know whether he has to take asthma drugs for the rest of his life.

Questions

1. What additional information is needed to answer the patient's question?
2. What environmental factors are important to consider in the management of asthma?
3. What are the three levels of prevention, and how do they apply to this patient?

* Supported in part by a Preventive Pulmonary Academic Award, K07-HL02474. National Heart, Lung and Blood Institute. National Institutes of Health.

Malignant and nonmalignant pulmonary diseases cause substantial morbidity and mortality in the United States. Approximately 25 million Americans suffer from chronic lung diseases, with chronic obstructive pulmonary disease (COPD) responsible for about 60% of cases. More than 3 million cases of pneumonia occur in children and adults annually, accounting for over 530,000 hospital admissions among persons 15 years of age and older. Environmental and occupational respiratory exposures also cause an enormous burden of potentially preventable disease. For example, cigarette smoking results in over 400,000 deaths annually, making it the single largest cause of death in the United States.

As a group, malignant and nonmalignant pulmonary diseases are the third leading cause of death in the United States, accounting for about 15% of all deaths in 1990. COPD and related conditions were the fifth leading cause of death, with pneumonia and influenza being the sixth.

Preventive interventions have traditionally been classified as primary, secondary, or tertiary. The aim of **primary prevention** is *to reduce the incidence of disease, usually by eliminating exposures (e.g., smoking cessation) or by providing specific immunizations.* **Secondary prevention** refers to screening for disease that is not clinically evident (e.g., PPD [purified protein derivative tuberculin] testing for occult tuberculosis infection) as well as early intervention to prevent the occurrence of the symptoms and signs of disease (e.g., chemoprophylaxis with isoniazid [INH] to prevent active tuberculosis). **Tertiary prevention** involves treatment of clinically evident disease to prevent or minimize complications (e.g., oxygen therapy for patients with COPD and chronic hypoxemia).

RISK FACTOR IDENTIFICATION

Identification of risk factors among patients is an essential starting point for all levels of pulmonary disease prevention (Table 14–1). Although clearly evident for primary prevention (e.g., smoking cessation), the importance of risk factor identification may be less obvious for secondary and tertiary prevention. Because risk factors influence the probability of developing disease, their presence or absence helps determine which patients are at highest risk for disease and thus should undergo screening. Similarly, for patients with established disease, removal of a risk factor may have therapeutic benefit (e.g., smoking cessation).

Careful review of a patient's medical history will enable identification of the major risk factors for pulmonary diseases. However, the traditional outline for the medical history makes recall of specific risk factors difficult and clouds their importance because they are scattered throughout the various components of the history (e.g., past medical history, family history, social history). To facilitate recall of risk factors and to emphasize their importance for making diagnoses and for preventing disease, Sheagren and coworkers have proposed a new outline for the medical database. This new outline emphasizes identification of fixed and acquired risks (see Table 14–1) as a key task when formulating the medical database for patients.

Although all components of fixed and acquired risks have potential relevance to pulmonary diseases, environmental and occupational risks are particularly important but often are overlooked. With daily inhalation of 10,000 to 20,000 liters of air, agents present even in low concentrations may be biologically significant in the causation of lung diseases. Therefore, knowledge about current and past exposures, particularly in the workplace and at home, may provide essential information for predicting future risk of disease and for making diagnoses.

PRIMARY PREVENTION

Avoiding Environmental and Occupational Exposures

A major focus for the primary prevention of pulmonary diseases should be eliminating or limiting exposures to environmental and occupational agents (see Table 14–1; Chapter 125). Elimination of tobacco smoking is the single most important preventive intervention that physicians can advise (see Chapter 105). The elimination of other agents from workplace or home environments may range from simple removal of the agent to expensive engineering controls. How to control

TABLE 14–1. Major Risk Factors for Pulmonary Diseases

Risk Factor Assessment	Risk Factor	Examples of Disease
Fixed risks		
Genetic	Family history of lung disease	Cystic fibrosis, COPD, asthma, lung cancer
Demographic	Age, sex, race/ethnicity	COPD, asthma, lung cancer
Acquired risks		
Environmental/ occupational	Biologic agents	Tuberculosis, asthma
	Environmental tobacco smoke	Lung cancer
	Other combustion sources	Carbon monoxide poisoning
	Inorganic dusts (e.g., asbestos)	Lung cancer, asbestosis
Life-style/behavioral	Smoking	Lung cancer, COPD
	Drug abuse, high-risk sex	HIV/opportunistic infections
Health maintenance habits	Lack of influenza and pneumococcal vaccination	Influenza and pneumococcal pneumonia/ sepsis
	Lack of PPD skin test	Active tuberculosis
Disease-associated	Obesity	Sleep apnea/cor pulmonale
	Immunosuppression	Opportunistic infections
Treatment-associated	Medications (e.g., angiotensin converting enzyme inhibitor, methotrexate)	Chronic cough, diffuse parenchymal lung disease
	Splenectomy	Pneumococcal pneumonia/sepsis

Reproduced, with permission, from J. N. Sheagren, A. J. Zweifler, and J. O. Woolliscroft. The present medical database needs reorganization. Arch Intern Med 150:2014–5, 1990. Copyright 1990, American Medical Assocation.

exposures to specific agents may require consultation with specialists in occupational medicine and industrial hygiene, safety and health personnel at the work site, and state and federal agencies concerned with environmental health and safety (e.g., the Occupational Safety and Health Administration [OSHA]).

For adults, occupational asthma is of special concern, with more than 200 causative agents identified to date. Early recognition of the relationship between an occupational exposure and asthma is important, since prompt removal from exposure correlates best with full resolution of asthmatic symptoms.

Receiving Influenza and Pneumococcal Vaccination

Although the efficacy of influenza and pneumococcal vaccines has been established and their administration has been repeatedly recommended, their overall use is low among persons for whom the vaccines are indicated. Numerous factors contribute to low use, including concerns about side effects and perceptions that they are not effective, both of which are unfounded. Physicians can play an important role in educating and motivating their patients to be vaccinated.

Influenza immunization is indicated for persons at high risk for influenza complications, including persons 65 years of age and older, patients with chronic cardiovascular or pulmonary disorders, patients with chronic metabolic diseases (e.g., diabetes mellitus, renal dysfunction), immunosuppressed patients, and residents of nursing homes. In addition, health care workers and household members in close contact with persons at high risk should be immunized. Absolute contraindications to the vaccine are a history of a significant hypersensitivity reaction to eggs or to previous influenza vaccines. Because infection peaks between December and March and antibody titers rise and fall rapidly, immunization should begin in September (when the most current vaccine usually becomes available), and all persons for whom the vaccine is indicated should be vaccinated by mid-November.

Although the indications for the pneumococcal vaccine are similar to those for influenza immunization, special indications include patients with splenic dysfunction and patients who will be undergoing splenectomy. Pneumococcal vaccine is not indicated for those in close contact with high-risk persons. There are no absolute contraindications to the use of this vaccine. The vaccine may be administered at any time and should be repeated at 6-year intervals.

SECONDARY PREVENTION

Compared with primary prevention, secondary prevention (e.g., screening for asymptomatic pulmonary diseases) has a relatively limited role in the prevention of lung diseases in the outpatient setting. For example, screening of cigarette smokers for lung cancer with periodic chest roentgenograms and sputum cytologies has not been shown to improve survival and therefore cannot be recommended. However, screening for tuberculosis, early airways obstruction, sleep-disordered breathing, and pneumoconioses may have a role in decreasing morbidity and mortality from these diseases.

Screening for Tuberculosis (TB)

With the rising incidence of TB since 1985 and the appearance of multidrug-resistant strains, a major priority of TB control is identification of infected individuals with PPD screening and provision of INH chemoprophylaxis to persons at low risk for INH-induced side effects. Persons at highest risk for TB infection and for whom PPD screening is indicated include (1) household contacts of, or others who are in close contact with, persons with TB; (2) recent immigrants from countries in which TB is common (e.g., Asia, Africa, Central and South America, Pacific Islands); (3) migrant workers; (4) residents of nursing homes, correctional institutions, and homeless shelters; and (5) persons with certain underlying medical disorders (e.g., HIV infection).

To decrease the likelihood of developing active TB, screening has to be followed by administration of INH chemoprophylaxis to persons with a positive skin test. Although there is some controversy about the relative benefits and risks (i.e., hepatotoxicity) of INH chemoprophylaxis, persons with a positive PPD who are less than 35 years of age should receive INH for 6 to 12 months after an evaluation for active TB. Because of an increased risk of hepatotoxicity with increasing age, INH should not be routinely offered to persons older than 35 years of age unless they have other characteristics associated with a high risk of developing active TB (e.g., recent close contact with a patient with active TB, radiologic evidence of inactive TB, or a medical condition associated with immunosuppression and increased risk of reactivation of TB). Patient adherence to a medication schedule requires frequent encouragement and use of multiple strategies (see Chapter 9). To maximize adherence, the primary care physician should consider consulting tuberculosis control experts associated with state public health departments for assistance.

Screening for Early Airways Obstruction

Asthma and COPD are two of the most common chronic respiratory diseases in the general population. Although data are limited on the effectiveness of screening for these diseases, current expert guidelines suggest that peak flow monitoring should be routine in the management of moderate to severe asthma. The rationale is to detect worsening air-flow obstruction before severe impairment develops and to institute early aggressive treatment (e.g., oral corticosteroids) to prevent hospitalization and death.

There is no consensus on screening for COPD, but current understanding about its development suggests that periodic spirometric screening of cigarette smokers may result in early identification of worsening lung function that is asymptomatic, thus offering the opportunity for early intervention. Data from epidemiologic studies suggest that COPD results from sustained loss of ventilatory function beyond that expected from aging alone. The rate of decline of lung function in smokers tends to increase with the number of cigarettes smoked, and former smokers generally revert to the rate of loss seen in nonsmokers. However, since only a minority of smokers develop COPD (15%–20%), a large number of smokers would have to be screened to detect the much smaller number who will exhibit an accelerated decline in function. Therefore, smoking cessation for all smokers remains the single most important method for preventing COPD.

Spirometric screening may have a role in detecting early impairment of lung function in certain occupational settings. However, as is the case for smoking, primary prevention by eliminating exposure is the preferred prevention strategy.

Screening for Sleep-Disordered Breathing

Breathing problems during sleep (snoring, hypopnea, and apnea) are common and may contribute to excess morbidity and mortality. One of the most severe complications of sleep-disordered breathing is nocturnal hypoxemia, which may lead to pulmonary hypertension and cor pulmonale. Although a limited amount of information is available on the utility of screening for these problems, increasing evidence suggests that (1) asking a few simple questions and (2) obtaining nocturnal home oximetry in high-risk patients may be useful for identifying persons in need of more comprehensive sleep studies.

The acronym "I SNORED" is a mnemonic for questions that identify patients at risk for sleep-disordered breathing.* The letters of the acronym correspond to questions related to insomnia/insufficient sleep?, snoring?, not breathing?, obesity?, restful/refreshing sleep?, excessive daytime sleepiness?, and drugs (sedatives, hypnotics, alcohol)? Persons who suffer from sleep apnea are likely to be obese, to snore, to have apneas, to lack restful sleep, and to have problems with excessive daytime sleepiness. For persons with symptoms that suggest sleep-disordered breathing, oximetry monitoring at home during sleep may be a useful screening tool and may prove diagnostic.

Screening for Pneumoconioses

Workers exposed to inorganic dusts (e.g., asbestos, silica, and coal dust) are at increased risk for pneumoconioses. Periodic screening with chest radiographs is offered to coal miners through a program conducted by the National Institute for Occupational Safety and Health (NIOSH) to detect asymptomatic pneumoconiosis in coal workers. Detection of early disease enables miners to transfer to a less dusty environment at the mine with the aim of preventing progression of the disease. For workers exposed to dusts, radiologic screening programs are not ideal, and primary prevention efforts to limit or remove exposure are preferred.

TERTIARY PREVENTION

Tertiary prevention is concerned with the management of established disease to prevent or minimize complications. Traditionally, management of diseases has focused on pharmacologic interventions. However, several nonpharmacologic methods have proved useful in the care of patients with asthma and COPD.

In recent years, patient self-management of asthma and pulmonary rehabilitation programs for patients with COPD have received increasing attention as treatment modalities that lessen morbidity and improve patients' quality of life. Patient education, both to increase knowledge about the disease and to develop skills for self-care, has been shown to be beneficial in the management of asthma and COPD. Self-help materials and physician counseling may be adequate for many patients, but referral to more formal programs may be indicated for selected and highly motivated patients.

For patients with COPD, pharmacologic management may provide symptomatic benefit, but only smoking cessation and 24-hour per day oxygen therapy (i.e., for patients with hypoxemia) have been shown to prolong life. With the availability of oximetry to noninvasively measure oxygenation, every patient with COPD should be evaluated for hypoxemia. If a patient's oxygen saturation is consistently less than 90% despite pharmacologic management of COPD for at least 1 month, an arterial blood gas measurement should be obtained to confirm and quantitate the degree of hypoxemia. Patients with a partial pressure of oxygen of 55 mm Hg or less will benefit from continuous oxygen therapy.

SUMMARY

Physicians have numerous opportunities to prevent pulmonary diseases, but the available literature suggests that many opportunities to detect environmental or occupational exposures, to help smokers quit, and to provide vaccinations are missed. Awareness of these opportunities is the first step toward accomplishing the goal of pulmonary disease prevention. Another key step is valuing prevention as highly as diagnosing and treating disease. Although practicing preventive medicine requires overcoming some barriers (e.g., lack of time, difficulty remembering, and lack of reimbursement), it is an effort that greatly benefits patients. Developing methods to improve our practice of preventive medicine in the outpatient setting is an active area of clinical investigation.

> **Research Questions**
>
> 1. Why are mortality rates from asthma disproportionately higher among African Americans?
> 2. Will the use of home peak flow monitoring decrease morbidity and mortality from asthma?

---

* Haponik, E. Personal communication.

Case Resolution

The occupational and environmental history of this young asthmatic revealed that his symptoms began several months after he started to work at an auto body and paint shop. The data sheets for materials he worked with at the shop were reviewed at a follow-up visit and indicated that several of the compounds contained toluene diisocyanate (TDI), a known cause of occupational asthma. He was told of this potential cause-and-effect relationship and advised to eliminate his exposure. He decided to quit his job and started work as a truck driver. His job change resulted in marked improvement in his symptoms, and he subsequently required only rare use of his metered dose inhaler. Furthermore, the state OSHA office was contacted to investigate and take appropriate action to prevent exposure among current and future workers at the shop.

Selected Readings

Chan-Yeung, M., and S. Lam. Occupational asthma. Am Rev Respir Dis 133:686-703, 1986.

Coultas, D. B., and W. E. Lambert. What you can do about air pollution and lung disease. J Respir Dis 14:905-20, 1993.

Ferguson, G. T., and R. M. Cherniack. Management of chronic obstructive pulmonary disease. N Engl J Med 328:1017-21, 1993.

Guidelines for the Diagnosis and Management of Asthma. U.S. Department of Health and Human Services. Publication No. 91-3042. Bethesda, Maryland, Public Health Service, National Institutes of Health, 1991.

Sheagren, J. N., A. J. Zweifler, and J. O. Woolliscroft. The present medical database needs reorganization. Arch Intern Med 150:2014-5, 1990.

U.S. Preventive Services Task Force. *Guide to Clinical Preventive Services: An Assessment of the Effectiveness of 169 Interventions.* Baltimore, Williams & Wilkins, 1989.

Young, T., M. Palta, J. Dempsey, et al. The occurrence of sleep-disordered breathing among middle-aged adults. N Engl J Med 328:1230-5, 1993.

C H A P T E R   1 5

PREVENTION OF CANCER

Thomas M. Becker, M.D., Ph.D.

H_x A 44-year old male shipbuilder presents for the first time for a routine physical examination as part of his employee health plan. Although his physical examination and laboratory studies are normal, his family history is significant for both lung and colon cancer in first-degree relatives. The patient reports a 15 pack-year history of cigarette smoking and remote exposure to asbestos on his job. He denies weight loss, hemoptysis, or change in his chronic cough. Further questioning indicates no changes in bowel habits or blood in the stool. He describes his health as "very good" but admits that some of his life-style choices are worrisome. He states that his eating habits are poor; since he lives alone, he eats most of his meals outside of the home and consistently orders only the foods that he likes most, namely, meat dishes and pastries. He occasionally skips meals. He consumes two or three beers most evenings, either with or after dinner. He does not exercise regularly, and his social life includes sexual encounters with different female partners. He reported two episodes of chlamydial urethritis over the past 10 years since his divorce.

Questions

1. For what cancers is the patient at increased risk based on family history and current life-style?
2. What modifiable cancer risks are suggested by the patient's history? How much can the patient reduce his risk for lung cancer, colon cancer, and oropharyngeal cancers?
3. How does the patient's sexual behavior influence his cancer risk?
4. How much does the patient's poor diet potentially contribute to development of cancers of various sites?

Cancer is an enormous public health problem in the United States and worldwide. Data published by the International Agency for Research on Cancer (Lyon, France) indicate that 7.6 million new cases of cancer occurred in 1985 alone. Worldwide, the highest incidence of cancer occurred in peoples of Africa, followed by the Caribbean, Central America, South America, and North America. In the United States, nearly 1.2 million new cases of cancer were reported in 1993, and almost 530,000 cancer-related deaths occurred the same year, making cancer the second leading cause of death nationwide. Although substantial research has been directed at secondary prevention of cancer (see Chapter 11), fewer studies have adequately evaluated primary prevention strategies for cancer control. This field is now rapidly developing, however, and ongoing prevention trials, in addition to etiologic research, promise to provide much needed data. Currently, however, clinicians are not armed with sufficient information to clearly support all "popular" ideas about cancer prevention. Some of the more convincing lines of evidence related to primary prevention strategies are summarized below.

CANCER EPIDEMIOLOGY IN THE UNITED STATES

Cancer rates vary by age, sex, and race, and temporal changes in incidence and mortality have been documented. Most data on cancer incidence come from the National Cancer Institute-sponsored Surveillance, Epidemiology, and End Results (SEER) program. This network of population-based registries provides surveillance for approximately 10% of the population. The SEER program periodically publishes incidence data for cancers of many sites. The data indicate that cancer occurs more frequently with advancing age; however, cancer is also the leading cause of death due to disease among children aged 1 to 14 years. Data collected by the SEER program show that the highest age-specific incidence rates are for the oldest age groups. The lowest age-specific rates are for children aged 5-9 years. Cancer epidemiologists have pointed out that as age advances from 25 to 75 years, cancer incidence increases dramatically—100-fold for men and 30-fold for women. The largest proportion of cancers, however, develops in persons aged 60 years and older.

Cancer occurs more frequently in men than in women. Sex-specific incidence rates vary dramatically by site, especially for cancers of the lung, stomach, bladder, and colon-rectum. In fact, for cancers of nongenital and nonsexual sites, incidence for males exceeds that for females for all sites except thyroid, gallbladder, and extrahepatic biliary ducts. For all ethnic groups and all cancer sites combined, the annual age-adjusted rate for males from 1987 to 1991 was 466 cases per 100,000 compared to a rate of 343 cases per 100,000 for females during the same time period.

Cancer risk varies by ethnic/racial group, with African Americans showing higher overall cancer incidence and mortality rates than members of other racial/ethnic groups. Rates for African Americans are higher than for whites for both sexes. The incidence rate differences are particularly apparent for cancers of the lung, pancreas, mouth, esophagus, larynx, liver, and cervix. Although Native Hawaiians also showed higher overall cancer incidence than did whites, other minority groups reported in the SEER data had lower cancer incidence than the white majority population. Asian Americans, southwestern Hispanics, and southwestern Native Americans had comparatively low cancer incidence rates for both sexes for all sites combined. On a site-specific basis, however, some of these minority groups with low overall rates showed some dramatic increases for several cancer sites. For example, southwestern Hispanics and Native Americans showed elevated rates for gallbladder, stomach, and cervical cancers. Within specific ethnic groups, furthermore, cancer incidence and mortality vary by geographic region. For example, Native Americans in many northern states (including Alaska) have higher cancer incidence and mortality for all sites combined compared to southwestern Native Americans. For Hispanics, overall and site-specific rates also vary substantially.

For the clinician, knowledge of the racial and ethnic differences in cancer rates can help guide screening practices and further help in establishing differential diagnoses in clinical workups of patients. Such knowledge may also be useful in designing targeted cancer prevention programs for specific racial or ethnic groups.

Cancer incidence and mortality have changed over the past 50 years. Mortality data, although subject to more bias than incidence data, have provided a long-term perspective of changing rates over the last half-century. In the 1930s, stomach cancer and uterine cancer were the most common causes of cancer death. Both have decreased markedly through the 1990s. Conversely, lung cancer mortality over the same period increased from approximately 7 deaths per 100,000 population per year to 49 deaths per 100,000 population per year for both sexes combined. For African Americans over the past quarter-century, mortality has increased at a higher rate than for whites. For southwestern Hispanics, site-specific mortality has increased for cancers of the breast and lung over a recent 30-year period (1958–1987), while mortality for other sites has remained stable or has decreased. Thus, within the span of one generation, cancer mortality can change dramatically: we can expect continued changes in future generations, particularly if prevention practices change and treatment options improve.

PATHOPHYSIOLOGY

Cancer refers to a diverse group of diseases characterized by abnormal growth and spread of cells. Cancers are classified according to organ or tissue of origin (site or topography code) and by their histologic features. They may also be classified according to their stage at diagnosis—the extent to which the cancer has grown locally or invaded other tissues or organs. Local, regional, or distant stage disease are the three classifications used to describe the spread of cancer.

The chain of events that connects undifferentiated cells with the later development of malignancy is not fully understood. Popular theories of carcinogenesis include two-stage and multistage models of neoplastic disease development. Our expanding knowledge base resulting from oncogene research and cancer genetics promises to modify models of disease development and lead to new theories of carcinogenesis.

Known or strongly suspected carcinogens include tobacco exposure, alcohol abuse, industrial exposures, drug exposures, radiation, exogenous sex hormones, DNA and RNA viruses, and dietary carcinogens such as nitrites. Dietary deficiencies of vitamins A, C, E, and folate represent additional risks for cancers of various sites, especially those of epithelial cell origin, and high-fat, low-fiber diets also represent risks for other cancers. Colon cancer, for example, has been associated

TABLE 15–1. Potentially Modifiable Risks for Cancers of Selected Sites

Cancer Site	Potentially Modifiable Risk Factors
Lung	Cigarette smoking; secondhand cigarette smoke inhalation; residential radon exposure; occupational exposures to asbestos, arsenic, polycyclic hydrocarbons, and radon; diets low in β-carotene
Colon-rectum	Diet high in saturated fat and low in vegetables, fruits, and fiber
Breast	Late age at first full-term pregnancy; radiation exposure; never having children; obesity after menopause; high fat diet; high doses of estrogens
Cervix	High number of sex partners; early age at first intercourse; acquisition of sexually transmitted diseases, especially human papillomavirus; cigarette smoking; nonuse of barrier contraceptives; low dietary intake of β-carotene and folate
Bladder	Cigarette smoking; occupational exposures
Oropharynx	Tobacco use; betel leaf chewing; high alcohol intake; occupational exposures; diets low in β-carotene and vitamin C
Melanoma	Sun exposure, especially repeated heavy burns
Kaposi's sarcoma	HIV infection
Hepatoma	HBV infection, especially in infancy; exposure to vinyl chloride
Prostate	Occupational exposure to cadmium; high fat diet
Pancreas	Cigarette smoking

with both of these dietary patterns, while breast cancer has been associated with high-fat diets. Substantial effort is now being directed at better understanding the relationship between diet and cancer; the many complexities of measuring nutritional intake complicate this area of research. While definitive studies of dietary deficiencies and excesses should be forthcoming, some already published data utilize prevention strategies related to dietary intake.

PREVENTION

Primary prevention of cancer is prevention of the initial development of a neoplasm or its precursor. Primary prevention can be accomplished if causes of a neoplasm are known and can be affected by reducing or preventing exposure to the causative agent. Determining causation is very difficult in epidemiologic studies. Most epidemiologic studies are aimed at identification of risk factors for development of various cancers; a risk factor can represent a cause of cancer whether or not the precise mechanism of carcinogenesis is known. From the viewpoint of primary prevention, it is not particularly important whether or not the mechanism of action of a carcinogen is known. However, primary prevention efforts will be better directed as our knowledge of cancer etiology progresses.

The National Cancer Institute has worked toward improvement of cancer mortality in the United States by promoting primary and secondary prevention strategies. The Institute has advocated as national goals the reduction of tobacco use, increase in consumption of fiber, decrease in percentage of total calories from fat, increase in cervical and breast cancer screening, and

provision of appropriate cancer treatment to all who would benefit from such treatment. Thoroughly convincing data do not support all these strategies (especially those related to diet and cancer), and data are lacking to strongly support some other prevention strategies presented in Table 15–1. Indeed, many of the potentially modifiable risk factors for cancers of various sites are just now being adequately evaluated in prevention trials.

Although a high proportion of all cancers may be related to genetic factors, a substantial fraction of all cancers (perhaps up to one half) are related to life-style factors that are modifiable (Table 15–2). Alteration of certain life-style factors may be a reasonable strategy to reduce the occurrence of cancers of selected sites. Clinicians can urge changes and suggest life-style modifications to patients in an attempt to reduce their cancer risk. In the list of potentially useful primary prevention strategies outlined below, clinicians can feel most confident about recommendations centered on decreasing tobacco use in all of its forms. Other well-directed advice may include the following:

1. Discouraging frequent and heavy alcohol consumption.
2. Encouraging intake of fruits and vegetables, as well as fiber, while reducing fat intake.
3. Avoiding foods that are salt-cured, smoked, or preserved with nitrites.
4. Decreasing exposures to known occupational or environmental carcinogens.
5. Avoiding becoming obese.
6. Encouraging use of barrier contraceptives.
7. Encouraging vaccination against hepatitis B virus (HBV) among sexually active, occupationally exposed, or neonatally exposed individuals.
8. Avoiding unnecessary exposure of patients to x-rays.
9. Avoiding drugs that may be carcinogens.
10. Limiting sunlight exposure.

Some data suggest that increasing physical activity may reduce cancer risk for cancers of certain sites, especially the colon, although mechanisms of preventive action for this strategy are not well established.

TABLE 15–2. Estimates of the Proportion of Cancer Deaths Attributed to Various Factors

Factor	Percent
Tobacco use	30
Diet	35
Infections	10
Reproductive/sexual history	7
Occupation	4
Geophysical (radiation)	3
Alcohol	3
Pollution	2
Medications/medical procedures	1
Industrial products	<1

Reproduced, with permission, from R. Doll and R. Peto. *The Causes of Cancer: Quantitative Estimates of Avoidable Risks of Cancer in the U.S. Today.* New York, Oxford Press, 1981, p. 1256.

Certainly, this issue warrants further examination with appropriately designed studies.

Case Resolution

The physician made several recommendations to this patient, including quitting smoking, ceasing or drastically decreasing alcohol consumption, and changing his diet to include less fat, more fruits and vegetables, and more fiber. He might further reduce his colon cancer risk by increasing his level of exercise. In addition, he could avoid AIDS-related cancers by modifying his sexual behavior. Other recommendations for primary prevention might be suggested by additional historical information.

Selected Readings

American Cancer Society. Cancer Facts and Figures—1993. Atlanta, American Cancer Society, 1993.

Bernstein, L., R. K. Ross, and B. E. Henderson. Prospects for the primary prevention of cancer. Am J Epidemiol 135:142-52, 1992.

Blot, W. J. Alcohol and cancer. Cancer Res 52:2119–23, 1992.

Doll, R., and R. Peto. *The Causes of Cancer: Quantitative Estimates of Avoidable Risks of Cancer in the U.S. Today.* New York, Oxford Press, 1981.

Greenwald, P., and E. J. Sondik (eds.). *Cancer Control Objectives for the Nation, 1985-2000.* National Cancer Institute Monograph No. 2. DHHS Publication No. 86-2880. Washington, D.C., U.S. Government Printing Office, 1986.

Page, H. S., and A. J. Asire. *Cancer Rates and Risks,* 3rd ed. NIH Publication No. 85-691. Bethesda, Maryland, National Cancer Institute, 1985.

Sternfeld, B. Cancer and the protective effect of physical activity: The epidemiologic evidence. Med Sci Sports Exerc 24:1195–1209, 1992.

Trock, B., E. Lanza, P. Greenwald. Dietary fiber, vegetables, and colon cancer: Critical review and metaanalysis of the epidemiologic evidence. J Natl Cancer Inst 82:650–61, 1990.

U.S. Department of Health and Human Services. *The Health Benefits of Smoking Cessation.* DHHS Publication No. CDC 90-8416. Rockville, Maryland, Centers for Disease Control, Office on Smoking and Health, 1990.

Willett, W. C., M. J. Stampfer, G. A. Colditz, et al. Relation of meat, fat, and fiber intake to the risk of colon cancer in a prospective study among women. N Engl J Med 323:1664–72, 1990.

CHAPTER 16

PREVENTION OF INJURIES

Christopher E. Urbina, M.D., M.P.H.

H$_x$ It is 2:00 AM when a paramedic calls in to the head nurse at the university hospital emergency room. The paramedic states that she has just arrived at the scene of a two-car head-on collision on a major roadway outside of town. The driver of a car that had been going the wrong way on a divided roadway is bleeding profusely from a head wound he sustained after being thrown 50 feet from the car. The paramedic reports that the driver is semiconscious; she is applying a MAST garment and is bringing him in. The driver of the second car is dead, and the three children in the back seat (who had been wearing their seat belts) are cut and badly shaken. Another paramedic is bringing the children in. The front-seat passenger of the second car is unconscious and pinned under the dashboard. Firefighters are prying open the door and attempting to remove her from the vehicle. The paramedic is requesting that a helicopter be sent to the scene. Several emergency room technicians immediately begin to prepare for the incoming trauma patients.

Questions

1. Is there a relationship between the location, timing, and severity of each patient's injuries?
2. What is the role of a primary care physician in the treatment and prevention of injuries?

This case history represents a common experience for physicians in almost every hospital emergency department in the United States. According to the

National Center for Health Statistics (NCHS), physicians manage more than 100 million trauma visits annually. Visits for trauma are second only to visits for respiratory conditions. Injuries represent 25% of all emergency room visits and account for nearly $3 billion in hospital costs each year. Annually, one quarter of the U. S. population sustains an injury that requires medical treatment and results in medical disability for a minimum of 1 day. The majority of these injuries are evaluated and treated by primary care physicians.

For children and adults aged 1–44 years, injuries are the number one cause of death and disability. Males are more likely to suffer from injuries than females. Some ethnic groups have higher rates of intentional injuries than others. The elderly are especially likely to incur morbidity and mortality after sustaining a fall. Motor vehicle fatalities occur more often in rural areas. Injuries are arguably the number one preventable cause of death and disability in the United States.

How is injury defined? The most common classification divides injuries into two categories: intentional and unintentional. The word "accident" has been eliminated by many injury experts because it implies that the event occurred by chance and could not have been prevented. Intentional injuries are injuries caused by one individual to another or to oneself, such as homicide and suicide. Unintentional injuries encompass motor vehicle-related injuries (including those where pedestrians are victims), burns, falls, poisonings, asphyxiation, and injuries that occur on the job or while playing sports.

Public health physicians and others have examined injuries using the classic public health model (Fig. 16–1). The host is the person involved in the injury, the agent is energy, and the environment is the physical setting. A motor vehicle injury, for example, occurs when there is a transfer of force from the impact of a host (driver or passenger) with an agent (energy passed through a steering wheel/windshield) in an environment (roadway), resulting in a negative outcome (motor vehicle injury). However, the public health model is limited because it does not adequately explain the sequence of events leading to the injury.

A different approach is to examine the injury on a time continuum. William Haddon was the first to analyze the mechanisms of injury using the public health model integrated with three phases of time, which he termed preinjury, injury, and postinjury. His matrix allows one

to focus on the sequence events that led to the injury, with an eye toward prevention. Haddon's work focused on motor vehicle injuries but has been used to study other types of injuries as well. Table 16–1 demonstrates how the Haddon matrix can be applied to a bicycle-related injury.

EVALUATION AND MANAGEMENT

The Haddon matrix allows the physician to evaluate and understand the mechanism of injury from a public health perspective. It enables the physician to focus on the pertinent physical symptoms and signs of an acute injury as well as long-term consequences such as rehabilitation.

In the case history at the beginning of this chapter, the occupants of the two vehicles sustained injuries differing in degree of severity. The driver of the first car (the car going the wrong way) was not wearing a seat belt. He was thrown from his vehicle and landed on his head. No history is available because he is semiconscious, so the physical examination becomes more important. The physician must first ensure that his cardiovascular/ pulmonary status is stable, with all visible bleeding controlled. A large-bore intravenous access must be established in case his cardiovascular status deteriorates. A careful examination of the skin, head, eyes, ears, mouth, face, neck, heart, lungs, abdomen, and extremities must be performed to ensure that no other significant injuries have occurred.

The three children in the second car pose a different problem. They appear at first glance to have sustained only superficial injuries. A complete review of systems should be obtained with an emphasis on areas of pain, impairment, or limitations in mobility. A thorough physical examination is essential. Equally important in the evaluation of the children is the identification of a family member, friend, or other designated adult to talk to and support each of them. The primary care physician can also play a significant role in encouraging the children to talk about what happened. Early attention to grieving and loss is important. The emotional trauma of a motor vehicle accident can be enormous for children, especially if they saw their parents become injured or die. Long-term emotional support and counseling are critical.

TABLE 16–1. The Haddon Matrix Illustrated for Bicycle-Related Injuries

Phase	Human	Vehicle	Environment
		Factors	
Preinjury	No bicycle helmet	No bicycle light	Narrow road, poor lighting, potholes
Injury	Head exposed	Hard and pointed bicycle frame	Hard cement
Postinjury	Bleeding from head injury	Rapidity of energy transfer	Emergency medical system

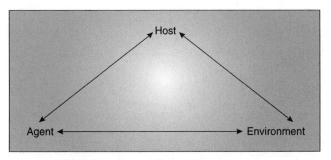

FIGURE 16–1. *The public health model of injury.*

TABLE 16–2. Strategies to Prevent Common Injuries Using the Haddon Matrix

Injury	Prevention Strategies		
	Human	*Vehicle*	*Environment*
Drowning	Swimming lessons	*	Fences around swimming pools
Burns	Fire-resistant clothing	Reduced hot water temperature	Smoke alarms
Carpal tunnel syndrome	Physical therapy	Ergonomic design of work station	Enforcement of worker protection laws
Childhood poisoning	Informed parents	Child-proof medication bottles	Removal of poisons from environment
Falls in elderly	Exercise programs	Soft carpet	Railings in hallways

*Often the vehicle cannot be altered. In the case of drowning, water cannot be altered.

EDUCATION

Efforts to prevent injuries can occur in many settings. Frequently, primary care physicians have the opportunity to provide health education as part of well-child visits, sports physicals, prenatal care, occupational screening examinations, and acute and chronic health care visits. The U. S. Preventive Services Task Force's *Guide to Clinical Preventive Services* provides health education guidelines for specific age groups. For example, parents of children aged 2–6 years should be reminded to (1) use safety belts/car seats, (2) have a smoke detector in the household, (3) reduce the hot water heater temperature, (4) have window guards, (5) make sure there is a fence of suitable height around swimming pools, (6) use bicycle safety helmets, (7) store drugs, toxic chemicals, matches, and firearms out of the reach of children, and (8) have syrup of ipecac and the local poison control telephone number handy.

In addition, primary care physicians can play a vital role in the community-based prevention of injuries. The primary care physician can participate in strategies that reduce injury at each of Haddon's matrix phases (preinjury, injury, and postinjury). For example, a physician could petition the school board to put soft sand under playground equipment at a local park. The physician could testify at a city council meeting on behalf of more street lights, a well-placed traffic light,

reduced automobile speed limits, and divided highways. The state legislature can be lobbied to eliminate drive-up liquor windows and to impose stiffer drunk driving laws. Elected officials and public institutions can be influenced by health experts who are motivated by prevention and patient welfare rather than financial or political gain. A list of common injuries and strategies to prevent them are presented using a Haddon matrix in Table 16–2.

Research Questions

1. What impact do primary care physicians currently have on the prevention of injuries at the local, state, and national level?

2. What is the cost of injuries to individual patients? What is the cost to families? What is the cost to society?

3. What types of injuries are most prevalent in individual communities, both urban and rural? What specific strategies can be implemented to prevent them?

Case Resolution

Although prompt medical treatment was provided to the driver of the car going the wrong way, he subsequently died of massive brain trauma. The passenger of the second car recovered without long-term physical disability. She remains depressed with a significant grief reaction secondary to the loss of her husband. She takes antidepressant medication and is seeking counseling. Two of the three children have been experiencing recurrent nightmares since the accident.

Selected Readings

Baker, S. P., B. O'Neill, M. J. Ginsberg, and G. Li. *The Injury Fact Book,* 2nd ed. New York, Oxford University Press, 1992.

Haddon, W., Jr. A logical framework for categorizing highway safety phenomena and activity. J Trauma 12:193–207, 1972.

Rice, D. P., E. J. MacKenzie, et al. Cost of injury in the United States: A Report to Congress. San Francisco, Institute for Health and Aging, University of California, and Injury Prevention Center, Johns Hopkins University, 1989.

U.S. Preventive Services Task Force. *Guide to Clinical Preventive Services: An Assessment of the Effectiveness of 169 Interventions.* Baltimore, Williams & Wilkins, 1989.

PREVENTION OF OSTEOPOROSIS

Lesley W. Janis, M.D.

Hx   A 68-year-old female comes in for a "get acquainted" visit. She is married, a retired teacher, and active both socially and physically. She is healthy and has no specific problems. Her gallbladder was removed a few years ago because of gallstones. She has had no other surgeries and takes no medication. She has three children, all of whom were delivered vaginally. Family history is unremarkable. A social drinker, she has a 25 pack-year history of cigarette smoking. She stopped menstruating at age 48 years. She took estrogen for approximately 10 years, then stopped for the past 10 years. She now wonders whether she should restart hormone replacement therapy.

Questions

1. What additional information do you need for consideration of hormone replacement?
2. Are any diagnostic tests needed?
3. What life-style issues would you address with this patient, and why?

Osteoporosis is primarily encountered in the elderly and is the most common metabolic bone disease in the United States, accounting for 1.2 million fractures each year. One of three white women over the age of 75 years will have a hip fracture as a result of osteoporosis, and approximately 10% of those women will ultimately die of their injuries. Most commonly, the cause of death is a postoperative pulmonary embolus. Although osteoporosis-induced fractures are a major cause of morbidity and mortality in the elderly, they are preventable.

PATHOPHYSIOLOGY

Normal bone has both cellular and extracellular components that are in a constant, dynamic cycle of bone formation and resorption. The extracellular component of bone consists of an organic phase (primarily type I collagen) and an inorganic phase (primarily calcium and phosphorus). The cellular component of bone consists of (1) osteoblasts, which secrete the organic matrix and regulate bone mineralization, (2) osteoclasts, which are responsible for bone resorption, and (3) osteocytes, which are the stable cells embedded in bone matrix. The activity of these cells is controlled by numerous factors and substances, such as parathyroid hormone, calcitonin, and vitamin D (Fig. 17–1).

The formed skeleton consists of trabecular (cancellous) bone and cortical (compact) bone. Osteoporosis

is defined as a decrease in the density of otherwise normally mineralized bone below the level required for mechanical support. When osteoporosis develops, the bone is weakened and more susceptible to fracture.

DIFFERENTIAL DIAGNOSIS

Secondary causes of osteoporosis must be ruled out (Table 17–1). Primary osteoporosis is of two types: postmenopausal (type I) and senile (type II). Type I is seen in middle-aged postmenopausal women or in women whose ovaries were removed surgically before the menopause. Type I osteoporosis predominantly affects the vertebral bodies, which are composed of trabecular bone, and develops more rapidly than type II osteoporosis. Lack of estrogen plays a major role in the pathophysiology of type I osteoporosis. Type II osteoporosis occurs in both men and women and is a more gradual, age-related loss of both cortical and trabecular bone.

EVALUATION

History

There are few early symptoms of osteoporosis. Older patients may notice a gradual decrease in height owing

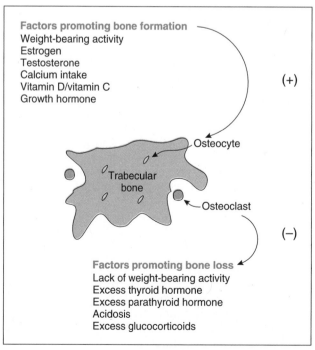

FIGURE 17–1. *Factors influencing bone formation (+) and bone loss (–).*

TABLE 17-1. Secondary Causes of Bone Loss

Hyperthyroidism
Hyperparathyroidism
Cushing's disease
Hypogonadism
Paget's disease
Diabetes mellitus
Renal disease
Rheumatoid arthritis
Multiple myeloma
Metastatic disease
Paralysis
Malabsorption
Chronic malnutrition
Alcoholism
Certain medications (e.g., anticonvulsants, glucocorticoids)

to vertebral fractures that may occur with trivial trauma. If the patient has an acute fracture, the chief complaint and presenting symptoms will be related to the bony structures involved.

A thorough review of the patient's past medical history and current medications should uncover any of the secondary causes of osteoporosis (see Table 17–1). Once secondary causes have been ruled out, management centers on determination of bone density and prevention of further decline of bone mass.

For asymptomatic patients, evaluation should focus on early detection and prevention, based on an understanding of the risk factors for osteoporosis (Table 17–2). A thorough risk factor assessment is essential. It improves the practitioner's ability to predict which patients are at particularly high risk for the development of osteoporosis, and it identifies potentially modifiable risk factors.

Physical Examination

The physical signs of developing osteoporosis are few. Once osteoporosis is established, the patient may present with gradually decreasing height or a dorsal kyphosis, or "dowager's hump," from loss of bone mass in the vertebral bodies.

Most commonly, patients present with acute fractures. The patient should be assessed for localized pain, muscle spasm, neurologic deficit, and loss of strength and range of motion in the affected area. Fractures most commonly occur in the vertebral bodies, wrist, humerus, hip, rib, and pelvis (in that order).

Additional Evaluation

Selection of other tests is guided by clinical suspicion. Since osteoporosis is a chronic problem that takes years to develop, it is often recognized for the first time on a plain x-ray (which may have been ordered to evaluate acute back pain, a common presentation, or to assess the patient for a possible fracture). Osteoporotic bones appear osteopenic on plain films. While hip and wrist

fractures are common, the most frequently occurring fractures are in the spine. X-rays will demonstrate either a wedge compression fracture of the thoracic vertebrae or a classic biconcave compression fracture of the lumbar vertebrae.

If osteopenia is seen on x-ray, a specific cause should be sought. Again, the choice of tests depends on the patient's history and clinical picture. Thyroid function tests will rule out hyperthyroidism. Hyperparathyroidism can be evaluated by serum calcium, phosphorus, and parathyroid hormone studies. Diabetes and renal disease are initially evaluated by obtaining a serum glucose and renal function tests, respectively. If cancer involving the bone is suspected, initial testing should begin with a CBC and serum alkaline phosphatase measurement. Male patients should be evaluated for hypogonadism by checking a serum testosterone level. Serious nutritional deficiencies secondary to malabsorption or wasting are rare and involve elaborate evaluations beyond the scope of this chapter.

Up to 30% of bone may have been lost before osteoporosis is picked up on plain x-rays. Newer, more sensitive radiologic techniques are available for measuring bone mineral density (BMD) and can provide information on baseline BMD. While dual-energy x-ray absorptiometry (DEXA) is currently the preferred modality, other types of scans are used when DEXA is unavailable. DEXA is ideal because of its low radiation dose, short scanning time (about 5 minutes), and precise, high-resolution imaging of both cortical and trabecular bone. Dual-photon absorptiometry (DPA) and quantitative computerized tomography (QCT) also measure both types of bone, but each requires much longer scanning time (about 20–30 minutes) and yields less accurate results. QCT also delivers a high radiation dose. SPA (single-photon absorptiometry) is rarely used, since it measures only the appendicular skeleton.

The use of these techniques in routine screening of all perimenopausal women is both promising and controversial. While more widespread screening may become more common in the future, current recommendations endorse bone density measurements in the following situations: (1) to aid in the decision to prescribe hormone replacement, (2) to verify the management of patients whose plain x-rays are interpreted as showing osteoporosis, (3) to evaluate patients on long-term glucocorticoid therapy for low bone mass, and (4) to identify patients with known primary hyperparathyroidism who are at risk for skeletal disease (and who therefore may need parathyroid surgery).

TABLE 17-2. Risk Factors for Osteoporosis

Elderly	Sedentary life-style
Female	Chronic low intake of dietary calcium
Thin frame	Cigarette smoker
Caucasian/Asian	Alcohol abuser
Early menopause	History of secondary amenorrhea
Positive family history	

MANAGEMENT

The key to management of osteoporosis is prevention. All women should be counseled as they enter their forties, including a thorough risk factor assessment.

The first step in prevention is life-style modification. Women who smoke or drink heavily should be encouraged to stop and supported in their efforts. Women with low body weight (those with eating disorders or competitive athletes) should receive appropriate evaluation, treatment, and dietary counseling. Excessive caffeine intake should be avoided. The importance of routine weight-bearing activities should be emphasized.

Adequate calcium intake should become a priority before women enter the menopause. While calcium is best obtained through dietary sources, most women will need supplementation. Beginning at age 40 years, women should supplement their diet with at least 1200 mg of calcium daily and increase to 1500 mg at the time of menopause. Studies show that calcium supplementation alone can retard bone loss. Adequate intake of vitamin D is also essential, but most people receive adequate amounts through exposure to sunlight. A patient who does not should supplement her diet with 400–800 IU of vitamin D daily.

While calcium supplementation and life-style modifications are important, estrogen replacement is the most effective method for preventing postmenopausal bone loss. Bone loss is most rapid in the first 5 years after menopause. Therefore, estrogen replacement should start immediately and continue for at least 10 years after menopause. Most research suggests that women should remain on hormone replacement indefinitely because bone loss resumes when the hormone is discontinued.

Not all women are candidates for hormone replacement, and some women prefer not to take the medication. The risks, benefits, and contraindications should all be reviewed with the patient (see Chapter 76). If the patient is unwilling or unable to take hormones, she should be counseled to aggressively modify other risk factors.

Progesterone must be added to the regimen if the patient has an intact uterus; its addition will not negatively impact the effect of estrogen on bone density.

The same basic approach should be used for men who are diagnosed with senile osteoporosis: risk factor modification, calcium supplements, and weight-bearing exercise. In addition, men who have low testosterone levels may benefit from testosterone replacement.

A few agents are currently being used to treat osteoporosis with varying degrees of success. Calcitonin may be especially helpful in treating painful vertebral fractures. Bisphosphonates have also been used. The advantage of bisphosphonates is that they are oral agents, whereas calcitonin must be inhaled nasally or injected.

PATIENT EDUCATION

Educating patients on specific ways they can modify their individual risk profile is a powerful preventive tool. While a woman has no control over her ethnicity or family history, she can control her level of activity, diet, and use of tobacco and alcohol.

Research Questions

1. Should all postmenopausal women be screened with a bone density measurement?
2. In patients with known osteoporosis, how can those who are at high risk of falling be identified?
3. What measures can be implemented to prevent fractures in this especially high-risk group?

Case Resolution

The patient received a thorough risk factor assessment and was counseled about risk factor modification as it pertains to the development of osteoporosis. The patient chose to stop smoking, take calcium supplementation, and increase the length of her daily walk. The risks and benefits of hormone replacement therapy were also discussed.

Selected Readings

Aloia, J. F., A. Vaswani, J. K. Yeh, et al. Calcium supplementation with and without hormone replacement therapy to prevent postmenopausal bone loss. Ann Intern Med 120:97–103, 1994.

Kellie, S. E. Diagnostic and therapeutic technology assessment (DATTA): Measurement of bone density with dual-energy x-ray absorptiometry (DEXA). JAMA 267:286–94, 1992.

Lufkin, E. G., H. W. Wahner, W. M. O'Fallon, et al. Treatment of postmenopausal osteoporosis with transdermal estrogen. Ann Intern Med 117:1–9, 1992.

Melton, J. Epidemiology of osteoporosis: Predicting who is at risk. Ann NY Acad Sci 592:295–306, 1990.

Prince, R. L., M. Smith, I. M. Dick, et al. Prevention of postmenopausal osteoporosis: A comparison study of exercise, calcium supplementation, and hormone replacement therapy. N Engl J Med 325:1189–95, 1991.

Riggs, M. The prevention and treatment of osteoporosis. N Engl J Med 327:620–7, 1992.

Tosteson, A. N., D. I. Rosenthal, J. Melton, et al. Cost effectiveness of screening perimenopausal white women for osteoporosis: Bone densitometry and hormone replacement therapy. Ann Intern Med 113:594–603, 1990.

PREVENTION OF ADVERSE DRUG REACTIONS

Michael T. Reed, Pharm.D.

H_x A 64-year-old female librarian presents to the urgent care clinic of her HMO with a chief complaint of pain in her left knee. She states that the pain is "so bad it makes me want to cry." She reports a similar episode 2 years earlier, diagnosed as acute gouty arthritis, and states that her regular physician gave her some pills that "turned my stomach inside out." No medical records are available, but a self-reported medication history on the "consent to be treated" form lists the following prescription drugs: captopril, 25 mg three times daily; verapamil, 240 mg once daily; furosemide, 20 mg daily; and digoxin, 0.125 mg daily. The treating physician makes the clinical diagnosis of recurrence of acute gouty arthritis and prescribes indomethacin, 50 mg every 6 hours for 24 hours, followed by 50 mg three times daily for 4 days, with follow-up by her primary care physician at the end of the treatment course. Three days later the patient presents to the emergency department with increasing dizziness, lethargy, and shortness of breath. Her blood pressure is 90/60 mm Hg, and her heart rate is 50–60 bpm with occasional 3- to 4-second pauses. Her laboratory tests are normal with the exception of a potassium of 5.4 mEq/L, BUN of 64 mg/dL, and serum creatinine of 4.2 mg/dL.

Questions

1. What additional information would you have liked to have had before prescribing any drug for this patient?
2. What drug-related factors should be considered before you prescribe medications for this patient?
3. What patient-related factors should be considered before you prescribe medications for this patient?
4. Working on the premise that the patient's presentation to the emergency department represents one (or several) adverse medication effects, what management strategies would you consider?

The U.S. Food and Drug Administration (FDA) considers all drugs to be "unavoidably unsafe." The wisdom behind this statement is evident in light of the fact that up to 7% of hospital admissions occur as the result of an adverse drug reaction (ADR); in addition, one of six hospitalized patients will experience at least one adverse drug reaction, of which 10% may be considered life-threatening. These figures are undoubtedly conservative, since adverse drug reactions and medication errors are consistently underreported in institutions and only rarely reported in community-based practices.

Accurate estimates of adverse drug reactions are further compromised by the lack of standardized criteria. While each institution accredited by the Joint Commission on Accreditation of Healthcare Organizations (JCAHO) is required to have (1) an operational definition of an adverse drug reaction and (2) a functional system for reporting ADRs to appropriate authorities (e.g., Pharmacy and Therapeutics Committee, FDA, United States Pharmacopeia [USP]), no universal criteria exist. Factors such as (1) inter- and intra-patient variability, (2) reporter bias, (3) use of multiple drugs, (4) presence of multiple disease states, and (5) delayed recognition of ADRs for newer drugs make the establishment of causation a difficult task. For the purposes of this discussion, an adverse drug reaction is defined as *any reaction to a drug that is noxious and unintended and occurs at a dosage that is appropriate for the diagnosis, treatment, or prophylaxis of a given disease state in a given patient, including drug-drug, drug-disease, and drug-food interactions, but excluding failure to accomplish the intended therapeutic purpose.*

To identify a potential ADR, the evaluator must address the questions listed in Box 18–1. In particular, the establishment of a temporal relationship, the determination of the relationship between the observed effect and the known pharmacologic profile of the drug, and the use of dechallenge and rechallenge are critical to the establishment of causation. The more questions that can be answered affirmatively, the greater the likelihood that causation exists.

BOX 18-1. Questions to Ask to Establish a Causal Relationship Between a Drug and an Observed Effect

1. Was there a temporal relationship between the administration of the drug and the observed effect?
2. Is the temporal relationship compatible with the drug's known pharmacokinetic profile (e.g., rate of absorption, time to peak plasma levels, achievement of steady-state concentration)?
3. Could the observed effect be reasonably explained by a known pharmacologic effect of the drug? (This does not preclude classification as an ADR but may support dose-related causality.)
4. Did the observed effect disappear after the drug was stopped or the dose was reduced (i.e., dechallenge)?
5. Did the observed effect reappear after the drug was restarted (i.e., rechallenge)?
6. Could the observed effect be reasonably explained by the patient's clinical state?

CLASSIFICATION

A number of classification systems have been developed for prospective and retrospective determinations of adverse drug reactions. The simplest and most commonly used classification separates ADRs into types A ("anticipated") and B ("bizarre"). Although there is considerable overlap in this system, it is usually helpful to the practicing clinician when making drug use decisions.

Type A reactions are those that could be anticipated or predicted by the known pharmacologic profile of the drug involved. They are usually dose-related, represent an extension of the known pharmacologic effects of the drug, and are not a manifestation of the intended use. For example, sedation due to an antihistamine prescribed for allergy symptoms is a type A adverse drug effect. Sedation from an antihistamine prescribed for sleep would *not* be considered an ADR, although dry mouth (i.e., an unintended effect) *would* qualify as a type A ADR. In summary, type A adverse drug reactions are generally a function of the dose of the drug and the intended use of the drug and can usually be anticipated on the basis of the known pharmacologic effects of the drug.

Type B ADRs represent unanticipated drug reactions. They are usually not dose-related, do not conform to the known pharmacologic profile of the drug, and are therefore unpredictable. Allergic reactions are the classic example of this type of reaction, but other effects (e.g., agranulocytosis due to NSAIDs) also fall into this category. Some authorities refer to these types of reactions as idiosyncratic (i.e., peculiar to an individual).

PREDISPOSING FACTORS

Drug-related Factors

An adverse drug reaction is frequently a function of the **dose** administered. The Greek physician Galen is quoted as having said, "Only the dose determines the poison." In other words, anything administered in sufficient quantity can produce an adverse effect. This principle applies not only to the overdosed patient or situations in which an excessive dose has been prescribed but also to situations in which a "normal" dose has been administered to a patient with an altered drug disposition. The simplest example is the prescribing of a drug (e.g., digoxin) in a usual dose to a patient who has decreased clearance of that drug (i.e., owing to impaired renal or hepatic function). In general, higher doses of a drug result in higher serum concentrations with resultant increased pharmacologic effects, whether desirable or undesirable.

The **route of administration** may influence the propensity for an ADR, primarily by influencing the serum concentration of the drug. Drugs administered by the parenteral route are generally more likely to produce ADRs because of (1) higher serum concentrations, (2) failure to adjust the dose for the difference in bioavailability, (3) too rapid administration, and (4) complications such as phlebitis or extravasation. Parenteral administration of drugs is also more commonly used in more seriously ill patients, a group that has been identified as being at greater risk for ADRs. In addition, drugs can irritate the gastrointestinal tract after oral administration, produce muscle necrosis after intramuscular administration, or produce cutaneous reactions after topical administration.

In general, practitioners tend to believe that the longer the patient has been on a drug and has tolerated it well, the less likely the chance of an ADR. However, **duration of therapy** can be an important factor in the development of an ADR. Drug accumulation may also occur, leading to a type A ADR. The duration of therapy may be excessive for the drug's indication (such as frequently occurs with H_2 antagonists for peptic ulcer disease), exposing the patient to risk without proven benefit. Although allergic reactions are most likely to occur early in therapy (especially with prior exposure to the drug or a related compound), they can develop at any time during therapy.

Adverse drug reactions, especially allergic drug reactions, can be caused by **drug formulations.** In the case of allergic drug reactions, dyes such as FD&C yellow No. 5 (tartrazine) or preservatives such as sulfites are commonly implicated. In addition, sustained-release preparations may be prescribed on standard-release schedules, resulting in excessive drug levels.

One of the most significant factors affecting the risk of adverse drug reactions is the **number of drugs administered**. Not only is the risk of drug-drug interactions increased geometrically with each additional drug, but multiple drug therapy usually reflects **multiple disease processes**, another factor increasing the likelihood of ADRs.

Patient-related Factors

The **age** of the patient is frequently overlooked as a cause of adverse drug reactions. While everyone recognizes that prescribing an adult dose for a pediatric patient can lead to problems, many clinicians fail to recognize that elderly patients also require dose adjustments to prevent type A ADRs. Alterations in (1) drug absorption, (2) renal and hepatic clearance, (3) the muscle-to-fat ratio, and (4) the ratio of ideal to actual body weight require that the elderly patient receive the same careful dosing consideration as the pediatric patient. Assessment of liver, renal, and cardiac function should be made to accurately determine optimal dosing requirements. In addition, the elderly patient is likely to suffer from multiple diseases (e.g., congestive heart failure, diabetes, hypertension, left ventricular hypertrophy) that may be adversely affected by, or require dose adjustments for, any prescribed regimen. Polypharmacy is also more common in the elderly, increasing the likelihood of drug-drug interactions.

Allergic reactions to drugs usually require **prior exposure** to the drug or related compounds. A knowledge of the patient's medication history and the chemical structure of prescribed compounds is required to avoid allergic challenges. For example, exposure to quinine in tonic water is sufficient to sensitize a patient to quinidine-induced thrombocytopenia, while patients with diabetes treated with NPH (neutral protamine Hagedorn) insulin have a 50-fold increase in allergic reactions to protamine sulfate. Similarly, a patient who relates having had an adverse effect from a β-blocker (e.g., propranolol) may experience a similar problem with another sympatholytic drug (e.g., clonidine).

Certain races or individuals may be predisposed to specific ADRs (particularly type A reactions) owing to **genetic factors.** The classic example is procainamide-induced lupus erythematosus. Genetically predisposed people who are slow acetylators of the parent compound (procainamide) to the active metabolite (N-acetyl-procainamide) have a greater chance of developing this drug-induced complication. Another example is the increased prevalence of alcoholic liver disease in Native Americans, many of whom have lower levels of alcohol dehydrogenase than most whites.

Increased serum concentrations of drugs are frequently associated with type A ADRs. Increased serum concentration may be due to the prescribing of normal doses of drugs to patients with **altered drug disposition.** In particular, the primary routes of drug elimination—hepatic metabolism, renal elimination—may be impaired by drug- or disease-induced dysfunction. Alcohol abuse is a frequent cause of hepatic dysfunction, while NSAIDs are recognized as a potential cause of acute renal dysfunction, particularly in patients with preexisting renal disease.

Another major factor contributing to the risk of ADRs is inadequate **patient education.** Regardless of who handles patient education, it is well documented that an informed patient is (1) more likely to comply with a prescribed regimen, (2) less likely to suffer the consequences of over- or undertreatment, and (3) more likely to inform the health-care provider of untoward reactions.

MANAGEMENT

Despite the best efforts of a coordinated team of physicians, pharmacists, and nurses, adverse drug reactions will still occur, especially when commonly offending drugs are prescribed (Table 18–1). When an ADR occurs, the team must design a management approach based on the most likely cause, the type and severity of the reaction, and the availability of treatment alternatives.

For type A reactions, the standard course of action is **dose reduction or discontinuation.** Neither of these approaches usually alters the course of a type B reaction. However, to determine causality for a type A reaction, the disappearance of an observed effect should correspond to the known pharmacokinetics of the drug in question. In general, discontinuation of the suspected offending agent (dechallenge)—with subsequent resolution of the observed effect—is considered a fairly reliable indicator of causality. While reinitiation of therapy at a lower dose may support the supposition

TABLE 18–1. Drug Classes Responsible for ADRs (in Decreasing Order of Frequency)

Antibiotics	Hypoglycemics
Chemotherapeutic agents	Insulin
Cardiovascular agents	Oral agents
Cardiac glycosides	Sedatives/hypnotics
Diuretics	Antidepressants
Antiarrhythmics	Analgesics
Antihypertensive agents	Antiasthmatics
Anticonvulsants	

of a dose-related effect, a true rechallenge requires that the same drug, at the same dose, be readministered. Informed consent may be required, depending on the nature of the reaction.

Antidotes are rarely required or effective for reversing ADRs. Few agents meet the criteria for an "ideal" antidote, including the ability to reverse only the undesirable effects of the suspected offending agent without producing any pharmacologic effect of its own. **Additional drugs** prescribed to prevent, minimize, or treat a recognized or expected ADR generally tend to complicate, rather than improve, the situation.

As the pharmacologic armamentarium continues to expand, there are more **therapeutic alternatives** at the clinician's disposal. There are very few situations in which a different drug from a different class (with a different chemical structure) is not available. However, selection of therapeutic alternatives requires that clinicians ascertain whether the effect they are trying to avoid is (1) a function of the class of drug (e.g., impotence secondary to β-blockers), (2) a function of the formulation of the drug (e.g., asthma due to tartrazine-containing products), (3) a function of the treatment strategy (e.g., hypotension due to afterload reduction for congestive heart failure), or (4) an isolated effect in a given patient (idiosyncratic reaction).

In addition to preventing or reacting to an ADR in a given patient, the prescriber must fulfill an obligation to future patients and the rest of the medical community by reporting a known or suspected ADR to the appropriate authorities and organizations. In the institutional setting, the Pharmacy and Therapeutics Committee, a medical staff committee, responds to all reports of adverse drug reactions. In addition, the clinician may report the ADR independently to either the FDA, through their Adverse Drug Reaction Report Form (FDA form No. 1639) or to the United States Pharmacopeial Convention PRN (Practitioners' Reporting Network) system. Practitioners are also encouraged to report known or suspected adverse drug reactions directly to the manufacturer.

PREVENTION

The old axiom "an ounce of prevention is worth a pound of cure" summarizes an important concept in the management of ADRs. Development of an appropriate patient data base, conscientious prescribing habits, careful monitoring, and focused patient education

TABLE 18–2. Components of a Detailed Medication History*
All current active medical problems
All previous medical problems and their treatments
All currently prescribed drugs and nondrug treatments, including indications for use, frequency, duration, and problems encountered (e.g., side effects, scheduling, compliance)
All currently used over-the-counter (OTC) drugs, including reason for use, frequency, quantity, and duration
All currently used natural or nontraditional (e.g., herbal) drugs and treatments, including reasons for use, frequency, quantity, and duration
Any previous medication problems including difficulty swallowing or administering certain formulations or dose forms, side effects that the patient (realistically or unrealistically) attributes to the medication, and issues related to medication costs
All documented or patient-reported drug allergies, including a description of the allergic reaction
All drug-induced sensitivities or side effects; e.g., gastrointestinal irritation due to erythromycin or nausea due to narcotics (these should be distinguished in the medical record from true drug allergies)

*Responses should be based on the use of open-ended questions.

by all health care providers will greatly reduce the likelihood of an ADR.

The patient data base should include a comprehensive history of past and current medical problems, as well as a detailed medication history (Table 18–2). With this information, the clinician can avoid the use of medications that might aggravate an existing medical condition, precipitate an allergic challenge, or produce side effects that might compromise patient compliance.

Another preventable source of ADRs is the prescription itself. Knowledge of the proper spelling of the drug, the patient-specific dose, the dose form, and the dose regimen is essential to assure that the patient receives the intended drug in the intended fashion. The use of manufacturers' trade names instead of generic or chemical names can result in filling or transcription errors. Another common source of prescription filling errors is illegible handwriting. Furthermore, the use of traditional Latin abbreviations (e.g., qid, QD) does not assure the accurate transmission of information. If the intended drug regimen is to be administered "four times daily," this information should be clearly written out rather than using "qid," which can be misread as "QD," or once daily.

Adverse drug reactions, as well as therapeutic failures, may go undetected without careful monitoring and frequent communication with the patient. Abnormalities in organ function that do not produce overt symptoms, such as elevated liver function tests, can be detected only if the clinician is aware of the possibility of these ADRs and monitors for them. While serum drug levels may be useful monitoring tools in certain situations, for most drugs there is little correlation between the serum drug level and therapeutic or toxic effects.

As noted above, the well-educated patient is likely to be more compliant and have fewer ADRs. However, education should involve not only the patient but also other family members or care givers. Certain ADRs might go unnoticed by the patient but be apparent to family members or care givers if they have been made aware of the possibility of this side effect.

Ultimately, the best method to avoid adverse drug reactions is to have a well-educated prescriber and well-educated patient. While patients will generally rely on the physician, nurse, and pharmacist for their drug information needs, physicians have the responsibility to never prescribe a drug without being fully informed of its appropriate use, pharmacokinetics, and therapeutic and toxic effects. Although drug company representatives are heavily relied upon by the medical community to provide information about specific products, other resources are available for objective, comparative information. These resources include the local drug information center, pharmacists, and a variety of texts such as *Drug Facts and Comparisons* (Facts and Comparisons, St. Louis, Missouri), *AHFS Drug Information* (American Society of Healthcare Pharmacists, Bethesda, Maryland), and *USP DI* (United States Pharmacopeial Convention, Rockville, Maryland).

Case Resolution

The patient's acute problems were attributed to acute renal failure precipitated by NSAID use. Bradycardia and heart block were secondary to digoxin toxicity, which in turn was caused by decreased renal clearance secondary to NSAID-induced renal failure. Hypotension was attributed to reduced cardiac output secondary to bradycardia and also to accumulation of a vasodilator metabolite of verapamil, which is cleared by the kidneys. The NSAID prevented the blood pressure from being lowered further by antagonizing the pressure-lowering effect of the angiotensin-converting enzyme (ACE) inhibitor. Hyperkalemia was attributed to the acute renal failure superimposed on hypoaldosteronism secondary to the ACE inhibitor.

Research Questions

1. What administrative or educational systems could be developed to minimize the risk of ADRs?
2. Who should be held responsible for ADRs—manufacturers, regulatory bodies, the prescriber, or the pharmacist?

Selected Readings

ASHP guidelines on adverse drug reaction monitoring and reporting. Am J Hosp Pharm 46:336–9, 1989.

Blaiss, M. S., and R. D. deShazo. Drug allergy. Pediatr Clin North Am 35:1131–47, 1988.

Jones, J. K. Adverse drug reactions in the community health setting: Approaches to recognizing, counseling and reporting. Fam Community Health 5:57–82, 1982.

Karch, F. E., and L. Lasagna. Adverse drug reactions: A critical review. JAMA 234:1236–41, 1975.

Leape, L. L., T. A. Brennan, N. Laird, et al. The nature of adverse events in hospitalized patients. N Engl J Med 324:377–84, 1991.

Simon, R. A. Adverse reactions to drug additives. J Allergy Clin Immunol 74:623–30, 1984.

Stafford, C. T. Adverse drug reactions. Med Times 116:31–42, 1988.

COMMON CONSTITUTIONAL SYMPTOMS

C H A P T E R   1 9

CHRONIC TIREDNESS

Bronwyn E. Wilson, M.D.

H$_x$ A 47-year-old female homemaker presents with a 3-month history of being tired all the time. She states she barely has any energy to do housework; in fact, she sits on the floor in order to do her vacuuming. She has to take a nap for 1 to 2 hours every afternoon after doing only a few household chores. She goes to bed around 10 PM and gets up around 8 AM. Her past medical history is remarkable for localized breast cancer that was treated by mastectomy 3 years ago. She has no sign of recurrent disease according to her oncologist, and she regularly keeps her follow-up appointments. She does not take any prescribed medications. She has had difficulty controlling her weight over the past year and has gained 7 kg (15 lb) since she quit smoking several months ago. The physical examination is normal except for her increased weight and a surgical scar on her left chest where her breast was removed.

Questions

1. Chronic tiredness can be a manifestation of many different conditions. How should the investigation be organized?
2. What additional history is important to elicit?
3. How do you decide which laboratory tests to order?

Chronic tiredness or fatigue is the seventh most common complaint among patients in the primary care setting. As many as 20% of patients list fatigue as one of their complaints when they visit their doctor. The primary care provider should have a plan of action ready to evaluate this condition.

The first step is to determine what the patient means by being tired. Is this condition mostly related to physical symptoms, such as muscle weakness during or after activity, mental symptoms, such as poor memory and difficulty concentrating, or an inability to cope with social stressors, reflected by a lack of motivation or energy to engage in the activities of daily living?

The next step is to ascertain what is meant by the term "fatigue" in the medical literature. There is much discussion about how to be more precise about this term so that studies of patients with fatigue can be fairly compared. In some studies, fatigue is categorized as acute (usually < 6 months' duration) or chronic (> 6 months' duration), with different causes and prognoses for each type. In other studies, fatigue is categorized by cause: fatigue as a consequence of organic disease versus fatigue related to functional or psychiatric disease. Some authors do not think that this division is appropriate, since many patients with chronic medical conditions are *not* fatigued and, therefore, the symptom of fatigue should be investigated separately from other conditions. Finally, the Centers for Disease Control and Prevention has described fatigue for the purpose of defining the chronic fatigue syndrome as "new onset of persistent or relapsing, debilitating fatigue in a person without a previous history of such symptoms that does not resolve with bed rest and that is severe enough to reduce or impair average daily activity to less than 50% of the patient's premorbid activity level for at least 6 months." In addition to having such fatigue, to qualify for the chronic fatigue syndrome patients must not have any other clinical conditions that could explain this degree of tiredness. They must also have eight of eleven related symptoms or six symptoms and two of three physical findings as listed in Table 19–1.

DIFFERENTIAL DIAGNOSIS

Once an understanding of what the patient means by chronic tiredness is established, how does one proceed to determine the underlying cause and best treatment? Few problems in medicine have as broad a differential diagnosis.

First, it is important to be familiar with the epidemiology of the most common causes of fatigue in both primary and tertiary care settings. In the tertiary care setting, there is a high prevalence (60%–80%) of lifetime or concurrent psychiatric disorders in patients presenting with fatigue. The most common of these disorders are depression (by far the most prevalent), anxiety, and somatization disorder.

In the primary care setting, however, the prevalence of lifetime or concurrent psychiatric disorders in

TABLE 19–1. Working Case Definition of the Chronic Fatigue Syndrome

Major Criteria (the patient must demonstrate both)
1. Fatigue for greater than 6 months
2. Absence of other clinical conditions that may explain such fatigue

Minor Criteria (the patient must have 8 / 11 symptoms or 6 / 11 symptoms and at least 2 signs)

Symptoms
Generalized headaches (different from any previous pattern)
Myalgias
Migratory arthralgias without swelling or redness
Mild fever or chills (temperature between 37.5 and 38.6° C [99.5–101.5° F])
Sore throat
Painful adenopathy—posterior or anterior cervical or axillary
Unexplained generalized muscle weakness
Prolonged (≥ 24 hours) generalized weakness after exercise at levels previously tolerated
Neuropsychologic symptoms (one or more of the following: photophobia, transient visual scotomata, forgetfulness, excessive irritability, confusion, difficulty thinking, inability to concentrate, depression)
Sleep disturbance (hypersomnia or insomnia)
Rapid onset of the main symptom complex (hours to days)
Signs (must be documented by a physician on two separate occasions at least 2 months apart)
Low-grade fever (between 37.5 and 38.6° C [99.5–101.5° F] orally)
Nonexudative pharyngitis
Palpable or tender cervical or axillary lymph nodes (<2 cm in diameter)

Modified and reproduced, with permission, from G. P. Holmes, J. E. Kaplan, N. M. Gantz, et al. Chronic fatigue syndrome: A working case definition. Ann Intern Med 108:387–9, 1988.

patients presenting with fatigue is lower, about 20%–50%. Estimates of the prevalence of undiscovered organic disease that may explain a patient's tiredness range from 10% to 45%. The most common organic conditions associated with fatigue are listed in Table 19–2. It is important to remember that chronic fatigue in patients with chronic medical conditions can be multifactorial in cause.

For up to one third of patients, no organic or psychiatric cause for fatigue can be identified. Whether these patients have been adequately questioned about social stressors is not always clear, since physicians are often unable or unwilling to take the time to investigate such issues during a routine office visit. The chronic fatigue syndrome as defined above is probably a relatively rare condition. There is controversy in the medical literature about whether such a discrete syndrome exists. Several surveys of patients presenting with chronic tiredness to special chronic fatigue clinics show that only about 6% of these patients meet all the criteria for diagnosis of this syndrome.

EVALUATION

History

A detailed medical, psychological, and social history is mandatory and will lead to the diagnosis in most cases. Hypotheses formed after gathering this data will lead to the selection of appropriate laboratory testing to confirm or narrow the list of probable causes. Investigating the cause of this problem can be quite time consuming, and several visits may be necessary to complete the evaluation.

It is important to carefully review the patient's current and past medical and psychiatric history. All medications, both prescribed and over-the-counter, should be listed as well as any herbal or home remedies. An in-depth social history should be done that reviews the patient's occupation, recreational activities, home situation, sexual history, and use of alcohol, cigarettes, and any other recreational drugs. The patient's diet, sleep habits, and exercise patterns should be reviewed. Any new or increased stressors should be documented.

Functional status should be assessed, especially in light of what the patient cannot do because of fatigue. A mental status examination should be performed. Finally, the physician should elicit the patient's explanation of his or her tiredness, in order to address the patient's worries and to form a good therapeutic relationship.

Because of the high prevalence of depression in these patients, a comprehensive interview to evaluate the patient for this condition should be done. Several self-administered screening scales are available, such as the Beck Depression Inventory and Zung Self-Rating Depression Scale. Although such scales can suggest that a person is depressed, they are not a substitute for a physician evaluation based on *DSM-IV* criteria (see Chapter 101).

TABLE 19–2. Organic Diseases Commonly Associated with Chronic Tiredness

Anemia

Cardiovascular Disease
Congestive heart failure
Valvular disease

Endocrinopathies
Hyperthyroidism or hypothyroidism
Pituitary insufficiency
Diabetes mellitus

Infections
Mononucleosis
Tuberculosis
Hepatitis
Chronic viral infections
Lyme disease

Inflammatory Diseases
Systemic lupus erythematosus
Polymyalgia rheumatica
Inflammatory bowel disease
Fibromyalgia/fibrositis

Malignancies

Medications
Antihistamines
Antiinflammatory agents
Antihypertensives, especially reserpine, α-methyldopa, clonidine, β-blockers
Anticonvulsants, especially phenobarbital
Sedatives
Antianxiety agents
Analgesics
Alcohol
Caffeine

Neurologic Conditions
Multiple sclerosis
Parkinson's disease

Sleep Disorders
Sleep apnea
Narcolepsy

Physical Examination

The physical examination can be guided by clues obtained during the medical history. In the absence of any specific findings, a thorough examination should be conducted with a special search for fever, pharyngitis, lymphadenopathy, hepatosplenomegaly, and neurologic deficits.

Controversy exists about performing routine screening laboratory tests in patients with fatigue who have no other signs or symptoms of a specific organic illness. The positive predictive value of random screening is very low when the index of suspicion for a given condition and the prevalence of that condition in the general population are low. In fact, most of the positive test results will not represent true disease but will be falsely positive (see Chapter 3). However, it is difficult to convince some patients that laboratory tests do not need to be done in the absence of physical and historical findings, and some authors feel that it is valuable to do limited testing to reassure such patients. Such testing might include a CBC, sedimentation rate, thyroid-stimulating hormone level, urinalysis, and blood chemistry profile.

MANAGEMENT

The management of these patients depends on the suspected or confirmed cause of the tiredness. For example, if the patient proves to be depressed, an evaluation for counseling and/or medication can be considered. Medical conditions should be treated as indicated. If the patient is able to identify a particular psychosocial stressor, counseling and behavior modification strategies can be used.

For many patients, a specific organic, psychiatric, or social cause for their tiredness may not be discovered. In that setting reassurance and watchful waiting are appropriate therapies.

PATIENT AND FAMILY EDUCATION

The patient should be informed about the many causes of fatigue and about how difficult it is to identify a cause in many cases. Patients should be encouraged to report any new symptoms or signs promptly.

NATURAL HISTORY/PROGNOSIS

Prospective studies that have looked at the outcome of patients with nonspecific fatigue show that 28%–66% still complain of fatigue after 1 year of follow-up. One variable that affects the prognosis is the duration of the fatigue at the time of presentation to the physician. If a patient has been chronically tired for more than 6 months, the prognosis is poor. Advanced age and having a large number of somatic symptoms also are associated with a poorer prognosis.

Research Questions

1. How can we more precisely define chronic tiredness or fatigue to better compare studies on this subject?
2. Can we develop a useful screening scale for social stressors that can be quickly administered by physicians during an office visit?
3. What are the long-term outcomes of patients with chronic fatigue? Is the current definition of the chronic fatigue syndrome a useful one?

Case Resolution

Further questioning revealed that the patient felt that her life had been completely altered by having had breast cancer. Although there was no sign of recurrence and her laboratory tests were normal, she felt that she was still sick and debilitated from this disease. She had minimal social support. She was referred for counseling and over the next few months became more active and less fatigued.

Selected Readings

Barofsky, I., and M. W. Legro. Definition and measurement of fatigue. Rev Infect Dis 13:594–7, 1991.

Cathebras, P. J., J. M. Robbins, L. J. Kirmayer, and B. C. Hayton. Fatigue in primary care: Prevalence, psychiatric comorbidity, illness behavior, and outcome. J Gen Intern Med 7:276–86, 1992.

Chen, M. K. The epidemiology of self-perceived fatigue among adults. Prev Med 15:74–81, 1986.

Elnicki, D. M., W. T. Shockcor, J. E. Brick, and D. Beynon. Evaluating the complaint of fatigue in primary care: Diagnoses and outcomes. Am J Med 93:303–6, 1992.

Katon, W., and J. Russo. Chronic fatigue syndrome criteria. Arch Intern Med 152:1604–9, 1992.

Kirk, J., R. Douglass, E. Nelson, et al. Chief complaint of fatigue: A prospective study. J Fam Pract 30:33–41, 1990.

Kroenke, K., D. R. Wood, A. D. Mangelsdorff, et al. Chronic fatigue in primary care: Prevalence, patient characteristics, and outcome. JAMA 260:929–34, 1988.

Manu, P., J. L. Lane, and D. A. Matthews. The frequency of the chronic fatigue syndrome in patients with symptoms of persistent fatigue. Ann Intern Med 109:554–6, 1988.

Matthews, D. A., P. Manu, and T. J. Lane. Evaluation and management of patients with chronic fatigue. Am J Med Sci 302:269–77, 1991.

GENERALIZED ACHINESS

Chi Chi Lau, M.D.

"There is only one pain that is easy to bear and that is the pain of others."

—Rene Leviche

H$_x$ A 59-year-old retired female teacher presents with a 4-month history of "hurting everywhere," as well as with chronic fatigue. On closer questioning, her pain is especially pronounced in the right shoulder region and is severe enough to keep her awake at night. She arises in the morning feeling unrested and stiff all over but is able to loosen up after 15–20 minutes. She has experienced increased constipation and a 4.5-kg (10-lb) weight gain over the past 8 months. Her past medical history is unremarkable. She denies any history of tick bites or travel outside her home town in southern California. She was widowed 1 year ago and currently lives alone. The physical examination reveals an elderly appearing woman with a depressed affect moving stiffly. There is (1) decreased abduction of the right shoulder secondary to pain and (2) tenderness to palpation over the trapezii, over the lateral tendon insertions at the elbows, and over the gluteal muscles. There are no joint effusions.

Questions

1. How can the physician differentiate between psychogenic pain and musculoskeletal pain?
2. What laboratory tests would yield significant information and also be cost-effective?

The large number of disease entities that can be associated with generalized achiness and the nonspecific nature of the complaint often leave the primary care provider feeling dismayed and frustrated. A systematic approach consisting of a detailed history and physical examination and several screening laboratory tests will help narrow down the possibilities.

PATHOPHYSIOLOGY

Musculoskeletal pain can usually be localized to intraarticular or periarticular structures. Intraarticular disease is discussed in Chapter 87; the present chapter deals primarily with the patient who presents with diffuse musculoskeletal pain *not* associated with joint swelling.

The periarticular anatomy comprises tendons, ligaments, muscles, and bursae. Pain may arise from inflamed tendon insertions, from the tendon sheaths (**tendinitis**), from the bursae or potential spaces between tendon and bone (**bursitis**), or from the muscles.

Arthralgia is pain originating from a joint without objective evidence of inflammation, while **arthritis** is present if joint swelling is observed. **Myalgia** is discomfort arising from muscle. Arthralgias and myalgias are the presenting symptoms in many systemic diseases, especially those in which immune complexes are generated. Discomfort arising from soft tissue regions can also be secondary to nerve impingement, pain emanating from a proximal joint, or pain referred from a diseased internal organ.

DIFFERENTIAL DIAGNOSIS

Disorders associated with generalized body pain are listed in Table 20–1. The most common causes of aches and pains in outpatients are those listed under the category of **nonarticular rheumatism**. Several nonarticular rheumatic conditions may present simultaneously to create a picture of "total body pain."

Fibromyalgia, a chronic condition seen most commonly in women, is characterized by widespread musculoskeletal pain and numerous tender points on physical examination. In addition, these patients frequently have unrestful sleep, chronic fatigue, headaches, symptoms of anxiety or depression, gastrointestinal complaints consistent with irritable bowel syndrome, and symptoms worsening with stress or changes in the weather. Laboratory tests are normal. Fibromyalgia is a

---

TABLE 20–1.   Disorders Associated with General Achiness

Common Disorders

Nonarticular rheumatism
Fibromyalgia
Myofascial pain
Tendinitis, bursitis
Nerve entrapment syndromes
Osteoarthritis
Viral infections
Metabolic or endocrine disorders
Psychogenic pain

Less Common Disorders

Bacteremia, Lyme disease, hepatitis
Myopathies
Neuropathies
Collagen vascular diseases
Cancer
Polymyalgia rheumatica/temporal arteritis

diagnosis of exclusion and may be associated with other disorders.

Myofascial pain is another tender point syndrome. Trigger points in muscles around the neck and low back give rise to pain in the surrounding soft tissue areas on muscle contraction. Most myofascial trigger points are initiated by injuries or overuse.

The generalized achiness felt by deconditioned patients following heavy **physical exertion** rarely lasts more than several days. Symptoms that persist beyond 4–5 days need to be further evaluated.

Low back pain (see Chapter 91) is a frequent component of generalized achiness. Mechanical lumbosacral sprain is the most common cause of low back pain in young healthy persons. Herniated disks or degenerative bone spurs in the spine of older patients may impinge on nerves with subsequent referred pain to soft tissue areas.

Repetitive strain conditions such as **tendinitis** and **bursitis** are common causes of pain and may result in generalized discomfort if several different regions of the body are affected at the same time. Shoulder pain that worsens at night and is associated with morning stiffness is typical of overuse injuries such as supraspinous tendinitis, bicipital tendinitis, or subacromial bursitis. Individuals complaining of lateral hip pain that radiates to the knee and prevents them from lying on the affected side should be examined for bursitis in the greater trochanter region.

Idiopathic **osteoarthritis** (see Chapter 87) is seen in the majority of people over age 50 years. This arthropathy is characterized by joint pain and deformity associated with cartilage degeneration and periarticular bony proliferation.

An acute illness associated with upper respiratory tract symptoms, low-grade fever, or diarrhea is most likely secondary to a **viral infection**. A patient with **influenza** has intense myalgias, has a high fever, and often appears quite ill. **Parvovirus B19** infection is a highly contagious disease that can be epidemic in both children and adults. In adults, arthralgias and rash may be the presenting symptoms. Although the illness is usually mild and self-limited, some patients develop a polyarticular inflammatory arthritis. An elevated parvoviral IgM titer is diagnostic of acute infection.

Acute hepatitis B infection can present with transient arthralgias that resolve once the patient becomes icteric. **Chronic hepatitis B** and **hepatitis C** are associated with circulating immune complexes that may cause chronic migratory joint pains. Liver function tests and hepatitis serologies are helpful in confirming these diagnoses.

Patients with **bacteremia** frequently experience diffuse arthralgias and myalgias. These patients appear ill, have high fevers often associated with shaking chills, and have a leukocytosis with a left shift. The source of infection and the responsible organism should be sought aggressively.

Lyme disease is an infection caused by the tick-borne spirochete *Borrelia burgdorferi* endemic to the Northeast, northern Midwest, and Pacific Coast states. Symptoms seen in the early stages of the illness include diffuse arthralgias, myalgias, fever, chills, and a characteristic "target-like" rash, erythema chronicum migrans. These initial symptoms may last for weeks. The diagnosis should be suspected in patients with diffuse musculoskeletal pain who have been in endemic areas. Many patients with Lyme disease are unable to recall an antecedent tick bite.

Metabolic disorders that can cause muscle discomfort include hyponatremia, hypocalcemia, and hypomagnesemia. **Hypothyroidism** is associated with diffuse arthralgias, myalgias, fatigue, stiffness, and elevated muscle enzymes (e.g., CPK, aldolase). An elevated thyroid-stimulating hormone (TSH) level will help make the diagnosis. **Hyperthyroidism** should be suspected in a patient who complains of migratory arthralgias, muscle weakness, weight loss (despite a preserved appetite), and painful swelling of the distal extremities.

Polymyalgia rheumatica (PMR) is a condition that is most prevalent in the elderly. It is characterized by pain and tenderness in the soft tissues of the shoulder and pelvic girdles, weakness proportionate to the pain, morning stiffness, fatigue, and a markedly elevated erythrocyte sedimentation rate (ESR) (often >100 mm/h). Muscle enzyme levels are normal. Patients respond dramatically to low-dose corticosteroids.

Cranial or **temporal arteritis** is a granulomatous vasculitis that may be associated with polymyalgia rheumatica. Clinical manifestations include new-onset headaches, visual disturbances, jaw claudication (jaw pain with chewing), stroke-like symptoms, and tender temporal arteries. If temporal arteritis is suspected, high-dose corticosteroids should be started to prevent vision loss, and a temporal artery biopsy should be obtained.

Collagen vascular diseases, such as rheumatoid arthritis, systemic lupus erythematosus, and the vasculitides, can present with diffuse musculoskeletal pain without joint swelling early in the course of the illness.

The **myopathies** are primary and secondary disorders of muscle. Myalgias at rest and proximal muscle weakness disproportionate to the degree of pain should lead to a workup for polymyositis. Inherited deficiencies of muscle enzymes can also result in exertional myalgias and fatigue that resolve with rest. Laboratory abnormalities seen in myopathies include elevated CPK and aldolase levels, an abnormal electromyogram, and an abnormal muscle biopsy.

Multiple myeloma or **malignancy** metastatic to bone can cause musculoskeletal pain if complicated by compression fractures. Paraneoplastic polyneuropathy associated with lung cancer or lymphoma can also result in diffuse aching and paresthesias.

Pain that is diffuse, variable, poorly described, and unaffected by activity or rest should raise suspicions of **psychogenic pain** as well as fibromyalgia. Patients with psychogenic pain do not have the characteristic tender points of fibromyalgia on examination. These patients may grimace and withdraw at the slightest touch, yet be able to move the affected parts of the body with little discomfort when distracted.

EVALUATION

History

The area of the body causing the most pain is identified by having the patient point to the spot. If the patient remains vague, the physician should ask about pain in specific regions. The history should characterize the areas of musculoskeletal pain, rapidity of onset, frequency and duration of pain, time of day the pain is worse, aggravating or relieving factors, and concomitant constitutional symptoms. The severity of the pain can be assessed by asking whether symptoms interfere with work, sleep, or other daily activities.

A thorough review of systems will help determine whether there is an underlying systemic or connective tissue disease. The interview should include questions about the presence of fever, chills, weight fluctuations, changes in bowel habits, and collagen vascular disease symptoms such as photosensitive rashes, dry eyes or dry mouth, oral ulcers, Raynaud's phenomenon, or pleuritic chest pain. If the history suggests a diagnosis of polymyalgia rheumatica, it is important to also inquire about the symptoms of temporal arteritis.

Fatigue is a common complaint in generalized achiness. Fatigue may be a consequence of lack of sleep due to chronic pain or related anxiety or depression. Patients with inflammatory joint disease are typically fatigued later in the day, while patients with fibromyalgia or depression awaken with a low energy level and give a history of poor-quality sleep.

Information about the patient's job, history of recent travel, prior transfusions, or past or current substance abuse can provide important diagnostic clues.

Physical Examination

Special attention should be paid to the back and peripheral joints. The patient's posture, stance, and gait may indicate the location and degree of pain. The physician should note whether the patient looks acutely ill, anxious, or depressed. Examination of the skin, mucous membranes, lymph nodes, and thyroid gland should also be carried out.

Sites of pain should be examined in detail for visible swelling, palpable tenderness, and limitation in range of motion. Swelling around a joint is always abnormal. Tenderness along tendon sheaths or over bony prominences is seen in tendinitis and bursitis, respectively. Pain on active (but not passive) range of motion indicates periarticular soft tissue inflammation. A careful search should be made for the tender points of fibromyalgia especially in those patients complaining of painful muscles, chronic fatigue, anxiety, or unrestful sleep. Such tender points are located in the soft tissues over the trapezii, distal to the lateral epicondyles, in the buttock regions, over the medial fat pads of the knee, and over the anterior chest wall. Myofascial trigger points are most frequent around the neck and upper back muscles and refer pain to surrounding areas when palpated.

A neurologic examination should be performed on all patients complaining of neck pain, low back pain, or paresthesias in one or more extremities. Back pain elicited on straight leg raising is seen in patients with sciatica. Tender muscles may reflect an underlying myopathic process, in which case muscle strength must be quantified.

Additional Evaluation

The extent of testing depends on the acuteness, severity, and chronicity of the patient's complaints. In general, nonarticular rheumatic conditions are diagnosed by physical findings; laboratory tests and x-rays usually are normal. If musculoskeletal pain persists beyond 6 weeks (the usual time allotted for healing of focal soft tissue injuries), the physician should screen for possible underlying disease (Table 20–2). Radiologic evaluation of joints is unrevealing if the condition is of a periarticular or soft tissue nature. Plain x-rays of musculoskeletal regions are useful when the pain has been chronic and is thought to originate from within the joint or bone. Bone scintigraphy (i.e., a bone scan) has relatively higher sensitivity but lower specificity and costs more than plain radiography. Bone scans should be reserved for those patients with arthralgias who, by history or laboratory screening, are suspected of having early inflammatory arthritis, metastatic malignancy, or osteomyelitis. CT scan and MRI are useful in identifying specific structural abnormalities, such a meniscal tear of the knee, rotator cuff tear of the shoulder, herniated disk with root impingement, or spinal stenosis.

Electromyograms and nerve conduction studies are indicated when suspicion exists for myopathies or neuropathies, respectively.

MANAGEMENT

In many cases, the diagnosis is unclear even after extensive evaluation; in these situations, close follow-up and observation for new symptoms or signs are essential. Patients with a negative workup should be reassured that, although they have chronic discomfort, there is no clinical evidence of systemic illness such as infection, malignancy, metabolic disease, or crippling inflammatory arthritis.

The foremost goal in the management of any musculoskeletal condition is to maintain the patient's level of

---

TABLE 20–2   Screening Laboratory Tests for Persistent General Achiness

CBC with differential
Electrolytes, liver enzymes
CPK
ESR
Urinalysis
Free T_4, TSH
Antinuclear antibody (ANA), rheumatoid factor (RF)
Blood cultures, viral titers, if indicated
Selected radiologic procedures (plain x-rays, bone scan, CT/MRI), if indicated

functioning. If the patient's daily activities are compromised by pain, analgesia in the form of acetaminophen or an NSAID can be prescribed. Narcotic medications should be used only when the presence of severe pain is accompanied by an established diagnosis and there are objective findings of disease. Empiric use of corticosteroids should be avoided unless the physician strongly suspects a diagnosis of polymyalgia rheumatica or temporal arteritis.

Physical therapy, rest, and ice or heat packs are first-line therapies for low back syndrome and overuse conditions. If conservative measures are ineffective in the management of repetitive strain disorders (e.g., tendinitis of the shoulder or trochanteric bursitis of the hip), local corticosteroid injections may prove useful. Myofascial trigger points can be treated by avoidance of activities that worsen the pain, regular stretching of the involved muscles, and local anesthetic injections.

Fibromyalgia can be a difficult condition to treat. Patients' symptoms may improve if they engage in a program of physical conditioning. Low-dose tricyclic antidepressants are often prescribed for use at bedtime, both to improve the quality of sleep as well as to reduce the level of chronic pain.

Persistent inactivity is to be discouraged, especially when objective findings are lacking. Rheumatologic consultation should be sought if a patient continues to have debilitating pain despite conservative therapy, if the diagnosis is unclear, or if a collagen vascular disorder is suspected.

PATIENT AND FAMILY EDUCATION

The majority of patients presenting to the primary physician with diffuse body pain will have osteoarthritis or nonarticular rheumatism. Although symptoms may recur and become chronic, patients with a negative workup should be reassured that their discomfort is not due to an inflammatory arthropathy or serious underlying disease. Patients with fibromyalgia often comply better with a therapeutic program if they are educated about their condition through pamphlets distributed by the Arthritis Foundation or by joining local support groups.

If NSAIDs are prescribed, patients should be warned about their potential adverse effects, which may include lethargy, tinnitus, dyspepsia, peptic ulcers, fluid retention, elevation of liver enzymes, and renal insufficiency.

NATURAL HISTORY/PROGNOSIS

Most outpatients with aches and pains have common musculoskeletal conditions that can be alleviated by conservative measures and that have a good prognosis. However, the practitioner must maintain a high index of suspicion and be vigilant about the possibility of an underlying systemic illness, since the earlier such illnesses are recognized and treated, the better the outcome.

Research Questions

1. What is the relationship between emotional stress and musculoskeletal pain?
2. How can detection of early inflammatory joint disease be improved, especially when the clinical examination is unrevealing?

Case Resolution

The patient's history and physical examination were very suggestive of fibromyalgia. CBC, sedimentation rate, and TSH level were all normal. The physician prescribed a low dose (25 mg) of amitriptyline to be taken at bedtime, and the patient reported moderate improvement in her symptoms when seen 3 weeks later.

Selected Readings

Block, S. R. Fibromyalgia and the rheumatisms: Common sense and sensibility. Rheum Dis Clin North Am 19(1):61–78, 1993.

Byrne, E. Chronic myalgia, a personal approach. Aust NZ J Med 16:745–748, 1986.

Ehrlich, G. E. Diagnosis and management of rheumatic diseases in older patients. J Am Geriatr Soc 30(suppl 11): 545–551, 1982.

McDermott, F. T. Repetition strain injury: A review of current understanding. Med J Aust 144:196–200, 1986.

FEVER

Lourdes Irizarry, M.D.

"Fever is a mighty engine which nature brings into the world for the conquest of her enemies."

—Thomas Sydenham

H$_x$ A 63-year-old heterosexual male route driver with a history remarkable for chronic obstructive pulmonary disease (COPD), rheumatic fever (RF), and a subtotal gastrectomy presents to the hospital with a 2-month history of dysphagia and odynophagia accompanied by a 27-kg (60-lb) weight loss over 6 months, coinciding with the appearance of painful oropharyngeal lesions. He also claims a 6-month history of fever, night sweats, and fatigue. He denies hoarseness, cough, hemoptysis, dyspnea, and urinary frequency. He has a 110 pack-year history of cigarette smoking. There is no history of intravenous drug abuse or alcohol abuse. He denies any recent travel or animal exposure. Although he currently lives in New Mexico, prior residences include Louisiana and Ohio. The physical examination is remarkable for a temperature of 38.3° C (101° F) and heart rate of 110 bpm. The patient appears ill, older than his stated age, and cachectic. Erythema of his palms and soles are noticeable. There are ulcerative, irregularly shaped lesions on his oral mucosa and tonsillar fossae. There is no lymphadenopathy. A II/VI systolic murmur is heard best at the aortic region with radiation to the carotids. The lungs are clear. The liver span is about 15 cm.

Questions

1. What additional questions would you ask this patient?
2. What is your differential diagnosis?
3. What would be your diagnostic strategy?
4. Based on the above data, would you start this patient on therapy? Explain.

From the time of the ancient Greeks, the beneficial role of fever as a mechanism of defense has been recognized. Although this concept went untested for millennia, contemporary studies documenting febrile responses of endothermic and ectothermic vertebrates to the injection of pyrogens and to the stress of captivity show that this adaptive behavior is an important host defense response.

Although we tend to think of fever as any elevation in body temperature above 37° C (±1), the accepted definition is an elevation of body temperature that occurs as a consequence of the hypothalamic thermal regulator being set at a higher temperature (as opposed to mere hyperthermia). During hyperthermic states, the body temperature is higher than the set point. Hyperthermic states are usually the result of environmental exposure or an adverse reaction to a drug. During a febrile state, the set point is elevated with or without a concomitant equivalent rise of the body temperature. This is the basis for the categorical division of fever into three stages: (1) a cold stage, when the body has not reached the set point and therefore is "hypothermic," requiring a variety of heat-conserving measures to facilitate reaching the set point; (2) a hot stage, which is the heat-maintaining stage; and (3) the defervescence stage, at which point the thermal regulatory set point is below the body temperature and the now hyperthermic individual uses a variety of heat-losing reflexes to dissipate heat.

PATHOPHYSIOLOGY

The role of the central nervous system (CNS) in body temperature regulation has been studied since the 1930s when experimental data in animals demonstrated that animals could not maintain normal body temperature when the hypothalamus was injured or removed. Heating of the anterior hypothalamus produced cutaneous vasodilatation, sweating, and a fall in body temperature; cooling induced shivering, vasoconstriction, and an increase in body temperature.

By the early 1960s, two types of neurons in the hypothalamus had been described: warmth-sensitive neurons, which increase their firing rates with high hypothalamic temperatures, and cold-sensitive neurons, which increase their firing rate with lower hypothalamic temperatures.

More recently, exogenous and endogenous pyrogens that function as fever mediators have been discovered. The list of known mediators includes prostaglandin E (PGE), interleukin 1α (IL-1α) and 1β (IL-1β), tumor necrosis factor (TNF), interferons α and γ, interleukin 6 (IL-6), and other cytokines.

Fever results from a myriad of host responses to inflammation; when an insult, such as a bacterial infection, activates blood monocytes and macrophages, a chain of events is triggered. Pyrogenic cytokines such as IL-1, IL-6, TNF, and interferon are released. The number of immature neutrophils released to the periphery is increased as a direct action of IL-1. Serum levels of zinc and iron are reduced. Hepatic synthesis of acute-phase proteins begins. Not only are new proteins produced, but an increase in normally circulating proteins is observed, including haptoglobin, some protease inhibitors, components of the complement cascade, fibrinogen, and ceruloplasmin. The synthesis

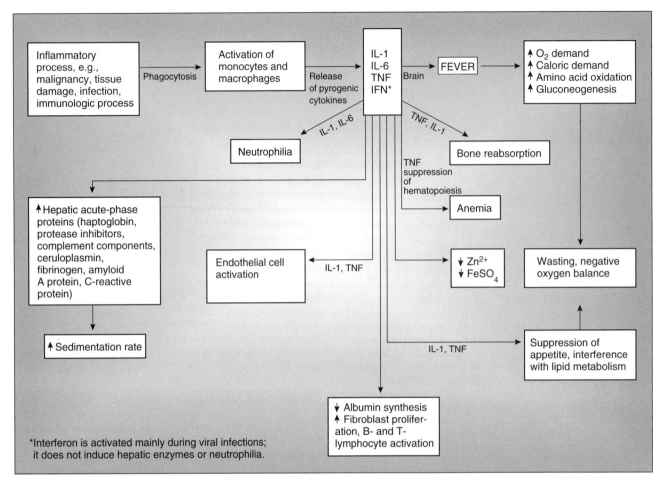

FIGURE 21–1. *Pathophysiology of fever.*

of albumin and cytokines is increased during this time. The catabolic state of the body is augmented. Muscle wasting occurs, and oxygen demands as well as caloric requirements increase. Negative nitrogen balance results from the oxidation of amino acids for immunologic reactions and the synthesis of new proteins (Fig. 21–1).

DIFFERENTIAL DIAGNOSIS

The most common cause of fever is infection. In adults, malignancies (especially lymphomas and leukemias) are the second most frequent cause of fever. Immune disorders such as systemic lupus erythematosus (SLE), rheumatoid arthritis, and vasculitis can also result in fever. Other causes are listed in Table 21–1.

Elevation of body temperature also occurs in non-pathologic circumstances. Exercise is an example. An increase in the core temperature that lasts for hours following strenuous exercise has been well-documented. Exercise causes the release of cytokines capable of inducing fever. Levels of IL-1 and interferon increase with physical activity. In a similar way, a woman's temperature is higher during the luteal phase of the menstrual cycle than during the follicular phase. Although many studies postulate that the high

plasma concentration of progesterone is responsible for this increase in temperature, high levels of IL-1 have been found after ovulation. Stress hyperthermia, observed in many species of animals in captivity, is also thought to be a fever mediated by prostaglandins, IL-1, IL-6, and TNF.

EVALUATION

History

The character of the fever pattern is rarely useful in determining the cause, with the exception of relapsing fevers, i.e., temperature elevations that recur after periods of normal temperature and that are frequently associated with tick-borne diseases.

Symptoms such as headache, photophobia, and confusion suggest a CNS process such as encephalitis or meningitis; confusion is more commonly associated with encephalitis, whereas lethargy is more frequently seen with meningitis. Cough, dyspnea, pleuritic chest pain, sputum production, and hemoptysis suggest a pulmonary process, such as lung cancer, pulmonary embolism or infarct, pneumonia, tuberculosis, or empyema, or a cardiac process, such as pericarditis. Abdominal pain suggests an intraabdominal process originating in the peritoneal or pelvic cavities, either a localized infection or inflammatory disease. Sometimes a vague complaint of abdominal pain may be the only clue to the presence of a lymphoma or an abscess.

Low back pain referred to the lower extremities in a febrile patient is suggestive of a paraspinal abscess,

---

TABLE 21–1. Causes of Fever

Infection

Malignancy

Lymphoma
Leukemia
Renal cell CA
Hepatoma
Lung CA
Atrial myxoma

Hypersensitivity/autoimmune diseases

Systemic lupus erythematosus
Polymyalgia rheumatica
Drug fever
Vasculitis
Polyarteritis nodosa
Erythema multiforme
Mixed connective tissue disease
Serum sickness
Dermatomyositis
Behçet's disease
Giant cell arteritis
Graft-vs-host disease
Juvenile rheumatoid arthritis
Sweet's syndrome (acute febrile neutrophilic dermatosis)
Toxic epidermal necrolysis
Wegener's granulomatosis
Gout

Central nervous system

Bleeding
Infection
Seizure
Neuroleptic malignant syndrome

Cardiovascular/pulmonary

Myocardial infarction
Dressler's syndrome
Pulmonary infarction/embolism
Pericarditis
Myocarditis
Atelectasis

Metabolic

Substance withdrawal
Fabry's disease
Hyperthyroidism
Adrenal insufficiency
Heat stroke

Hematologic

Deep vein thrombosis
Bleeding
Sickle cell disease

Gastrointestinal

Pancreatitis
Cholecystitis
Hepatitis (infectious, noninfectious)
Inflammatory bowel disease
Ischemic colitis

Other

Burns
Familial Mediterranean fever
Postoperative
Trauma (including injections)
Procedure-related (e.g., bronchoscopy)
Toxins
Sarcoidosis

---

psoas abscess, diskitis, osteomyelitis, or metastasis to the spine. Urinary frequency, urgency, hesitancy, dysuria, flank pain, or hematuria may be indicative of cystitis, pyelonephritis, renal tuberculosis, or renal cell carcinoma. A history of a rash associated with fever may indicate a viral etiology, such as the enteroviruses, rubella, rubeola, or varicella zoster, and drug reactions, autoimmune disorders, atypical mycobacterial infections, or fungal infections. As a rule, patients with acute febrile illnesses present with symptoms that help target the body organ or system affected, whereas chronic febrile illnesses tend to require a more extensive history and investigational workup as well as the use of technologic aids.

A travel history is mandatory, since some infections are endemic to specific geographic areas. Malaria, filariasis, hemorrhagic fevers, and protozoal infections are endemic to parts of the world outside North America. Within the United States, there are areas endemic for plague, Lyme disease, blastomycosis, coccidioidomycosis, histoplasmosis, and so on.

Animal exposure is significant because animals can be vectors of multiple infectious agents. The exposure may be difficult for the patient to remember. A short exposure to a dog may be all that is needed for an individual to develop tick fever. Q fever has occurred after exposure to parturient cats and after exposure to a truck transporting sheep.

A history of intravenous drug use may suggest endocarditis, osteomyelitis, or hepatitis as the cause of fever. People with alcoholism develop infections due to *Mycobacterium tuberculosis* and gram-negative organisms more frequently than does the general population, and therefore an accurate alcohol history should be sought.

A sexual history is necessary to assess for sexually transmitted diseases that may account for fever, such as lymphogranuloma venereum, disseminated gonorrhea, syphilis, and HIV infection.

Ethnic background is important, since certain groups are more prone to specific malignancies and autoimmune disorders than others. An occupational history to assess possible biohazard exposure should be sought.

Physical Examination

No laboratory test can substitute for a comprehensive physical examination. From the texture and quality of the hair, which can be altered by autoimmune disorders and infections such as syphilis, to the finding of a skin rash, which may represent a fungal disease, mycobacterial infection, viral exanthem, rickettsial infection, bacterial sepsis, or connective tissue disorder, *all* physical findings are important in determining the etiology of the fever (Table 21–2).

Additional Evaluation

A CBC is required for any febrile patient considered to have significant disease requiring evaluation. An el-

TABLE 21–2. Common Physical Findings

Organ System	Finding	Likely Cause
Vital signs	Pulse-temperature dissociation	Intracellular infection
	Pulsus paradoxus	Cardiac tamponade secondary to pericarditis
	Hypotension	Dehydration/volume depletion, sepsis, adrenal insufficiency
Skin	Rash	Infection (viral, bacterial, fungal, mycobacterial)
		Malignancy (leukemia)
		Sarcoidosis
		Systemic lupus erythematosus (SLE)
		Ulcerative colitis
		Crohn's disease
		Still's disease
		Behçet's disease
		Drug reaction
	Petechiae	Disseminated intravascular coagulation
		Infective endocarditis
		Neisseria meningitidis
	Jaundice	Hepatitis
		Cholangitis
	Darkening	Addison's disease
	Malar rash/photosensitivity	SLE
Lymph nodes	Generalized lymphadenopathy	Infection
		Viral (CMV, EBV, rubella, rubeola, HIV, hepatitis)
		Syphilis
		Brucellosis
		Microbacterial Infection
		Fungal infection (histoplasmosis; coccidioidomycosis)
		Protozoa (toxoplasmosis, leishmaniasis)
		Lymphoma
		Sarcoidosis
		Collagen vascular disease
		Hyperthyroidism
		Myeloproliferative/lymphoproliferative disorders
	Localized lymphadenopathy	Drug side effects (e.g., phenytoin, isoniazid, hydralazine)
	Axillary	Upper extremity bacterial infection
		Sporotrichosis
		Cat-scratch disease
		Plague
		Tularemia
		Lymphoma
		Breast cancer
	Epitrochlear	Infection of hand or forearm
		Syphilis
		Lymphoma
	Inguinal	Lower extremity infection
		Sexually transmitted disease
		Plague
		Tularemia
		Cat-scratch disease
		Melanoma
		Lymphoma
		Pelvic cancer
	Supraclavicular	Mycobacterial infection
		Thoracic or abdominal cancer
	Cervical	Pharyngitis
		Tuberculous cervical lymphadenitis
		Disseminated mycobacterial or fungal infection
		Lymphoma
		Sarcoidosis
		Lymphoproliferative disorder
Neck	Stiffness	Meningitis
	Goiter	Hypothyroidism
	Tender thyroid	Thyroiditis
Head	Tender temporal area	Temporal arteritis
	Alopecia	SLE
		Syphilis
		Tinea capitis
		Hyperthyroidism

TABLE 21–2. Common Physical Findings *Continued*

Organ System	Finding	Likely Cause
Eye	Raccoon's eye	Trauma with possible basilar skull fracture leading to meningitis
	Proptosis	Hyperthyroidism
		Lymphoma of the orbit
		Retro-orbital granulomatous disease
		Neurofibroma
		Metastasis
	Dry eye	Rheumatoid arthritis
		SLE
	Band keratopathy	Still's disease
		Sarcoidosis
	Corneal ulceration	Enteritis
		Infection
	Conjunctival lesion	Erythema multiforme
		Erythema nodosum
		Infection (e.g., tuberculosis, syphilis, tularemia, histoplasmosis, cat-scratch fever, infectious endocarditis)
	Uveitis	SLE
		Vasculitis
		Serum sickness
		Sarcoidosis
		Toxoplasmosis
		Syphilis
		Tuberculosis
		Still's disease
	Discharge	Conjunctivitis
	Purulent	Bacterial
	Clear	Viral
	Fundoscopic	
	Roth's spots	Infective endocarditis
	Cotton wool exudates/hemorrhage	Retinitis (CMV)
	Chorioretinitis	Toxoplasmosis
	Posterior uveitis	Tuberculosis
		Syphilis
		Ocular histoplasmosis
	Endophthalmitis	Infection
		Bacteria (aerobic/anaerobic)
		Syphilis
		Fungi *(Candida, Aspergillus, Coccidioides, Histoplasma, Mucor)*
		Viruses (herpes, CMV)
		Parasites *(Toxoplasma, Toxocara)*
	Keratitis	Bacteria
		Chlamydia
		Viruses (herpes simplex, adenovirus)
		Parasites *(Trypanosoma, Leishmania, Acanthamoeba)*
		Mycobacteria
		Fungi
Ears	Erythema of the canal skin	Otitis externa
	Bulging tympanic membrane/exudate/erythema/hearing loss	Otitis media
	Displacement of the pinna; swelling, tenderness, and erythema over mastoid bone	Mastoiditis
Nose	Red and swollen nasal mucosa, discharge	Rhinitis
	Tender sinuses/absence of glow upon transillumination	Sinusitis
Mouth	Labial sore/ulcer	Herpes simplex infection/exacerbation
	Labial chancre	Syphilis
	Oral thrush	*Candida*
	Oral ulcer	Infection (e.g., tuberculosis, histoplasmosis, herpes simplex)
		Behçet's disease
		Cancer
	Koplik's spots	Measles
	Mild redness and swelling of the pillars with lymphoid patches on the posterior pharynx	Viral pharyngitis
	Erythema, swelling of tonsils, pillars and uvula with white or yellow patches of exudate on the tonsils	Bacterial pharyngitis (streptococcal)
	Swollen uvula and pillars, dark gray exudate over tonsils, uvula, or soft palate	Diphtheria
	Uvula, displacement; red, tense, bulging tonsil/pillar	Tonsillar/peritonsillar abscess
Heart	Friction rub	Pericarditis (viral, bacterial, collagen-vascular disease)
	Murmur	Endocarditis

TABLE 21–2. Common Physical Findings *Continued*

Organ System	Finding	Likely Cause
Lungs	Localized crackles, increased bronchial sounds, dullness to percussion, increased tactile fremitus	Pneumonia

	Dullness to percussion, decreased breath sounds, decreased tactile fremitus	Effusion
		  Malignant
		  Rheumatoid arthritis
		  SLE
		  Pulmonary embolism

	Lack of cough with decreased breath sounds at the bases during postoperative period	Atelectasis
	Persistent single monophonic wheeze	Partial obstruction of bronchus by tumor

	Friction rub	Pleurisy
		  Malignant
		  Infectious (tuberculosis, viral)

	Resonant lungs, crackles with expiratory wheezes	Bronchitis
	Normal to hyperresonant lungs with decreased or absent breath sounds	Pneumothorax (spontaneous pneumothorax in HIV infection often caused by *Pneumocystis carinii*)
Back	Costovertebral angle tenderness	Pyelonephritis Trauma
	Spinal tenderness	Osteomyelitis Localized abscess
Abdomen	Splenomegaly	Malignancy (lymphoma, leukemia) Infection (EBV, CMV, intracellular bacteria, *Chlamydia pneumoniae*, *Mycoplasma*, *Legionella*, *Coxiella*)
	Hepatomegaly	Hepatitis Malignancy Sarcoidosis Hepatic abscess Schistosomiasis Bacterial, viral, fungal infections
	Ascites	Spontaneous bacterial peritonitis Tuberculosis
	Diffuse tenderness, involuntary rigidity of abdominal muscles, rebound, abdominal pain with cough or light percussion	Peritoneal inflammation
	Epigastric tenderness, rebound but soft abdominal wall	Pancreatitis
	Right upper quadrant tenderness	Localized abscess Hepatitis Cholecystitis/cholangitis
	Positive Murphy's sign	Cholecystitis/cholangitis
	Right lower quadrant tenderness/guarding, rebound, right rectal tenderness, positive psoas sign	Appendicitis
	Guarding, tenderness above the inguinal ligaments, tender uterus	Acute salpingitis Pelvic inflammatory disease
	Left lower quadrant tenderness	Diverticulitis Bowel infarction
	Enlarged palpable kidney	Hydronephrosis Cyst Tumor
	Suprapubic tenderness	Urinary tract infection
Genital/pelvic, and rectal	Ulcers	Herpes simplex Chancroid Syphilitic chancre Behçet's disease
	Cervical discharge	Sexually transmitted disease
	Painful adnexa	Pelvic inflammatory disease
	Tender prostate	Prostatitis
	Enlarged, nodular prostate	Cancer
	Tender perirectal area, fluctuance	Perirectal abscess
Extremities	Edema, erythema	Deep venous thrombosis Septic thrombophlebitis Skin and soft tissue infections
	Joint deformity	Arthritis
	Osler's nodes	Infectious endocarditis
	Janeway lesion	Infectious endocarditis
	Arthritis	Septic joint SLE Gonorrhea Rheumatic fever Gout
	Splinter hemorrhage	Infective endocarditis Trauma
	Ulcer	Tularemia Diabetic foot ulcer Osteomyelitis

evated white blood cell (WBC) count is often associated with serious bacterial infection. Leukemoid reactions—leukocyte counts ≥25–30,000/L—are often seen with infections such as tuberculosis, empyema, and abscesses as well as with leukemias and other malignancies. Leukopenia is frequently seen with viral diseases. The presence of atypical lymphocytes historically has been related to Epstein-Barr virus (EBV) or cytomegalovirus (CMV) mononucleosis, yet may occur with any viral infection. White blood cell counts <2500 in the acutely ill person with fever may be a harbinger of imminent death due to bacterial sepsis. Patients whose bone marrow has been suppressed by either chemotherapy or infection involving the marrow (such as HIV infection) and who present with absolute granulocyte counts ≤500 and fever are likely to have bacteremias or fungal infections. The peripheral blood smear can be helpful; the presence of toxic granulation is strongly associated with infection. The presence of Howell-Jolly bodies is a sign of asplenia. People without a spleen are predisposed to develop serious infections due to encapsulated organisms such as *Haemophilus influenzae, Streptococcus pneumoniae,* and *Neisseria meningitidis.* Malaria is diagnosed by seeing the parasites on the blood smear.

The hemoglobin and hematocrit are useful measurements. Low hematocrits are often seen in chronic diseases. Low platelet counts may be seen in patients with serious infections complicated by disseminated intravascular coagulation (DIC). Thrombocytopenia can be seen in people with alcoholism or may represent an adverse reaction to a medication. Thrombocytosis, on the other hand, is often observed with empyemas, abscesses, and malignancies.

Cultures and stains of body fluids may be diagnostic. Sputum culture with predominant growth of a particular or specific bacterium may indicate the real pathogen causing a pneumonia. A urine culture with significant bacteriuria (≥10^5 cfu/mL) is associated with urinary tract infection. The growth of organisms from presumably sterile sites such as ascitic fluid, cerebrospinal fluid (CSF), or pleural fluid is almost always diagnostic. Tissue biopsies may be helpful in determining the cause of fever. For example, bone cultures and histopathologic studies are necessary for the diagnosis of osteomyelitis. Any tissue that can be studied (skin, pleura, bone marrow, brain, etc.) ought to be obtained when the etiology is in doubt and the therapy is not trivial.

Blood chemistries are of assistance in assessing the general state of health of the patient and the status of organ function. Radiologic imaging often complements the physical examination and laboratory evaluation. The workup of a chronic febrile illness may at times require all the previously mentioned studies.

MANAGEMENT

The management of a febrile person consists of symptomatic, supportive, and definitive treatment of the cause of the fever using the most appropriate chemo-

therapeutic agents. Once definitive therapy is initiated, most patients diagnosed with an infectious disease exhibit a temperature drop within 24 to 96 hours.

Supportive measures, such as hydration, are necessary to compensate for the insensible losses of fluid. Although antipyretic agents are commonly used to treat febrile children, adults can tolerate fever better unless they have cardiovascular compromise and cannot withstand the usual increase in cardiac output that accompanies fever. If antipyresis is desired for the patient's comfort, it is helpful to know the cause of the fever or to have observed its pattern before these agents are used. The preferred antipyretic for children is acetaminophen. Salicylates should be avoided owing to the risk of Reye's syndrome. Adults can be treated with acetaminophen or NSAIDs such as aspirin or ibuprofen.

Research Questions

1. What is the role of fever in host defense?
2. What are the effects of the physiologic alterations secondary to fever on drug pharmacokinetics?

Case Resolution

This patient presented with a chronic febrile illness with associated systemic symptoms but few other clues to the diagnosis. The diagnosis of disseminated histoplasmosis with endocarditis was made by liver biopsy, biopsy of the oral ulcers, and discovery of *Histoplasma* antigen in the urine. A transesophageal echocardiogram demonstrated a large aortic valve vegetation, which also grew out *Histoplasma capsulatum* on culture of the surgically removed valve.

Selected Readings

Brush, J., and L. Weinstein. Fever of unknown origin. Med Clin North Am 75:1247–61, 1988.

Chang, J. Neoplastic fever: A proposal for diagnosis. Arch Intern Med 149:1728–30, 1989.

Clarke, D. E., J. Kimelman, and T. A. Raffen. The evaluation of fever in the intensive care unit. Chest 100: 213–20, 1991.

Heymann, W. R. Noninfectious causes of fever and a rash. Int J Dermatol 28(3):145–53, 1989.

Kluger, M. J. Fever: Role of pyrogens and cryogens. Physiol Rev 71:93–127, 1991.

Knockaert. D. C., L. J. Vanneste, and H. J. Boffaers. Recurrent or episodic fever of unknown origin: Review of 45 cases and survey of the literature. Medicine 72(3):184–95, 1993.

Knockaert, D. C., L. J. Vanneste, and S. B. Vanneste. Fever of unknown origin in the 1980s: An update of the diagnostic spectrum. Arch Intern Med 152:51–5, 1992.

MacKowiak, P. A. Influence of fever on pharmacokinetics. Rev Infect Dis 11(5):804–6, 1989.

Riedel, W. Mechanisms of fever. J Basic Clin Physiol Pharmacol 1(1-4):291–322, 1990.

Saper, C. B., and D. C. Breder. Endogenous pyrogens in the CNS: Role in the febrile response. Prog Brain Res 93(28):419–29, 1992.

INVOLUNTARY WEIGHT LOSS

Gregory G. Fotieo, M.D.

H_x A 50-year-old female accountant presents with a complaint of a 7-kg (15-lb) weight loss over the past 6 months. The weight loss has been unintentional and gradual. She has not been dieting and has had no significant increase in her activity level. She denies having had fever, chills, or night sweats but has been feeling quite fatigued over the past few months. She does not feel that her mood has changed. For the past 10 months, she has been experiencing hot flashes. Her menstrual periods have been irregular, and her last menstrual period was 3 months ago. Her past medical history is significant for two vaginal deliveries. Otherwise, she has not seen a physician for 20 years. She has a 30 pack-year history of cigarette smoking. She rarely drinks alcohol and denies illicit drug use. She has been married for 28 years but has been separated from her husband for the past 10 months and now lives alone. Her physical examination is unremarkable, although she refuses a pelvic examination. She weighs 63.5 kg (140 lb).

Questions

1. Is the weight loss clearly documented? How might you verify it?
2. What are possible causes of this patient's weight loss?
3. What further history would you like from the patient? What questions might you ask family and friends?
4. Would you order any diagnostic tests at this point?

Weight problems are frequently encountered in the ambulatory care setting. Although obesity is a significant health concern, it rarely has a clearly defined organic cause. Conversely, unintentional weight loss may be the presenting sign of numerous pathologic conditions.

PATHOPHYSIOLOGY

Adults maintain a stable body weight when caloric intake and caloric expenditure are matched. An alteration in either variable will result in a change in weight. Caloric intake is dependent on many factors. Availability of food, attractiveness of food, and the ability to digest and absorb food are all essential to maintain caloric intake. Intake of calories can be hampered for a variety of reasons. Some examples include ill-fitting dentures, medication-induced nausea, and intestinal malabsorption.

Caloric expenditure is the sum of the calories expended to maintain the basal metabolic rate and the calories spent to perform physical activity. Basal metabolic needs generally account for about half an individual's caloric expenditure. The amount of calories expended as a result of physical activity varies greatly between individuals. Many athletes expend well over 50% of their calories on physical activity, whereas sedentary individuals may use less than 40% for physical activity. The clearest example of a disease state that causes weight loss through increased metabolic rate and caloric expenditure is hyperthyroidism. Most diseases that cause weight loss do so through varying degrees of both impaired caloric intake and excessive caloric expenditure.

DIFFERENTIAL DIAGNOSIS

The complaint of unintentional weight loss is not uncommon in primary care clinical practice. Despite the frequency of this complaint, only a limited number of studies have addressed the prevalence of the various conditions that cause involuntary weight loss (Table 22–1).

The majority of these studies found that in patients with documented involuntary weight loss, the most frequent "diagnosis" was that the weight loss was **idiopathic**. The cause of weight loss remains undetermined in over 25% of cases despite exhaustive workups in either the inpatient or the outpatient setting. Fortunately, patients with idiopathic weight loss tend to have a significantly better outcome than those who are found to have a physical cause of weight loss.

When a cause of involuntary weight loss is uncovered, the three most common diagnoses are cancer, gastrointestinal (GI) disease, and psychiatric disorders. A variety of less common causes account for the remainder of cases.

TABLE 22–1. Causes of Involuntary Weight Loss

Common Causes
Idiopathic
Malignancy (lung, lymphoma, GI tract)
Gastrointestinal disease (peptic ulcer disease, malabsorption, dysmotility)
Psychiatric disorders (depression, anxiety)

Less Common Causes
Cardiovascular disease (congestive heart failure)
Pulmonary disease (chronic obstructive lung disease)
Endocrine (hyperthyroidism, poorly controlled diabetes mellitus)
Infection (tuberculosis, lung abscess)
Medication-induced (levothyroxine, theophylline, procainamide)
Substance abuse
Inflammatory diseases (rheumatoid arthritis, sarcoidosis)
Neurologic (cerebrovascular events, Alzheimer's disease)

The most worrisome concern in the patient with unintentional weight loss is that the weight loss is secondary to malignancy. Although **cancer** is found in 20%–36% of patients with involuntary weight loss, the degree of weight loss usually does not become significant until late in the disease process. In most cases, the diagnosis of neoplasm can be made through the history, physical examination, and a few selected laboratory tests. It is uncommon for cancer to be diagnosed in a patient with weight loss who has no other localizing signs or symptoms related to the malignancy.

The relationship between cancer and weight loss is well established and is frequently referred to as "cancer cachexia." The reason for the weight loss is poorly understood but is believed to be multifactorial. Patients with malignancy can experience anorexia secondary to taste derangements, nausea, or various humoral anorectic factors released by the malignant cells. In addition to reduced intake, cancer patients often have abnormalities of energy metabolism: studies have demonstrated increased energy expenditures to meet the increased basal metabolic rate. Inefficient energy utilization has also been demonstrated in cancer patients. Both these factors contribute to increased caloric expenditure that, coupled with decreased nutritional intake, results in weight loss.

Gastrointestinal diseases are responsible for 11%–17% of cases of involuntary weight loss. The most common disorders include malabsorption, peptic ulcer disease, esophageal motility disorders, cholelithiasis, and inflammatory bowel disease.

Psychiatric diagnoses are occasionally associated with weight loss. The most common is depression, in which the mechanism of weight loss is usually decreased food intake. The outcome for patients with weight loss from a psychiatric cause is better than for those with a physical cause of weight loss. Weight gain usually follows treatment of the underlying psychiatric disorder.

Less common causes of involuntary weight loss are also listed in Table 22–1. Since HIV infection has become more prevalent, HIV-associated wasting and weight loss should be considered in the differential diagnosis of unintentional weight loss, particularly in patients with HIV risk factors.

EVALUATION

History

A complete history, with special attention to the questions listed in Box 22–1, is essential in the evaluation of the patient with weight loss.

Before embarking on an exhaustive workup to evaluate weight loss, the loss must be confirmed. One study group found that half the patients considered for enrollment did not actually have weight loss that could be reasonably documented. The best way to confirm weight loss is through serial weight measurements over time. Unfortunately, prior weights may not have been recorded. Other means to confirm weight loss are to seek evidence of change in clothing size, to corroborate

---

BOX 22–1. Questions to Ask Patients with Involuntary Weight Loss

1. How much weight have you lost and over what period of time?
2. Can the weight loss be verified?
3. Has there been a decrease in caloric intake? If yes, why?

   Nausea?
   Poor dentition or oral pain?
   Dysphagia or odynophagia?

4. Are there any associated symptoms?

   Change in bowel habits, melena, hematochezia?
   Fever, chills, or night sweats?
   Shortness of breath, paroxysmal nocturnal dyspnea, or orthopnea?
   Depressed mood, sleep disturbances, tearfulness?
   Heat intolerance, palpitations, anxiety?

5. Do you smoke? If so, has a new cough developed, or has there been a change in the usual cough? Hemoptysis?
6. Do you take any medications (particularly thyroid replacement, theophylline, digoxin, antiarrhythmics)?

---

weight loss with friends or family, or to assess the ability of the patient to give a numerical estimate of the amount of weight lost.

A dietary history also is essential. For example, a patient with weight loss despite an increase in dietary intake would be suspected of having hyperthyroidism. If there has been a decrease in intake, then the patient should be asked why he or she is eating less. The reason can help focus the workup. For instance, if the patient has anorexia secondary to nausea, the differential diagnosis might include gastritis, medication-induced nausea, or gastric dysmotility.

The use of prescription and over-the-counter medications should be assessed, since many drugs can result in weight loss via several mechanisms. An attempt should be made to identify patients who abuse alcohol or other substances because these patients frequently are malnourished. A smoking history is important, since smokers are at risk for a variety of diseases and malignancies, particularly lung cancer.

A thorough social history may uncover social or psychological factors that can cause weight loss. These factors include poverty, social isolation, lack of transportation, immobility, functional disabilities, and bereavement.

Physical Examination

Weight loss is a systemic complaint. For this reason, the examination needs to be very thorough to assess all organ systems.

The evaluation should begin with an assessment of the general appearance of the patient. Evidence of wasting, poorly fitting clothes, and signs of hyperthyroidism should be sought. The head and neck examination should include a search for oral lesions, assessment of dentition, thyroid palpation, and evaluation for adenopathy. The cardiovascular and pulmonary examinations should focus on evidence of congestive heart failure, obstructive pulmonary disease, or localized wheezes (which may suggest airway obstruction due to an endobronchial tumor). The abdomen should be palpated for masses, organomegaly, or tenderness. A rectal examination should be done in all patients and is particularly important in older men, who have a high incidence of prostate cancer. In women, a breast examination, pelvic examination, and Pap test need to be performed.

Additional Evaluation

If no explanation for the involuntary weight loss is apparent on the history and physical examination, a screening set of laboratory tests is appropriate. A reasonable screen would include a CBC, chemistry profile (including liver function tests), urinalysis, and test of the stool for occult blood. One study conducted at a Veterans Administration (VA) hospital found that a chest x-ray was a high-yield test; however, this finding may be particular to the VA hospital patient population with its high rate of lung disease and lung cancer. Certainly, a chest radiograph should be performed in all long-term smokers with unexplained weight loss.

Other diagnostic tests should be performed only if indicated based on the history and physical examination. Upper and lower GI endoscopy, barium enema, upper GI series, and thyroid function tests are high-yield, cost-effective tests when performed in selected patients. Screening CT scans, on the other hand, are of limited diagnostic value. A "shotgun" approach to ordering diagnostic tests is costly and of little diagnostic use. In a patient with weight loss that cannot be explained after the history, physical examination, and appropriate laboratory and radiographic studies are performed, a period of watchful waiting is appropriate. The patient should be reevaluated at frequent intervals and monitored for further weight change.

MANAGEMENT

The treatment plan for patients with involuntary weight loss depends on the underlying disease. Certain diseases respond well to treatment, while others are characterized by progressive weight loss regardless of therapeutic intervention.

When weight loss is secondary to depression, patients tend to gain weight as their psychiatric disorder is treated. If the primary care physician is managing the care of a depressed patient with anorexia and weight loss, fluoxetine and the other serotoninergic agents should be used with caution because of their potential anorectic side effect. In such individuals, a tricyclic antidepressant may be more appropriate. Weight loss associated with hyperthyroidism also responds well to treatment of the underlying disorder.

The cancer patient with weight loss poses a particularly difficult management problem. It has been clearly established that in the cancer patient both morbidity and mortality increase if the individual is malnourished. Protein malnutrition results in diminished cellular and humoral immunity. In addition, patients undergoing oncologic surgery or chemotherapy fare better if they are not malnourished. There is no evidence that improved nutrition promotes tumor growth.

Both the enteral and parenteral routes are efficacious in supplying the nutritional needs of the patient with cancer. While the parenteral route may provide more rapid repletion, the enteral route is preferred if the GI tract is functioning normally, since nutrition via this route is more physiologic, less expensive, and has fewer complications. The approach to the malnourished cancer patient should begin with a precise evaluation of the patient's nutritional status. Detailed nutritional counseling should be implemented to improve oral caloric intake. The normal diet often needs to be supplemented with high-protein, high-calorie preparations to maintain an adequate nutritional state.

Individuals with severe anorexia or upper GI tract neoplasms may require enteral tube feeding if they are unable to take in adequate calories via the oral route. Nasogastric or nasoduodenal feeding tubes can be used in these cases effectively and with minimal complications. If long-term (>6 weeks) enteral feeding is required, a gastrostomy or jejunostomy tube should be considered. Gastrostomy tubes can be placed endoscopically using mild sedation and a local anesthetic.

If a patient cannot be nutritionally supported by the enteral route, parenteral nutrition may be indicated (particularly if the tumor is considered to be potentially responsive to therapy). The parenteral route usually requires central venous access to deliver the hypertonic solution necessary to provide adequate calories and amino acids.

PATIENT AND FAMILY EDUCATION

Patients with involuntary weight loss and their families need to have a clear understanding of the disease process responsible for the weight loss. Both patient and family need to meet with a nutritionist to assess the patient's nutritional requirements and establish an appropriate dietary plan to meet those requirements. They also need to understand the prognosis and treatment plan for the underlying disease.

NATURAL HISTORY/PROGNOSIS

Involuntary weight loss often is a symptom of an underlying disease process, and it is this disease process which determines the outcome in a particular patient. The prognosis is most favorable for psychiatric disorders, endocrinologic disorders, GI diseases, and idiopathic weight loss. Cancer has the worst prognosis.

Research Questions

1. How should a weight loss evaluation differ between a 20-year-old and a 70-year-old?
2. How much weight loss should be considered significant and over what period of time?
3. What are the various mechanisms by which medications can cause weight loss?

Case Resolution

At the next visit, the patient agreed to a pelvic examination, which was normal. On further discussion, she revealed a sense of loneliness and isolation, along with anhedonia and early-morning awakening. She was started on nortriptyline for depression, and her weight loss resolved.

Selected Readings

Fischer, J., and M. A. Johnson. Low body weight and weight loss in the aged. J Am Diet Assoc 90:1697–1706, 1990.

Holdcraft, C. Evaluating involuntary weight loss in older adults. Nurse Pract 13(3):9–15, 1988.

Marton, K. I., H. C. Sox, Jr., and J. R. Krupp. Involuntary weight loss: Diagnostic and prognostic significance. Ann Intern Med 95:568–74, 1981.

Rabinowitz, M., S. D. Pitlik, M. Leifer, et al. Unintentional weight loss: A retrospective analysis of 154 cases. Arch Intern Med 146:186–7, 1986.

Thompson, M. P., and L. K. Morris. Unexplained weight loss in the ambulatory elderly. J Am Geriatr Soc 39:497–500, 1991.

COMMON EYE, EAR, NOSE, AND THROAT PROBLEMS

CHAPTER 23

THE RED EYE

Denise A. Farnath, M.D.

H$_x$ A 32-year-old female employment counselor was poked in the left eye by her 2-year-old daughter this morning. She complains of blurred vision, redness, tearing, pain, photophobia, and a foreign body sensation. There is no history of ocular disease or prior injury, and she is not presently using any ocular medication.

Questions

1. What diagnoses come to mind?
2. What information in the history provides clues to the diagnosis?
3. What further information is needed?
4. What would you look for during the examination to make the diagnosis?

Primary care physicians frequently encounter patients with a red eye. Although there are many possible etiologies, it is fairly easy to narrow the differential diagnosis by performing a focused history and ocular examination. Several causes of red eyes can be managed in the primary care setting. Most important is to know how urgent a particular condition is and when referral to an ophthalmologist is indicated.

PATHOPHYSIOLOGY

A red eye occurs when there is injury to or inflammation of the anterior aspect of the globe or orbit (Table 23–1). The inflammation may be localized to the eyelid, orbit, conjunctiva, sclera, cornea, or anterior chamber and iris (Fig. 23–1).

DIFFERENTIAL DIAGNOSIS

The conjunctiva is the thin, transparent mucous membrane that lines the posterior surface of the lids (the palpebral conjunctiva) and the anterior surface of the sclera (the bulbar conjunctiva). **Conjunctivitis** is inflammation of the conjunctiva with resultant vascular dilatation, cellular infiltration, and exudation (Fig. 23–2).

A **subconjunctival hemorrhage** occurs when a conjunctival blood vessel ruptures, causing a sudden bright red eye (Fig. 23–3). The appearance is striking and often alarms the patient. There usually are no associated symptoms such as blurred vision or discomfort. Examination with a penlight reveals a deep red hemorrhage under the conjunctiva that may be severe enough to cause elevation of the conjunctiva.

A **corneal abrasion** is an area where the corneal epithelium has been removed (Fig. 23–4). The epithelium forms the anterior surface of the cornea and serves as a barrier to infection of the underlying stroma. Corneal abrasions most commonly occur as a result of minor

---

TABLE 23–1. Causes of Red Eye

Common Causes

Eyelid problems (stye, chalazion, cellulitis, blepharitis)
Conjunctivitis (infectious, allergic, toxic)
Pterygium
Subconjunctival hemorrhage
Corneal abrasion
Corneal foreign body
Iritis
Chemical injury

Less Common Causes

Corneal ulcer
Keratoconjunctivitis sicca
Herpes simplex or herpes zoster ophthalmicus
Contact lens overwear
Corneal exposure
Corneal dystrophy
Hyphema
Endophthalmitis
Lacerated or ruptured globe
Orbital inflammatory disease
Carotid cavernous fistula
Acute angle closure glaucoma

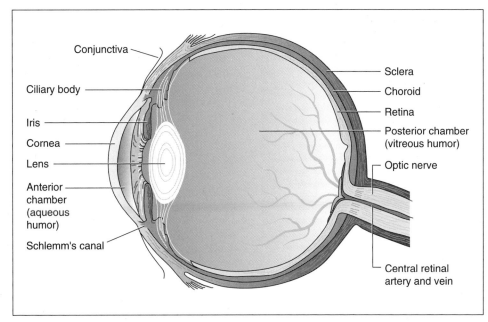

FIGURE 23-1. *Anatomy of the eye.*

trauma, such as being poked in the eye or getting a foreign body in the eye.

Iritis or anterior uveitis is inflammation of the iris or anterior uveal tract. It is usually unilateral and often occurs spontaneously, although it may occur a few days after blunt traumatic injury. The differential diagnosis for iritis is a long one and includes infectious, autoimmune, and posttraumatic etiologies.

Patients with **chemical injuries** typically call or come in stating that they splashed or sprayed something in their eye.

EVALUATION

History

The duration and severity of symptoms should be elicited. It is also important to ask about a history of trauma or recent contact with others who had "red eyes." Trauma is often associated with subconjunctival hemorrhage, corneal abrasion, or after a few days, iritis. A patient who says he or she "has something in the eye" is likely to have a corneal foreign body, corneal abrasion, or chemical injury.

A history of previous ocular problems or a family history of ocular disease should be sought. Iritis and herpes simplex keratitis may be recurrent. Less common corneal dystrophies may be hereditary.

The symptoms of **conjunctivitis** are irritation and a mucoid or mucopurulent discharge. Often, the eyelids are "stuck together" in the morning upon awakening as a result of the discharge. There may be a burning sensation, tearing, and occasionally a foreign body sensation, but true pain, which implies corneal involve-

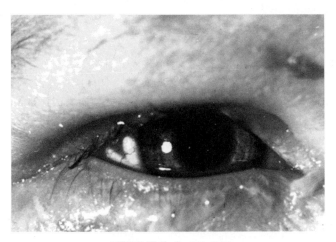

FIGURE 23-2. *Conjunctivitis.*

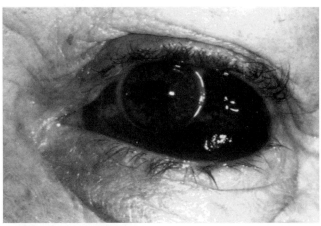

FIGURE 23-3. *Subconjunctival hemorrhage. Hemorrhages are often less extensive than this one, which extends 360 degrees. (Courtesy of M. L. Schluter, M.D.)*

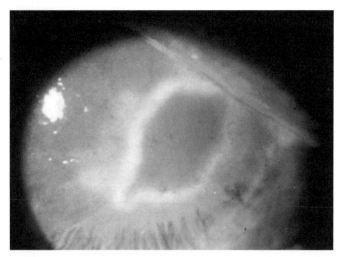

FIGURE 23–4. *Corneal abrasion. This is the appearance of an abrasion when viewed with a cobalt blue light after fluorescein staining. (Courtesy of M. L. Schluter, M.D.)*

ment, is uncommon. Frequently, there is a history of recent exposure to others with "pink eye," since viral conjunctivitis is highly contagious.

Subconjunctival hemorrhages are often associated with a Valsalva maneuver such as coughing or sneezing, or they may be spontaneous. Other associated disorders include hypertension and blood dyscrasias.

The patient with a **corneal abrasion** generally gives a history of minor trauma such as being poked in the eye or getting a foreign body in the eye; typical symptoms include pain, photophobia, a foreign body sensation, and tearing. There may be blurred vision if the abrasion involves the central cornea.

Patients with **iritis** typically complain of blurred vision, pain, photophobia, and tearing.

Physical Examination

The physical examination is needed to make a definitive diagnosis. Much of the examination can be done without specialized equipment. Visual acuity must be checked in every patient with an ocular complaint. Attention should be initially directed to the eyelids and external eye. Proptosis, injection, erythema, and abnormal extraocular movements should be noted.

The nature of conjunctival injection can indicate the source of inflammation. Is the conjunctival injection diffuse, concentrated at the limbus, or localized? Conjunctivitis generally results in diffuse injection, whereas corneal disorders and iritis lead to perilimbal injection.

The cornea must be examined with fluorescein staining using a cobalt blue light or Wood's lamp. Finally, the cornea and anterior chamber should be examined with a slit lamp for evidence of infection or inflammation.

Funduscopy is an important part of any ophthalmic examination; however, most causes of red eyes are evident upon examination of the anterior segment.

Evaluation of the typical patient with **viral conjunctivitis** can be performed without a slit lamp. In most cases of conjunctivitis, vision will be unaffected or mildly decreased. The signs of conjunctivitis are diffuse conjunctival injection, discharge, and preauricular lymphadenopathy (in viral conjunctivitis). Diffuse conjunctival injection refers to hyperemia that involves the palpebral and bulbar conjunctiva equally. It is helpful to rule out a corneal abrasion by instilling fluorescein dye in the eye and checking for fluorescence with a cobalt blue light or Wood's lamp. If this examination is negative and the signs and symptoms are classic for conjunctivitis, the diagnosis can be made.

The diagnosis of a **corneal abrasion** is made by placing fluorescein dye in the eye and looking for an area of fluorescence with a cobalt blue light or Wood's lamp. The corneal stroma takes up the dye and fluoresces, whereas intact epithelium does not. A slit lamp is not generally needed to visualize moderate to large abrasions. Redness of the eye will be evident and will be most intense at the limbus. The pupil is often more miotic on the affected side. Topical anesthetics such as proparacaine typically relieve the symptoms dramatically but should be used only for diagnostic purposes. The patient should never be given a supply of proparacaine, because it is toxic to the epithelium.

Examination of a patient with **iritis** reveals a mild to severe decrease in visual acuity, a miotic pupil, and ciliary injection (redness concentrated at the limbus). These symptoms and signs are nearly identical to those associated with corneal abrasion. The important difference is the absence of corneal staining with fluorescein. The diagnosis of iritis is made with a slit lamp by visualizing white blood cells floating in the anterior chamber.

Additional Evaluation

The workup for a **subconjunctival hemorrhage** consists of only a blood pressure check. Recurrent subconjunctival hemorrhages require further investigation to rule out an underlying blood dyscrasia.

Workup for **iritis** includes a full, dilated examination by an ophthalmologist to rule out posterior segment involvement.

MANAGEMENT

Conjunctivitis may be infectious, allergic, or toxic. Viral conjunctivitis is most common, is extremely contagious, and typically has a 2-week course. Most forms of viral conjunctivitis are self-limited. Less common forms, however, can have severe permanent sequelae. Since many forms of viral conjunctivitis are highly contagious, it is important to minimize contact with others during the first week and to keep the hands washed and away from the eyes as much as possible.

Bacterial conjunctivitis is associated with a more purulent discharge and usually resolves quickly with topical antibiotics (e.g., erythromycin). For this reason, many ophthalmologists prescribe topical antibiotics for all conjunctivitis patients, recognizing that conjunctival cultures are often unhelpful and that a certain percentage of cases will be treated unnecessarily with this approach.

Allergic conjunctivitis is usually associated with itching, and there is often a history of seasonal allergies. Management includes topical antihistamines and cold compresses. More severe cases may require topical cromolyn if available, but topical corticosteroid use is probably best left to the ophthalmologist.

The inflammation of toxic conjunctivitis is due to a chemical irritant such as soap, hair spray, makeup, smog, or eye drops. Treatment requires identification and removal of the irritant.

There is no treatment for a **subconjunctival hemorrhage** other than to reassure the patient that the blood will resolve within 2 weeks.

The treatment of a **corneal abrasion** is straightforward. First, it is important to rule out the presence of a corneal foreign body or a corneal infection. A corneal infection has a white appearance on penlight examination, whereas a simple abrasion appears clear. A simple abrasion is treated with a cycloplegic agent, topical antibiotic, and pressure patch. A cycloplegic agent, such as cyclopentolate 1%, dilates the pupil and relieves ciliary muscle spasm causing pain. A topical antibiotic such as erythromycin ointment prevents infection, and a pressure patch speeds healing. The patient is reexamined daily until the abrasion has resolved. If at any time there is evidence of infection, immediate referral to an ophthalmologist is indicated. A moderate abrasion should heal completely in 1–3 days.

Treatment of **iritis** consists of topical corticosteroids and dilating drops to prevent scarring, and is probably best left to an ophthalmologist. Long-term topical steroid use may lead to cataracts or glaucoma.

A **chemical injury** is a true ophthalmic emergency, and immediate irrigation is essential. If the patient calls in, have the patient irrigate the eye before leaving for the emergency room. In the emergency room, a quick pH check is helpful, followed by immediate irrigation with sterile isotonic saline. Topical anesthetic drops will facilitate irrigation. Several liters per eye is required if the pH is abnormal. The fornices should be swept with a cotton swab and the lid flipped to check for particles. The pH should be neutral 30 minutes after discontinuing irrigation to ensure that there is no retained particulate matter. After lavage, examination for corneal staining or haziness can be carried out. Alkali is much more damaging to the eye than acid because it penetrates tissue more readily. Acids form a barrier of precipitated tissue that tends to limit further damage.

Mild chemical injuries resulting in small corneal epithelial defects should be treated as corneal abrasions. If corneal clouding or conjunctival blanching is noted, immediate referral to an ophthalmologist is indicated once the pH has been neutralized. Severe acid or alkali burns can lead to permanent visual loss or loss of the eye.

PATIENT EDUCATION

It is extremely important to ensure that contact lenses are fitted properly by an ophthalmologist or optom-etrist. Lenses should not be overworn or placed in the mouth. Regular cleaning and disinfection with the appropriate solutions will minimize the risk of infection. Overwear and inadequate care of lenses can result in bacterial or amebic keratitis. Patients who wear contact lenses must be evaluated promptly for pain or redness.

NATURAL HISTORY/PROGNOSIS

Conjunctivitis is generally self-limited and will run its course in 1–2 weeks.

Corneal abrasions heal quickly if treated appropriately. There may be a mild permanent stromal scar if the abrasion has violated the epithelial basement membrane (Bowman's membrane). Unless the scar lies in the visual axis, there are no visual sequelae. The primary risk associated with a corneal abrasion is infection (bacterial keratitis). This can result in permanently decreased vision or loss of the eye.

There are no visual sequelae of a **subconjunctival hemorrhage**. The discoloration resolves within 2 weeks.

Iritis may be a benign, self-limited disease, as in posttraumatic anterior uveitis, or it may lead to severe recurrent episodes of inflammation with permanent visual loss.

Severe acid or alkali **burns** can lead to permanent visual loss or loss of the eye.

Research Questions

1. How can patients be more effectively persuaded to wear protective goggles to prevent sports- and work-related injuries?
2. How can we determine the etiology of iritis in a greater percentage of cases?
3. How can recurrent corneal erosions be prevented?

Case Resolution

The patient's history and presentation are typical of a corneal abrasion. A fluorescein dye examination (using cobalt blue light) demonstrated loss of epithelial cells, and the patient was treated with an eye patch, an antibiotic ophthalmic ointment, and a cycloplegic agent. She was carefully followed in the outpatient clinic, and the corneal abrasion resolved entirely in 2 days' time.

Selected Readings

Arffa, R. C. Conjunctivitis I and II. *In* R. C. Arffa (ed.). *Grayson's Diseases of the Cornea,* 3rd ed. St. Louis, Mosby–Year Book, 1991.

Howes, D. S. The red eye. Emerg Med Clin North Am 6:43–56, 1988.

Larrison, W. I., P. S. Hersh, T. Kunzweiler, et al. Sports-related ocular trauma. Ophthalmology 97:1265–9, 1990.

Lubeck, D., and J. S. Greene. Corneal injuries. Emerg Med Clin North Am 6:73–94, 1988.

McCully, T. P. Chemical injuries. *In* G. Smolin and R. A. Thoft (eds.). *The Cornea: Scientific Foundations and Clinical Practice,* 2nd ed. Boston, Little, Brown, 1987.

O'Connor, G. R. Factors related to the initiation and recurrence of uveitis. Am J Ophthalmol 96:577–99, 1983.

Shingleton, B. J. Eye injuries. N Engl J Med 325:408–13, 1991.

Silverman, H., L. Nunez, and D. B. Feller. Treatment of common eye emergencies. Am Fam Physician 45:2279–87, 1992.

Wagoner, M. D., and K. R. Kenyon. Chemical injuries of the eye. *In* B. J. Shingleton, P. S. Hersh, and K. R. Kenyon (eds.). *Eye Trauma.* St. Louis, Mosby, 1991.

Yanofsky, N. N. The acute painful eye. Emerg Med Clin North Am 6:21–42, 1988.

CHAPTER 24

COMMON DISORDERS OF VISION

Denise A. Farnath, M.D.

H$_x$ A 62-year-old male broadcast technician with diabetes complains of decreasing vision in his right eye. He states that objects appear blurred and that his vision has been declining over the past 4 months. He last saw an ophthalmologist 1 year ago who told him he had mild background diabetic retinopathy that did not require laser treatment. His glucose levels have been well controlled, running between 100 and 130 during the past 6 months. There is no history of cataracts, glaucoma, or macular degeneration. On ocular examination, the visual acuity is 20/60 in the right eye and 20/20 in the left eye. Funduscopic examination reveals multiple scattered dot and blot hemorrhages as well as several hard exudates in the macula of the right eye.

Questions

1. What diagnostic possibilities are you considering?
2. What additional questions would be important to ask?
3. What other tests may be helpful?
4. Is the serum glucose level relevant? Why or why not?

Patients frequently consult their primary care physician when they notice a change in vision. Although the differential diagnosis of blurred vision is extremely long, a few conditions occur commonly and should be familiar to the general practitioner. It is also important to be able to distinguish between emergent and routine visual disorders. A directed history and physical examination usually provide the necessary information.

PATHOPHYSIOLOGY

In order for a person to see, a clear image must be projected onto the retina. Light rays must pass through the cornea, aqueous humor, lens, and vitreous humor on their way to the retina. Thus, all these structures must be transparent to provide a clear retinal image. In addition, the retina and optic nerve must be healthy in order to transmit an accurate image to the visual cortex in the occipital lobe. When the eye sees an object in the distance, essentially parallel rays of light enter the cornea. In an eye with no refractive error, the light rays are bent by the cornea and lens to converge in the retina. The macula of the retina is responsible for central visual acuity and therefore is the most important portion of the retina. This is the region of the retina that is used for reading and distinguishing detail. When the light rays do not come to a point on the retina, the patient perceives a blurred image. If the light rays converge in front of the retina, the patient is said to be nearsighted, or myopic. Conversely, if the light rays converge posterior to the retina, the patient is farsighted, or hyperopic. If the light rays focus to two lines rather than a single point, the patient has astigmatism. Patients with refractive errors will experience blurred vision unless corrective lenses are used to bring light rays to a single point on the retina.

DIFFERENTIAL DIAGNOSIS

In addition to refractive error, decreased vision can be caused by any opacity within the cornea, aqueous, lens, or vitreous. It can also be caused by abnormalities of the retina, optic nerve, visual pathways in the brain or visual cortex. The list of possible etiologies is extensive; the most common are listed in Table 24–1.

Refractive Errors

Approximately 45% of the population has a refractive error, many of which are not corrected or are incompletely corrected. This is by far the most common cause of visual disorders. Interestingly, a person who has good vision in one eye may not be aware of having

TABLE 24–1. Common Causes of Decreased Vision

	Improves with Pinhole	Red Eye	Pain	Sudden Onset	Requires Urgent Treatment
Refractive error	+	−	−	−	−
Amblyopia	−	−	−	−	−
Keratitis (corneal inflammation, edema or scarring)	may	+	+	+	+
Iritis	+	+	+	+	+
Hyphema	may	+	+	+	+
Cataract	may	−	−	−	−
Uncontrolled serum glucose	+	−	−	+	−
Vitritis	may	may	may	+	+
Vitreous hemorrhage	−	−	−	+	+
Retinitis	−	−	−	+	+
Diabetic retinopathy	−	−	−	−	usually not
Macular de-generation	−	−	−	usually not	usually not
Glaucoma	−	−	may	−	−
Optic neuritis/ neuropathy*	−	−	−	may	+
Stroke	−	−	−	+	+
Head trauma	−	−	−	+	+

*Disorders of the optic nerve may lead to visual field defects with or without decreased central vision.

poor vision in the other eye. If something happens to the "good eye," such as trauma or inflammation, the person may suddenly realize that the vision is blurred in the other eye.

Large, uncorrected refractive errors or media opacities in childhood may lead to a lazy eye, or amblyopia. Amblyopia typically affects one eye only. If a child reaches the age of 8 or 9 years without treatment for amblyopia, the visual loss is generally permanent. For this reason, it is important to screen visual acuity in children.

Disorders Unrelated to Refractive Error

Broad categories of visual disorders unrelated to refractive error that are encountered frequently in primary care are cataracts, diabetic retinopathy, macular degeneration, and glaucoma.

A **cataract** is defined as any opacity of the natural lens of the eye (Fig. 24-1). It may involve a small part of the lens or the entire lens. The degree of opacification is also variable. Mild opacities occurring in the periphery of the lens may not affect vision at all. Most commonly, cataracts occur as a result of the natural aging process, although the precise pathophysiology has not been determined. Although not everyone develops cataracts, some degree of lens opacity is expected over age 70. This type of cataract is usually bilateral but not necessarily symmetrical.

Traumatic cataracts, congenital cataracts, and cataracts secondary to medication use (including chronic corticosteroid use) are less common and are often unilateral.

Glaucoma is a condition in which the intraocular pressure is elevated enough to cause damage to the optic nerve. Loss of central vision occurs very late in the disease. Early on, peripheral visual field defects occur and often go unnoticed by the patient. Because glaucoma is asymptomatic until late in its course, it is advisable to screen all people over age 40.

The prevalence of glaucoma over the age of 40 years is approximately 0.7%, and it is three times more prevalent in blacks than in whites. Glaucoma is usually bilateral and probably multifactorially inherited. The vast majority of glaucoma patients have open angle glaucoma. Acute angle closure glaucoma constitutes less than 5% of all cases. A third type, congenital glaucoma, is usually autosomal recessive.

Diabetic retinopathy is the leading cause of blindness in the United States in people aged 20–60 years. The frequency of diabetic retinopathy increases with the duration of the disease. It is a progressive microangiopathy characterized by small vessel damage and occlusion. The earliest changes are thickening of the capillary endothelial basement membrane and a loss of pericytes. Background diabetic retinopathy reflects the incompetence of the vascular walls. Microaneurysms form as well as retinal hemorrhages. Leaking capillaries cause edema of the retina and a decrease in central vision if the macula is involved. In areas where the fluid is resorbed, a lipid precipitate called hard exudate is left behind (Figure 24–2).

With progressive microvascular occlusion, retinal ischemia develops, causing cotton wool spots and possible macular ischemia. Finally, ischemia may stimulate the growth of new blood vessels, or neovascularization. This is called proliferative diabetic retinopathy and often leads to vitreous hemorrhage or retinal detachment (due to traction) if untreated.

Age-related **macular degeneration** is the leading cause of blindness in the United States in people over age 60. It is characterized by slowly progressive atrophy

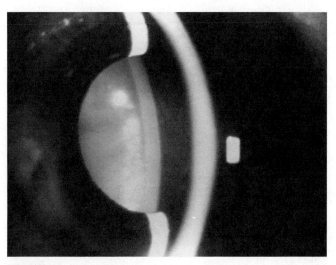

FIGURE 24–1. *Cataract. The cloudy lens is visible posterior to the iris in this slit lamp photograph.*

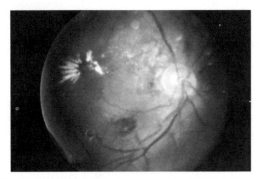

FIGURE 24–2. *Background diabetic retinopathy with clinically significant macular edema. Light-colored hard exudate is clearly evident in a "star" pattern around the fovea. Intraretinal dot and blot hemorrhages are also present.*

and degeneration of the outer retina (Fig. 24–3). This condition is termed "dry" macular degeneration. Occasionally, new blood vessels develop under the retina in the macula, causing a sudden distortion or loss of central vision. This condition is known as "wet" age-related macular degeneration.

The cause of macular degeneration is not known, but risk factors include age, race (usually white), and family history.

EVALUATION

History

The history is extremely important when patients complain of visual changes. Although the history alone may not lead to the definitive diagnosis, it allows the physician to determine whether the condition is emergent or routine.

Perhaps the most important question is whether the visual loss was acute or occurred gradually over a period of weeks or months. The severity of the visual loss is also important. Acute severe visual loss often heralds a serious condition and should be evaluated immediately. Vitreous hemorrhage, retinal detachment, and vascular occlusion generally present as a sudden severe loss of vision. A gradual progressive change is more likely with changing refractive error, cataract, glaucoma, diabetic retinopathy, and macular degeneration.

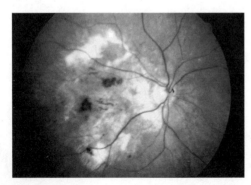

FIGURE 24–3. *Advanced, age-related macular degeneration. A large area of chorioretinal atrophy involves the entire macula. Areas of hypopigmentation are visible as well as "clumps" of pigment.*

The patient should be asked about a history of recent trauma. Corneal abrasion, hyphema, and ruptured globe should be considered in such instances. Past ocular history is helpful. A history of diabetes, iritis, or recent ocular surgery may suggest the most likely diagnosis. Diabetic retinopathy can lead to acute or slowly progressive visual loss. Acute monocular visual loss with sudden floaters in a diabetic suggests a vitreous hemorrhage. In contrast, a person with diabetes whose glucose is poorly controlled usually experiences painless blurred vision in both eyes. Iritis is associated with pain, photophobia, and red eye and may be recurrent. Recent ocular surgery may result in iritis but can also be complicated by a ruptured wound, an infection, or acutely elevated intraocular pressure.

Other symptoms that should be addressed specifically include pain, redness, flashing lights, and floaters. Refractive error, cataracts, diabetic retinopathy, macular degeneration, and vascular occlusion generally do not cause pain. Retinal detachment also is not painful and is often associated with flashing lights and floaters as well as a visual field defect. Pain and redness suggest corneal problems, intraocular inflammation, or blood in the anterior chamber. Acute angle closure glaucoma is extremely painful because the rise in intraocular pressure is rapid and causes corneal edema.

Physical Examination

The ophthalmic examination will provide the definitive diagnosis, and at times, referral to an ophthalmologist is necessary. However, a primary care physician familiar with the slit lamp examination and direct ophthalmoscopy can often make the diagnosis.

All patients with visual disturbance must have their visual acuity documented. Patients should wear their distance prescription (eyeglasses or contact lenses) if available. If the vision is less than 20/20, it should be checked with a pinhole. Improvement in vision with a pinhole implies an uncorrected refractive error. Patients with a central corneal abrasion or iritis may also experience an improvement in vision with a pinhole.

The external examination includes evaluation of the lids, conjunctiva, pupils, and extraocular movements. An unreactive pupil is present in acute angle closure glaucoma, and a Marcus Gunn pupil (afferent pupillary defect) implies damage to the optic nerve. Conjunctival injection is noted with corneal problems, trauma, iritis, hyphema, and acute angle closure glaucoma.

The slit lamp examination is used to evaluate the cornea, anterior chamber, lens, and intraocular pressure (IOP). Alternatively, a Schiotz tonometer or tonopen can be used to measure pressure. Acute angle closure glaucoma is characterized by a markedly elevated IOP. A corneal abrasion involving the visual axis will stain brightly with fluorescein when viewed with a Wood's lamp or cobalt blue light. A corneal ulcer also stains with fluorescein but appears white when viewed with a white light. The diagnosis of iritis is made by viewing white blood cells floating in the aqueous humor. A hyphema will be seen as blood layered out in the anterior chamber. Cataracts may appear as a white lens opacity, a yellow or yellow-brown discoloration of the lens, or a plaque on the posterior surface of the lens.

A funduscopic examination using the direct ophthalmoscope should be undertaken. Attention should be directed to the optic disk, blood vessels, and macula. On occasion, indirect ophthalmoscopy by an ophthalmologist may be required to view the peripheral retina. A normal funduscopic examination would be expected if the visual disturbance were due to cataract or a refractive error. If the cataract is dense, it may be difficult to obtain a clear view of the retina. Patients with glaucoma have increased cupping of the optic disk. A normal cup-to-disk ratio is 0.5 or less, meaning that the cup should be one half the size of the disk or less. Any patient with increased cupping should be referred for a nonemergent ophthalmic evaluation. Diabetic retinopathy is characterized by retinal hemorrhages, hard exudate, cotton wool spots, or neovascularization. Vitreous hemorrhage may be noted in diabetics with sudden visual loss. Typically, the fundus is difficult or impossible to view in the presence of a vitreous hemorrhage.

Clumps of pigment irregularly interspersed with depigmented areas of atrophy in the macula are typical of macular degeneration. Early in the disease, yellowish round spots (drusen) may be the only noticeable macular change.

Additional Evaluation

Frequently, the history and ocular examination are all that are required to make a diagnosis. Additional tests are indicated for specific disorders, however.

In a patient who is suspected of having a refractive error, a nonemergent refraction by an ophthalmologist or optometrist is indicated to confirm the diagnosis. Before referring a diabetic patient for refraction, be sure the serum glucose has been relatively well controlled for at least 2 weeks. Patients with suspected glaucoma also require visual field testing, which is generally ordered by an ophthalmologist. Patients with suspected optic nerve disease or neurologic disorders often require visual field testing. A confrontational visual field is a useful preliminary test in these situations. Optic nerve disorders often result in diminished color vision, which is easily tested with Ishihara's color plates. Patients who present with proptosis, orbital inflammation, or trauma often require an orbital CT scan. It is important to obtain coronal views if an orbital fracture is suspected. Finally, certain cases of diabetic retinopathy and macular degeneration require fluorescein angiography; this determination should be made by an ophthalmologist.

MANAGEMENT

In many cases, treatment is left to the ophthalmologist. Any sudden marked decline in vision should be evaluated immediately and the patient referred if a diagnosis cannot be made. Visual loss that has occurred gradually over a period of several weeks or months is less likely to be emergent but should be evaluated in a timely manner. Patients who complain of seeing flashing lights should be evaluated immediately for retinal tear or detachment. Likewise, patients who have visual loss associated with recent ocular surgery or trauma must be evaluated promptly.

Patients with refractive errors are referred nonemergently for refraction and a prescription for eyeglasses. Patients with cataracts also require a nonemergent referral for evaluation and possible surgery.

Open angle glaucoma is generally not urgent unless the intraocular pressure is above 30. Treatment is initiated by an ophthalmologist and consists of topical pressure-lowering agents, oral carbonic anhydrase inhibitors, laser therapy, or surgery if the condition is not adequately controlled. Acute angle closure glaucoma is an ocular emergency, and treatment should be started in the emergency room once the diagnosis has been made.

All patients with diabetes should be referred to an ophthalmologist yearly for a dilated funduscopic examination. Diabetics with sudden visual loss must be evaluated immediately, whereas those with gradual visual loss should be seen in a timely but nonemergent fashion. Uncontrolled serum glucose must be corrected. Treatment for diabetic retinopathy consists of laser therapy, surgery, or both.

Most cases of macular degeneration result in a gradually progressive deterioration of central vision that is generally not treatable. Oral vitamins have not been proved to improve the course of the disease. Low vision aids are helpful for those with poor visual acuity. Sudden visual loss or distortion of vision in a patient with macular degeneration requires emergent referral for evaluation of a subretinal neovascular membrane (wet macular degeneration). If the membrane is treatable by laser, it must be done immediately to prevent severe permanent loss of central vision.

PATIENT AND FAMILY EDUCATION

Patients should be encouraged to seek evaluation immediately for any sudden decrease in vision. Glaucoma patients should generally be seen by an ophthalmologist several times per year. Patients with macular degeneration should be encouraged to monitor their vision daily with an Amsler grid and are generally evaluated at least twice yearly. Diabetics should have a dilated funduscopic examination at least yearly.

Research Questions

1. How can we better educate patients about visual disorders and the importance of ophthalmic screening over the age of 40?

2. What other factors (e.g., renal failure, smoking, diet) contribute to the progression of diabetic retinopathy?

3. What is the mechanism by which elevated intraocular pressure damages the optic nerve?

Case Resolution

The history, gradual onset of symptoms, and well-controlled glucose all suggest worsening of this patient's background diabetic retinopathy. His examination is typical of diabetic macular edema. He underwent focal argon laser treatment of the right eye, which successfully decreased leakage of fluid and plasma constituents from macular microaneurysms. His vision remained stable at 20/60.

Selected Readings

Ferns, F. L., and A. Patz. Macular edema: A complication of diabetic retinopathy. Surv Ophthalmol 28:452–61, 1984.

Gottlieb, L. K., B. Schwartz, and S. G. Parker. Glaucoma screening: A cost-effective analysis. Surv Ophthalmol 28:206–26, 1983.

Jaritt, J. C., J. K. Canner, F. G. Frank, et al. Detecting and treating retinopathy in patients with type I diabetes mellitus. Ophthalmology 97:483–95, 1990.

Klein, B. E., and R. Klein. Cataracts and macular degeneration in older Americans. Arch Ophthalmol 100:571–3, 1982.

Klein, R, and B. E. K. Klein. Vision disorders in diabetes. *In* National Diabetes Data Group. *Diabetes in America: Diabetes Data Compiled, 1984.* Bethesda, Maryland, U. S. Department of Health and Human Services, 1985, Chapter XIII.

Levi, L., and B. Schwartz. Glaucoma screening in the health care setting. Surv Ophthalmol 28:64–174, 1983.

Marshall, G. S. K. Garg, W. E. Jackson, et al. Factors influencing the onset and progression of diabetic retinopathy in subjects with insulin-dependent diabetes mellitus. Ophthalmology 100:1133–9, 1993.

Nelson, W. L., F. T. Fraunfelder, J. M. Sills, et al. Adverse respiratory and cardiovascular events attributed to timolol ophthalmic solution, 1978-1985. Am J Ophthalmol 102:606–11, 1986.

Singer, D. E., D. M. Nathan, H. A. Fogel, et al. Screening for diabetic retinopathy. Ann Intern Med 116:660–71, 1992.

Vaughan, D., T. Asbury, and P. Riordan-Eva (eds.). *General Ophthalmology,* 13th ed. Norwalk, Connecticut, Appleton & Lange, 1992.

CHAPTER 25

EAR PAIN

Fred S. Herzon, M.D.

Hx A 48-year-old male music video producer presents with a 2-week history of left ear pain. The pain is worse at night but does not keep him awake. He denies any recent hearing loss but feels his hearing is "not what it used to be." He denies dizziness, ear drainage, head trauma, drug use, or loud noise exposure. He is an admitted "workaholic," has a 30 pack-year history of cigarette smoking, and describes himself as a "social drinker." The physical examination reveals tympanic membranes that are scarred bilaterally. A 3-mm dry perforation of the left tympanic membrane is noted. The Weber test is midline, and the noise from a 512-Hz tuning fork is heard better by air conduction than bone conduction in both ears. The rest of the physical examination is normal.

Questions

1. Should any additional noise exposure questions be pursued? If so, why?
2. What conditions, other than primary ear disease, may cause otalgia?
3. What additional testing would you recommend?

Ear pain (otalgia), either acute or chronic, is a common presenting symptom in patients of all ages. Although the source of the pain can frequently be found within the middle or external ear, it is not unusual for it to originate elsewhere in the head and neck, especially in adults.

PATHOPHYSIOLOGY

Primary otalgia can result from inflammation of the middle ear, tympanic membrane, or external canal. These structures are innervated by the fifth, seventh, ninth, and tenth cranial nerves. Acute bacterial infection of the middle ear space is the most common cause of ear pain. Acute or chronic loss of normal middle ear aeration caused by eustachian (auditory) tube dysfunction is another frequent cause of ear pain, especially in infants and young children. Abnormal middle ear pressure in adults is usually secondary to barotrauma from flying or scuba diving misadventures. Inflammation of the external canal from any cause is extremely uncomfortable, since the lack of subcutaneous tissue between the skin and the underlying periosteum does not allow room for swelling. The pinna itself may be the site of painful inflammatory, traumatic, or neoplastic conditions.

Secondary otalgia is most commonly associated with temporomandibular joint (TMJ) disorders. Ear pain also may be the first sign of either acute inflammatory or neoplastic disease of the mouth or pharynx. In these cases, pain is referred to the ear via the auriculotem-

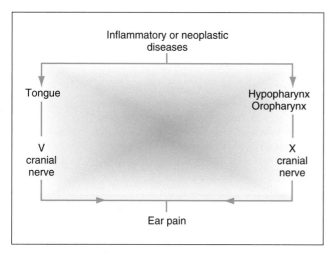

FIGURE 25–1. *Referred ear pain.*

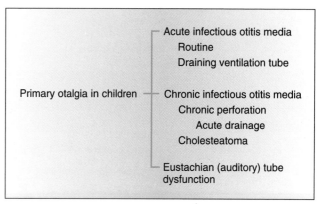

FIGURE 25–3. *Differential diagnosis of primary otalgia in children.*

poral branch of the fifth cranial nerve or by a small branch of the tenth cranial nerve that innervates a portion of the external canal (Fig. 25–1).

DIFFERENTIAL DIAGNOSIS

Primary Otalgia

Inflammation of the external ear, tympanic membrane, or middle ear is the most frequent source of primary ear pain. In adults, external otitis is probably as common a cause of primary otalgia as is acute infectious otitis media. In children, however, middle ear disease (including effusion) accounts for most ear pain.

Middle ear effusion in children is usually due to acute inflammation or eustachian tube dysfunction and is rarely a sign of serious disease. Unilateral middle ear effusion in an adult or teenager, however, requires a thorough evaluation of the nasopharynx for possible neoplasia. Pressure-induced middle ear pathology secondary to inadequate pressurization of the middle ear space during flying or diving is common (Figs. 25–2 and 25–3).

A draining ear often accompanies primary otalgia and may be a sign of acute or chronic infection of either the external or the middle ear (Fig. 25–4).

Secondary Otalgia

Secondary otalgia is a symptom predominantly found in adults. Diseases of the temporomandibular joint, mouth, and naso-, oro-, and hypopharynx often present initially with otalgia. If ear pain continues for several weeks and remains unexplained after a screening otologic evaluation, a complete head and neck examination is required. The most common cause of secondary otalgia in adults is temporomandibular joint syndrome

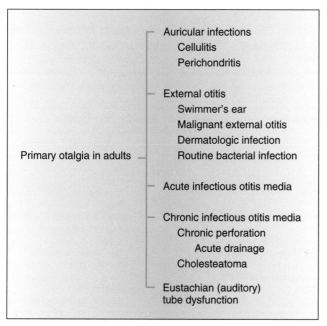

FIGURE 25–2. *Differential diagnosis of primary otalgia in adults.*

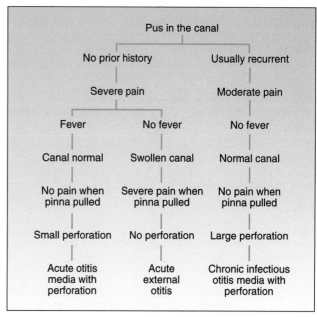

FIGURE 25–4. *The draining ear.*

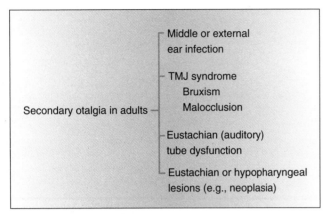

FIGURE 25–5. *Differential diagnosis of secondary otalgia in adults.*

secondary to either malocclusion or nightly grinding of the teeth (bruxism) (Fig. 25–5).

EVALUATION

History

Initial questioning should attempt to differentiate between primary and secondary otalgia. Questions should be asked about ear function, including hearing and balance. If there is no problem with hearing or balance (and no report of drainage from the ear), it is unlikely that the otologic apparatus is the disease site. Additional inquiry should be made about dysphagia, hoarseness, pain while chewing or swallowing, and the patient's smoking and drinking habits. Information related to the duration and intensity of the pain as well as the patient's occupation and recreational habits also should be explored.

Physical Examination

Attention should first be directed to examining the otologic apparatus, beginning with the **auricle** and **external canal**. Direct inspection of the auricle may reveal signs of inflammation and swelling (e.g., auricular cellulitis or perichondritis). If severe pain is elicited when a normal-appearing auricle is tugged, an acute infection of the external canal is the most likely diagnosis. Inspection of the **tympanic membrane** with a hand-held otoscope should be carried out as well as "palpation" of the tympanic membrane using a pneumatic attachment. Screening **hearing tests** using a 512-Hz tuning fork—including the Weber test (stimulating in the midline and then noting whether the sound lateralizes) and the Rinne test (comparing bone conduction with the normally louder air conduction)—may reveal additional information about the status of the middle ear space and cochlea.

If the physical examination of the ear is normal, attention should be directed to possible causes of secondary otalgia, beginning with the temporomandibular joint. Palpation while the jaw is in motion, first in front of the ear and then with a finger in the external canal, will often elicit pain when there is a TMJ abnormality. A complete oral examination should then be performed to look for tumor or infection of the tongue or floor of the mouth. If no source of otalgia is found, referral for a complete hypopharyngeal inspection is indicated (i.e., an examination with a mirror or flexible fiberoptic endoscope by a qualified otolaryngologist).

Additional Evaluation

Perhaps the only test that a primary care physician might consider requesting for evaluation of **primary otalgia** is a complete audiogram (including tympanometry). This test provides an objective evaluation of the middle ear space including hearing acuity. The workup of **secondary otalgia** may sometimes include extensive radiologic evaluation of the temporomandibular joint and oral and hypopharyngeal structures; consultation with an otolaryngologist is usually advisable to help guide the evaluation process.

MANAGEMENT

Tables 25–1, 25–2, and 25–3, respectively, outline the management of primary otalgia in adults and children and the management of secondary otalgia in adults.

TABLE 25–1.   Management of Primary Otalgia in Adults

Diagnosis	Medical Treatment	Surgical Treatment
Auricular cellulitis	Oral antbiotics	None
Auricular perichondritis	Oral antibiotics, intravenous cephalosporins (2nd or 3rd generation)	None
External otitis—routine ("swimmer's ear")	Antibiotic ear drops, pain medication*	Ear wick
External otitis—dermatologic	Corticosteroid drops or cream	None
External otitis—malignant	Anti-*Pseudomonas* intravenous antibiotics	May need surgical debridement
Acute infectious otitis media	Oral amoxicillin, pain medication	Rare myringotomy
Chronic infectious otitis media—perforation	Antibiotic ear drops,† systemic antibiotics may be of help†	Tympanoplasty
Chronic infectious otitis media—cholesteatoma	Antibiotic ear drops,† systemic antibiotics may be of help†	Tympanomastoidectomy
Auditory tube—primary dysfunction	None	Ventilating tube
Auditory tube—allergy	Nasal steroids,† oral antihistamines,† desensitization†	None
Auditory tube—barotrauma	Nasal steroids,† oral decongestants†	Myringotomy
Auditory tube—neoplastic disease	None	Specific treatment of neoplasia

*Narcotic-level analgesia is frequently necessary for patient comfort.
†Treatment recommendations have limited prospective studies proving their effectiveness.

TABLE 25–2.   Management of Primary Otalgia in Children

Diagnosis	Medical Treatment	Surgical Treatment
Acute infectious otitis media—routine	Oral antibiotics	Rare myringotomy for pain relief or diagnosis
Acute infectious otitis media—draining pressure-equalization tube	Oral antibiotics*, ear drops*	Remove pressure-equalization tube
Persistent middle ear effusion—after infection	Oral antibiotic for 2–4 weeks	Myringotomy and tubes if no resolution, adenoidectomy if >3 years
Persistent middle ear effusion—chronic auditory tube dysfunction	None that is effective	Myringotomy and tubes, adenoidectomy if >3 years
Persistent middle ear effusion—allergic	Antihistamines,* decongestants,* nasal corticosteroids,* desensitization*	Myringotomy and tubes if no resolution
Chronic infectious otitis media—perforation	Antibiotic ear drops*	Tympanoplasty
Chronic infectious otitis media—cholesteatoma	Antibiotic ear drops,* oral antibiotics*	Tympanomastoidectomy
Auditory tube—primary dysfunction	Normal growth and development	Adenoidectomy and ventilating tubes
Auditory tube—barotrauma	Nasal steroids,* oral decongestants*	Myringotomy

*Treatment recommendations have limited prospective studies proving their effectiveness.

Secondary Otalgia in Children

Except for pharyngitis, children are rarely subject to the same oral or hypopharyngeal pathology that can lead to secondary otalgia in adults. A child with severe tonsillitis or pharyngitis may complain of referred ear pain secondary to oropharyngeal inflammation. Such referred pain is also common after tonsillectomy.

Draining Ear

The draining ear requires a specific (and accurate) diagnosis for proper therapeutic intervention. Once external otitis has been ruled out, the diagnostic approach illustrated in Figure 25–4 should be utilized. If acute infectious otitis media is diagnosed, an appropriate systemic antibiotic covering *Streptococcus pneumoniae, Haemophilus influenzae,* and *Moraxella catarrhalis* should be prescribed. If, however, there is drainage from the middle ear space through a tympanic membrane perforation and no accompanying fever or malaise, local treatment with antibacterial ear drops (e.g., Cortisporin) is appropriate. The use of systemic antibiotics in this situation is controversial.

PATIENT AND FAMILY EDUCATION

Patients and adult care givers should be counseled not to ignore a draining ear. This finding frequently occurs in isolation (unaccompanied by pain or fever) and therefore is sometimes disregarded by the patient or parent. A draining ear should always be evaluated by a physician.

NATURAL HISTORY/PROGNOSIS

Acute Inflammation

Most acute inflammatory disorders causing otalgia are self-limited. However, the use of antimicrobial therapy helps prevent such infrequent—but potentially devastating—complications such as mastoiditis.

Chronic Inflammation

The goal of treating an acute infectious or inflammatory condition is to prevent the development of a chronic inflammatory process, which is often destructive and sometimes irreversible. Chronic infectious otitis media with perforation cannot be reversed by medical therapy and thus often requires a surgical procedure (tympanoplasty) to restore normal function. Left untreated, chronic infectious otitis media may develop into a cholesteatoma (squamous epithelial invasion of the middle ear or mastoid space), which can destroy ossicles and erode bone to the point of endangering the central nervous system.

Research Questions

1. Are there any interventions that can prevent the occurrence of TMJ syndrome?
2. Can any medical therapy be developed that will be effective in managing chronic eustachian tube dysfunction?

TABLE 25–3.   Management of Secondary Otalgia in Adults

Diagnosis	Medical Treatment	Surgical Treatment
Temporomandibular joint syndrome—malocclusion	Soft diet, NSAID	Orthodontia may help; surgery on joint is difficult
Temporomandibular joint syndrome—bruxism	Soft diet, NSAID	Bite blocks
Oropharyngeal lesions	Rarely primary treatment	Specific surgery or radiation therapy

Case Resolution

The patient's perforation of the left tympanic membrane was "dry" with no evidence of infection. He had no tenderness of the temporomandibular joint. He was given ibuprofen for pain, and a return visit was scheduled for 3 weeks. At the time of the return visit, however, there was no improvement in the patient's symptoms and the physical examination was unchanged. The patient was referred to an otolaryngologist. Indirect mirror examination revealed a small ulcerated lesion on the left side of the epiglottis, which on biopsy proved to be squamous cell carcinoma.

Selected Readings

Klein, J. O., D. V. Teele, and B. Rosner. Epidemiology of acute otitis media in Boston children from birth to seven years of age. *In* G. Mogi et al. (eds.). *Recent Advances in Otitis Media.* New York, Kugler, 1994.

Kraus, D. H., and S. E. Kinney. Necrotizing external otitis. *In* G. Gates (ed.). *Current Therapy in Otolaryngology—Head and Neck Surgery,* 4th ed. St. Louis, Mosby–Year Book, 1993.

Mandel, E. M., H. E. Rockette, C. D. Bluestone, et al. Efficacy of amoxicillin in effusion. N Engl J Med 316:432, 1987.

Pelton, S. E., and J. O. Klein. The draining ear: Otitis media and externa. Infect Dis Clin North Am 2(1):117, 1988.

Senturia, B. H., M. D. Marcus, and F. E. Lecente. *Disease of the External Ear.* New York, Grune & Stratton, 1980.

CHAPTER 26

HEARING LOSS AND TINNITUS

Fred S. Herzon, M.D.

H_x A 54-year-old female dental hygienist has noted the gradual onset of decreased hearing bilaterally as well as noise in her right ear. These problems have been occurring for several months and have recently gotten worse. She has no pain, discharge, dizziness, or history of significant head trauma. Her ears feel "stuffed." She is healthy and takes no medication. Her mother developed hearing loss in her forties, but the rest of the medical history is unremarkable. Both tympanic membranes appear normal on physical examination of the ears; however, they do not move normally on pneumatic otoscopy. The rest of the head and neck examination is normal. On the Weber test, sound is heard in the midline, and sound from a 512-Hz tuning fork is transmitted better by bone conduction than by air conduction in both ears.

Questions

1. What additional information should be obtained about her mother's hearing loss?
2. Would any other historical information be useful?

Hearing loss is one of the most commonly occurring physical disabilities in the United States. More than 25 million people have hearing loss serious enough to interfere with communication. Hearing loss is described as **conductive** (a defect in the tympanic membrane or middle ear structures) or **sensorineural** (a defect in the peripheral or central neural pathways). A combination **(mixed)** of these two categories sometimes is found in the same patient (Fig. 26–1). Tinnitus may accompany hearing loss and is especially common with a sensorineural deficit.

PATHOPHYSIOLOGY

Sound is conducted through the external canal, tympanic membrane, and ossicular chain to the inner ear (cochlea). Any abnormality that interferes with sound transmission may result in **conductive** hearing loss. Such abnormalities can range from simple occlusion of the external ear with cerumen (earwax) to a rare congenital fixation of the stapes. Any of the basic pathologic processes—traumatic, mechanical, inflammatory, autoimmune, metabolic, or neoplastic—can interfere with the normal conduction of sound to the inner ear.

Acute infectious otitis media is the most common entity causing transient conductive hearing loss in children (see Chapter 120). Untreated or severe infections may progress to a chronic state, resulting in

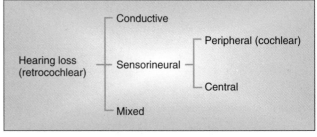

FIGURE 26–1. *Hearing loss.*

damage to the tympanic membrane (e.g., perforation) or middle ear structures (e.g., ossicular fixation or necrosis), thereby causing secondary conductive hearing loss.

Sensorineural hearing loss occurs when there is damage to the peripheral neural end organ (cochlea), eighth nerve, or brain. The more proximal the abnormality is to the central nervous system, the greater its effect on function. A lesion affecting the eighth nerve, for example, usually interferes with hearing to a greater degree than does a lesion in the cochlea. Cochlear pathology is the most common cause of sensorineural hearing loss. Age-related hearing loss (presbycusis) accounts for most cases. The exact pathophysiology is uncertain, but histopathologic studies of the temporal bone reveal deterioration of the neural elements found in the cochlea.

Prelingual hearing loss refers to an auditory deficit identified prior to the development of oral speech. Such hearing loss can be identified within days of birth.

Tinnitus has subjective and objective forms. Subjectively perceived noise can be associated with any type of hearing loss but is most frequently associated with a sensorineural problem. Objective tinnitus is almost always vascular in nature.

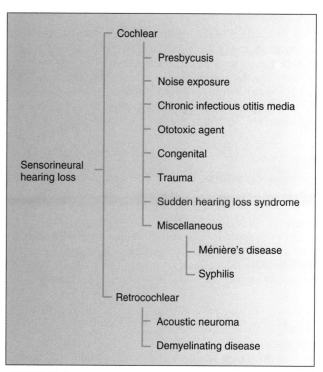

FIGURE 26–3. *Differential diagnosis of sensorineural hearing loss.*

DIFFERENTIAL DIAGNOSIS

The initial determination to make when a patient complains of hearing loss is whether a true auditory deficit is present. The answer is not always clear cut, especially in children. Once it is established that a hearing loss exists, the next step is to distinguish between a **conductive** and **sensorineural** deficit. If **sensorineural** impairment is diagnosed, an attempt should be made to establish whether the site of pathology is cochlear or more proximal (retrocochlear). Establishing the exact type of **conductive** hearing loss is even more critical because these deficits are more likely to be reversible. It should also be recognized that hearing loss can be **mixed,** with elements of both conductive and sensorineural dysfunction.

The following are the most common entities encountered in clinical practice (Figs. 26–2 and 26–3).

Conductive Hearing Loss
External Canal

Cerumen impaction is the most common reversible cause of mild conductive hearing loss in adults. Simple inspection of the external canal will confirm the diagnosis.

Otitis externa is characterized by a swollen, narrowed external canal, often with whitish debris. Pain is a prominent feature and is typically increased by applying traction to the pinna. Otitis externa is frequently associated with swimming and is commonly referred to by patients as "swimmer's ear."

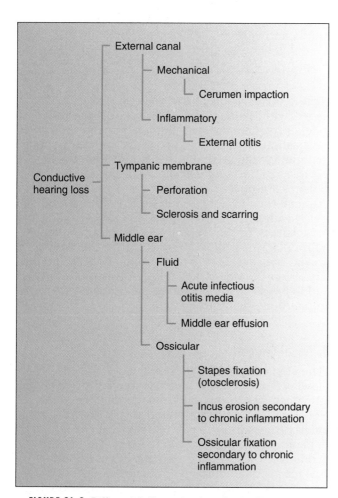

FIGURE 26–2. *Differential diagnosis of conductive hearing loss.*

Tympanic Membrane

Abnormalities of the eardrum are diagnosed by direct observation using an otoscope. In the case of a large **perforation,** confusion may result because of the absence of easily identifiable landmarks. This condition is often misdiagnosed as a "thickened tympanic membrane." Severe **sclerosis or scarring** of the drum also may interfere with hearing.

Middle Ear

A **fluid** collection behind the tympanic membrane may be either acute (e.g., infection, barotrauma) or chronic (e.g., eustachian [auditory] tube dysfunction, low-grade infection, allergy).

The **ossicles** may become fixed (e.g., otosclerosis, chronic inflammation, congenital abnormality) or discontinuous (e.g., trauma, acute or chronic inflammation, cholesteatoma).

Sensorineural Hearing Loss

Most cases (90%) of sensorineural hearing loss are due to pathology within the cochlea. Making a specific diagnosis is usually more helpful in establishing the prognosis than in reversing the dysfunction.

Cochlear

With advancing age, a gradual decrease in cochlear function occurs in many people **(presbycusis),** making this the most common cause of sensorineural hearing loss in the United States.

A history of significant exposure to either chronic or acute **noise** is valuable in making this diagnosis. Does the patient report a history of working in a noisy environment? Military veterans frequently have significant hearing loss secondary to weapons-fire exposure. Loud noise exposure during recreation or hobbies can also take its toll; the extraordinarily high volume of today's popular music may leave a legacy of premature sensorineural hearing loss in a generation of young people.

Chronic infectious otitis media is more commonly associated with a conductive hearing loss, but if perforation occurs, a sensorineural component also may develop.

Ototoxic pharmacologic agents can lead to significant hearing loss. Such medications include aminoglycosides, loop diuretics (e.g., furosemide), and cisplatin.

Several conditions (e.g., trisomy defects and maternal rubella) may result in **congenital** deafness.

Head **trauma** is a common cause of acquired sensorineural hearing loss in both children and adults.

Sudden hearing loss syndrome is defined as the sudden (developing within 24 hours) onset of a sensorineural hearing loss. The incidence in the general population is approximately 10/100,000. Etiologic theories range from viral infections to autoimmune disease.

Commonly thought of, but less often diagnosed, is **endolymphatic hydrops (Ménière's disease).** The classic triad of symptoms consists of vertigo, tinnitus, and hearing loss.

Sexually transmitted diseases (e.g., syphilis and AIDS) may be accompanied by sensorineural hearing loss.

Retrocochlear

Acoustic neuroma, an uncommon benign tumor of the eighth nerve, most often presents as *unilateral* hearing loss.

Demyelinating diseases such as **multiple sclerosis** are relatively uncommon causes of sensorineural hearing loss.

EVALUATION

History

Certain historical features are helpful in distinguishing between conductive and sensorineural hearing loss. Children more often have conductive losses, while older adults are more likely to present with a sensorineural problem. The difficulty associated with conductive pathology is primarily volume (i.e., sound intensity) related, whereas sensorineural hearing loss usually presents with deficits in both volume and understanding.

If the patient has a history of prior or ongoing ear infections, a conductive deficit should be suspected. It is also important to ask about a history of noise exposure, ototoxic drug exposure, head trauma, kidney disease, HIV risk factors, and a family history of hearing loss. Inquiry should be made about symptoms such as tinnitus and vertigo.

Physical Examination

Direct observation of the ear can easily be accomplished with a hand-held otoscope. Newer fiberoptic models provide increased illumination and thus better visualization. Pneumatic "palpation" of the tympanic membrane (using a rubber bulb attached to the head of the otoscope) is a skill that should be mastered by every primary care physician.

Tuning fork evaluation of hearing should be performed with a 512-Hz (or higher) frequency tuning fork. The accuracy of the Weber lateralization test depends on firm placement of the tuning fork on the skull of the patient. The same is true when comparing air and bone conduction (Rinne test). It takes at least a 20- to 30-db conductive loss for sound to be transmitted better through bone than through air.

Additional Evaluation

The standard audiometric evaluation consists of the following tests: (1) bone and air thresholds (which help distinguish sensorineural from conductive loss), (2) discrimination (understanding words), and (3) tympanometry (measuring pressure-induced movement of the tympanic membrane and middle ear). Except for tympanometry, these tests are **subjective** in nature but allow for adequate hearing evaluation in all but a small percentage of patients. In the case of acoustic neuroma, audiometric evaluation characteristically shows a hearing loss that interferes with the patient's understanding to a greater degree than would a cochlear abnormality.

The brain stem auditory evoked response (BAER) test has made it possible to **objectively** evaluate hearing in children under 6 months of age. Even neonates can be successfully screened and diagnosed with this methodology. *No child is too young to have a suspected hearing loss evaluated!* This test can also be used in adults to localize the site of a central nervous system audiologic defect.

A CT scan of the temporal bone is helpful in diagnosing cholesteatomas, congenital syndromes, and acoustic neuromas. If a CT scan is equivocal, an MRI study should be performed.

MANAGEMENT

Medical Therapy for Conductive Hearing Loss

Any acute or chronic infection causing a conductive hearing loss should be treated according to the guidelines set forth in Chapter 25. Chronic middle ear effusion that does not respond to antibiotic management may resolve with vigorous antiallergy therapy (e.g., antihistamines, decongestants).

Surgical Therapy for Conductive Hearing Loss

Any mechanical defect of the tympanic membrane or middle ear is potentially reversible with an appropriate reconstructive procedure.

Hearing deficits secondary to a persistent middle ear fluid collection are easily reversed with short-term (i.e., over months) aeration of the middle ear with ventilating tubes. These procedures are especially helpful in children.

Medical Therapy for Sensorineural Hearing Loss

In general, there are no effective treatments for the disorders that cause sensorineural hearing loss.

The sudden hearing loss syndrome may respond to a course of high-dose corticosteroids tapered over 7–10 days.

Surgical Therapy for Sensorineural Hearing Loss

A cochlear implant is a computerized device that can be implanted in the temporal bone and cochlea to provide limited hearing to patients with profound sensorineural hearing loss. This treatment is restricted to individuals with severe hearing loss refractory to the use of hearing aids. Cochlear implantation is controversial within the deaf community, where some assert that deaf children who receive a cochlear implant may not easily assimilate into hearing society.

Rehabilitation

Hearing aids can correct most conductive losses when medical or surgical therapy fails to improve hearing. They can also provide help for (although not "cure") many sensorineural disorders.

Schools and rehabilitation resources are available for children with severe hearing impairment. Controversy exists, however, within both the health care community and the deaf community as to what constitutes appropriate rehabilitation.

Major medical centers are already engaged in screening high-risk neonates. Intervention in the form of hearing aids and rehabilitative programs is more effective when initiated earlier rather than later.

Tinnitus

Tinnitus often is difficult to treat, although some management strategies have proved beneficial for individual patients. At the present time, **biofeedback** is the most widely available treatment modality. Selected patients may subjectively improve by using **tinnitus maskers,** which provide a competing (and more tolerable) noise.

PATIENT AND FAMILY EDUCATION

Acute or chronic exposure to intense noise can lead to sensorineural hearing loss. It is important to use hearing protection when firing a weapon (e.g., while hunting or target shooting) or when attending rock concerts.

Many older people have a sensorineural hearing loss that can interfere with their ability to communicate. This may lead to social isolation and even depression. Families need to be aware that a parent or grandparent who is hard of hearing should be evaluated for aural rehabilitation.

NATURAL HISTORY/PROGNOSIS

Conductive Hearing Loss

The wide array of available medical, surgical, and rehabilitative interventions has resulted in an excellent prognosis for the majority of patients with conductive hearing loss.

Sensorineural Hearing Loss

Most sensorineural hearing loss problems cannot be cured or even significantly improved with medical therapy. Rehabilitation of the hearing handicap is, at best, moderately successful.

Tinnitus

Despite extensive research in this area, most patients with chronic tinnitus continue to have persistent symptoms with only slim chance of "cure." The resolution of tinnitus is usually directly related to correction of the hearing loss, which rarely occurs in sensorineural dysfunction.

Case Resolution

A hearing evaluation revealed a bilateral 40-db conductive hearing loss. The presumptive diagnosis was otosclerosis. The patient was offered the choice of a hearing aid or surgical reconstruction. Surgery corrected the hearing loss in one ear, and the other ear will be reevaluated for reconstructive surgery in a year's time if the hearing improvement in the first ear remains stable.

Selected Readings

Goodhill, V. *Ear Diseases, Deafness, and Dizziness.* Hagerstown, Maryland, Harper & Row, 1979.

Northern, J. L. *Hearing Disorders.* Boston/Toronto, Little, Brown and Company, 1984.

Northern, J. L., and M. P. Downs. *Hearing in Children.* Baltimore, Maryland, Williams & Wilkins, 1991.

Wilson, R. W., F. M. Byl, and N. Laird. The efficacy of steroids in the treatment of idiopathic sudden hearing loss. Arch Otolaryngol 106:772–6, 1980.

CHAPTER 27

RHINORRHEA AND NASAL STUFFINESS

Fred S. Herzon, M.D.

Hx   A 56-year-old male systems analyst presents complaining of a 2-year history of periodic nasal stuffiness, postnasal drip, and "sinusitis." The symptoms seem to be worse in the spring. Periodically he has noted bilateral maxillary pain associated with greenish nasal discharge. He has no other major medical problems and denies smoking. Over-the-counter "allergy remedies" occasionally ameliorate his symptoms. Examination of the nose reveals a mild deviation of the septum to the right and bilateral nasal congestion with glistening, large inferior turbinates. No polyps are seen. The remainder of the head and neck examination is unremarkable.

Questions

1. Is the smoking history described above adequate?
2. What environmental factors should you ask about?
3. What further diagnostic testing, if any, is needed?

Rhinorrhea and nasal stuffiness are symptoms that virtually every adult experiences on a recurring basis. Many patients will seek medical attention for the complaint of "sinusitis," a term often used to describe any acute or chronic problem involving rhinorrhea, stuffy nose, or facial pain. Physicians seeing these patients should recognize that the complaint of "sinusitis" does not necessarily mean that the patient has sinusitis in any of its standard pathophysiologic forms (i.e., infectious, allergic, or neoplastic). Frequently, in fact, the disorder is confined to the nose without *any* involvement of the paranasal sinuses.

PATHOPHYSIOLOGY

The nose serves several functions including olfaction, respiration, protection, and humidification. The protective and humidification functions are mediated through a dynamic mucous blanket that is replaced approximately every 10 minutes. Up to 1 L of water is added to inspired air every 24 hours. Any inflammatory or mechanical process interfering with normal nasal function can result in increased or altered secretions. This change in secretions, whether an increase in volume or a thickening of viscosity, is readily and negatively perceived by the individual. Alteration of the nasal secretions may be secondary to mechanical or biochemical (e.g., histamine) stimulation of the mucus-secreting glands. In addition, nasal secretions may be affected by the autonomic innervation of the nose. A major determination to be made is whether the rhinitis is primary or is secondary to sinusitis or nasopharyngeal disease.

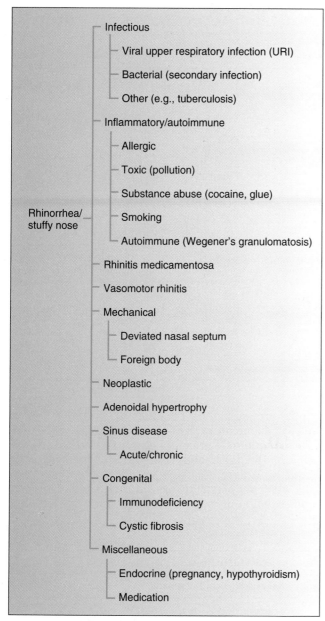

FIGURE 27–1. *Differential diagnosis of rhinorrhea.*

DIFFERENTIAL DIAGNOSIS

The most common causes of rhinorrhea/nasal stuffiness are listed in Figure 27–1.

EVALUATION

History

Table 27–1 illustrates how a careful history can help differentiate among the various causes of rhinorrhea and nasal stuffiness.

Smoking is the most common environmental cause of **chronic** rhinologic symptoms, while **upper respiratory infections and allergic disease** (with its seasonal variation) are the two most common causes of **episodic** symptoms. A careful inventory of a person's

exposures and surroundings, including hobbies and pets, is helpful in making the diagnosis of allergic rhinitis. Periodic facial pain associated with fever and discolored nasal discharge suggests infectious sinusitis, while trauma—followed by complaints of unilateral nasal obstruction—points to a mechanical problem within the nose.

Nasal obstruction (whether secondary to environmental, allergic, or mechanical problems) can lead to either acute or chronic infectious sinusitis. Careful history taking often reveals symptoms of both allergy and infection. **Unilateral purulent rhinitis in a child** is a foreign body until proved otherwise. Chronic use of nasal decongestant sprays (e.g., phenylephrine) can cause nasal obstruction and rhinorrhea—symptoms that these sprays were originally intended to relieve.

Physical Examination

Anterior rhinoscopy using the nasal speculum or hand-held otoscope should be performed in all patients complaining of rhinorrhea. Unilateral or bilateral **congestion** of the nasal mucosa can be assessed using this technique. The characteristics of the mucus (clear or purulent) help in establishing a diagnosis. **Masses** such as polyps, neoplasms, or foreign bodies can also be identified. **Complete rhinoscopy** requires referral to a specialist, who can visualize the entire nasal cavity by performing nasal endoscopy.

A thorough examination of the face and neck should be carried out. Facial tenderness, erythema, or swelling can be seen in acute sinusitis, and cervical lymphadenopathy often accompanies acute rhinologic infections.

Additional Evaluation

Further evaluation in the form of allergy testing or radiologic imaging is sometimes useful.

The simplest and least expensive test for allergic rhinitis is a **nasal smear for eosinophils.** If positive, this test provides objective evidence of allergic disease. The specific allergens to which the patient is sensitive can then be determined through skin or blood testing.

The most common imaging techniques used in the evaluation of nasal or sinus disease are (1) plain sinus x-rays, (2) a limited CT scan, and (3) a complete CT scan of the paranasal sinuses.

Plain x-rays of the sinuses are the traditional—and still useful—screening tool. They are especially helpful when (1) the clinical diagnosis is unclear, (2) CT scanning is not available, or (3) the diagnosis of acute frontal sinusitis (which requires either hospitalization or very close follow-up) is suspected. Plain x-rays are also useful in documenting the persistence of acute sinusitis after an antibiotic course of appropriate length (usually 2 weeks) has been completed. Plain sinus x-rays are limited in their ability to show (1) the exact extent of the disease, (2) evidence of bony erosion, (3) differences between disease in the anterior and posterior ethmoid sinuses, and most importantly (4) ad-

TABLE 27–1. Differential Diagnosis of Rhinorrhea/Stuffy Nose: History and Physical Examination Findings

Disease or Condition	Duration	Seasonal	Adult vs. Child	Discharge	Obstruction	Systemic
Viral upper respiratory infection	Acute	No?	Both	Clear/thin	Bilateral	Yes
Bacterial rhinitis	Usually acute	No	Both	Purulent	Bilateral	?
Miscellaneous (e.g., tuberculosis)	Chronic	No	Both	Purulent	Bilateral	Yes
Allergy	Variable	Yes	Both	Clear	Bilateral	No
Toxic (pollution)	Acute	No	Both	Clear	Bilateral	No
Substance abuse	Chronic	No	Adult	Clear	Unilateral	No
Smoking	Chronic	No	Adult	Clear/thick	Bilateral	No
Autoimmune (Wegener's granulomatosis)	Chronic	No	Adult	Variable	Bilateral	Yes
Rhinitis medica-mentosa	Chronic	No	Adult	Clear	Bilateral	No
Vasomotor rhinitis	Chronic	No	Adult	Clear	Bilateral	No
Deviated nasal septum	Chronic	No	Both	None	Unilateral	No
Foreign body	Chronic	No	Child	Purulent	Unilateral	No
Cancer	Chronic	No	Both	Purulent	Variable	No
Adenoiditis and/or hypertrophy	Chronic	No	Child	Variable	Bilateral	No
Acute sinusitis	Acute	No	Both	Purulent	Variable	Yes
Chronic sinusitis	Chronic	No	Both	Variable	Variable	No
Immunodeficiency	Chronic	No	Both	Purulent	Variable	Yes
Cystic fibrosis	Chronic	No	Child	Purulent	Variable	Yes
Endocrine disease	Chronic	No	Child	Clear	Bilateral	Yes
Medication use	Chronic	No	Both	Clear	Bilateral	No

equate information about the "osteomeatal complex," the approximately 1-cm³ area just behind the anterior portion of the middle turbinate into which the frontal, maxillary, and anterior ethmoidal sinuses drain.

The **limited CT scan** provides an excellent, detailed picture of the nose and paranasal sinuses. Although the limited CT scan affords only coronal views, these usually are sufficient to diagnose most acute and chronic inflammatory disorders of the nose and sinuses.

The **complete CT scan** includes both coronal and axial views of the nose and sinuses. This imaging study should be ordered in more complex situations, especially when neoplastic disease, a congenital disorder, or a complication of infectious sinusitis is suspected.

TABLE 27–2. Management of Rhinorrhea/Stuffy Nose

Disease or Condition	Antibiotic Therapy	General Medical Treatment	Surgical Treatment
Viral upper respiratory infection	None	Decongestants, oral and topical	None
Bacterial rhinitis	Penicillin, amoxicillin, or a cephalosporin	Decongestants, oral and topical	None
Tuberculosis	Multiple drugs	Saline rinse	None
Allergy	None	Antihistamines, decongestants, cortico-steroid sprays	None
Toxic (pollution)	None	Saline rinse, corticosteroid sprays	None
Substance abuse	None	Stop using	None
Smoking	None	Stop smoking, saline rinse, corticosteroid sprays	None
Autoimmune disorder	None	Corticosteroids, antineoplastic agents	None
Rhinitis medicamentosa	None	Stop using drug; saline rinse, corticosteroid sprays	None
Vasomotor rhinitis	None	Saline rinse, corticosteroid sprays	Rarely
Deviated nasal septum	None	None	Yes
Foreign body	May be infected	Saline rinse	Yes
Cancer	None	Saline rinse	Possibly
Adenoid hypertrophy	None	None	Yes
Acute sinusitis	Amoxicillin, amoxicillin/clavulanate	Oral decongestants, pseudoephedrine spray	Possibly
Chronic sinusitis	Amoxicillin, amoxicillin/clavulanate	Decongestants	Possibly
Cystic fibrosis	As needed	Specific medication	Possibly
Pregnancy	None	Decongestants if approved by obstetrician	Normal delivery
Thyroid disease	None	Specific medication	None
Medication use	None	Stop using drug; saline rinse, corticosteroid spray	None

MANAGEMENT

Table 27–2 summarizes the management of common causes of rhinorrhea/stuffy nose.

Research Questions

1. What is the relationship between air pollution and chronic rhinorrhea?
2. Do nasal decongestants improve the outcome in acute sinusitis?

Case Resolution

Further history taking revealed that the patient had two cats and a dog. A nasal smear for eosinophils was positive.

A corticosteroid nasal spray was prescribed, and the patient was counseled to have his wife wash his cats and dog weekly. He returned 2 months later, reporting a significant decrease in his symptoms.

Selected Readings

King, H. C., and R. L. Mabry. *A Practical Guide to the Management of Nasal and Sinus Disorders.* New York, Thieme Medical Publishers, 1993.

Mackay, I. S. (ed.). *Rhinitis: Mechanisms and Management.* London, Royal Society of Medicine Services, 1989.

Maran, A. G., and V. J. Lund. *Clinical Rhinology.* New York, Thieme Medical Publishers, 1990.

Rice, D. H. (ed.). Inflammatory diseases of the sinuses. Otol Clin North Am 26(4), 1993.

C H A P T E R   2 8

EPISTAXIS

Fred S. Herzon, M.D.

H$_x$ A 46-year-old male minister presents to the emergency room of a major metropolitan hospital complaining of a nosebleed. The bleeding started while he was watching television about 4 hours earlier. There is no history of trauma. He has no history of hypertension or other significant medical problems, and he takes no medication. There is no personal or family history of easy bleeding or bruising. He denies smoking and alcohol use. Physical examination reveals a well-nourished male with blood dripping down his face, oozing around a large clot in the right nostril. His blood pressure is 180/90 mm Hg, and his pulse is 100/min.

Questions

1. Which over-the-counter medications should the patient be asked about?
2. Which additional physical examination maneuvers (relevant to his vital signs) would be important to perform?

Epistaxis is a relatively common problem in both adults and children. Most nosebleeds can be controlled with simple measures and have an easily defined etiology. Occasionally, however, they can be life threatening or the manifestation of a serious underlying disease. Epistaxis represents a clinical situation in which the symptom itself may have to be controlled prior to establishing a definitive diagnosis.

PATHOPHYSIOLOGY

The respiratory functions of the nose include humidification, temperature control, and cleaning of inspired air. Inspired air reaches body temperature in the pharynx and a humidity of 85% or more upon entering the trachea. An extensive blood supply to the mucosal lining of the nose is necessary for these functions to occur (Fig. 28–1). This vascular mucosal layer is under constant stress from environmental insults and diseases (e.g., upper respiratory infection), which may lead to breakdown of the mucosa and subsequent rupture of the underlying vascular bed, resulting in epistaxis.

DIFFERENTIAL DIAGNOSIS

Anterior epistaxis is the most common form of nosebleed and is named for its anterior location on the septum of the nose, with bleeding usually arising from Kiesselbach's area. The diagnosis is made by observing the bleeding point on the anterior septum.

Posterior epistaxis represents bleeding with no easily observable anterior source, often from high posterior

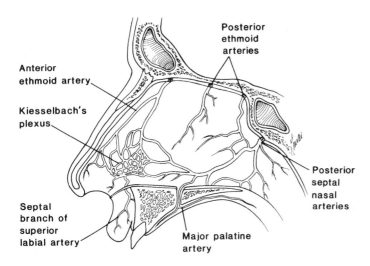

FIGURE 28–1. *Nasal septal blood supply. (Reproduced, with permission, from L. R. Boies et al. Fundamentals of Otolaryngology, 4th ed. Philadelphia, W.B. Saunders Company, 1964, p. 304.)*

spurs (small cartilage shelves lying perpendicular to the septum) or from under the inferior turbinate. Bleeding occasionally may be due to a posteriorly located neoplasm. Frequently, a specific diagnosis is not made, the only determination being that the bleeding emanates from the posterior part of the nose.

Diffuse points of bleeding from multiple sites on the nasal mucosa are suggestive of a **systemic coagulopathy.** In such cases, the patient's medical (or medication) history frequently points to the correct diagnosis.

Hereditary hemorrhagic telangiectasia is associated with significant recurrent epistaxis.

Patients living in a dry environment (e.g., a desert climate, winter home heating) are at risk for nasal bleeding due to **desiccation of the nasal mucosa** ("chapped" nasal mucosa).

Nasal trauma due to **external injury** (e.g., a blow sustained during an athletic activity or a motor vehicle accident) is a common precursor of nasal bleeding, while **self-inflicted trauma** is especially prevalent in the pediatric age group.

Any acute or chronic **inflammation** of the nose (e.g., due to allergy, upper respiratory infection, or sinusitis) can lead to increased nasal vascularity and a friable nasal mucosa from which bleeding can originate.

Primary benign or malignant **neoplasia** of the nose may present as epistaxis. New, severe nasal bleeding in an adolescent male with no signs or symptoms of the previously described disease processes should be considered nasopharyngeal angiofibroma until proved otherwise.

Sniffing cocaine can severely irritate the nasal mucosa and may even result in septal perforation. **Foreign bodies** can also lead to bleeding either by a direct irritant effect or because of secondary infection.

Any major **surgical procedure** involving the nose may be associated with varying degrees of postoperative bleeding.

EVALUATION

The initial evaluation should be carried out promptly so that treatment can be instituted as soon as possible.

The full diagnostic evaluation must often be postponed until the bleeding is controlled.

History

The physician should ask about recent trauma, underlying medical problems, medication use, substance abuse, and the onset and duration of the epistaxis. Specific inquiry should be made about use of anticoagulants (e.g., warfarin) and NSAIDs.

Physical Examination

Universal precautions, including the use of gowns, masks, gloves, and eye protection, must be followed by all health care personnel during the physical examination. The paramount task is to identify the site of bleeding. Using adequate light and suction as needed, the physician should examine the nose with the patient seated in a mildly head-forward position (to prevent blood from going back into the pharynx and interfering with respiration). Nasal spurs, septal deviations, excoriated mucosa, and masses should be searched for and documented.

The physician should also check the patient's blood pressure and assess the skin and mucosal surfaces for signs of easy bruising and petechiae.

Additional Evaluation

Once the bleeding has been controlled, a CBC, coagulation profile, and liver function tests should be ordered if warranted by the history and physical examination. If a mass lesion is suspected, a CT scan may be needed for further delineation. Angiography is occasionally necessary if a vascular abnormality is suspected (e.g., an angiofibroma in an adolescent male).

MANAGEMENT

The management of epistaxis is outlined in Figure 28–2.

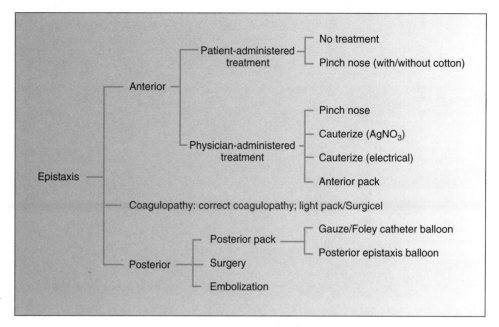

FIGURE 28–2. *Algorithm for the management of epistaxis.*

Because the inside surface of the nose is extremely tender, topical anesthesia should be applied as extensively as possible. Tetracaine 0.5% or cocaine 5% will help numb the nasal mucosa. Intravenous analgesics are often necessary as well.

Anterior Bleeding

Either silver nitrate ($AgNO_3$)or electric cautery usually stops the bleeding. If these fail, an anterior pack utilizing petrolatum gauze or Surgicel packing should be inserted. Packs should be left in place for 2 to 3 days (Fig. 28–3).

FIGURE 28–3. *Anterior nasal packing. (Reproduced, with permission, from G. L. Adams, L. R. Boies, Jr., and P. A. Hilger (eds.). Boies Fundamentals of Otolaryngology, 6th ed. Philadelphia, W.B. Saunders Company, 1989, p. 235.)*

Posterior Bleeding

A posterior nosebleed usually requires packing. The classic approach is to obstruct the choanae with a device such as a gauze pack or the balloon of a 30-mL Foley catheter and then insert petrolatum gauze packing anteriorly to control the hemorrhage. A number of balloon products have been successfully used to stem the bleeding (Fig. 28–4).

Posterior epistaxis may also be controlled *without* packing by using one or a combination of the following techniques: (1) cauterization of the bleeding site using direct endoscopic visualization, (2) surgical ligation of the vessels supplying the nose, and (3) angiographic embolization of the bleeding vessel.

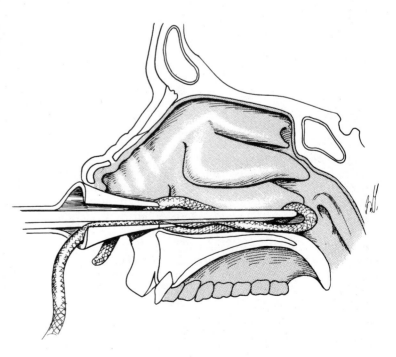

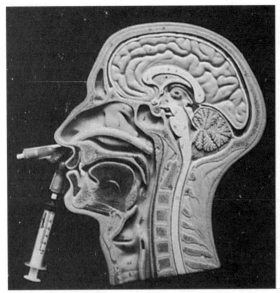 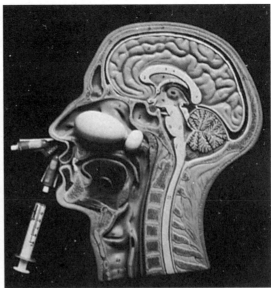

FIGURE 28–4. *Balloon device used to control posterior epistaxis. (Reproduced, with permission, from G. L. Adams, L. R. Boies, Jr., and P. A. Hilger (eds.). Boies Fundamentals of Otolaryngology, 6th ed. Philadelphia, W.B. Saunders Company, 1989, p. 235.)*

If the patient has a **blood dyscrasia,** the bleeding usually arises from multiple mucosal sites. Light Surgicel packing throughout the nose may be sufficient to control the hemorrhage until the primary coagulation deficit can be corrected.

Complications of Nasal Packs

Toxic shock syndrome induced by *Staphylococcus aureus* has been associated rarely with the use of nasal packing. To avoid this complication, a systemic anti-staphylococcal antibiotic should be administered throughout the duration of the packing.

Since nasal packing is **painful,** adequate oral or parenteral analgesia should be provided.

Both **hypoxia** and **hypercapnia** may result from bilateral nasal packing. The administration of narcotic analgesics further increases the risk of respiratory depression. It is therefore appropriate to hospitalize and closely monitor any patient with a posterior pack.

PATIENT AND FAMILY EDUCATION

Most nosebleeds in adults and children (1) are anterior and minor, (2) stop spontaneously, and (3) do not require the services of a physician. Bleeding rarely lasts longer than 5 minutes and usually can be controlled by the patient. The patient should wait 5–6 minutes for normal clotting to take place before calling a physician. If the bleeding continues, the patient should be instructed to pinch the nose for 5 minutes. If that measure fails, a piece of cotton soaked in phenylephrine (the "active ingredient" of several over-the-counter nasal sprays) should be placed into the front of the nostril from which the blood is oozing (bleeding usually is unilateral unless a coagulopathy is involved) and then held

for an additional 5 minutes. If this measure is unsuccessful, the patient should seek attention from a health care professional.

Research Questions

1. Can simple nonpacking treatment modalities for posterior epistaxis be developed?
2. How do environmental factors such as smoking, air pollution, and weather contribute to epistaxis?

Case Resolution

Initial evaluation of the patient revealed posterior bleeding from the right nostril. A posterior pack was placed, and the patient was hospitalized. The pack was removed 4 days later, and bleeding did not recur. Laboratory tests to rule out a systemic coagulopathy were unremarkable, as was posthospitalization examination of the head and neck.

Selected Readings

Fairbanks, D. N. Complications of nasal packing. Otolaryngol Head Neck Surg 94:412–5, 1986.

Hueston, D. K., and R. L. Mabry. Epistaxis. In *A Practical Guide to the Management of Nasal and Sinus Disorders.* New York, Thieme Medical Publishers, 1993.

Jacobson, J. A., and E. N. Kasworm. Toxic shock syndrome after nasal surgery. Arch Otolaryngol Head Neck Surg 112:329–32, 1986.

Meyerhoff, W. L., and D. H. Rice (eds.). Epistaxis. In *Otolaryngology: Head and Neck Surgery.* Philadelphia, W.B. Saunders Company, 1992, pp. 507–17.

SORE THROAT

Peter G. Stein, M.D.

H$_x$ A 22-year-old car salesman presents with the chief complaint of a "sore throat" of 1 day's duration. He states that he has some diffuse muscular aches but specifically denies nasal congestion or cough. His companion states that ciprofloxacin has worked well for her in the past, and she wonders whether that might work for her friend's condition. Physical examination reveals a low-grade fever and diffusely injected pharynx without tonsillar exudates or tender anterior cervical lymph nodes.

Questions

1. What are the three most likely causes of this patient's sore throat?
2. What diagnostic tests should you order?
3. What epidemiologic and personal history data would be important to obtain in deciding on a treatment plan for this patient?

Acute sore throat (pharyngitis) is a frequent presenting problem in general medicine. Practitioners often consider it a straightforward clinical problem requiring little time or mental effort. The availability of rapid tests for group A streptococcal antigen and the ability to prescribe penicillin, an inexpensive and relatively safe drug, have simplified diagnosis and treatment. However, the large number of recent articles in the medical literature on the subject of pharyngitis are testimony to ongoing concern about appropriate diagnosis and management of this entity. Additionally, serious sequelae of streptococcal pharyngitis, especially rheumatic valvular disease, underlie the importance of thoughtful management of patients with sore throat.

PATHOPHYSIOLOGY

The pain of sore throat may originate from mucosal inflammation in several anatomic areas: nasopharynx, oropharynx, hypopharynx, or larynx. Odynophagia (painful swallowing) may occur when mucosal inflammation involves the pharyngeal musculature. Suppuration may occur in the peritonsillar or retropharyngeal spaces, causing difficulty in swallowing and airway compromise.

Viruses cause varying degrees of inflammatory response. Rhinovirus infections bring about bradykinin release, stimulating pain receptors but causing little inflammation. Hyperemia and edema are prominent features of other viral infections.

Infection with Group A β-hemolytic streptococci (GABS) causes intense mucosal inflammation owing to bacterial extracellular factors such as pyrogenic exotoxin (formerly, erythrogenic toxin) and streptolysin O. A major virulence factor is the streptococcal cell wall M protein (with 80 serotypes), which has antiphagocytic properties; particular serotypes appear to correlate with the occurrence of rheumatic fever and glomerulonephritis.

DIFFERENTIAL DIAGNOSIS

Rhinovirus, coronavirus, adenovirus, and group A β-hemolytic streptococci cause approximately 50% of cases of acute pharyngitis. A cause cannot be identified in 40% of cases. Both respiratory viruses and GABS have higher attack rates in the fall and winter, the "respiratory disease season." Group A streptococcal disease is primarily a disease of children aged 5–15, but young adults are also susceptible and epidemic outbreaks commonly occur in military training facilities. GABS occurs sporadically in older adults. *Corynebacterium diphtheriae* may be a serious cause of pharyngitis in an unimmunized person. It is rare in nonepidemic settings because of high rates of immunity and the low rate of the asymptomatic carrier state of the bacterium. *Neisseria gonorrhoeae* pharyngitis may mimic other acute infectious pharyngitides but is relatively rare, and its diagnosis should be pursued on the basis of the sexual history. *Mycoplasma* and *Chlamydia* species have been implicated in acute respiratory illness associated with a sore throat.

Pharyngitis associated with common cold viruses is characterized by a sore or scratchy throat with associated nasal symptoms (nasal discharge, nasal obstruction) or cough. Sore throat may not be the primary complaint, and systemic complaints (fever, myalgias, malaise) may be absent. Signs of inflammation are mild, and there is no prominent adenopathy. The presentation of sore throat due to influenza virus or adenovirus is often more severe, demonstrating prominent erythema and edema of the pharynx. In adenovirus infection, an exudate may be present. Systemic complaints are more prominent. Moderately severe sore throat, exudative tonsillitis, adenopathy, and fever are common in infectious mononucleosis caused by the Epstein-Barr virus (EBV). Acute herpetic pharyngitis is manifested as vesiculation, ulceration, and exudate of the pharyngeal mucosa, mimicking adenovirus or GABS pharyngitis.

The onset of sore throat associated with GABS is abrupt and accompanied by malaise, fever, and headache. The posterior pharynx may demonstrate marked erythema and edema, and the tonsils may show a grayish white exudate. Cervical lymph nodes are often enlarged and tender. Not all patients with GABS have the classic presentation with all these findings. The appearance of a rash on the trunk and extremities together with a strawberry-like appearance of the tongue suggests scarlet fever caused by a GABS strain producing pyrogenic exotoxin.

Gonococcal pharyngitis may produce an exudative pharyngitis but is often asymptomatic.

While most cases of acute sore throat are caused by viruses or GABS, other causes of acute pain in the throat such as laryngitis, gastroesophageal reflux, and postnasal drip from sinusitis should be considered. Severe sore throat with a normal pharyngeal examination suggests the possibility of epiglottiditis. Agranulocytosis and mucosal ulceration due to chemotherapeutic agents may also cause sore throat although the onset is more likely to be subacute. Disease of the thyroid may first manifest itself to the patient as throat discomfort. Acute pain in the neck or jaw may be a manifestation of cardiac ischemia.

EVALUATION

History

Certain key symptoms should be elicited in the history. What is the severity of the sore throat? Are there associated nasal, laryngeal, or bronchial symptoms such as stuffiness, hoarseness, chest pain, or cough? Do systemic symptoms such as fever, myalgias, and malaise figure in the patient's history? Is anyone else at the patient's home experiencing similar symptoms?

Physical Examination

The focused physical examination includes inspection of the anterior nasal passage for edema of the turbinates and discharge. The fauces are examined for edema, erythema, and uvular deviation. The palatine tonsils between the faucial folds are examined for enlargement, exudate, and ulceration. Tense swelling of the soft palate and anterior fold above the tonsil indicates peritonsillar cellulitis or abscess. The posterior oropharyngeal wall should be inspected for erythema and edema as well as for the presence of a membrane. This brief, directed examination is completed by palpation of the cervical lymph nodes. If cough is present, auscultation of the lungs should be done.

Additional Evaluation

The laboratory evaluation in acute sore throat is generally limited to the identification of GABS. Diphtheritic and gonococcal pharyngitis are rare and tested for only if indicated by the history or examination. All other etiologies generally cause brief, self-limited illnesses for which laboratory evaluation is (with the exception of the mononucleosis test for EBV antibodies) neither readily available nor indicated. It is important to diagnose GABS pharyngitis because it is treatable and prompt intervention prevents the serious sequelae of peritonsillar abscess and rheumatic fever.

Tests for GABS include rapid assays for extracted streptococcal cell wall carbohydrate antigen that use immunologic methods to identify GABS in less than an hour. Standard culture techniques have a turnaround time of 1 day. Older rapid antigen assays had relatively low sensitivities, but a newer generation test (involving an optical immunoassay) compares favorably with culture in both sensitivity and specificity although it is substantially more expensive.

The throat culture remains the practical "gold standard" against which the rapid assays are measured. The sensitivity is about 90% and the specificity 99%. When a negative rapid assay for streptococcal antigen is coupled with a negative throat culture at 48 hours, then GABS is ruled out for all practical purposes. Acute and convalescent antibody titers (ASO titers) are impractical for making routine treatment decisions but are sometimes used for documenting GABS infection. The leukocyte count is neither sensitive nor specific for GABS infection. If *Neisseria gonorrhoeae* or *Corynebacterium diphtheriae* is being sought, the former culture should be obtained using appropriate transport media and the latter should be sent to the laboratory with a specific request for the isolation of diphtheria.

MANAGEMENT

The principles of management of the patient with a sore throat are to (1) formulate a practical and focused differential diagnosis, (2) rule out GABS infection, and (3) come to an understanding with the patient about the likely causes of and indicated treatments for the condition.

An extensive literature deals with the first and second principles. The clinician's ability to diagnose streptococcal pharyngitis on clinical examination is neither sensitive nor specific. The combination of tonsillar exudate, anterior cervical lymphadenopathy, and temperature of >37.8° C (100° F) confers a probability of a positive culture of 42% (when the overall prevalence of GABS in the population seeking care is approximately 10%). Conversely, the absence of these findings in a patient with sore throat confers a probability of a positive culture for GABS of 3.4%. Thus, for practical purposes, 58% of adult patients presenting with the "classic" symptoms of GABS pharyngitis cannot be shown to be infected by the standard culture method. While there is no explicit standard of care for the evaluation and management of acute pharyngitis, current data and expert opinion suggest that, when reasonably suspected, GABS infection should be ruled out with a rapid antigen assay. If it is positive, the patient is treated without follow-up cultures. If it is negative, then a throat swab is cultured. Optimally the throat swab should make contact with both tonsillar regions as well as with the posterior pharyngeal wall to ensure maximal recovery of GABS.

Whether to treat the patient with a negative rapid assay pending the results of culture is a judgment call on the part of the clinician and the patient. Given the false-negative rate of rapid assays, a patient who is more than moderately ill may value the earlier resolution of symptoms (a fraction of a day) conferred by the early administration of antibiotics. A less ill patient may decide to await culture results. Since acute rheumatic fever appears to be prevented by the administration of penicillin within 10 days of infection, a 24- to 48-hour delay in initiation of treatment confers no added risk. When the rapid assay is not available or when cost factors figure prominently, clinical judgment may be substituted, recognizing that in the United States, the bias is to treat with antibiotics under conditions of uncertainty. Controversy exists about whether to forego laboratory examination and treatment in a subgroup of patients thought to be at very low risk for GABS on clinical grounds. Some authors emphatically state that no lower threshold for laboratory testing exists, arguing that there is always a risk of GABS infection. Others conclude that the absence of fever, tonsillar exudate, and tender adenopathy in a patient with a cough or clearly viral prodromal symptoms makes GABS infection unlikely.

A small percentage of the adult asymptomatic population is colonized by GABS, a phenomenon known as pharyngeal carriage or a carrier state. When these individuals develop viral pharyngitis, their laboratory evaluation may be positive for GABS despite a lack of serologic response indicating infection. Practically, it is not possible to sort out these patients from those with symptomatic streptococcal infection, and their condition should be treated as acute streptococcal pharyngitis.

Penicillin is the drug of choice in treating GABS, given either orally or intramuscularly. Penicillin VK, 250 mg, is prescribed three times per day for 10 days; if compliance is difficult, benzathine penicillin G is administered intramuscularly. Erythromycin may be given to patients who are allergic to penicillin. "Treatment failure" refers to persistently positive throat cultures after completion of a course of penicillin; it may be a result of failure of medication compliance, a reinfection, a reflection of the chronic carrier state, or a true treatment failure. Routine reculture of the patient who becomes asymptomatic is not indicated. Treatment with a β-lactamase-resistant antibiotic may be considered in the patient who remains symptomatic despite evidence of medication compliance, but support for this course of action remains anecdotal. To date, there is no evidence for GABS resistance to penicillin. Symptomatic management of the patient includes the prescription of over-the-counter analgesics, lozenges, or troches and salt-water gargles.

PATIENT EDUCATION

The encounter with the patient who presents with pharyngitis provides an opportunity for the clinician to explain the difference between viral and bacterial infections and to address appropriate indications for the administration of antibiotics. When antibiotics are administered without testing, the clinician should briefly explain the rationale for treatment. Indiscriminate use of antibiotics in the treatment of sore throat may result in patients' concluding that antibiotics are indicated for all sore throats.

NATURAL HISTORY/PROGNOSIS

Streptococcal and viral sore throats are generally self-limited illnesses lasting about 5 to 7 days. Low-grade fever may persist for the duration of the illness. In cases of GABS infection, the probability of peritonsillar abscess is about 2% among untreated patients. A septic syndrome involving GABS that is associated with a case fatality rate of 20%–30% has been reported recently; however, the pharynx does not appear to be the initial site of infection.

A delayed sequela to pharyngeal infection with GABS known as acute rheumatic fever (ARF) is a rare complication in the United States. The risk of acute rheumatic fever after untreated GABS pharyngitis is estimated at about 0.01%. Prompt treatment of individuals with GABS is thought to markedly decrease their risk of acquiring acute rheumatic fever and certainly lowers the attack rate in epidemic situations. Acute poststreptococcal glomerulonephritis may also occur and also appears to be immunologically mediated. Antibiotics do not seem to prevent this complication of GABS infection.

Research Questions

1. To what extent do β-lactamase-producing organisms in the pharynx neutralize penicillin and cause true treatment failure?

2. Rheumatic fever causes substantial disease in socioeconomically depressed areas of the world. Could a multivalent M protein vaccine protect against rheumatogenic serotypes?

Case Resolution

Closer questioning of the patient revealed that several of his coworkers had had similar illnesses recently. Although they all had been "treated for strep throat," this patient's optical immunoassay was negative for Group A β-hemolytic streptococci. A few minutes of explanation convinced him that he had no need for antibiotics, and he agreed to symptomatic treatment only, with follow-up in a few days if there was no improvement.

Selected Readings

Bisno, A. L. *Streptococcus pyogenes. In* G. L. Mandell, R. G. Douglas, Jr., and J. E. Bennett (eds.). *Principles and Practice of Infectious Diseases,* 3rd ed. Vol. 2. New York, Churchill Livingstone, 1990.

Bisno, A. L. Group A streptococcal infections and acute rheumatic fever. N Engl J Med 325:783–93, 1991.

Centor, R. M., F. A. Meier, and H. P. Dalton. Throat cultures and rapid tests for diagnosis of group A streptococcal pharyngitis in adults. *In*

H. C. Sox (ed.). *Common Diagnostic Tests: Use and Interpretation,* 2nd ed. Philadelphia, American College of Physicians, 1990.

Gerber, M. A. Treatment failures and carriers: Perception or problems? Pediatr Infect Dis J 13:576–9, 1994.

Gwaltney, J. M., Jr. The common cold. *In* G. L. Mandell, R. G. Douglas, Jr., and J. E. Bennett (eds.). *Principles and Practice of Infectious Diseases,* 3rd ed. Vol. 1. New York, Churchill Livingstone, 1990.

Gwaltney, J. M., Jr. Pharyngitis. *In* G. L. Mandell, R. G. Douglas, Jr., and J. E. Bennett (eds.). *Principles and Practice of Infectious Diseases,* 3rd ed. Vol. 1. New York, Churchill Livingstone, 1990.

Harbeck, R. J. U., J. Teague, R. Grossen, et al. Novel rapid optical immunoassay technique for detection of group A streptococci from pharyngeal specimens: Comparison with standard culture methods. J Clin Microbiol 31:839–44, 1993.

COMMON PULMONARY PROBLEMS

CHAPTER 30

CHRONIC COUGH

Richard H. Rubin, M.D.

H$_x$ A 59-year-old male supermarket manager presents with a 2-month history of nonproductive cough. The cough occurs throughout the day and is made worse by walking, especially in cold weather. In addition, it has awakened him almost nightly for the past 2 weeks with resultant daytime tiredness. He denies shortness of breath, wheezing, pleuritic chest pain, hemoptysis, fever, chills, night sweats, recent weight loss, postnasal drip, or heartburn. He has no history of asthma, tuberculosis, or known tuberculosis exposure. He has never smoked and denies exposure to chemicals, fumes, or dusts. In fact, the patient reports good general health except for mild hypertension and glaucoma, for which he takes unknown medications. His physical examination, including examination of the lungs, is normal.

Questions

1. What possible diagnoses are you considering?
2. What other questions might you want to ask the patient?
3. Do you think he needs further testing? If so, which tests would you recommend?
4. Would it be important to find out what medications he is taking for hypertension and glaucoma? If so, why?

PATHOPHYSIOLOGY

Most nonsmokers cough relatively infrequently; in healthy people, the mucociliary mechanism lining the tracheobronchial tree serves to sweep mucus and particulate matter upward to the pharynx, where this material can be either swallowed or expectorated. In the presence of infection or inflammation, the functioning of the mucociliary mechanism is often impaired; in addition, it may be overwhelmed by the sheer volume of secretions produced. In these cases, coughing serves the protective function of clearing the tracheobronchial tree of debris.

Coughing is a complex act: in essence, it is a reflex that can also be initiated voluntarily. Like all reflexes, the cough reflex arc (Fig. 30–1) is composed of the following components arranged in specific sequence: (1) **receptor sites** in the periphery that, after appropriate stimulation

(by inflammation, mechanical or chemical irritation, or extremes of temperature), generate a series of nerve impulses; (2) **afferent nerve fibers** that carry these impulses centrally; (3) a **"cough center" in the medulla,** which can also be influenced by higher brain centers in the cerebral cortex; (4) **efferent nerve fibers** that convey impulses from the medulla back to the periphery; and (5) **effector muscles** whose contractions lead to the cough itself.

DIFFERENTIAL DIAGNOSIS

Acute cough is most often due to a self-limited viral upper respiratory infection. Chronic cough, variably defined as a cough persisting longer than 3–8 weeks, can have many causes (Table 30–1), although a small number of conditions are responsible for over 80%–90% of cases.

Cigarette Smoking

Cigarette smoking is the leading cause of chronic cough in the general population. Smoking induces cough via two mechanisms: (1) by a direct irritant effect on the tracheobronchial cough receptors, and (2) by causing an inflammatory response within the mucosal lining of the airways, which also leads to increased mucus production. The likelihood of a smoker's having a chronic cough is directly related to the average number of cigarettes smoked per day: approximately 25% of those who smoke a half-pack a day report a chronic cough, while over 50% of those who smoke more than two packs daily have a chronic cough. Many smokers, however, grow so accustomed to their chronic cough that they eventually come to regard it as normal and do not seek medical attention for it.

Smoking cessation usually leads to a dramatic decrease in cough. In one survey of 224 patients who stopped smoking, 77% reported complete disappearance of their cough while another 17% noted marked improvement. Most improved within 1 month after quitting.

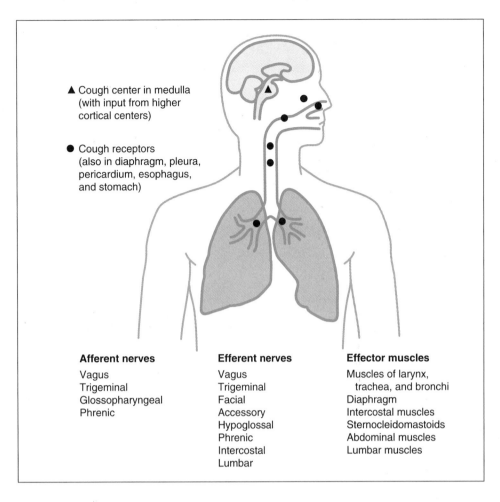

▲ Cough center in medulla
(with input from higher
cortical centers)

● Cough receptors
(also in diaphragm, pleura,
pericardium, esophagus,
and stomach)

Afferent nerves	Efferent nerves	Effector muscles
Vagus	Vagus	Muscles of larynx,
Trigeminal	Trigeminal	trachea, and bronchi
Glossopharyngeal	Facial	Diaphragm
Phrenic	Accessory	Intercostal muscles
	Hypoglossal	Sternocleidomastoids
	Phrenic	Abdominal muscles
	Intercostal	Lumbar muscles
	Lumbar	

FIGURE 30–1. *Components of the cough reflex.*

Chronic cough may also develop in nonsmokers exposed to environmental smoke, a phenomenon seen especially in the children of smokers. Some studies suggest an association between chronic cough and other air pollutants as well.

TABLE 30–1. Causes of Chronic Cough

Common Causes
Smoking (and other environmental irritants)
Transient airway hyperresponsiveness (e.g., after viral URI)
Asthma
Postnasal drip
Gastroesophageal reflux
Chronic bronchitis

Less Common Causes
Lung cancer
Interstitial lung disease
Bronchiectasis
Lung abscess
Tuberculosis and other chronic lung infections
Cystic fibrosis
Recurrent aspiration
Aspirated foreign body
Congestive heart failure
Pressure from extrinsic mass (thyromegaly, aortic aneurysm, etc.)
Irritation of cough receptors in ear (due to cerumen, hair, etc.)
Psychogenic cough
Pneumocystis carinii and other opportunistic infections in immunosuppressed patients (e.g., those who are HIV-positive)

Chronic Postnasal Drip, Asthma, and Gastroesophageal Reflux

Chronic cough in nonsmokers is most often due to one (or a combination) of three causes.

Chronic postnasal drip is a somewhat ill-defined condition felt to be related most often to chronic sinusitis, allergic rhinitis, or nonallergic (so-called vasomotor) rhinitis. It is postulated that cough results from the repeated stimulation of receptors in the nose, sinuses, or pharynx. The presumed causal relationship between postnasal drip and chronic cough is based, at least in part, on the cough's disappearance following specific treatment for the postnasal drip.

Although **asthma** symptomatology has traditionally been regarded as a triad of wheezing, cough, and shortness of breath, it is now known that some patients with asthma can present with cough as their sole symptom. The cause of chronic cough in asthma is not entirely clear. Most investigators believe it is related to the airway hyperresponsiveness (i.e., bronchospasm) seen in asthma as well as a lower "set point" for activation of the tracheobronchial cough receptors.

Gastroesophageal reflux presumably causes chronic cough by stimulation of the cough receptors in the esophagus and pharynx. In addition, repeated bouts of "mini-aspiration" may occur, stimulating cough receptors in the larynx and tracheobronchial tree. Although most patients with gastroesophageal reflux will admit to heartburn, nocturnal choking spells, or a sour taste in the mouth on awakening, as many as 43% of reflux patients will present with cough alone.

Medications

The use of certain medications can result in chronic cough. Approximately 5%–20% of patients treated with **angiotensin-converting enzyme (ACE) inhibitors** (e.g., for hypertension or congestive heart failure) experience cough as a side effect. The cough is typically dry, with many patients complaining of an associated "tickle" in the throat; it usually disappears within 2 weeks after stopping the medication. The mechanism of this cough is not fully known; however, it may be related to the accumulation of prostaglandins, kinins (e.g., bradykinin) or substance P.

β-**Blockers** are another class of medication associated with chronic cough. This is an especially important consideration in the elderly, since bronchospasm (and cough) have been associated with β-blocker eye drops used to treat glaucoma as well as with oral β-blockers used to manage hypertension and angina.

Other Causes

Other less common causes of chronic cough are listed in Table 30–1. For patients who are immunosuppressed (e.g., those who are HIV-positive), diagnosis is even more extensive and includes *Pneumocystis carinii* and other opportunistic infections. Mention should also be made of psychogenic cough; this condition, primarily found in children and adolescents, characteristically disappears during sleep and increases during periods of emotional stress. In adults, it is best regarded as a diagnosis of exclusion.

EVALUATION

History

A thorough history (Box 30–1) leads to the correct diagnosis in 60%–80% of patients. The patient should be asked about the **character** of the cough. Some patients, for example, may refer to repetitive clearing of the throat, a symptom that is actually more suggestive of a chronic postnasal drip, as a "cough." It is often helpful to have patients demonstrate their cough. "Wet" and "dry" coughs can be distinguished by their respective sounds, and patients whose "cough" actually represents a clearing of the throat can also be identified in this manner.

The **duration** of the cough should also be ascertained, as well as whether it began after an **upper respiratory infection (URI).** A cough of less than 8 weeks' duration that developed after a URI probably represents postviral airway hyperresponsiveness.

Inquiry should also be made about the **timing** of the cough. A morning cough suggests chronic bronchitis or a postnasal drip, while cough with a prominent nocturnal component is consistent with asthma, congestive heart failure, or gastroesophageal reflux.

BOX 30–1.   Questions to Ask the Patient with Chronic Cough

1. How long has the cough been present?
2. Is sputum being produced? If so, what are its characteristics?
3. Under what circumstances does the cough occur?

   Primarily at night
   With exercise
   After meals
   Certain seasons of the year

4. Are there any associated symptoms?

   Hemoptysis
   Involuntary weight loss
   Wheezing
   Chronic postnasal drip
   Chest pain
   Frequent throat clearing
   Shortness of breath
   Heartburn or other reflux symptoms
   Fever, chills, or night sweats

5. Was the cough preceded by an upper respiratory infection?
6. Do you smoke (or have you ever smoked)? Do you have (or have you ever had) exposure to other environmental irritants?
7. Do you take any medication (specifically, ACE inhibitors or β-blockers, including β-blocker eye drops used in the treatment of glaucoma)?

The presence or absence of **sputum** provides a valuable clue. A chronic cough productive of copious amounts of foul-smelling sputum suggests bronchiectasis or a lung abscess. A chronic productive cough associated with persistent fever, chills, or night sweats should bring tuberculosis to mind.

Since **smokers** can become accustomed to their chronic cough, it is important to routinely ask whether their cough has recently worsened, since a change could be due to the development of bronchogenic cancer.

Exacerbating factors may reveal additional useful information. The cough in asthma, for example, is made worse by exertion or cold exposure, while cough due to gastroesophageal reflux or aspiration is worse after eating.

Associated symptoms need to be assessed as well. Wheezing or shortness of breath suggests asthma. Patients with cough due to postnasal drip may complain of persistent nasal stuffiness, sinus pain or pressure, or a sense of mucus "dripping" down the back of the throat. Gastroesophageal reflux is often associated with heartburn, regurgitation, nocturnal choking, or a sour taste in the mouth on awakening. Congestive heart failure is typically accompanied by dyspnea on exertion, orthopnea, and pedal edema. Cough in conjunction with hemoptysis or weight loss would make bronchogenic cancer a possibility.

Lastly, **exposure to possible lung "toxins"** should be assessed. This includes a detailed smoking and medication history as well as questions about occupational or leisure-time exposure to dust, fumes, and chemicals.

Physical Examination

The physical examination should focus on careful assessment of the ears, nose, throat, lymphatic system, lungs, cardiovascular system, and extremities.

The **ears** should be checked for foreign bodies, cerumen, or hair lodged against the tympanic membrane. The **nose** and **throat** should be inspected for mucus discharge, a finding consistent with postnasal drip. A pale, boggy nasal mucosa and a "cobblestone" appearance of the oropharynx suggest chronic rhinitis. An enlarged supraclavicular **node** raises the possibility of lung cancer.

Patients with chronic cough frequently have a normal **lung** examination. However, certain "clues" should be searched for systematically. Bibasilar rales, for example, could represent congestive heart failure or interstitial lung disease. Generalized wheezing, especially with forced expiration, is suggestive of asthma, although it is important to remember that some patients with asthma will have an entirely normal lung examination. A *localized* wheeze, on the other hand, should bring to mind partial obstruction of a single airway, as might be found in endobronchial cancer or an aspirated foreign body.

The **cardiovascular** examination should define whether valvular heart disease or congestive heart failure is present. Careful auscultation for murmurs (including the sometimes subtle diastolic rumble of mitral stenosis) should be carried out. An S_3 gallop, jugular venous distention, and lower extremity edema are findings that point to congestive heart failure.

The presence or absence of **clubbing** should be noted, since this may be a clue to a number of underlying chronic pulmonary disorders, including lung cancer, bronchiectasis, tuberculosis, and lung abscess.

Additional Evaluation

Sometimes the history and physical examination are so suggestive of a specific diagnosis that no further testing is necessary. A 4-week history of cough in a young, nonsmoking patient with a recent upper respiratory infection and a normal physical examination probably represents a postviral tracheobronchitis. In this situation, watchful waiting is reasonable, with further evaluation if the patient does not improve over the next few weeks.

If additional evaluation is deemed appropriate, a **chest x-ray** is usually the next step. Although exceptions exist, the chest x-ray will almost always be abnormal in the patient with lung cancer, lung abscess, bronchiectasis, pulmonary tuberculosis, interstitial lung disease, or congestive heart failure. Most patients with chronic cough will have a normal chest x-ray; however, a negative study helps narrow the diagnostic possibilities and also serves to reassure the patient.

If the chest x-ray is normal, the next diagnostic step should be guided by clues obtained from the history and physical examination. A chronic cough worsened by exertion or by exposure to cold, for example, suggests asthma; **spirometry** (performed before and after the use of an inhaled bronchodilator) can help confirm this diagnosis. However, asthmatic patients presenting with cough as their sole symptom will have normal spirometry 30%–60% of the time.

If, after normal spirometry, asthma is still highly suspected, either a trial of inhaled bronchodilator can be attempted or a methacholine challenge test can be performed. Methacholine is an inhaled cholinergic agent that causes bronchoconstriction preferentially in asthmatics; a "positive" test is one in which the post-methacholine spirogram shows a greater than 20% decrease in function compared with the baseline spirogram. There is no reason, however, to perform this test in patients already known to have asthma or chronic obstructive lung disease.

Other testing also depends on the clinical situation. If sputum is being produced, it should be sent for **Gram's stain and culture, AFB (tuberculosis) studies,** and **cytologic studies. Sinus x-rays** can be requested if the history suggests chronic sinusitis. Patients with reflux symptoms can be evaluated with an **upper GI series, upper GI endoscopy,** or **esophageal pH monitoring.** When the chest x-ray is normal, **bronchoscopy** tends to have an extremely low yield in the evaluation of chronic cough; it should probably be reserved for patients who (1) complain of additional symptoms (e.g., hemoptysis), (2) have a significant smoking history, or (3) are over 50 years of age, especially when no explanation for the chronic cough can be found through less invasive testing.

MANAGEMENT

Specific Treatment

Treatment should be directed at the diagnosis uncovered during the evaluation process and should be as specific as possible. Occasionally, treatment is started based on a *presumptive* diagnosis, e.g., in a patient felt to have asthma based on the history or physical examination. This approach is reasonable if prompt control of symptoms is achieved; if not, further studies are advised.

Asthma (see Chapter 33) usually responds to a regimen of inhaled bronchodilators as well as inhaled antiinflammatory agents (either corticosteroids or cromolyn sodium). Sometimes a short course of oral steroids is needed to gain rapid control of symptoms.

Patients with **gastroesophageal reflux** (see Chapter 51) can be managed with a stepwise approach. Antacids and "antireflux" measures (elevation of the head of the bed, avoidance of late evening meals, etc.) should be tried first, with the subsequent addition of medications like H_2-blockers or omeprazole if necessary.

Postnasal drip often requires prolonged treatment for several weeks (or even months) before improvement is seen. Some patients seem to respond to oral decongestants or decongestant-antihistamine combinations; others appear to do better with chronic use of inhaled nasal steroids. Decongestant nasal sprays may help relieve symptoms acutely but, if used for more than 1 week, can

TABLE 30–2.   Complications of Cough

Common Complications

Strain of intercostal muscles
Sleep disturbance (and resultant daytime tiredness)
Irritation of normal larynx and trachea
Retching and vomiting

Less Common Complications

Rib fracture (if this occurs, rule out pathologic fracture secondary to metastatic cancer, multiple myeloma, or osteoporosis)
Tear of intercostal or rectus abdominis muscle
Provocation or exacerbation of low back pain
Rupture of subconjunctival or nasal veins
Pneumothorax
Pneumomediastinum/subcutaneous emphysema
Urinary incontinence (stress incontinence)
Wound dehiscence (after surgery)
Bradycardia
Cough syncope

result in "rebound" nasal congestion (known as rhinitis medicamentosa) if abruptly discontinued.

General Treatment

By ridding the airways of secretions and debris, cough performs an important protective function. Suppression of a *productive* cough, therefore, usually is not in the patient's best interest. Severe or persistent coughing, however, can result in complications (Table 30–2). **Cough suppressants** are thus reasonable to prescribe when a cough-related complication develops or when the cough is clearly accomplishing nothing useful. They may also provide symptomatic relief when no specific cause of the cough can be identified.

Cough suppressants are classified as being either centrally or peripherally acting. Central cough suppressants affect the medullary cough center and include codeine and dextromethorphan. The less well studied peripheral cough suppressants include a variety of over-the-counter syrups and lozenges that are thought to temporarily anesthetize or "coat" the cough receptors in the pharynx, larynx, or upper airway.

Expectorants such as guaifenesin can be found in many over-the-counter products, but their effectiveness has never been reliably demonstrated.

PATIENT AND FAMILY EDUCATION

Smokers should be encouraged to quit smoking, and a specific plan of action to accomplish this goal should be discussed and agreed upon (see Chapter 105). For nonsmokers, a precise diagnosis and treatment regimen should be established.

Research Questions

1. How can we more effectively persuade patients to stop smoking? How can we more effectively *dissuade* younger patients from starting smoking?
2. What is the precise mechanism of the cough associated with ACE inhibitor therapy? Since ACE inhibitors are valuable in the treatment of hypertension and congestive heart failure, how can this cough be prevented or managed short of stopping the medication?

Case Resolution

The patient's chest x-ray was normal, but spirometric studies demonstrated a mild obstructive defect that improved following administration of an inhaled bronchodilator. The physician learned that the patient was taking a low dose of metoprolol for his hypertension and timolol eye drops—another β-blocking agent—for his glaucoma. The physician substituted diltiazem for metoprolol and, after consulting with the patient's ophthalmologist, changed his eye drops to betaxolol, a β-blocker that is less likely to cause bronchospasm. An albuterol metered-dose inhaler (to use on an "as needed" basis) was also prescribed. After several days, the patient reported marked improvement in his cough and after 3 weeks reported that it had all but disappeared.

SELECTED READINGS

Braman, S., and W. M. Corrao. Cough: Differential diagnosis and treatment. Clin Chest Med 8:177–88, 1987.

Corrao, W. M., S. S. Braman, and R. S. Irwin. Chronic cough as the sole presenting manifestation of bronchial asthma. N Engl J Med 300:633–7, 1979.

Fuller, R. W., and D. M. Jackson. Physiology and treatment of cough. Thorax 45:425–30, 1990.

Irwin, R. S., W. M. Corrao, and M. R. Pratter. Chronic persistent cough in the adult: The spectrum and frequency of causes and successful outcome of specific therapy. Am Rev Respir Dis 123:413–7, 1981.

Irwin, R. S., F. J. Curley, and C. L. French. Chronic cough: The spectrum and frequency of causes, key components of the diagnostic evaluation, and outcome of specific therapy. Am Rev Respir Dis 141:640–7, 1990.

Israili, Z. H., and W. D. Hall. Cough and angioneurotic edema associated with angiotension-converting enzyme inhibition therapy. Ann Intern Med 117:234–42, 1992.

Poe, R. H., R. V. Harder, R. H. Israel, and M. C. Kallay. Chronic persistent cough: Experience in diagnosis and outcome using an anatomic diagnostic protocol. Chest 95:723–8, 1989.

Poe, R. H., R. H. Israel, M. J. Utell, and W. J. Hall. Chronic cough: Bronchoscopy or pulmonary function testing? Am Rev Respir Dis 126:160–2, 1982.

Pratter, M. S., T. Bartter, S. Akers, and J. DuBois. An algorithmic approach to chronic cough. Ann Intern Med 119:977–83, 1993.

Stulbarg, M. Evaluating and treating intractable cough. West J Med 143:223–7, 1985.

HEMOPTYSIS

Richard E. Crowell, M.D.

H$_x$ A 50-year-old female hospital administrator presents with a 2-day history of coughing up blood. She states that she noted yellowish sputum and began to experience low-grade fever about 4 days ago. Over the past 2 days she has noticed blood streaking of the sputum. She denies feeling dizzy or weak and denies chest or leg pain or sweats. She has a 50 pack-year history of cigarette smoking and usually produces about 1–2 teaspoons of clear sputum every morning. For the last 15 years, she has worked in a chronic care hospital and has had exposure to patients with tuberculosis. Her vital signs and physical examination are normal.

Questions

1. Do specific aspects of the patient's history help focus on a few especially likely diagnoses?
2. Which diagnostic tests would help sort out the differential diagnosis for this patient?

Hemoptysis refers to expectoration of blood from the lower respiratory tract, including expectorated material that contains blood. Hemoptysis is often categorized by the volume and rapidity of bleeding. Massive hemoptysis, the coughing up of large amounts of grossly bloody material, can be life-threatening but is seen infrequently. Submassive hemoptysis, which includes slight bloody streaking of sputum, is much more common.

PATHOPHYSIOLOGY

The mechanism of hemoptysis depends on the site of bleeding within the lower respiratory tract and the underlying pathologic process. Hemoptysis may occur as a result of necrosis of lung parenchyma (e.g., tumor, pulmonary infarction) or direct damage to the alveolar-microvascular interface (e.g., pulmonary hemorrhage syndromes, inhaled toxins). However, in most cases hemoptysis occurs as a result of erosion of blood vessels within the bronchial mucosa owing to an underlying pathologic process (e.g., ongoing bronchiectasis, infection of parenchymal cavities, tumor invasion). Occasionally, the pathologic process results in either (1) replacement of the airway vasculature with vessels originating from the bronchial circulation or (2) anastomoses between the bronchial and pulmonary circulations. Since intrinsic flow pressures are much higher in the bronchial circulation (which originates from the aorta) than in the pulmonary vasculature, erosion of these vessels tends to result in bleeding that is much more brisk and copious.

DIFFERENTIAL DIAGNOSIS

Although a large number of causes of hemoptysis have been described, most cases can be explained by a limited number of disorders (Table 31–1).

Infection involving the airways or lung parenchyma is the leading cause of hemoptysis worldwide and causes the majority of cases of massive hemoptysis. Prior to the antibiotic era, bronchiectasis was a leading cause of hemoptysis arising from the bronchial tree. Although seen less frequently now, hemoptysis can still be a major problem in patients with bronchiectasis due to cystic fibrosis or chronic infection such as tubercu-

---

TABLE 31–1. Causes of Hemoptysis by Location Within the Lower Respiratory Tract

Airway

Infection
  Bronchitis*
  Bronchiectasis*
    Cystic fibrosis
Malignancy
  Primary lung cancer*
  Metastatic cancer
  Bronchial adenoma
Other
  Broncholithiasis

Lung Parenchyma

Infection*
  Pneumonia
  Primary cavitary disease
    Tuberculosis*
    Lung abscess
  Colonization in preexisting cavitary disease
    Aspergillus, other fungi (mycetoma)*
    Bacterial
    Tuberculosis
Diffuse pulmonary hemorrhage
  Pulmonary-renal syndromes

Vascular

Pulmonary vascular disorders
  Pulmonary embolism
  Systemic lupus erythematosus, other rheumatologic diseases
  Primary pulmonary hypertension, pulmonary veno-occlusive disease, amyloidosis
Cardiac disorders
  Mitral stenosis
  Congestive heart failure
Vascular anomalies
  Arteriovenous malformations
  Telangiectasias
  Aneurysms

Miscellaneous

Trauma
Aspiration, toxic inhalation
Bleeding disorders

*Signifies most common causes of hemoptysis (80% as a group).

losis. Bleeding can be brisk in these patients owing to communication between the bronchial mucosa and the systemic vasculature.

As the cases of bronchiectasis have decreased over the years, chronic bronchitis has assumed a more prominent role as a cause of hemoptysis originating from the airways. Usually seen in cigarette smokers, hemoptysis in chronic bronchitis is also due to erosion of mucosal vessels. However, bleeding in these patients tends to be less brisk than that occurring with bronchiectasis, since chronic bronchitis tends to involve only the superficial mucosa and does not result in bronchopulmonary anastomoses.

Hemoptysis can also originate from infectious processes within the lung parenchyma. Pneumonia due to organisms capable of causing necrosis of lung tissue (e.g., *Pneumococcus, Staphylococcus, Pseudomonas,* or anaerobes) is associated with hemoptysis, as is infection of preexisting blebs, bullae, or cavities within the lung. Ongoing infection of such cavities due to bacteria or fungi progresses to involve the cavity wall, leading to bleeding from vessels from either the pulmonary or bronchial circulations.

The role of tuberculosis (TB) as a cause of hemoptysis deserves special mention. Although TB was a common cause of hemoptysis through the 1960s, its significance waned as the number of TB cases dropped; over the last several years, however, TB has reemerged, especially in patients who are infected with HIV. Hemoptysis in TB patients can be related to the erosion of mucosa within bronchiectatic sites or within superinfected cavities, both of which can develop during the course of tuberculous infection. Alternatively, residual calcified peribronchial lymph nodes from tuberculous infection can erode bronchial walls, causing significant hemoptysis.

The other major cause of hemoptysis in the United States is primary endobronchial lung cancer. Cancers that are metastatic to the lung from other organs (e.g., kidney, colon, and breast) also can cause hemoptysis, particularly if the metastases are endobronchial in location. However, hemoptysis from metastases occurs much less frequently than that due to primary lung cancers. In addition, bronchial adenomas can cause brisk hemoptysis, since they tend to be vascular in composition.

While infectious processes and tumors account for the majority of cases of hemoptysis, several noninfectious, nonneoplastic disorders can induce significant bleeding in the lower respiratory tract. Of disorders related to the pulmonary vascular system, pulmonary thromboembolism is one of the more common causes of hemoptysis. Vasculitic disorders and other pulmonary hemorrhage syndromes, including Goodpasture's syndrome and systemic lupus erythematosus, can lead to hemoptysis, as can agents that directly injure the pulmonary parenchyma, such as aspirated acids or toxic gases. Bleeding from the airways is not uncommon in patients with systemic coagulation abnormalities (severe cirrhosis, coagulation factor deficiencies, etc.) although severe hemoptysis is unusual unless the patient has other disorders of the airways or pulmonary parenchyma.

EVALUATION

History

First, it must be established that the blood is indeed coming from the lower respiratory tract. Blood originating from the upper airways or regurgitation of bloody stomach contents can be misinterpreted by both patient and physician as being hemoptysis. Bleeding from other sites requires different diagnostic and therapeutic measures.

Second, the severity of the hemoptysis episode must be quickly assessed, since the approach to the patient is influenced by the total volume of blood coughed up, how long the episode has lasted, and whether the hemoptysis is recurrent. Although several definitions of "massive hemoptysis" are used in the literature, anyone with hemoptysis resulting in blood loss of > 300 mL over a 6-hour period deserves careful monitoring and an aggressive strategy for evaluation and management.

Finally, a thorough search for clues to the cause of the hemoptysis should be instituted. Inquiry should be made about cigarette smoking, inherited disorders such as bleeding diatheses or cystic fibrosis, and exposures to possible carcinogens or infectious agents.

Physical Examination

The examination should be directed at (1) confirming the lower respiratory tract as the site of bleeding, (2) looking for evidence of illnesses that can lead to hemoptysis, and (3) assessing the effects of the bleeding on intravascular hemodynamics and gas exchange within the lungs.

Although sometimes difficult, every attempt should be made to ensure that the bleeding is originating from below the larynx. For example, simple observation may indicate that coughing is followed by the expectoration of blood. A thorough inspection of the mouth and upper airways helps rule out these sites as the origin of bleeding.

Upper airway examination may also help determine the presence of sinusitis (as is often seen in Wegener's granulomatosis), and inspection of the extremities and skin may provide evidence of vasculitis. The presence of clubbing may indicate bronchiectasis or other chronic lung infection but may also be seen in patients with lung cancer. Peripheral edema may indicate underlying congestive heart failure, whereas unilateral lower extremity edema, tenderness, and Homan's sign may indicate the presence of a deep vein thrombosis.

The effects of hemoptysis on hemodynamic stability and gas exchange should be assessed. The presence of orthostatic changes in blood pressure and pulse suggests intravascular volume depletion and a significant amount of blood loss. Pale skin color suggests severe anemia, possibly from chronic blood loss. However, tachypnea and peripheral cyanosis may indicate that gas exchange has been impaired, either by the underlying disease process or by bleeding severe enough to spill into adjacent lung tissue.

Examination of the lungs may not be helpful in detecting the cause of hemoptysis. However, signs of focal consolidation may suggest pneumonia or bleeding severe enough to flood a large region of alveoli and to impair gas exchange. Crackles heard throughout the lungs bilaterally may be due to severe bleeding but could also represent congestive heart failure or pulmonary edema if other signs of left ventricular dysfunction are present.

Additional Evaluation

Laboratory Tests

Routine laboratory studies may be helpful in determining the etiology of hemoptysis. Leukocytosis may point toward infection, although pulmonary hemorrhage syndromes and pulmonary emboli may also cause small increases in the white blood cell count. A prothrombin time, partial thromboplastin time, and platelet count are mandatory to rule out coagulation disorders. In addition, arterial blood gases are useful in determining whether intrapulmonary bleeding is severe enough to endanger gas exchange.

Chest X-ray

A chest x-ray (CXR) evaluation is crucial in the workup of patients with hemoptysis. Not only can the CXR suggest the origin of the hemoptysis, but it may also help determine the amount of parenchyma affected by severe bleeding. Alternatively, a normal CXR will narrow the differential diagnosis significantly. If a focal lesion is responsible for the hemoptysis, a normal chest film implies either that the lesion is extremely small or that it lies within a large airway. In addition, hemoptysis due to chronic bronchitis is not associated with focal CXR abnormalities, although changes consistent with underlying chronic obstructive pulmonary disease may be seen. Nevertheless, evaluation of hemoptysis in patients with a normal CXR often is inconclusive.

Although any pattern of CXR abnormality can be seen in patients with hemoptysis, some patterns are more suggestive of specific diagnoses. For example, a large hilar mass or parenchymal nodule suggests primary lung cancer. Cavitary masses may be due to cancer, tuberculosis, fungal disease, or pyogenic lung abscesses. Focal infiltrates suggest pneumonia, but can also result when bleeding from a focal lesion spills into surrounding lung parenchyma. Diffuse, bilateral infiltrates suggest pulmonary hemorrhage syndromes, congestive heart failure, or toxic inhalations.

Special Tests

Since the cause of hemoptysis in many patients is not obvious from the history, physical examination, initial laboratory testing, and CXR, further assessment is often required using specialized techniques. Bronchoscopy is safe and easy to perform and easily identifies the site of bleeding if it originates within the larger airways or from a specific lobe or segment. If the patient's CXR is abnormal, bronchoscopy should be strongly considered, es-

pecially if the CXR suggests a tumor or if a focal infiltrate does not clear with appropriate therapy. Most pulmonary physicians prefer to perform this procedure as early as possible to pinpoint the bleeding site, although some studies have suggested that the timing of bronchoscopy has no effect on therapeutic decision making.

If the CXR is normal, the history will help determine the need for bronchoscopy. For example, hemoptysis in a nonsmoking 40-year-old patient with signs and symptoms strongly suggestive of bronchitis may not require bronchoscopic evaluation. Alternatively, a 60-year-old cigarette smoker with constitutional symptoms and stridor may have a tracheal tumor that was not visualized on a routine CXR. However, it should be remembered that if the patient's CXR is normal, bronchoscopy is usually not helpful in determining the cause of hemoptysis.

A CT scan of the chest can provide a comprehensive assessment of lung masses, and may demonstrate areas of cavitation not previously appreciated on CXR. A "thin cut" CT scan is extremely helpful as a method for diagnosing bronchiectasis. For vascular anomalies such as arteriovenous malformations and anastomoses between bronchial and pulmonary circulations, angiographic evaluation of selected areas of lung parenchyma is a valuable diagnostic tool. Pulmonary angiography is the "gold standard" for diagnosing acute pulmonary thromboembolism, although assessment of ventilation-perfusion matching by radioisotope scanning is usually performed as the initial screening test.

MANAGEMENT

Acute management of hemoptysis depends on whether the episode is life-threatening owing to intravascular blood loss or, more commonly, to spillage of blood throughout the lung parenchyma or diffuse parenchymal bleeding resulting in severe gas exchange abnormalities. Massive hemoptysis has been associated with > 50% mortality. Maintenance of central airway patency, aggressive suctioning, and emergency evaluation are crucial. Bronchoscopy may visualize the site of bleeding, but massive or continuous bleeding may preclude positive identification by this method. In such situations, however, the bronchoscope can often be used as a tamponade against the bleeding site. Alternative therapeutic approaches include (1) selective angiography and embolization of the artery leading to the bleeding site and (2) surgical resection of the bleeding site. Surgery in unstable patients, however, is associated with high mortality.

If the amount of expectorated blood is not massive or if the bleeding has stopped, the patient should be kept in a quiet environment and coughing should be suppressed. The patient's gas exchange status should be monitored continuously and supplemental oxygen provided as needed. If the initial evaluation suggests an infectious cause, appropriate therapy should be instituted. Selective angiography and embolization have been used to treat hemoptysis, particularly for patients with recurrent episodes due to arteriovenous malformations or bronchiectasis or when the bleeding originates from the walls of infected pulmonary cavities.

PATIENT AND FAMILY EDUCATION

Patients with hemoptysis due to treatable diseases should be counseled about optimizing their therapy. This would include smoking cessation in patients with chronic bronchitis and the need to complete the course of therapy in infectious diseases, especially tuberculosis.

PROGNOSIS

Most cases of hemoptysis that are not massive in nature tend to be self-limited, although in certain instances recurrences are common. In particular, hemoptysis due to tumors often recurs unless definitive therapy is undertaken, and patients with bronchiectasis or other chronic parenchymal abnormalities frequently have hemoptysis during acute flares. Massive hemoptysis >50% can be associated with mortality rates depending on the cause of the bleeding.

Research Question

1. What is the most cost-effective approach to the evaluation of a patient with recurrent mild hemoptysis?

Case Resolution

The patient was able to produce a sputum sample while in the office that confirmed streaks of blood. A chest x-ray revealed signs of hyperinflation but was otherwise normal. Her laboratory data, including CBC, PT, and PTT, were all within normal limits. A culture and sensitivity of the sputum revealed mixed flora. The patient responded to a 10-day course of trimethoprim-sulfamethoxazole. A presumptive diagnosis of acute bronchitis was made. The patient has subsequently given up smoking, and there has been no recurrence of symptoms.

Selected Readings

Adelman, M., E. F. Haponik, E. R. Bleeker, and E. J. Britt. Cryptogenic hemoptysis: Clinical features, bronchoscopic findings, and natural history in 67 patients. Ann Intern Med 102:829–34, 1985.

Conlan, A. A., S. S. Hurwitz, and L. Krige. Massive hemoptysis: Review of 123 cases. J Thorac Cardiovasc Surg 85:120–4, 1983.

Heimer, D., J. Bar-Ziv, and S. M. Scharf. Fiberoptic bronchoscopy in patients with hemoptysis and nonlocalizing chest roentgenograms. Arch Intern Med 145:1427, 1985.

Poe, R. H., R. H. Israel, M. G. Marin, et al. Utility of fiberoptic bronchoscopy in patients with hemoptysis and a non-localizing chest roentgenogram. Chest 93:70–5, 1988.

Wolfe, J. D., and D. H. Simmons. Hemoptysis: Diagnosis and management. West J Med 127:383, 1977.

CHAPTER   3 2

DYSPNEA

Betty Newville, M.D.

H$_x$ A 70-year-old female presents to the clinic stating she feels short of breath. She first noticed the symptom approximately 2 weeks ago while playing with her grandchildren. She lives by herself and has a sedentary life-style but is able to care for herself. Her longest daily walk is 15 m (50 ft) to the mailbox, which she performs without difficulty. Her daughter, who has accompanied her to the clinic, reminds her that last year she regularly took walks around the neighborhood. The patient responds that she stopped this activity 4 months ago because she didn't have the energy for trips outside the house. She has not experienced fever, chills, chest pain, or weight loss. Over the past 2 weeks, she has been awakened almost nightly by shortness of breath; in addition, she has experienced shortness of breath during activities such as playing ball with her grandchildren and doing strenuous household chores. She has a nonproductive morning cough, which she thinks might have become worse over the past several months. She was hospitalized 5 years ago for pneumonia and has been treated for bronchitis on many occasions. She has a 50 pack-year history of smoking, and she still smokes one pack of cigarettes daily despite advice to stop.

Questions

1. Does the patient have risk factors that would help you differentiate between cardiac and pulmonary disease?
2. Why does she continue to smoke despite her physician's warnings?
3. How can you help her remain independent?

Shortness of breath, breathlessness, and dyspnea all refer to an abnormal awareness of breathing. This complaint is frequently associated with anxiety, fatigue, and sometimes a vague chest discomfort. Although shortness of breath is a common presenting complaint in the outpatient setting, it is sometimes difficult for the patient to precisely describe the duration, severity, or quality of the symptoms. Depending on the etiology of the shortness of breath, its onset can be insidious (e.g., in chronic obstructive pulmonary disease [COPD]) or abrupt (e.g., with pulmonary embolism).

PATHOPHYSIOLOGY

Given the frequency with which patients present with dyspnea, it might seem surprising that the exact mechanism has not been clearly elucidated. Most likely, there are a multitude of "dyspnea mechanisms." Dyspnea is experienced primarily because of increased stimulation of the brain-stem respiratory center. This area of the medulla consists of three coordinating centers: the pneumotaxic center, which controls the rate and pattern of respiration; the dorsal respiratory group, which controls inspiration; and the ventral respiratory group, which modulates inspiration and expiration. There also is a chemosensitive area very close to the ventral respiratory group and located on the ventral surface of the medulla. This area is highly responsive to the carbon dioxide (CO_2) level in the blood, and to a lesser extent it is responsive to the hydrogen ion (H^+) concentration. CO_2 or H^+ activates neural pathways in the chemosensitive area to stimulate the dorsal respiratory group, thereby effecting inspiration. Other chemoreceptors are located in the aortic body and the carotid body. "Stretch" receptors are located in the lung and are aroused by the expansion, or "stretch," of the lungs during deep inspiration. The reticular activating system, the part of the brain activated during attention and consciousness, also seems to play a role in the awareness of breathing or dyspnea. Additionally, activation of the brain respiratory center comes from afferent somatic nerves and the vagus nerve through intrathoracic receptors (Fig. 32–1).

DIFFERENTIAL DIAGNOSIS

By far the most common causes of shortness of breath are related to abnormal cardiac or pulmonary function, although various systemic disorders such as anemia, cancer, hypothyroidism, and neuromuscular diseases also can cause dyspnea. The differentiation between primary cardiac disease and primary pulmonary disease is not always easy, and some patients will have symptoms caused by disease in both organ systems ("cardiopulmonary disease"). Despite the reality of combined organ system disease, a definitive diagnosis should be pursued in all patients. Pulmonary pathology includes asthma, bronchitis, upper or lower airway obstruction, pulmonary embolism, and pulmonary parenchymal disease (e.g., pneumonia, pneumoconiosis). Anxiety and other psychiatric conditions can also cause the sensation of dyspnea.

EVALUATION

History

The patient's age, pulmonary risk factors, cardiac risk factors, past medical history, and family history must be

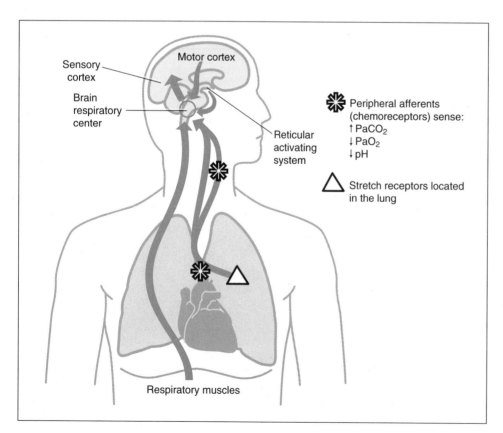

FIGURE 32–1. *"Anatomy" of dyspnea.*

considered. Occupational history should be included as a part of the pulmonary evaluation; a detailed history regarding previous exposures to inhaled toxins (e.g., silica) frequently yields important information that patients may fail to volunteer spontaneously.

Symptoms suggestive of a primary pulmonary disorder include those precipitated by exposure to relatively extreme temperature changes. Allergens, pollutants, or other inhaled substances that provoke shortness of breath also suggest primary pulmonary disease. If the shortness of breath is associated with chest, arm, or neck discomfort, cardiac disease should be placed higher on the differential. This determination is not always straightforward, since a pulmonary embolism or pneumonia can also cause chest pain, and inhalants that compromise oxygen delivery can aggravate cardiac disease and thus precipitate angina.

Many symptoms are nonspecific. For example, exertional dyspnea may be a feature of asthma or intestitial pulmonary disease, but also can be present in heart failure. Furthermore, the absence of certain symptoms does not necessarily rule out a disease. For example, some patients with cardiac ischemia present without chest pain. In this syndrome, called "silent ischemia," shortness of breath can be the sole presenting complaint. Diabetic patients are especially prone to this syndrome, making the diagnosis of coronary artery disease and cardiac ischemia in this group especially challenging.

Physical Examination

The most important step in the initial evaluation of the dyspneic patient is to look at the patient. The patient's color, respiratory rate, respiratory pattern, and overall degree of distress must be assessed immediately. If the patient appears uncomfortable, is pale or cyanotic, or has an abnormal respiratory rate or pattern, the physician should assess oxygen saturation by means of pulse oximetry or arterial blood gas (ABG) measurement. If the patient is hypoxemic, supplemental oxygen must be provided promptly. Additionally, if chest pain is a feature of the patient's initial presentation or if cardiac disease is high on the differential, then an electrocardiogram (ECG) should be obtained immediately as well. If there is evidence of ischemia or a change from a previous ECG, the patient should be admitted to an inpatient bed and cardiology consultation obtained. In this situation, the patient needs supplemental oxygen therapy as well as cardiac monitoring even while arrangements are being made for further evaluation.

An increase in respiratory rate or in heart rate is not specific for dyspnea, although both signs are fairly sensitive and therefore should not be discounted when present. Cardiac, pulmonary, hematologic, metabolic, infectious, and psychiatric disorders all can result in tachypnea and tachycardia. A reduced respiratory or heart rate can portend respiratory failure, heart block, or cardiorespiratory arrest. Central cyanosis, a blue discoloration of mucosal membranes or skin, is caused

by elevated levels of circulating unsaturated hemoglobin. It may result from hypoxemia due to respiratory failure or from a right-to-left cardiac or pulmonary shunt. Peripheral cyanosis, manifesting as blue-appearing fingertips, is more likely caused by nonrespiratory disease such as congestive heart failure or vasoconstriction. Patients with long-standing COPD often appear "barrel-chested." This physical characteristic is caused by chronic hyperinflation of the lungs, resulting in an increase in the anteroposterior (AP) diameter of the chest wall. Examination of the heart and lungs is critical in the evaluation of the dyspneic patient.

Additional Evaluation

If the patient appears comfortable, is without chest pain, and has no evidence of cyanosis or tachypnea, the initial evaluation can proceed at a slower pace. The history and physical examination help focus the workup. If pulmonary disease heads the differential, a chest x-ray, spirometry, and an ABG will help establish the diagnosis and direct therapy. Asthma, COPD, restrictive lung disease, and upper airway obstruction are readily diagnosed by spirometry and flow volume loops. These tests are complementary to the chest x-ray and ABG in the initial evaluation of these disorders.

The chest x-ray also is helpful in the evaluation of cardiac and skeletal abnormalities that may contribute to breathlessness. An enlarged heart suspected by history or physical examination can be confirmed by the chest x-ray. Cardiomegaly can be further evaluated by echocardiogram, which more accurately assesses the degree of cardiac enlargement, presence or absence of valvular disease, or pulmonary hypertension. The ECG is another mainstay of the initial cardiac evaluation. Information regarding heart rate, rhythm, axis, previous injury, ongoing injury, and ischemia is readily obtained by this fast and inexpensive test. Further testing for rhythm disturbances with Holter monitoring or evaluation for ischemic heart disease with exercise treadmill testing can be pursued depending on the information obtained from the initial ECG assessment.

Other useful diagnostic tests in the assessment of dyspnea are the ventilation-perfusion (V/Q) scan, CT scan, and bronchoscopy. These specialized tests may be indicated after the initial investigation has narrowed the differential diagnosis and focused the evaluation. For example, if the history suggests pulmonary embolism (i.e., a history of prolonged immobilization, unilateral leg swelling associated with sudden onset of chest pain, or a hypercoagulable state), a V/Q scan in conjunction with a chest x-ray and ABG is appropriately obtained early in the evaluation of a dyspneic patient. The V/Q scan does not always definitively confirm or rule out a pulmonary embolism (Table 32–1). If the clinician suspects a pulmonary embolism and the V/Q is "intermediate," further testing with lower extremity duplex scanning or pulmonary angiography must be pursued. A CT scan is useful to investigate suspicious abnormalities detected by chest x-ray. Bronchoscopy, used to obtain tissue from endobronchial lesions, is ordered and

TABLE 32–1. Interpretation of V/Q Scan

V/Q Report	Percentage of Patients with Pulmonary Embolism
Normal	Essentially 0
Low probability	Up to 10%–15%
Intermediate probability	20%–40%
High probability	> 85%

performed by a pulmonary specialist, who should be consulted if this procedure seems indicated.

MANAGEMENT

Appropriate initial management and triage of the dyspneic patient should begin when the patient arrives at the clinic. Patients who are visibly dyspneic, cyanotic, or confused, as well as those with significantly abnormal vital signs, should be evaluated by a physician without delay. The decision to administer oxygen or to order a chest x-ray usually is not difficult. The challenge generally is to decide where to proceed with the workup— should the patient be an inpatient, an outpatient, or in an intermediate observation unit? Patients whose vital signs are normal and stable and who are not hypoxemic can generally be managed on an outpatient basis. Patients with hypotension, profound hypoxemia, or electrocardiographic changes require admission to an inpatient bed.

There are a few guidelines to help with these decisions. For cardiac patients who present with chest pain but have a normal ECG—and whose chest pain resolves promptly with oxygen or nitroglycerin, or spontaneously—observation with cardiac monitoring is appropriate. Such patients usually require a 24-hour hospital stay for serial monitoring of vital signs, cardiac enzymes, ECGs, arrhythmias, and symptoms. If monitoring suggests cardiac instability, the patient must immediately be transferred to an inpatient ICU. Patients with exacerbations of heart failure can be managed similarly. These patients require diuresis as well as cardiac monitoring as described above. If there is a good explanation for the congestive heart failure exacerbation (e.g., excessive salt ingestion, noncompliance with medications) and the patient does not have new electrocardiographic changes or hypoxemia, outpatient management is reasonable. Close outpatient follow-up is required for this approach to be successful; therefore, issues such as transportation and patient reliability must be considered.

Triage of pulmonary patients is not always so straightforward. Evaluation of COPD and asthma exacerbations is more efficient and simpler if results of recent baseline pulmonary function tests are available. The best method to assess the acuity and severity of the exacerbation is to perform bedside spirometry in the clinic and compare the results to those of baseline testing. Mild exacerbations usually can be managed on an outpatient basis by administration of inhaled bronchodilators and sometimes oral corticosteroids. Patients with new or worsening hypoxemia need more aggressive treatment and therefore require observation and hospitalization. Severe dyspnea, initial unresponsiveness to therapy, cyanosis, hypoxemia, or hypercapnia that is worsening despite initial care warrants prompt inpatient admission—to an ICU if respiratory failure necessitating intubation seems likely. The patient who "looks good" (i.e., has none of the above) and whose previous exacerbations responded promptly to therapy should be considered for treatment in an observation area.

Comparatively, the management of pneumonia is simple. Patients who have no major medical problems, are less than 65 years of age, and are not hypoxemic or immunosuppressed can be safely managed as outpatients, assuming that close outpatient follow-up is possible. The exception is patients whose pneumonia involves two or more lobes; these patients require admission. Patients with involvement of three or more lobes generally require even closer monitoring.

PATIENT AND FAMILY EDUCATION

Dedicating a few minutes of each office visit to patient education can make the difference between a productive, rewarding patient-physician relationship and a confusing, frustrating one. For patients with pulmonary illness, the importance of clean air cannot be overemphasized. This means avoidance of cigarette smoke (even when it is passive exposure), avoidance of known allergens, and a heightened awareness of substances that cause symptoms to flare. Whenever possible, families should be involved in these discussions, since their behaviors can dramatically influence the health of the patient.

The importance of compliance with medication needs to be addressed frequently. If the patient perceives that the medications are not important enough for the doctor to inquire about, the patient may conclude that taking them is not important. A discussion of the proper use of medications is especially important for patients with pulmonary disease. On at least one occasion, the patient should be asked to demonstrate use of the inhaler to assure proper administration of the medication. Regular home monitoring of pulmonary function with a hand-held peak flow meter is also useful. Patients who use this technique are able to identify trends in their breathing, and will be more likely to contact their physicians at an early stage of an exacerbation. With early intervention, serious morbidity and hospitalization may be avoided.

Patients and families should be made aware of local and national organizations such as the American Lung Association, American Cancer Society, and American Heart Association, all of which provide reading materials and information about specific support groups.

NATURAL HISTORY/PROGNOSIS

Prognosis depends on the diagnosis and severity of illness at the time of diagnosis. Perhaps equally significant is the patient's understanding of the illness and willingness to adhere to exercise, diet, and pharmacologic prescriptions. These life-style modifications are often difficult but should not be presumed impossible by the patient or physician.

Coronary artery disease can be stabilized and sometimes reversed by aggressive control of risk factors such as hypertension, hyperlipidemia, diabetes, smoking, and sedentary life-style. Although many patients with coronary artery narrowing are managed with medication, some are advised to undergo percutaneous transluminal coronary angioplasty (PTCA) or coronary artery bypass grafting. Patients and physicians must remember that unless risk factors are controlled, the disease will likely recur.

The prognosis for COPD differs. Although symptoms can be controlled and exacerbations treated, there is no surgical or medical cure for this disease. However, patients should be encouraged to stop smoking, since disease progression is slowed after smoking cessation is accomplished.

Research Questions

1. What factors hinder smoking cessation in patients who are diagnosed with heart or lung disease?How much does family education enhance the COPD patient's quality of life and compliance?

Case Resolution

On evaluation, the patient had a normal blood pressure and temperature. Her respiratory rate was 24/min, heart rate 96 bpm, and O_2 saturation 94% on room air. The only abnormal findings on physical examination were the presence of crackles at the bases of both lung fields and an S_3 on cardiac auscultation. A chest x-ray showed an enlarged cardiac silhouette and mild pulmonary venous congestion. Her physician made the diagnosis of congestive heart failure, and oral diuretic therapy was instituted.

Selected Readings

Isselbacher, K. K. (ed.). *Harrison's Principles of Internal Medicine,* 13th ed. New York, McGraw-Hill Book Company, 1994, pp. 174–7.

Murray, J. F., and J. A. Nadel. *Textbook of Respiratory Medicine,* 2nd ed. Philadelphia, W.B. Saunders Company, 1994.

CHAPTER 33

ASTHMA AND CHRONIC OBSTRUCTIVE PULMONARY DISEASE

David S. James, M.D.

H$_x$ A 56-year-old female accountant presents to her family physician with a 3-day history of worsening cough and shortness of breath. She has a 70 pack-year history of cigarette smoking. For the past 4 years she has noticed progressive shortness of breath that worsens with exertion. She used to be able to walk for several miles without difficulty but now becomes short of breath after only a few blocks. In addition, she avoids taking stairs because of breathlessness. For the past 2 years, she has had a productive cough, usually worse in the morning. Her respiratory rate is 24/min, and she is afebrile. Her throat is normal in appearance, there is no adenopathy, and the breath sounds are diminished over both lung fields. The cardiac examination is normal, and there is no peripheral edema.

Questions

1. What are the possible causes of acute and chronic shortness of breath and cough?
2. What is the chance of an individual's developing emphysema with a 70 pack-year smoking history?
3. What illnesses is this woman at greater risk of developing because of her smoking history?
4. What additional diagnostic tests are needed to evaluate the cough and shortness of breath?

Emphysema and chronic bronchitis affect approximately 15 million people in the United States, and approximately 20 million people, or 9% of the population, suffer from asthma. A common denominator in these conditions is expiratory airflow obstruction or limitation. Because there is similarity in their pathophysiology, diagnosis, and treatment, emphysema and chronic bronchitis are often grouped together as chronic obstructive pulmonary disease (COPD).

CLINICAL PRESENTATION

Dyspnea is the most common presenting symptom in asthma and COPD. Dyspnea is frequently intermittent in asthma and is typically slow in onset in COPD. Cough can occur in both disorders. A history of cigarette smoking will be obtained in 80%–90% of patients with COPD. On examination, wheezing or diminished breath sounds can occur in either asthma or COPD.

PATHOPHYSIOLOGY

Airflow limitation in emphysema, chronic bronchitis, and asthma involves several different mechanisms, one or more of which predominate in each condition. Loss of alveolar walls with decrease in elastic recoil is the primary defect in emphysema, whereas narrowing of airways by thickening of airway walls and accumulation of secretions occurs in both asthma and chronic bronchitis. Reversible bronchoconstriction caused by smooth muscle spasm is a hallmark of asthma. Another critical component of asthma is inflammation of the airways, which can be triggered by a variety of factors including infection, pollen, exercise, and dust; such inflammation can also lead to airway hyperresponsiveness and bronchoconstriction.

Risk factors for developing chronic airflow limitation are given in Table 33–1. Of these, cigarette smoking accounts for approximately 80%–90% of the cases of COPD and may also play a role in the development of asthma. The risk of developing COPD for a 45-year-old man is 20% if he smokes one pack of cigarettes a day and 40% if he smokes two packs of cigarettes a day. Factors that can acutely exacerbate chronic airflow limitation include cigarette smoke, respiratory infections, pollens, weeds, dusts, animal dander, perfume, fumes and vapors from hydrocarbons, outdoor and indoor air pollution, and exercise.

TABLE 33–1.   Risk Factors for Developing Chronic Airflow Obstruction

---

Asthma

Respiratory infections
Atopy or family history of atopy or asthma
Occupational exposure to animal waste, diisocyanates, wood dust, or grain dust

Chronic Obstructive Pulmonary Disease (COPD)

Cigarette smoke
Chronic dust exposure
Family history of COPD
Air pollution
α_1-Protease inhibitor deficiency

D$_x$ Asthma/COPD

- History of cigarette smoking (patients with COPD).
- Dyspnea (especially on exertion), wheezing, cough.
- Airflow obstruction documented by spirometry or peak expiratory flow monitoring.
- Bronchial provocation with methacholine may be necessary to diagnose asthma if initial evaluation (including spirometry) is inconclusive.

DIFFERENTIAL DIAGNOSIS

Airflow limitation can occur at different locations in the airway (Fig. 33–1). A history probing for risk factors (e.g., cigarette smoking) is particularly helpful in differentiating the causes of airflow limitation. **Documentation of airflow limitation** is the most important measurement for the diagnosis of COPD. The **duration of symptoms** is important in differentiating acute causes of airflow limitation from chronic causes. Acute causes of airflow limitation include (1) infection of the airways and (2) obstruction due to a foreign body. Flattening of the expiratory or inspiratory flow-volume loop on the spirometry tracing can be helpful in diagnosing large airway obstruction (e.g., from a foreign body or mass). Chronic causes of airflow limitation include chronic bronchitis, asthma, emphysema, cystic fibrosis, bronchiectasis, and α_1-protease inhibitor deficiency leading to emphysema.

EVALUATION

Distinguishing between asthma, chronic bronchitis, and emphysema may be difficult because they can have similar historical, physical, and laboratory findings and because the same causative agent (such as cigarette smoke) can cause more than one condition (e.g., emphysema and chronic bronchitis). Emphysema is a pathologic diagnosis that can be diagnosed with certainty only by documenting alveolar wall destruction and dilated airspaces. Asthma is an inflammatory condition of the airways characterized by variable airflow obstruction. Chronic bronchitis is diagnosed clinically by the presence of a productive cough for more than 2–3 years. Because of the difficulty in separating these three causes of airflow obstruction, COPD is frequently used as the diagnosis in individuals with emphysema, chronic bronchitis, and sometimes even asthma.

History

Dyspnea is the most common symptom; it is typically slow in onset in patients with COPD and is usually intermittent in patients with asthma. Dyspnea is frequently worsened by physical exertion in COPD and may occur only during or after exercise in some cases of asthma. Wheezing is frequent in asthma but can also

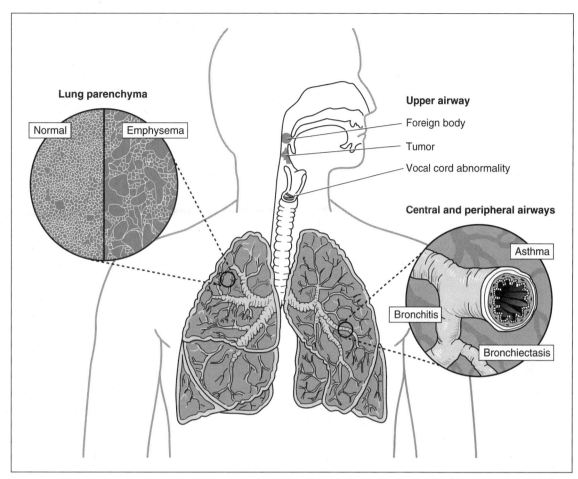

FIGURE 33–1. *Location of different causes of airflow limitation.*

occur in COPD. The associated cough can be dry and nonproductive, as is often seen in asthma, or productive of clear or discolored sputum, as is usually the case in chronic bronchitis.

Physical Examination

An increased anteroposterior chest diameter sometimes occurs in COPD. In addition, the expiratory phase of the respiratory cycle is typically prolonged. Auscultation of the lungs may reveal normal breath sounds in mild disease or diffusely diminished sounds in more advanced airflow obstruction. Diffuse wheezing can be heard in several conditions but is a frequent physical finding in asthma. Localized wheezing suggests a foreign body, large airway obstruction, or pneumonia. Absence of wheezing in someone who is having an exacerbation of asthma may indicate poor airflow and impending respiratory failure. On cardiac examination, elevated pulmonary pressures may cause the pulmonic valve portion of the second heart sound (P_2) to be louder than the aortic valve portion (A_2) in areas other than the pulmonic valve site. Right heart failure (cor pulmonale) can cause distention of neck veins, hepatic enlargement, and pitting lower extremity edema.

Additional Evaluation

Spirometric measurement of expiratory airflow and volume is the single most important test in the diagnosis of COPD (Table 33–2). Lack of an obstructive defect on spirometry makes the diagnosis of COPD unlikely. Because the airflow limitation in asthma can be variable, spirometry initially may be normal; serial tests using spirometry or peak expiratory flow meters are then required to document airflow limitation. Peak flow meters are inexpensive and can be used at home or at the work site. If asthma is suspected clinically but no airflow obstruction is present on spirometry or peak flow monitoring, bronchial provocation with agents such as methacholine may help in making the diagnosis. The chest x-ray is often useful to exclude tumors, pneumonia, or foreign bodies. Measurement of the serum α_1-protease inhibitor level should be considered in individuals with a family history of COPD, especially when affected family members have never smoked.

MANAGEMENT

The primary steps to follow in the management of COPD and asthma are shown in Table 33–3. Smoking cessation education is an important task of the primary care physician (see Chapter 105). Smoking cessation

TABLE 33–2. Spirometry Interpretation in Obstructive Lung Disease

FEV$_1$ % predicted	Decreased
FVC % predicted	Normal
FEV$_1$/FVC	Decreased
PEFR	Decreased

FEV$_1$—forced expiratory volume in 1 second (L); FVC—forced vital capacity (L); PEFR—peak expiratory flow rate (L/min).

can slow the rate of decline in airflow in patients with COPD.

For the pharmacologic treatment of asthma, a stepwise approach has been developed. In cases of mild asthma, the first step is the use of bronchodilators, such as inhaled β-agonists (e.g., albuterol), on an "as needed" basis. For mild to moderately severe asthma, inhaled β-agonists are continued and an inhaled antiinflammatory agent is added (e.g., corticosteroids or cromolyn). Metered-dose inhalers are the most effective method of delivering medication to the airways; they help prevent overdosing and keep systemic absorption of medication to a minimum, avoiding such systemic side effects as tachycardia secondary to β-agonists and immune suppression secondary to corticosteroids. For more severe asthma, theophylline or an inhaled anticholinergic agent (e.g., ipratropium bromide) may be added to the β-agonist and antiinflammatory therapy already in place. Although theophylline should not be used as a first-line medication, because of its long half-life it may be useful for controlling nocturnal symptoms. In cases of severe refractory asthma, oral corticosteroids and sometimes methotrexate are tried in addition to two or three inhaled agents. Antibiotics and short courses of a systemic corticosteroid such as prednisone may be useful for treating acute exacerbations.

The pharmacologic approach to the treatment of COPD is similar to that for asthma. Inhaled agents are the mainstay of therapy, and β-agonists alone are frequently used for mild cases. For more severe disease, an inhaled anticholinergic or corticosteroid is added. For individuals having a chronic productive cough as their major symptom, an inhaled anticholinergic may be par-

TABLE 33–3. Management of Conditions with Airflow Limitation

Measure Airflow Obstruction Objectively.
Peak expiratory flow rate (PEFR)
Spirometry (FEV$_1$, FVC)
Control or Eliminate Causative Agents.
Smoking, respiratory infections, causes of occupational asthma
Control Exacerbating Conditions.
Avoidance of exposure to smoke and dust
Treatment of heart failure, esophageal reflux, etc.
Administration of vaccinations for influenza and pneumococcus
Control Airflow Limitation.
β-Agonists, antiinflammatory agents (corticosteroids, cromolyn), anticholinergics, theophylline
Educate Patient and Family.
Monitoring of objective measurements of airflow limitation
Avoidance of exacerbating conditions

ticularly helpful and should be considered at an early stage of disease. Cromolyn and theophylline may also be useful in selected individuals. In cases of severe disease, oral corticosteroids are occasionally necessary.

The administration of continuous oxygen (i.e., for as close as possible to 24 hours a day) can improve survival in selected patients with COPD, including those with (1) PaO$_2$ < 55 mm Hg at rest, with exercise, or during sleep; (2) right heart failure (including peripheral edema due to right heart failure); and (3) polycythemia. Cardiopulmonary rehabilitation programs for COPD patients can improve exercise tolerance and decrease the number of hospital days per year but have not been shown to improve survival or slow the decline in the FEV$_1$.

PATIENT AND FAMILY EDUCATION

Patients and their families should be educated about the chronic nature of COPD and asthma and the stepwise approach to management. Instruction on the proper use of metered-dose inhalers (MDIs) should be provided on a regular basis; patients experiencing difficulty with MDIs should be given a spacer device, which is less dependent on patient coordination. In cases where airflow obstruction is variable (e.g., asthma), airflow can be measured at home with a peak expiratory flow monitor. The patient should be advised to avoid exposure to allergens (e.g., dust, pollen, animal dander) capable of exacerbating airflow obstruction.

NATURAL HISTORY/PROGNOSIS

Asthma will resolve or show improvement in 30%–70% of individuals who acquire the disease in childhood. A varying percentage of these individuals will become symptomatic later in life. Risk factors for higher mortality in asthma include (1) increasing age, (2) African American or Hispanic ethnicity, (3) previous life-threatening asthma exacerbation, (4) hospitalization for asthma within the last year, (5) psychosocial problems such as alcohol abuse and depression, and (6) lack of access to medical care.

Spirometry is useful in grading the severity of asthma and COPD and provides a guide to prognosis in COPD: an FEV$_1$ less than 1 L is associated with 5- and 10-year survival rates of 50% and 25%, respectively. In COPD, right heart failure and oxygen dependence are associated with a poor prognosis.

Research Questions

1. Between 1980 and 1987, the prevalence of asthma and the mortality from asthma each increased by approximately 30%. Why?

2. How do occupational and environmental factors cause and exacerbate emphysema, chronic bronchitis, and asthma?

3. How can physicians better educate patients, families, and fellow physicians on the management of asthma?

Case Resolution

The patient's chest x-ray revealed flattened diaphragms as well as hyperinflation. Spirometry demonstrated a moderately severe obstructive defect, with an FEV_1 of 1.33 L (48% of predicted), an FVC of 3.35 L (95% of predicted), an FEV_1/FVC ratio of 0.40, and a PEFR of 203 L/min (45% of predicted). The diagnosis of chronic obstructive pulmonary disease was made, and the patient was started on an albuterol metered-dose inhaler as well as a 10-day course of amoxicillin for probable acute bronchitis. The physician discussed smoking cessation with her, but she elected to try to cut down "on her own," declining a referral to a formal smoking cessation program.

Selected Readings

Anthonisen, N. R., J. Manfrada, C. P. W. Warren, et al. Antibiotic therapy in exacerbations of chronic obstructive pulmonary disease. Ann Intern Med 106:196–204, 1987.

Becklake, M. R. Occupational exposures: Evidence for a causal association with chronic obstructive pulmonary disease. Am Rev Respir Dis 140:S85–S91, 1989.

Chan-Yeung, M., and S. Lam. Occupational asthma. Am Rev Respir Dis 133:686–703, 1986.

Crapo, R. O. Pulmonary function testing. N Engl J Med 331:25–30, 1994.

Coultas, D. B., and J. M. Samet. Respiratory disease prevention. In J. M. Last and R. B. Wallace (eds.). *Maxcy-Rosenau Public Health and Preventive Medicine.* Norwalk, Connecticut, Appleton & Lange, 1992, pp. 885–94.

Ferguson, G. T., and R. M. Cherniack. Management of chronic obstructive pulmonary disease. N Engl J Med 328:1017–22, 1993.

Goldstein, R. A., W. E. Paul, D. D. Metcalfe, et al. Asthma. Ann Intern Med 121:698–708, 1994.

McFadden, E. R., and I. A. Gilbert. Asthma. N Engl J Med 327:1928–37, 1992.

National Asthma Education Program. *Guidelines for the Diagnosis and Management of Asthma.* Bethesda, Maryland, National Heart, Lung, and Blood Institute, 1991.

C H A P T E R   3 4

BRONCHITIS AND PNEUMONIA

Ronald W. Quenzer, M.D.

H$_x$ A 68-year-old female retired cook who has been in good health develops fever to 38° C (100.4° F) and rigors followed the next day by a productive cough, a sensation of breathlessness, and left-sided pleuritic chest pain. She does not smoke and has no history of lung disease. She recently traveled by automobile for 3 days to visit her daughter and grandchildren. Because of worsening of symptoms over the next 2 days she seeks care from her primary care physician.

Questions

1. What epidemiologic information is useful to determine the diagnosis?
2. Which clinical features suggest infectious versus noninfectious respiratory disease?
3. Which criteria are useful to determine whether or not to hospitalize the patient?
4. Which laboratory tests are most useful to determine the cause of the patient's complaints?

Respiratory tract infection is the most common infectious disease seen by primary care physicians. In adults, lower respiratory tract infections (LRTI) include acute bronchitis, acute exacerbation of chronic bron-

chitis (AECB), and pneumonia. Children may experience acute bronchiolitis as well. Pneumonia is the most serious of these infections, accounting for significant morbidity and mortality. More than 500,000 patients are hospitalized with pneumonia each year in the United States at a cost of over $5 billion. In addition, pneumonia is the leading cause of infection-related mortality in hospitalized patients.

CLINICAL PRESENTATION

The presenting symptoms and signs vary with airway infection and with pneumonia. However, cough, either dry or productive of sputum, is almost always present, and fever, vague chest tightness, dyspnea, tachypnea, and rales or rhonchi on chest examination are frequently present.

PATHOPHYSIOLOGY

Acute bronchitis is an acute inflammatory condition of the trachea and bronchi, usually resulting from infection. It is characterized by edematous mucous membranes, increased bronchial secretions, and diminished mucociliary function. One of several viruses is usually responsible. Influenza A and B viruses, adenovirus, rhinovirus, coronavirus, parainfluenza virus, coxsackievirus, and respiratory syncytial virus (RSV) are all important viral pathogens. Whereas influenza and adenoviruses predominate in adults, RSV is more common in infants and children and is responsible for significant morbidity and mortality in that age group. Only infrequently are bacteria solely responsible for acute bronchitis. The three chief bacterial pathogens are *Streptococcus pneumoniae, Haemophilus influenzae,* and *Moraxella catarrhalis,* particularly in the middle to older age group. *Bordetella pertussis* (whooping cough) is a problem in nonimmunized children, and in older children and young adults *Mycoplasma pneumoniae* and *Chlamydia pneumoniae* may cause acute bronchitis.

Chronic bronchitis is characterized by several changes in the lung: increased number of mucus-secreting goblet cells, hypertrophy of mucous glands, airway edema, mucosal inflammation, and mucus plugging. Infection does not initiate chronic bronchitis but may cause acute exacerbations (AECB) characterized by mucopurulence of sputum and increase in the amount of bronchial secretions. Infection is attributable to *S. pneumoniae, H. influenzae, M. catarrhalis,* and the respiratory viruses. AECB may also be precipitated by cigarette smoking and inhalation of environmental pollutants.

Bronchiolitis, or wheezing-associated respiratory infection (WARI), is an acute viral infection of infants and children in which necrosis of cilia and respiratory epithelium, marked edema, and mucus secretion cause obstruction of small airways. The production of IgE increases with the severity of the illness. Respiratory syncytial virus is the predominant pathogen associated with bronchiolitis in infants. In children, *M. pneumoniae* may be more common. Coinfection with other bacteria may be more common than previously thought. In one recent study, approximately one third of the 90 children with RSV infection demonstrated serologic evidence of *S. pneumoniae* and nontypable *H. influenzae.*

Acute pneumonia is an acute inflammation of the terminal airways, alveoli, and interstitium, usually a result of infection. There are three primary mechanisms by which pneumonia may develop: aspiration, aerosolization, and hematogenous spread. Aspiration of oropharyngeal secretions colonized by respiratory pathogens is the most common mechanism; aspiration of gastric contents occurs less frequently. The hematogenous route is the least common.

Pneumonia is often classified by microbial etiology, anatomic site, host, and clinical course. The list of microbes that can cause acute pneumonia is long, and the likelihood of a given organism's being present depends primarily on selected demographic, epidemiologic, and host factors (Table 34–1). In adults, community-acquired pneumonia is most often due to *S. pneumoniae, H. influenzae, M. pneumoniae, C. pneumoniae,* and respiratory viruses. Many of the microorganisms responsible for community-acquired pneumonia are difficult if not impossible to detect by conventional microbiologic techniques (e.g., Gram's stain and culture on routine media) and therefore may go undiagnosed.

TABLE 34–1. Causes of Pneumonia

Host	Pathogen(s)
Newborn	Group B *Streptococcus*
	Herpes simplex virus
2–6 weeks	*Chlamydia trachomatis*
< 2 years	RSV
	Rhinovirus
	H. influenzae
	S. pneumoniae
2–5 years	Parainfluenza virus
	Influenza A and B virus
> 5 years	*M. pneumoniae*
	S. pneumoniae
	B. pertussis
Adults	*S. pneumoniae*
	M. pneumoniae
	C. pneumoniae
	Adenovirus
	Influenza A and B virus
	Measles virus
	Atypical infection with measles virus
	Varicella
	H. influenzae
Alcohol abuser	*S. pneumoniae*
	Gram-negative bacilli
	Mixed anaerobes
	M. tuberculosis
Intravenous drug abuser	*S. aureus*
	Fungi
Hospitalized patient	Gram-negative enteric bacilli
	Pseudomonas aeruginosa
	S. aureus
	Candida spp.
	Anaerobes
Asplenic patient	*S. pneumoniae*
	H. influenzae
Patient with COPD	*S. pneumoniae*
	H. influenzae
	M. catarrhalis
	Legionella spp.
HIV-positive patient	*Pneumocystis carinii*
	M. tuberculosis
	Mycobacterium avium-intracellulare
	S. pneumoniae
	H. influenzae

Examples are *M. pneumoniae, C. pneumoniae, Legionella pneumophila,* and respiratory viruses. Hospital-acquired (nosocomial) pneumonia is principally due to partially antibiotic-resistant gram-negative bacilli (e.g., *Klebsiella* spp., *Enterobacter* spp., *Pseudomonas* spp.), *Staphylococccus aureus,* anaerobes, and occasionally fungi. Anaerobic bacteria are frequent pathogens in pneumonia. Ten percent of community-acquired and approximately 35% of nosocomial pneumonias are probably anaerobic infections. Immunocompromised individuals are at risk for pneumonia caused by opportunistic organisms, including bacterial, viral, protozoal, and fungal organisms.

DIFFERENTIAL DIAGNOSIS

Patients presenting with clinical features of lower respiratory tract infections, particularly pneumonia, must be considered for several noninfectious disorders (Table 34–2). Noninfectious conditions mimicking bac-

Dx   Lower Respiratory Tract Infection

ACUTE BRONCHITIS
- Antecedent upper respiratory tract infection.
- Acute cough.
- Low-grade fever and fatigue.
- Coarse rhonchi.

ACUTE PNEUMONIA
- Acute or subacute onset of fever, cough, and tachypnea.
- Vague chest discomfort or pleuritic chest pain.
- Leukocytosis.
- Pulmonary infiltrates on chest x-ray.

TABLE 34–2. Mimics of Infective Pneumonia

Foreign body or chemical aspiration
Pulmonary embolism and infarction
Mitral stenosis
Adult respiratory distress syndrome
Hypersensitivity pneumonias
Collagen vascular disease
Molar pregnancy (choriocarcinoma)
Pulmonary hemorrhage
Congestive heart failure
Pulmonary alveolar proteinosis
Allergic bronchopulmonary aspergillosis
Drug reaction
Lung cancer
Eosinophilic pneumonias
Atelectasis
Pleural effusion

terial pneumonia may have similar radiographic findings, requiring bronchoscopy or thoracotomy with biopsy for definitive diagnosis.

EVALUATION

History and Physical Examination

Patients with acute bronchitis generally present with a history of an antecedent upper respiratory tract infection, followed in a few days by an acute cough, usually dry. Low-grade fever and fatigue are common. The chest examination reveals coarse rhonchi and occasionally scattered crackles.

Patients with underlying chronic lung disease have more bothersome symptoms and signs. Initially, patients with AECB will notice an increase in the amount of sputum as well as a change in the color and consistency of the sputum. Accompanying this will be a low-grade fever, fatigue, dyspnea, increase in cough, and often vague chest tightness; cyanosis may also occur. Coarse rhonchi and moist crackles without signs of consolidation are frequent physical findings.

Infants and children with bronchiolitis will have a progressive illness developing over 3 to 5 days with fever, coryza, and cough. Physical examination generally reveals tachypnea, suprasternal and intercostal retractions, cyanosis, and high-pitched wheezing.

The clinical features of acute pneumonia vary depending on the causative microorganism and host factors. A thorough history to determine underlying conditions that may place the patient at increased risk for certain pathogens and to identify epidemiologic and geographic exposures is critical to the evaluation and cannot be replaced by laboratory tests. A properly done history narrows the list of causative agents to a few and directs testing and treatment. Typically, the patient with pneumococcal pneumonia complains of acute onset of symptoms with high fever, rigors, cough productive of purulent sputum, and pleuritic chest pain. On physical examination, the patient appears acutely ill, tachypneic, and modestly tachycardic with fever. Signs of consolidation are usually present. Nonpneumococcal, or atypical, pneumonia has more variable features. The onset of symptoms is gradual over a few days, with a low-grade fever and a paroxysmal, nonproductive cough. Signs of

consolidation are uncommon, but localized or generalized rales are often present. The patient appears less acutely ill. Patients who have anaerobic pleuropulmonary infections present with a wide variety of symptoms, ranging from acute pneumonia to a chronic syndrome with low-grade fever, chronic cough, and weight loss, suggesting tuberculosis or bronchogenic neoplasm.

Clinical features are especially variable in the very young, the aged, the hospitalized, and the immunocompromised. Significant weight loss (>10% of body weight), weakness, chronic diarrhea, organomegaly, and generalized lymphadenopathy may be clues to underlying disease, debilitation, or an immunocompromised state.

Additional Evaluation

To differentiate the patient with pneumonia from those with other types of lower respiratory tract infections may require additional laboratory or radiographic tests (Table 34–3). Because of the predictability of microbial etiology, unreliability of sputum analysis, and favorable prognosis of patients without pneumonia, the appropriate evaluation of patients with acute bronchitis or AECB is simple and inexpensive. In almost every circumstance, a diagnostic workup for the causative pathogen is not necessary. An assessment of oxygen saturation is important in all AECB patients to exclude significant respiratory insufficiency.

To prescribe appropriate therapy for pneumonia, however, a genuine effort should be made to determine

TABLE 34–3. Diagnostic Evaluation for Pneumonia

Gram's stain and culture of sputum
Blood cultures
Oxygen saturation/arterial blood gas
Complete blood count (CBC)
Serology
    Mycoplasma (ELISA-IgM, complement fixation test)
    Legionella (indirect fluorescent antibody test)
    Chlamydia, viral, fungal, *Coxiella*
Tuberculin skin test
Chest x-ray

the cause. Nonetheless, approximately 55% of all acute community-acquired pneumonia cases have an undetermined etiology. The essential laboratory tests for patients with pneumonia include a CBC, chemistry profile to determine liver and renal function, Gram's stain and culture of sputum, blood cultures, oxygen saturation or arterial blood gas measurement, and a chest x-ray. All patients suspected of having acute pneumonia should have a chest x-ray, which will show new or changing infiltrates. Adults with acute bronchitis or AECB will not have new infiltrates; however, young children and infants with bronchiolitis may show fleeting, interstitial infiltrates without consolidation.

MANAGEMENT

The first decision is whether to treat the patient in the hospital or as an outpatient. Outpatient care is appropriate for many, but hospitalization must be considered for pneumonia in infants, the elderly, the immunocompromised, and those meeting the other criteria listed in Table 34–4.

Acute bronchitis is often a self-limited disease not requiring antibiotic usage. If the clinician elects to institute therapy, appropriate agents are erythromycin, tetracycline, amoxicillin, and trimethoprim-sulfamethoxazole. A 7- to 10-day course of therapy is usually sufficient.

Therapy for acute exacerbations of chronic bronchitis involves elimination of underlying causes (e.g., smoking), aerosolized bronchodilators, oxygen supplementation if hypoxemia is present, systemic corticosteroids in responsive patients, and 7–10 days of empiric antimicrobial therapy. Amoxicillin, trimethoprim-sulfamethoxazole, tetracycline, and erythromycin are good first-line agents.

The most valued therapy for bronchiolitis is oxygen and mist therapy. Antibiotics have no value unless bacterial coinfection is a consideration. Ribavirin aerosol is recommended in children who are seriously ill or have congenital heart disease, bronchopulmonary dysplasia, prematurity, or immunodeficiency.

In pneumonia, early initiation of appropriate therapy is associated with reduced morbidity and mortality. Treatment decisions are related to the status of the host, severity of illness, and most likely microbial cause (Table 34–5). Seldom is the causative pathogen identified prior to the need to initiate antimicrobial therapy.

TABLE 34–4. Indications for Hospitalization in Pneumonia

Multilobe infiltrates
Splenectomy
Hypoxemia
Sepsis
Poorly responding disease
Chronic lung disease
Infant
Elderly
Immunodeficient status

TABLE 34–5. Antibiotic Therapy of Lower Respiratory Tract Infections

Type of Disease	Initial Therapy	Second-line Therapy
Acute bronchitis	Antibiotics seldom indicated	
AECB	Amoxicillin	Newer macrolides
	Trimethoprim-sulfamethoxazole (TMP/SMX)	Second-generation cephalosporin
	Erythromycin	
	Tetracycline	
Bronchiolitis	Ribavirin (for RSV infection)	
Pneumonia, community-acquired		
Mild-to-moderate	Erythromycin	Newer macrolides
	Tetracycline	Cephalosporins
Severe	Third-generation cephalosporin	Ampicillin/sulbactam
	+	or
	Erythromycin or tetracycline	Ticarcillin/clavulanate
	±	+
	Gentamicin	Erythromycin or tetracycline
		±
		Gentamicin
Pneumonia, hospital-acquired	Third-generation cephalosporin	Imipenem or piperacillin
	+	+
	Gentamicin	Gentamicin
Pneumonia, aspiration		
Community setting	Penicillin	Clindamycin
Hospital setting	Clindamycin	Ticarcillin/clavulanate
	+	+
	Gentamicin	Gentamicin

Therefore, empiric therapy is the acceptable standard of care pending definitive etiologic diagnosis; frequently, empiric treatment is continued for the total course of therapy if definitive etiologic diagnosis is not made.

Choice of antibiotic is guided by such considerations as spectrum of activity, serum and tissue levels, efficacy, safety profile, and cost. Other factors may influence the physician's selection, such as personal experience and familiarity with agents, patients' previous reaction or response to agents, and dosing convenience (e.g., frequency of dosing, size of pill). The selection of pharmacologic agents, anti-infectives in particular, is now strongly influenced by pharmacy budgets and not necessarily by cost-effectiveness.

An appropriate empiric antibiotic for outpatient treatment of individuals with mild community-acquired pneumonia is erythromycin or tetracycline. Patients requiring hospitalization with community-acquired pneumonia should be given intravenous antibiotics, often in combination. Erythromycin or tetracycline given with a third-generation cephalosporin provides broad coverage.

Since the etiology of nosocomial pneumonia is generally a partially antibiotic-resistant gram-negative bacillus, *S. aureus,* an anaerobe, or several microbes in combination, the initial treatment should be broad spectrum and intravenous.

Treatment of immunocompromised patients with opportunistic lung infections is beyond the scope of this chapter and requires consultation with infectious disease specialists.

PATIENT AND FAMILY EDUCATION

Patients should be discouraged from seeking and using antibiotics for most cases of acute bronchitis. By explaining the cause and natural history of the disorder, the physician can usually allay these demands. On the other hand, when antibiotics are prescribed, it is imperative that the patient or care givers understand the importance of taking the drug exactly as prescribed to maximize efficacy.

Allergic or other adverse reactions to antibiotics are common, (in the range of 5% to 10%), so general information, preferably in writing, should be shared with the patient and family. Patients need to know that if side effects develop or improvement is not appreciated, they should return for further evaluation.

Immunization against several serious lower respiratory pathogens—*S. pneumoniae*, influenza A and B viruses, *H. influenzae, Bordetella pertussis,* and measles virus—is available. The physician and patient share responsibility for vaccination. Widespread vaccination will diminish the prevalence of respiratory infections.

NATURAL HISTORY/PROGNOSIS

Nearly all cases of acute bronchitis resolve over 7 to 10 days without sequelae. Sometimes a dry cough lingers for several weeks.

Patients with chronic obstructive pulmonary disease (COPD) are almost certain to have recurring episodes of AECB. Again, with appropriate treatment and time, these exacerbations resolve. As the underlying chronic disease worsens, infectious exacerbations increase morbidity and the need for hospitalization or home support.

Infants and young children with bronchiolitis may show signs of air hunger and require hospitalization for a few days. The duration of illness is usually short, with full recovery in 5–7 days. The outcome is considerably worse for those infants with underlying disease, as discussed above. The mortality rate may reach 70% in infants with congenital heart disease.

The natural history and prognosis vary widely in pneumonia and do not permit many generalizations. Morbidity and mortality are lowest in healthy adults with mild illness and greatest in the young, the aged, and the immunocompromised with more serious disease. Patients with community-acquired pneumonia who require hospitalization may have a mortality rate as high as 20%. The mortality rate for nosocomial pneumonia ranges from 40% to 70%, depending on host factors, microbial etiology, severity, and therapy. The approach to pneumonia should not be taken lightly by the physician or patient.

Research Questions

1. What modifications can be made in the pneumococcal and influenza vaccines to elicit an improved antibody response in those patients at greatest risk for serious infections, such as the elderly and immunocompromised?

2. Can more rapid, sensitive, and specific noninvasive tests be devised to guide initial therapy in patients with pneumonia?

Case Resolution

The physician was able to determine that the patient had not been immunized for influenza or *S. pneumoniae*; her trip had been uneventful in that her relatives had not been ill, and she had no leg swelling, hemoptysis, or history of deep vein thrombosis. She had lung consolidation on examination, her sputum revealed gram-positive diplococci on Gram's stain, and the chest x-ray showed a dense left lower lobar infiltrate. Thus, the presumptive diagnosis was pneumococcal pneumonia. She was hospitalized and treated with intravenous penicillin and recovered fully.

Selected Readings

Bartlett, J. G. Anaerobic bacterial pneumonitis. Am Rev Respir Dis 119:19–23, 1979.

Brown, R. B. Acute and chronic bronchitis. Postgrad Med 85(8):249–54, 1989.

DiNubile, M. J. Antibiotics: The antipyretics of choice? Am J Med 89:787–8, 1990.

Fang, G. D., et al. New and emerging etiologies for community-acquired pneumonia with implications for therapy: A prospective multi-center study of 359 cases. Medicine 69:307–16, 1990.

Fine, M. J., D. N. Smith, and D. E. Singer. Hospitalization decision in patients with community-acquired pneumonia: A prospective cohort study. Am J Med 89:713–21, 1990.

Levy, M., F. Dromer, N. Brion, et al. Community-acquired pneumonia: Importance of initial non-invasive bacteriologic and radiographic investigations. Chest 92:43–8, 1988.

Mulholland, E. D., A. Olinsky, and F. A. Shann. Clinical findings and severity of acute bronchiolitis. Lancet 335:1259–61, 1990.

Pachon, J., et al. Severe community-acquired pneumonia. Am Rev Respir Dis 142:369–73, 1990.

Toews, G. B. Nosocomial pneumonia. Clin Chest Med 8:467–79, 1987.

Turner, R. B., et al. Pneumonia in pediatric outpatients: Cause and clinical manifestations. J Pediatr 111:194–200, 1987.

COMMON CARDIOVASCULAR PROBLEMS

CHAPTER 35

CHEST PAIN

Glen H. Murata, M.D.

H_x A 64-year-old male real estate agent presents with chest pain of 2 hours' duration. The pain is described as a "pressure-like" sensation in the left anterior chest radiating to the left side of his neck and left shoulder. He is nauseated but denies shortness of breath or vomiting. The patient has had "heartburn" in the past for which he has taken antacids. However, he denies a history of cardiac or other gastrointestinal disease and has never experienced similar symptoms. The physical examination reveals an obese, somewhat anxious patient in no acute distress. The pulse is 90/min, respiratory rate 16/min, and blood pressure 150/100 mm Hg. There is no jugular venous distention, and the carotid pulses are strong bilaterally with a normal contour. The chest examination reveals no dullness to percussion and no rales on auscultation. The cardiac examination shows that the point of maximal impulse (PMI) is in the fourth intercostal space in the midclavicular line and is not sustained. S_1 is of normal intensity, and S_2 is physiologically split with a soft P_2. There is a soft, midsystolic murmur heard best at the lower left sternal border and in the second right intercostal space. There is no pedal edema.

Questions

1. Should the patient be hospitalized on the basis of the current information?
2. What is the differential diagnosis at this point?
3. What additional history would you obtain?
4. What laboratory tests would you order, and why?

Chest pain is one of the most difficult symptoms to evaluate in the outpatient setting. The diagnostic possibilities range from a life-threatening problem such as myocardial infarction to a process as trivial as muscular strain. Myocardial infarction (MI) is a leading cause of death in the United States and accounts for more than 500,000 fatalities annually. Over half these deaths occur outside of the hospital, usually within 2 hours of the onset of symptoms. The case-fatality rate for patients who reach the hospital has substantially declined over the past three decades because of early antiarrhythmic therapy, cardiac resuscitation for ventricular arrhythmias, and thrombolytic therapy. It is therefore important to evaluate patients with chest pain in an expeditious manner, to have a systematic approach to the problem, and to identify those who have a serious medical condition.

PATHOPHYSIOLOGY

Somatic chest pain usually arises from the stimulation of pain fibers in the skin, subcutaneous tissues, muscles, and bones of the chest wall. Such pain is usually well localized and easily described by the patient. On the other hand, visceral pain results from stimulation of chemo- and mechanoreceptors in thoracic viscera, is not well localized, and is often described by the patient in vague terms. Stimulation of visceral pain fibers can cause pain in the somatic distribution of the spinal segments that receive these fibers. For example, the heart gives rise to afferent fibers that pass through sympathetic plexuses and enter the lower cervical and upper thoracic spinal segments. As a result, cardiac pain can be perceived as discomfort in the neck, shoulder, or arm.

The pain of pleuritis, pericarditis, or pulmonary infarction arises from irritation of the parietal pleura. Since the dome of the diaphragm is innervated by the phrenic nerve, lesions involving the diaphragmatic surface can result in pain referred to the shoulder. Although the innervation of certain organs has not been well defined, it is possible that the heart and other thoracic viscera share common afferent pathways. There is therefore little justification for the concept that cardiac pain differs from other types of visceral pain in terms of quality or radiation. On the other hand, pathophysiologic processes involving the heart, pericardium, esophagus, pulmonary vessels, and aorta respond differently to exercise, motion or change in position, swallowing, and medications. These differences can be used to pinpoint the cause of a patient's discomfort.

TABLE 35–1. Differential Diagnosis of Chest Pain

Diseases of the Skin, Nerves, Bone, and Muscle of the Chest Wall
Contusions of the chest wall
Fractures of the sternum or ribs
Injury or inflammation of the muscles of the chest or upper extremities
Neuropathies such as herpes zoster
Diseases of the Lungs or Pleura
Pulmonary infarction
Pneumonia
Infections of the pleural space
Pleuritis associated with connective tissue disease
Pneumothorax
Diseases of the Pericardium
Infectious diseases
Involvement by malignant processes
Trauma
Postinfarction pericarditis
Endocrinopathies
Renal failure
Pericarditis associated with connective tissue disease
Diseases of the Myocardium
Myocardial infarction
Angina
Vasospastic coronary syndromes
Mitral valve prolapse
Cardiomyopathies such as IHSS
Diseases of the Pulmonary Vessels
Pulmonary embolism
Primary pulmonary hypertension
Diseases of the Aorta
Dissecting aortic aneurysm
Diseases of the Esophagus
Reflux esophagitis
Esophageal motility disorders
Esophageal perforation or rupture

DIFFERENTIAL DIAGNOSIS

The systematic approach to the patient with chest pain is based upon a complete differential diagnosis. The most efficient method of generating such a differential is based upon the anatomy of the chest. As different structures are considered, different diseases come to mind. Thus, the evaluation consists of generating hypotheses about different diseases and testing each hypothesis by asking appropriate questions and eliciting certain physical findings.

Moving from front to back, the principal structures of the chest are the skin, bones, muscles, and nerves of the chest wall; the pericardium; the pleural cavities and lungs; the myocardium; the aorta; the pulmonary arteries and veins; and the esophagus. It is a simple matter to think of diseases involving these structures that could give rise to chest pain (Table 35–1). When using this approach, it should be kept in mind that diseases in the abdomen can also occasionally cause chest discomfort.

EVALUATION

History

Patients with chest pain usually belong to one of two groups—those with acute or worsening chest pain and those with recurrent chest pain and a relatively stable course. In either case, the nature of the patient's chest pain should be thoroughly investigated. These attributes include quality, location and radiation, severity, rapidity of onset, changes over time, factors that provoke or alleviate the pain, changes in functional status because of the pain, and associated symptoms.

Pain that arises from the **bones and muscles of the chest, parts of the pleural cavity,** and **pericardium** is often described as "sharp." Very intense, "tearing" type pain is also seen in patients with **aortic dissection.** It is unclear whether other qualities, such as "pressure," "aching," or "heartburn," can be used to differentiate the various causes of chest pain. For instance, one study showed that these qualities are seen in both cardiac and noncardiac disease. Moreover, radiation of pain to the left side of the neck, left shoulder, or left arm is seen in a substantial proportion of patients hospitalized with pain of esophageal origin.

The mode of onset is often used to distinguish different causes of pain, although this feature has not been the subject of much study. There is no reason to believe that pain that develops to a great intensity over a few seconds is due to an **inflammatory process** (which would occur more slowly). Sudden, severe chest pain is more compatible with a **vascular event** (such as coronary occlusion or aortic dissection), **pneumothorax, perforation of a viscus** (such as Boerhaave's syndrome), or **esophageal dysmotility** or **obstruction.**

Perhaps the most useful information comes from a survey of the factors that precipitate, aggravate, or alleviate the patient's symptoms, particularly for patients with recurrent or chronic chest pain, because they have had opportunity to experience the effects of certain activities, food intake, and medications. Pain that is worsened by certain positions, movement of the thorax or arms, coughing, or taking a deep breath is likely to be caused by **pericarditis, pleuritis,** or **diseases of the chest wall.** However, a small proportion of patients with **acute ischemic heart disease** have these features as well. Reflux esophagitis is often worsened by bending/stooping or recumbency, and esophageal dysmotility or obstruction is worsened by swallowing. On the other hand, the pain of myocardial ischemia arises from an imbalance between myocardial oxygen supply and demand. For patients with fixed coronary obstruction, factors that increase myocardial work will often precipitate angina. These factors include exercise, exposure to cold, eating, or emotional distress. Symptoms that occur at rest or at night are particularly worrisome because of the suggestion that limitations in oxygen delivery have become critical.

The physician should also identify the factors that alleviate the patient's discomfort. Rest alleviates the pain of myocardial ischemia in those with fixed coronary obstruction. Rest also reduces symptoms in some patients with pain of esophageal origin. A response to antacids increases the likelihood that the pain is due to esophagitis, although this finding is occasionally seen in patients with ischemic heart disease. Nitroglycerin reduces the pain of myocardial ischemia but, because of its actions on esophageal smooth muscle, reduces the pain of esophagospasm and may even worsen the pain of esophageal reflux.

Box 35-1 summarizes the most important questions to ask when the information has not already been volunteered by the patient.

The history should conclude with a brief survey of etiologic factors, again based upon an anatomically oriented differential diagnosis. Has the patient had trauma to the chest or unusually severe muscular activity? Has the patient experienced cough, an increase in sputum production, or fever? Is there an infection, collagen vascular disease, or malignancy that might have caused a pericardial effusion? Is there a family history of connective tissue disease that predisposes to aortic dissection? Does the patient have diabetes, hypertension, hypercholesterolemia, a history of smoking, or a family history of coronary disease? Has the patient suffered a myocardial infarction or angina in the past? Has an upper GI series been performed in the past? Is there a history of prolonged immobilization, calf pain, or a hypercoagulable state that might suggest the possibility of pulmonary embolism? The answers to these questions can be used to eliminate many diseases from the differential diagnosis and rank-order the remaining possibilities. The tests to order can then be inferred from this abbreviated list.

Physical Examination

The physical examination may not be helpful for patients with chest pain. The patient should be evaluated for cardiac murmurs and gallops, pleural and pericardial rubs, magnitude and symmetry of peripheral pulses, and rales and evidence of pleural effusion. Estimation of central venous pressure is most useful. Patients with clearly elevated central pressures should be considered to have a serious illness, since this finding is seen with myocardial infarction, pericardial effusion, tension pneumothorax, and pulmonary embolism. Tenderness of the chest wall does not always imply that the patient's pain is musculoskeletal in origin, since a small proportion of those with acute ischemic heart disease have their symptoms reproduced by palpation.

MANAGEMENT

The management of chest pain depends upon whether the patient's symptoms are acute and progressive or chronic. Acute ischemic heart disease (AIHD) should be considered in patients with new onset of chest pain or with angina that is progressively more severe, more frequent, longer in duration, more easily evoked, less easily relieved with rest or nitroglycerin, or associated with dyspnea or syncope. AIHD is a medical emergency, and patients with compatible symptoms should be referred to an emergency department for evaluation. On the other hand, patients with recurrent chest pain and a relatively stable course can be evaluated on an outpatient basis.

Acute Chest Pain

Enzyme Tests. Cardiac enzyme tests are usually ordered for patients with severe or progressive symptoms. The rationale is based on the presumption that the most ominous disease is myocardial infarction and that random measurement of cardiac enzymes is sufficient to exclude that possibility. The latter assumption is not necessarily true. Creatine kinase (CK) is an enzyme that catalyzes the transfer of high-energy phosphate from creatine phosphate to adenosine diphosphate. It comprises two enzymatically active subunits—the M and B types. MM is the isoenzyme found in skeletal muscle, whereas BB occurs predominantly in brain tissue. Cardiac muscle consists of 85% MM and 15% MB and is the only important source of MB in most clinical circumstances. The sensitivity of CK measurements depends on the time that has expired since the onset of symptoms and the assay that is used. CK does not peak until several hours after a myocardial infarction has occurred. Assays of CK-MB done by ion exchange column chromatography or electrophoresis are not as reliable as the double-antibody techniques that measure enzymatic mass. Recent studies have shown that the latter assays are more sensitive for MI if sampling is done repeatedly over several hours.

Electrocardiogram (ECG). An ECG is usually obtained in patients with chest pain. However, its role in the management of such patients should be carefully defined. A number of studies have shown that the ECG is positive for MI in only half the patients eventually given this diagnosis. In addition, a significant proportion of patients are incorrectly selected for thrombolytic therapy when ECG criteria are used. Thus, the ECG is unreliable for making the diagnosis of MI because of poor sensitivity and moderate specificity.

The ECG is far more useful as a method of stratifying patients according to the risk of cardiovascular complications. Patients with ST or T wave changes consistent with ischemia, infarction, or strain; new pathologic Q waves; left bundle branch block; left ventricular hypertrophy; or a paced rhythm are at greater risk of complications than those without such features. Patients with a normal ECG are at low risk for complications. On the other hand, those whose ECG has changed from a previous tracing are at higher risk of complications, even if those changes are not highly suggestive of cardiac ischemia.

Even when MI is excluded with certainty, there remains the possibility that the patient is suffering from another life-threatening disease for which hospitalization is indicated. A significant proportion of patients with unstable angina develop myocardial infarction within 48 hours of hospitalization and are at risk for ventricular arrhythmias. Patients hospitalized with chest pain not due to myocardial infarction may have a wide variety of disorders for which treatment is necessary, including pulmonary embolism, pericarditis, aortic dissection, and gastric ulcer. Since it is not practical to evaluate these possibilities in the outpatient setting, most patients with undiagnosed chest pain should be hospitalized. Cardiac enzymes and the ECG should only be used to determine whether a patient should be admitted to the coronary care unit or to a less intensive setting for monitoring.

Patients thought to have unstable angina or myocardial infarction should be given sublingual or intravenous nitroglycerin if they have persistent pain and a reasonable blood pressure. Thrombolytic therapy should be considered for patients with electrocardiographic evidence of acute myocardial infarction. A cardiologist should be consulted to assess the need for cardiac catheterization or revascularization procedures.

Recurrent and Chronic Chest Pain

Patients with recurrent chest pain can be evaluated on an outpatient basis if their episodes are not prolonged, frequent, or progressive. Since **chronic stable angina** is the most important disease to consider, it is reasonable to start with a cardiac evaluation and to proceed with other studies if ischemic heart disease has been ruled out. Most physicians begin with an exercise tolerance test (ETT). Patients selected for this study should be capable of vigorous exercise and should not have baseline ECG abnormalities (such as a conduction defect or left ventricular strain) that would make interpretation of ST segment changes difficult. The ETT has relatively low sensitivity and specificity, particularly for young women. Patients who have baseline ECG abnormalities or a positive ETT should undergo radionuclide evaluation of cardiac perfusion or function and/or cardiac catheterization.

Younger patients with atypical chest pain might benefit from two-dimensional echocardiography. Idiopathic hypertrophic subaortic stenosis and mitral valve prolapse can cause chest discomfort and are easily detected by this study. In addition, the presence of segmental wall motion abnormalities should be taken as evidence that the patient has an ischemic cardiomyopathy.

Esophagitis and the esophageal motility disorders can produce symptoms that resemble angina pectoris. Esophageal spasm is often confused with angina because the location and quality of the pain are similar for the two disorders, and both respond to nitrates and calcium-channel blockers. Patients suspected of having esophageal disease can be evaluated by several different tests, including an upper GI series, upper GI endoscopy, acid-perfusion tests, or esophageal manometry. The first two studies are particularly useful for patients who have dysphagia. Esophageal manometry is not widely available but can provide evidence that the patient's symptoms are due to dysmotility.

PATIENT AND FAMILY EDUCATION

The type of counseling given to the patient and family depends upon the diagnosis. For instance, patients with pulmonary embolism should be cautioned about the hazards of prolonged immobilization, while those with reflux esophagitis should be told to avoid substances that decrease esophageal sphincter tone, to take antacids before retiring, to avoid late-night snacks, and to elevate the head of their bed with blocks. The counseling of patients with AIHD should be incorporated into a formal program of cardiac rehabilitation.

Special precautions should be taken for patients undergoing outpatient evaluation for stable, recurrent chest pain. These patients should be given sublingual nitroglycerin until ischemic heart disease can be excluded with certainty. If an episode is particularly severe or prolonged, the patient should take nitroglycerin. If no response is obtained within 5 minutes, a second dose should be taken. If no response occurs with the second dose, the patient should be instructed to call "911" for transport to the nearest emergency facility.

Research Questions

1. What characteristics of chest pain distinguish serious diseases (such as AIHD) from those that are more benign?
2. To what extent do these characteristics raise or lower the probability of AIHD?
3. Can the history, physical examination, and ETT be used to derive a probability of coronary disease?

Case Resolution

The patient was admitted to the hospital, where a diagnostic evaluation failed to confirm the presence of MI. He then underwent an exercise stress test, which was negative. He was discharged with the presumptive diagnosis of reflux esophagitis, and H_2-blocker therapy was initiated.

Selected Readings

American Heart Association. *Textbook of Advanced Cardiac Life Support.* Dallas, 1987, pp. 1–10.

Brush, J. E. Jr., D. A. Brand, D. Acampora, et al. Use of the initial electrocardiogram to predict in-hospital complications of acute myocardial infarction. N Engl J Med 312:1137–41, 1985.

Davies, H. A., D. B. Jones, J. Rhodes, and R. G. Newcombe. Angina-like esophageal pain: Differentiation from cardiac pain by history. J Clin Gastroenterol 7:477–81, 1985.

Lee T. H., E. F. Cook, M. Weisberg, et al. Acute chest pain in the emergency room: Identification and examination of low-risk patients. Arch Intern Med 145:65–9, 1985.

Murata, G. H. Evaluating chest pain in the emergency department. West J Med 159(1):61–8, 1993.

CHAPTER 36

CORONARY ARTERY DISEASE

Craig Timm, M.D.

Hx A 60-year-old female judge presents with a 1-year history of exertional chest tightness. The tightness comes on only with activity such as playing tennis or running up the steps of the courthouse. The discomfort radiates to the left shoulder and arm and is associated with mild nausea. It is always relieved within 5 minutes by resting. There has been no recent change in the pattern of the patient's chest discomfort. She had not sought medical attention previously because of a busy work schedule and because the symptoms were not particularly bothersome. She has had hypertension and hypercholesterolemia for several years but is not currently being treated. Her mother died of a "heart attack" at age 55 years, and a brother recently underwent coronary bypass surgery at age 62 years. There is no history of diabetes or tobacco use. Menopause occurred at age 45 years, and she has not been on hormonal replacement. She takes no prescription or over-the-counter medications. Her blood pressure is mildly elevated at 170/100 mm Hg. The rest of the cardiovascular examination is unremarkable.

Questions

1. What tests are useful in establishing the diagnosis of coronary artery disease?
2. What are the benefits and risks of commonly used medications for angina (i.e., chest discomfort due to myocardial ischemia)?
3. When should a patient with ischemic chest pain be admitted to the hospital?

Coronary artery disease is a common and chronic process that develops and progresses over many years. Consequently, it is the source of many outpatient clinic visits. The goals in this setting include establishing the diagnosis, controlling symptoms, and preventing disease progression as well as myocardial infarction and sudden death.

Improved understanding of the pathophysiologic processes that cause ischemic heart disease, better pharmacologic agents, and greater interest in a healthy life-style by the general population have all led to significant progress in the management of coronary artery disease.

CLINICAL PRESENTATION

The typical presentation of stable coronary artery disease in the outpatient setting is exertional angina. Classically, angina is described as a pressure sensation in the anterior chest, relieved by rest or nitroglycerin. Common associated symptoms include radiation of the discomfort to the left jaw and arm, nausea, shortness of breath, and light-headedness.

PATHOPHYSIOLOGY

Chapter 13 describes our current understanding of how atherosclerosis develops. Once an area of atherosclerotic narrowing develops in a coronary artery, it is the balance of oxygen supply and demand that determines whether myocardial ischemia occurs. Oxygen supply is determined by (1) the cardiac output, (2) the oxygen content of the blood (i.e., the hemoglobin level and its degree of saturation with oxygen), and (3) the presence of any obstruction to flow in the coronary arteries. Oxygen demand is determined primarily by the (1) heart rate, (2) ventricular wall tension (related to blood pressure and ventricular size and thickness), and (3) contractile state of the heart. Considering the multiple factors that affect oxygen supply and demand, it is clear that myocardial ischemia can develop in a variety of ways from either inadequate supply or excessive demand. In an otherwise healthy patient with atherosclerosis, however, the usual cause of myocardial ischemia is oxygen demand exceeding supply. This situation is typically due to the higher heart rate, blood pressure, and myocardial contractility that occur during exercise or stress. Chest pain or discomfort due to myocardial ischemia is called angina pectoris, or simply angina.

The syndromes of unstable angina, myocardial infarction, and ischemic sudden death are due to "rupture" of an atherosclerotic plaque, which causes platelet aggregation, thrombus formation, and complete or nearly complete occlusion of the artery. These syndromes, therefore, have a much different pathophysiology (i.e., acute or subacute loss of oxygen supply) from that of chronic stable angina.

DIFFERENTIAL DIAGNOSIS

The differential diagnosis of chest pain is covered in Chapter 35. Since patients with coronary artery disease

Dx **Coronary Artery Disease**

- History of typical angina.
- Presence of risk factors for coronary artery disease.
- Cardiac ischemia documented by stress testing.

BOX 36–1. Important Questions in the CAD History

1. Is the pain occurring more frequently? Has the use of nitroglycerin increased? (Most clinicians find it helpful to *quantify* nitroglycerin use; i.e., on average, how many tablets are used each week?)
2. Does the pain come on with less activity than previously? Does it occur at rest?
3. Is the duration of pain longer? What is the longest amount of time the pain has lasted?
4. Has the patient experienced any bleeding, are there any symptoms of respiratory problems that might have caused hypoxia, or has anything else occurred that could have affected oxygen supply?
5. Is the patient taking prescribed medications as directed?

can develop other disorders associated with chest pain syndromes, it is especially important to identify any *changes* in symptoms that could represent a new and possibly nonatherosclerotic problem.

EVALUATION

History

The key historical points are different in the patient with known or strongly suspected coronary artery disease than in the patient presenting with undiagnosed chest pain/discomfort (see Chapter 35). Once the diagnosis of coronary artery disease has been established, the history should focus on identifying changes in pattern that may suggest progression of disease or possibly unstable angina. Useful questions appear in Box 36–1.

A significant change in symptoms, e.g., prolonged pain not easily relieved by nitroglycerin or chest pain occurring at rest, is worrisome. Such patients should be considered for hospital admission for more intensive therapy and further evaluation.

Patients also should be asked about symptoms of left ventricular dysfunction as well as symptoms of vascular disease in other areas (e.g., cerebral and peripheral circulations). Many patients with coronary artery disease have reduced left ventricular function due to prior myocardial infarction. A history of new-onset or worsening heart failure (dyspnea on exertion, shortness of breath, paroxysmal nocturnal dyspnea, orthopnea, peripheral edema) suggests deteriorating ventricular function, possibly due to intercurrent infarction.

Since atherosclerosis is a diffuse process, patients with coronary artery disease also have a much higher incidence of peripheral vascular disease and cerebrovascular disease than does the general population. Patients with angina should be routinely asked about symptoms suggesting vascular insufficiency in these areas, i.e., intermittent claudication or transient ischemic attacks.

Physical Examination

The physical examination in a patient with stable angina should focus on the cardiovascular system, assessing for evidence of (1) prior myocardial infarction (e.g., abnormal apical impulse due to left ventricular aneurysm), (2) left ventricular dysfunction, (3) other vascular disease, and (4) risk factors that may be modifiable such as hypertension, diabetes, hyperlipidemia, or tobacco use.

Patients with stable symptoms and normal or well-compensated left ventricular function may demonstrate few abnormal physical findings. If the left ventricle is enlarged, however, the point of maximal impulse (PMI) is often laterally displaced. In addition, the presence of elevated jugular venous pressure, pulmonary congestion, or an S_3 gallop rhythm suggests decompensated heart failure that requires further evaluation and treatment (see Chapter 40).

Since atherosclerosis is a diffuse process, important pathologic changes may occur in other vascular beds. Carotid bruits may indicate cerebrovascular disease, while femoral bruits, diminished peripheral pulses, and evidence of arterial insufficiency (e.g., loss of toe hair, poor capillary filling, cool extremities) are all suggestive of coexisting peripheral vascular disease.

Additional Evaluation

Risk factors in patients with coronary artery disease require aggressive management to minimize the risk of disease progression and the development of complications. The lipid profile should be evaluated on a regular basis in all adult patients and the blood glucose carefully monitored in patients with diabetes.

When symptoms remain unchanged, the value of periodic **electrocardiography** is controversial. Nonetheless, a relatively recent ECG is often valuable for comparison purposes, especially when a patient presents urgently with symptoms suggesting an unstable coronary syndrome.

Specialized cardiac testing (e.g., echocardiography, stress testing, or other functional assessments) is not generally recommended on a routine basis in patients with stable symptoms who have previously been evaluated to a sufficient degree to establish the diagnosis.

In contrast, the initial diagnostic evaluation of patients with *suspected* coronary artery disease usually should include an exercise tolerance test. The purpose of this test is to establish the diagnosis (if it is in doubt) and to identify patients with a "markedly positive" result. Such "markedly positive" results include (1) severe ischemia, (2) ischemia early in exercise or lasting well into recovery, (3) ischemia in multiple vascular territories, and (4) hypotension with exercise, each of which points to severe multivessel or severe left main coronary artery disease. These patients should undergo further evaluation including cardiac catheterization.

Additional testing may also be warranted if the history reveals a change in the pattern or type of chest pain. Similarly, the onset of new or different symptoms that may reflect other diagnoses (e.g., gastrointestinal or pulmonary problems or cardiac problems not related to ischemia) should prompt the physician to carry out additional testing as appropriate.

A patient may experience a change in the pattern of angina without becoming truly "unstable." For example, an increase in nitroglycerin use from once a month to twice a week raises the question of disease progression. In these situations, an exercise stress test (or another type of stress testing) can be beneficial to (1) evaluate the response to intensified therapy and (2) identify patients with "markedly positive" tests (see above).

MANAGEMENT

Risk factor modification (see Chapters 13, 38, 77, 79, and 105) includes (1) aggressive lowering of lipids, (2) strict control of blood glucose in patients with diabetes, (3) optimal antihypertensive therapy, (4) smoking cessation, and (5) development of a life-style characterized by regular, appropriate exercise, stress reduction, and a healthy diet.

Pharmacologic agents (Table 36–1) are useful to control symptoms and prevent subsequent adverse events. **Nitrates** are available in many forms and routes of administration. They act primarily as coronary vasodilators (improving myocardial blood flow) and secondarily by decreasing preload (venodilation), which decreases ventricular wall tension and therefore oxygen demand. Since nitrate tolerance occurs with chronic use, nitrates should be given in a way that provides a nitrate-free interval of 12 hours to prevent tolerance from developing. Headache is the most common adverse effect of nitrate administration.

Calcium channel blockers are more heterogeneous than nitrates. The dihydropyridines (e.g., nifedipine, nicardipine, amlodipine, felodipine) have prominent vasodilatory properties and therefore increase coronary blood flow. Reflex tachycardia is common (except with amlodipine) and may limit their utility unless a β-blocker is used concomitantly. Diltiazem and verapamil are the other calcium channel blockers used for treating myocardial ischemia. They have prominent negative inotropic and chronotropic effects. These actions lead to decreased blood pressure, heart rate, and contractility, which together help reduce myocardial oxygen consumption. Their mild vasodilatory effect is less pronounced than that produced by the dihydropyridines. Adverse effects of diltiazem and verapamil are related primarily to their mechanism of action and include development of congestive heart failure, symptomatic bradycardia, and heart block (the last related to their AV node blocking effect).

β-Blockers are commonly used in treating chronic coronary artery disease and are available in many preparations. β-Blockers differ in their metabolism as well as in their β_1 selectivity (e.g., atenolol and metoprolol are β_1 selective, whereas propranolol is nonselective). All β-blockers decrease oxygen consumption by reducing heart rate, blood pressure, and myocardial contractility, effects mediated by antagonism of adrenergic activity. Side effects are related to these actions and include hypotension, excessive bradycardia, heart block, and worsening of heart failure.

Aspirin is recommended for all patients with known coronary artery disease who do not have strong contraindications to its use (e.g., active peptic ulcer disease, renal disease, bleeding diathesis). The antiplatelet effect of aspirin is useful in stabilizing plaques and preventing development of unstable coronary syndromes.

PATIENT AND FAMILY EDUCATION

Unquestionably the most important contribution a primary care physician can make in the care of patients who have (or are at risk of developing) coronary artery disease is to educate them about the role of risk factor modification in the prevention of coronary artery disease. Risk factor modification often requires changing lifelong patterns of eating, smoking, and exercise. Developing the required degree of motivation will occur only if the patient is educated regarding the expected benefits of such changes. Words of encouragement and support from care providers are also helpful in the motivation process.

The patient should understand the indications for (and possible adverse effects of) all prescribed medications. Open communication between patient and physician ensures that patients will feel free to report side

TABLE 36–1. Pharmacologic Therapy of Angina

Medication	Usual Dose	Adverse Effects
Nitrates		
Isosorbide dinitrate	20–40 mg three times daily	Headache, tolerance
Nitroglycerin patch	0.2–0.4 mg/h	Same as for isosorbide
Nitroglycerin, sublingual	0.4 mg as needed	Headache
Calcium Channel Blockers		
Nifedipine	30–90 mg/d	Peripheral edema, light-headedness, headache, reflex tachycardia
Amlodipine	5–20 mg/d	Peripheral edema, light-headedness
Diltiazem	120–300 mg/d	Heart failure, hypotension, excess bradycardia, heart block
Verapamil	180–240 mg/d	Same as for diltiazem, constipation
β-Blockers (Nonselective)		
Propranolol	10–80 mg four times daily	Same as for diltiazem, bronchospasm
Timolol	10–30 mg twice daily	Same as for propranolol
β-Blockers (β_1 or Cardioselective)		
Atenolol	50–100 mg/d	Same as for diltiazem
Metoprolol	25–100 mg twice daily	Same as for diltiazem

effects rather than unilaterally stopping medications if they believe side effects are occurring. Patients should be aware that alternative medications are available if adverse effects require discontinuation of a specific drug.

Finally, patients should be instructed regarding when to seek medical attention. Some changes in anginal pattern may require only an adjustment in medication, while others may require further testing or admission to the hospital (e.g., suspected unstable angina or acute myocardial infarction).

Family members who learn about risk factors for coronary artery disease will likely become interested in identifying and modifying their own risk factors. Efforts to prevent cardiovascular disease have the greatest impact when begun at an early age. Family education is also helpful in fostering a cooperative team effort. Family members can encourage each other in developing an exercise program, eating a healthier diet, and stopping smoking.

NATURAL HISTORY/PROGNOSIS

Coronary artery disease is a chronic condition that is likely to progress slowly but inexorably unless the risk factor profile is significantly improved. Recent studies indicate that it may be possible to halt progression of disease if not actually cause regression. The currently available treatments for coronary artery disease—including medications, percutaneous revascularization (most commonly coronary angioplasty), and coronary artery bypass surgery—are palliative. In certain circumstances, they can even prolong life (e.g., bypass surgery in patients with multivessel or left main coronary artery disease and reduced left ventricular function). However, unless the milieu that leads to atherosclerosis develop-

ment and progression is favorably altered, these treatments only delay the inevitable.

Research Questions

1. At a biochemical/molecular level, what inherited or acquired characteristics make some people more susceptible than others to the development and progression of coronary artery disease?

2. How can we improve our ability to noninvasively identify patients who are at higher risk for plaque rupture and development of unstable coronary syndromes?

Case Resolution

The patient underwent an exercise tolerance test. Her typical chest pain—as well as ischemic changes on the ECG—developed at a high level of exercise. Therapy was initiated with isosorbide dinitrate, aspirin, and sublingual nitroglycerin. Lipid analysis revealed an elevated total cholesterol with an elevated low-density lipoprotein (LDL) and a decreased high-density lipoprotein (HDL). Initial management of her hyperlipidemia included encouragement of regular exercise and instruction on how to decrease her dietary intake of total fat and saturated fat.

Selected Readings

Rutherford, J. D., and E. Braunwald. Chronic ischemic heart disease. *In* E. Braunwald (ed.). *Heart Disease*, 4th ed, Philadelphia, W.B. Saunders Company, 1992.

Selwyn, A. P., et al. Pathophysiology of ischemia in patients with coronary artery disease. Prog Cardiovasc Dis 35:27–39, 1992.

C H A P T E R   3 7

PALPITATIONS AND ARRHYTHMIAS

Gary M. Greenberg, M.D.

H$_x$1 A 25-year-old female law student presents with a several-year history of "heart thumping" and "pounding." These sensations last only seconds at a time and can occur several times during the day without known precipitating or alleviating factors. There is no associated dizziness, syncope, shortness of breath, or chest pain. The sensations make her feel anxious and she wants to know what they are due to and if they represent "something serious." She is taking no medications, and her medical history and

review of systems are unremarkable. The physical examination and 12-lead ECG are both normal.

H$_x$2 A 62-year-old male retired telephone installer presents with a complaint of "rapid, regular heart pounding" that occurs suddenly without warning, makes him feel dizzy, and lasts up to 1 hour. He has had five such spells in the past 2 years. He now seeks medical attention because the last spell was associated with brief syncope, an event he found especially frightening. He is taking an angiotensin converting enzyme (ACE) inhibitor for hypertension and had a myocardial infarction 7 years ago. However, he states that he has not experienced chest pain since that time and also denies shortness of breath, orthopnea, and paroxysmal nocturnal dyspnea. His physical examination is unremarkable, and his 12-lead ECG shows Q waves in the inferior leads suggestive of an old inferior wall myocardial infarction.

Questions

1. What other questions might you want to ask these patients?
2. What physical examination findings might be especially important to search for and document?
3. Do these patients' symptoms represent a potentially serious condition or are they medically inconsequential?
4. Which tests or procedures can assist you in the evaluation of palpitations?

Palpitations are a ubiquitous anxiety-provoking symptom that may represent a benign process requiring little more than patient education and reassurance. Often they represent only an acute awareness of the normal heartbeat in otherwise healthy individuals. However, in individuals with underlying structural heart disease, palpitations may be associated with syncope or be a harbinger of sudden death, and in this setting they usually require intensive evaluation and therapy.

PATHOPHYSIOLOGY

In most otherwise healthy people, palpitations are due only to an enhanced perception of the normal heart rate. When a primary sustained bradycardiac or tachycardiac rhythm disturbance is present, the perceived palpitation can be due to the change in heart rate or rhythm (i.e., irregularity), or it can be due to changes in cardiac function, especially contractility (force of contraction) or stroke volume (volume of contraction). In addition, a variety of cardiac and noncardiac conditions (e.g., medications, thyroid disease, anemia) may secondarily affect cardiac rhythm or function and thus result in palpitations (Table 37–1).

Sporadic palpitations described as a heart "skip" or "stop" are often due to simple ventricular or supraventricular ectopic beats. The symptoms are related to (1) the "compensatory" pause after the ectopic beat and (2) the subsequent sinus beat, which usually is characterized by increased volume and increased contractility.

The palpitation perceived during an episode of primary sustained tachycardia is usually due to the change in rate (and sometimes rhythm) of the ventricles. The atria do not have sufficient mass or stroke volume to evoke palpitations, although a "flutter" sensation in the neck is often perceived during atrial tachyarrhythmias. Primary atrial arrhythmias are often associated with

underlying heart (e.g., valvular, myocardial, pericardial) or lung disease (e.g., emphysema). Other supraventricular arrhythmias—such as atrioventricular (AV) nodal reentrant tachycardia and AV reciprocating tachycardia associated with the presence of accessory pathways (Wolff-Parkinson-White syndrome)—usually are not associated with structural heart disease. These tachyarrhythmias typically present with sudden onset and offset, as well as rapid and regular palpitations.

Ventricular tachycardias occur most often in survivors of myocardial infarction; the perceived palpitations are similar to reentrant supraventricular tachycardias although they tend to be more hemodynamically unstable and therefore may have more serious associated symptoms such as syncope, chest pain, and shortness of breath. More importantly, they have the potential to degenerate into ventricular fibrillation and result in sudden death. A special type of polymorphic ventricular tachycardia called torsades de pointes can occur in normal hearts and is associated with a long QT interval on the ECG. Torsades de pointes can be either (1) reversibly produced by an electrolyte abnormality, toxin, or

---

TABLE 37–1. Differential Diagnosis of Palpitations

Primary Arrhythmic Causes
Sinus tachycardia or arrhythmia
Premature supraventricular or ventricular ectopic contractions
Tachy-brady syndrome (sick sinus syndrome)
Supraventricular tachycardia
    Multifocal atrial tachycardia
    Atrial fibrillation/flutter/tachycardia
    AV nodal reentrant tachycardia
    AV reciprocating tachycardia (Wolff-Parkinson-White syndrome)
    Accelerated junctional rhythm
Ventricular tachycardia
Bradycardia due to advanced AV block or sinus node dysfunction

Other Cardiac Causes
Changes in contractility or stroke volume
    Valvular disease such as aortic insufficiency or stenosis
    Atrial or ventricular septal defect
    Congestive heart failure
    Cardiomyopathy
    Congenital heart disease
Pericarditis
Pacemaker-mediated tachycardia
Pacemaker syndrome

Extracardiac Causes
Changes in contractility, heart rate, or stroke volume
    Fever
    Hypovolemia
    Anemia
    Hypoglycemia
    Pulmonary disease
    Pheochromocytoma
    Thyrotoxicosis
    Vasovagal episodes
Drugs
    Vasodilators
    Substance abuse (cocaine, alcohol, tobacco, caffeine)
    Digitalis
    Phenothiazines
    Theophylline
    β-Agonists
    Antiarrhythmics

Psychiatric Causes
Panic attack
Hyperventilation

drug (e.g., quinidine) or (2) due to a congenital electrical disorder that prolongs ventricular repolarization.

Primary bradyarrhythmias (e.g., sinus node dysfunction or paroxysmal high-grade AV block) can result in palpitations owing to changes in heart rate, contractility, or stroke volume. Sick sinus syndrome may cause palpitations either from the atrial tachyarrhythmia component or from the long sinus pauses that often follow the spontaneous cessation of the atrial tachycardia.

Patients with implanted pacemakers can feel palpitations due to a variety of mechanisms: many patients can perceive the change in heart contractility or the AV dissociation produced when a demand ventricular pacemaker is intermittently used, while dual chamber pacemakers are susceptible to induction of a pacemaker-mediated tachycardia.

A variety of drugs can cause palpitations including prescription medications, such as β-agonists, antiarrhythmics, vasodilators, and psychotropics, and recreational drugs such as cocaine, alcohol, caffeine, and nicotine. Drugs can cause palpitations via several mechanisms including increases in heart rate, changes in rhythm (e.g., ectopic beats), and changes in contractility. In addition, certain drugs (e.g., antiarrhythmic agents) have the potential to be proarrhythmic.

Other extracardiac conditions can similarly cause palpitations via changes in contractility, stroke volume, or heart rate. These include fever, sepsis, anemia, hypovolemia, thyroid disease, and pulmonary disease.

Finally, palpitations may be nothing more than an increased awareness of the normal heartbeat and may sometimes have a psychiatric basis. Complaints of palpitations are frequent in patients who have panic or anxiety attacks and in those who hyperventilate. In these cases, the palpitation usually is not a primary arrhythmia, underlying heart disease usually is not present, and the attacks do not typically result in serious associated symptoms.

DIFFERENTIAL DIAGNOSIS

When interviewing patients, it is helpful to remember that the differential diagnosis of palpitations can be divided into four major categories: primary arrhythmic, cardiac, extracardiac, and psychiatric (see Table 37–1).

EVALUATION

History

Palpitations often pose a diagnostic challenge because of (1) the broad range of descriptive terms used by patients, (2) the subjective nature of the symptomatology, and (3) the typically infrequent, episodic nature of the experience. Adjectives such as "fluttering," "skipping," "stopping," "pounding," "regular" or "irregular," and "heavy" are used by patients to describe their symptoms. A difficult-to-explain paradox is that some patients with "benign" dysrhythmias are highly symptomatic while other patients with more serious, incessant dysrhythmias are completely unaware of them.

Patients must be thoroughly questioned regarding

(1) the nature of their symptoms, (2) how frequently they occur, (3) how much these symptoms bother them or interfere with their life, and (4) what associated complaints and underlying medical conditions are present. Patients should also be asked about events that preceded the palpitations and how the palpitations resolved. Inquiry should be made about the use of caffeine, alcohol, cigarettes, illicit drugs (e.g., cocaine), and sympathomimetic medications (e.g., β-agonists, over-the-counter "diet" or "cold" pills).

Sometimes it is helpful to have the patient attempt to "tap out" the palpitation to gain insight into its rate and regularity. If the episode starts and ends abruptly and is associated with a rapid and irregular rhythm, paroxysmal atrial fibrillation is suggested. If the rhythm is rapid and regular, other supraventricular arrhythmias (such as AV nodal or AV reciprocating reentrant tachycardias) are suggested. A history of termination with vagal maneuvers (e.g., Valsalva maneuver, a cold splash to the face, carotid sinus massage) also is suggestive of a reentrant supraventricular tachycardia. Severe associated symptoms such as shortness of breath, syncope, dizziness, diaphoresis, and chest pain are suggestive of ventricular tachycardia, especially when there is a history of coronary artery disease. However, severe associated symptoms can occur with sustained reentrant supraventricular arrhythmias when the rate is sufficiently fast or when other medical illnesses are present (e.g., significant cardiac, pulmonary, renal, or hematologic disease).

A history of palpitations associated with rapid breathing, anxiety, and perioral numbness is highly suggestive of panic attacks or hyperventilation. Gradual onset of dizziness associated with nausea, a "hot feeling," and diaphoresis in an environment of anxiety, fear, or pain (e.g., venipuncture) strongly suggest a vasovagal spell. These spells are characterized by rapid, spontaneous, and complete resolution when the patient assumes a supine posture.

The past medical history and social history can provide information about (1) the use of prescription, over-the-counter, and illicit drugs; (2) the use of caffeine, alcohol, and nicotine; (3) underlying structural heart disease; (4) other significant medical diagnoses; and (5) any previously documented rhythm disturbances. A family history of structural heart disease, arrhythmia, syncope, or sudden death may be important. Some conditions such as hypertrophic cardiomyopathy, congenital long QT syndrome, and Wolff-Parkinson-White syndrome occur in inherited familial patterns.

Careful observation of the patient's mental and emotional status should be made during history taking. Issues of financial, job-related, family-related, or other social stresses should be thoroughly explored to assess for primary psychiatric diagnoses as well as functional symptoms.

Physical Examination

The physical examination usually is normal, especially when performed when the patient is asymptomatic. However, it is important to document the presence (and severity) of any underlying condition that may be associated with palpitations.

A thorough cardiovascular examination needs to be performed starting with the pulse. Ectopic beats are suggested if the pulse is irregular; however, an ECG is needed to verify the type of ectopy (e.g., atrial, junctional, or ventricular). A very slow pulse might suggest sinus node dysfunction or AV block. A bounding "water hammer" pulse is suggestive of aortic insufficiency. Pulsus alternans (a pulse that alternates between strong and weak) is suggestive of congestive heart failure.

Assessment of other vital signs may provide clues. Orthostatic blood pressure readings should be performed to rule out volume depletion. Accompanying pallor may suggest anemia. Fever due to any cause may be responsible for a rapid pulse, i.e., a sinus tachycardia.

The neck examination should include a search for thyroid enlargement or bruits suggestive of hyperthyroidism. An elevated jugular venous pressure is suggestive of increased right-sided filling pressure due to congestive heart failure (CHF), lung disease, pericardial tamponade, or restrictive cardiomyopathy. Careful examination of the jugular venous pulsation may show evidence of atrial fibrillation if the a wave is absent (also, the pulse will be irregularly irregular). Cannon a waves occur when AV dissociation is present, and their presence suggests either ventricular tachycardia or complete heart block. Atrial flutter may be diagnosed if "flutter" waves are present.

Cardiac auscultation needs to be carefully performed to look for underlying structural heart disease. An S_3 is suggestive of both hyperdynamic states (e.g., anemia, high-output congestive heart failure, thyrotoxicosis) and low-output congestive heart failure. An S_4 is suggestive of hypertension or myocardial disease (e.g., ischemic or dilated cardiomyopathy). Murmurs of valvular regurgitation or stenosis may be present. Lateral displacement of the point of maximum impulse is suggestive of an enlarged and weakened left ventricle. Rales on lung examination are suggestive of congestive heart failure. Wheezes, purse-lipped breathing, and altered chest shape (with increased anteroposterior diameter) suggest chronic obstructive pulmonary disease.

Additional Evaluation

The usually transient nature of palpitations can make it difficult to pinpoint the diagnosis, and ECG documentation at the time of the event is almost always needed to determine whether a primary rhythm disturbance is present. A search for underlying structural heart disease should be undertaken, since its severity usually determines the prognosis.

The **noninvasive tests** have relatively low cost and fair yield. All the tests can be performed on an outpatient basis. The decision to hospitalize depends on a number of clinical variables. Hospitalization is more likely to be necessary when associated severe symptoms such as syncope have occurred, especially when there is significant underlying structural heart disease. Since palpitations in such individuals may be a marker of a serious rhythm disturbance (e.g., ventricular tachycardia), a more expeditious workup, often including invasive testing, is indicated. In this way, serious rhythm disturbances can be quickly diagnosed (or ruled out); if present, such rhythm disturbances can be aggressively treated to prevent syncope and possibly sudden death.

Basic laboratory tests such as a CBC and chemistry panel usually are normal; however, they sometimes are helpful in screening for underlying conditions such as anemia or electrolyte abnormalities (e.g., hypokalemia, hypomagnesemia). If endocrine dysfunction (e.g., hyperthyroidism, hypoglycemia, or pheochromocytoma) is suspected, then additional laboratory testing should be performed.

A **12-lead ECG** probably should be performed in most, if not all, patients who complain of palpitations. However, the primary cause of palpitations is only rarely diagnosed with a single ECG. Clues that may be apparent on an ECG include (1) a delta wave suggesting the presence of an accessory pathway in Wolff-Parkinson-White syndrome, (2) q waves consistent with a previous myocardial infarction, (3) ST-T wave changes suggesting an electrolyte disturbance or coronary artery disease, (4) enhanced voltage indicative of left ventricular hypertrophy, and (5) a prolonged QT interval due to drugs, an electrolyte disturbance, or a congenital repolarization abnormality.

In making a definitive diagnosis, there is no substitute for ECG or rhythm strip documentation during a palpitation episode. Such a recording will show either a primary dysrhythmia or a normal heart rhythm that is perceived as a palpitation by the patient. If palpitations occur frequently (i.e., daily), a **24- to 48-hour ambulatory monitor**—often referred to as a Holter monitor—may suffice. The patient should be instructed to write down the exact time any symptom occurs so that the tape during those times can be carefully scanned. Some Holter systems have a button that can be pushed when symptoms occur; this "labels" the recording so that the scanners can more easily print out the corresponding rhythm strip. Ambulatory monitors are most useful when (1) an arrhythmia is documented at the exact time symptoms are being experienced or (2) normal sinus rhythm is consistently found at the time of symptoms, thus ruling out a primary arrhythmia as the cause. Ambulatory monitoring is more difficult to interpret if the patient experienced no symptoms but one or more "benign" arrhythmias are present on the recording. "Benign" arrhythmias commonly documented in the ambulatory recordings of normal healthy individuals include (1) premature atrial, junctional, and ventricular contractions; (2) sinus arrhythmia; (3) sinus bradycardia; (4) pauses up to 3 seconds (especially when sleeping); and (5) second-degree Wenckebach AV block.

A limitation inherent in Holter monitoring is that episodes of palpitations sometimes occur only infrequently. Transtelephonic **event recorders** with continuous memory loop allow for more prolonged monitoring.

These can be kept by the patient for extended periods of time (weeks to months). Some are worn all the time, while others can be attached to the fingers or chest when an event occurs. They are activated when the patient presses a button so the rhythm can be recorded at the precise time that an episode of palpitations occurs. Continuous memory-loop monitors are especially useful for the patient with episodic syncope. The monitor is worn all the time and is activated after awakening from a syncopal event, thus retroactively recording the rhythm that occurred during syncope.

Exercise stress testing is most valuable when the reported palpitation is associated with (or occurs just after) exercise. It is also useful in that it may suggest underlying ischemic coronary artery disease (CAD). Such CAD may be the cause of the palpitations; even if it is not, however, it may still require further evaluation and management in its own right.

Echocardiography is useful to confirm the presence—and gauge the severity—of underlying structural heart disease. It probably is not cost effective if the cardiac physical examination is entirely normal. The **head-up tilt table test** can provoke vasovagal spells (i.e., hypotension with sinus bradycardia producing dizziness or frank syncope) in susceptible individuals.

Invasive tests are generally performed on an inpatient basis. **Electrophysiologic study** (EPS) is best reserved for those in whom a sustained supraventricular or ventricular tachycardia is suspected; examples include a young patient with Wolff-Parkinson-White syndrome but an otherwise normal heart or an elderly patient with coronary artery disease and a previous myocardial infarction. EPS utilizes several multielectrode pacing catheters inserted percutaneously and advanced to various positions in the heart under fluoroscopic guidance. The catheters can be used to (1) electrically induce arrhythmias in susceptible individuals, (2) diagnose the arrhythmia mechanism, (3) cure arrhythmias by application of radiofrequency energy to "ablate" (scar) the portion of the heart responsible for the arrhythmia circuit, and (4) test the efficacy of drugs used to treat the arrhythmia. EPS can also be used to diagnose brady-arrhythmias, although Holter monitoring is usually more sensitive and specific. **Cardiac catheterization** is utilized to assess the extent of underlying coronary artery disease and to help with management decisions (e.g., medical therapy, angioplasty, or surgery).

MANAGEMENT

Treatment is aimed at (1) controlling the primary dysrhythmia, (2) managing the underlying cardiac or noncardiac condition responsible for the patient's symptoms, or (3) providing reassurance to the patient whose symptoms do not represent a life-threatening process.

In young healthy patients, often all that is needed is reassurance that the condition is not life-threatening possibly accompanied by behavior modification to facilitate cessation of tobacco, alcohol, or recreational drug use. Some patients may benefit from counseling or anxiolytic therapy, especially when the palpitations are associated with stress and a suitable evaluation finds no arrhythmia or other organic pathology. Healthy patients with a delta wave or long QT interval on the ECG should be referred to a cardiologist who specializes in treatment of arrhythmias.

Underlying medical disorders should be treated. Primary rhythm disorders can usually be managed with (1) antiarrhythmic drugs, (2) devices such as pacemakers (for symptomatic bradyarrhythmias) or defibrillators (for life-threatening ventricular arrhythmias), (3) angioplasty or coronary bypass surgery in the case of severe CAD, or (4) radiofrequency catheter ablation. The management of primary arrhythmias is best left to a cardiologist, since antiarrhythmic drug therapy can be quite complex; antiarrhythmic drugs, for example, sometimes *cause* new arrhythmias such as torsades de pointes.

PATIENT AND FAMILY EDUCATION

Most otherwise healthy patients presenting with palpitations will not have a life-threatening condition and often need nothing beyond reassurance, education, or perhaps behavior modification or emotional counseling. The same reassurance and education should be provided to family members, preferably at the same time, in order to dispel the often-held assumption that a life-threatening heart condition is present.

NATURAL HISTORY/PROGNOSIS

Prognosis is directly related to the degree of underlying illness, especially structural heart disease. Patients with poor left ventricular function secondary to previous myocardial infarctions have the substrate for developing sustained ventricular arrhythmias, which could degenerate into ventricular fibrillation and subsequent sudden death. Conversely, those without underlying myocardial, valvular, or electrical heart disease usually have a better prognosis even if a specific dysrhythmia is documented.

Survivors of myocardial infarction who have frequent ventricular ectopic beats represent a particularly thorny therapeutic problem, since ventricular ectopic beats appear to be associated with increased mortality. Prior to the results of the Cardiac Arrhythmia Suppression Trial (CAST) published in 1989, the widely held belief was that prognosis could be improved if these ectopic beats were suppressed with antiarrhythmic drugs. In the CAST, however, successful suppression of frequent ventricular ectopic beats with the antiarrhythmic drugs encainide and flecainide resulted in a significantly higher sudden death rate and total mortality rate than was found in a comparable group of post-myocardial infarction patients who were given placebo. Thus, post-myocardial infarction patients with ventricular ectopy may face an increased risk of death if the ectopy is treated with primary antiarrhythmic drugs. Such patients probably should be referred to a cardiologist for guidance in clinical decision making.

Research Question

1. Compared to other available diagnostic tests, what is the incremental yield of continuous memory-loop event recorders in the diagnostic evaluation of palpitations?

Case Resolutions

The first patient was evaluated using a 24-hour ambulatory monitor and was found to have isolated premature ventricular contractions. She was reassured that her palpitations were "benign," and she declined further testing as well as anxiolytic treatment.

The nature of the second patient's symptoms (as well as his known history of coronary artery disease) made ventricular tachycardia a leading diagnostic consideration. An exercise stress test was negative for ischemic changes or arrhythmia induction. A Holter monitor was also negative, and the patient failed to have symptoms during the 2-week period when he used an event monitor. Subsequent EPS, however, showed inducible ventricular tachycardia. He eventually received an internal defibrillator, and to date

he has experienced no shocks from his device nor has he had any further syncopal episodes.

Selected Readings

Brown, A. P., K. D. Dawkins, and J. G. Davies. Detection of arrhythmias: Use of a patient-activated ambulatory electrocardiogram device with a solid-state memory loop. Br Heart J 58:251, 1987.

Cardiac Arrhythmia Suppression Trial (CAST) Investigation. Preliminary report: Effect of encainide and flecainide on mortality in a randomized trial of arrhythmia suppression after myocardial infarction. N Engl J Med 321:406–12, 1989.

Ducasse, R., and E. E. Hardman. Transtelephonic cardiac monitoring: A comprehensive review of clinical applications. Crit Care Nurs 8:44–51, 1988.

Goldman, L., and E. Braunwald. Chest discomfort and palpitation. In J. D. Wilson et. al. (eds.). Harrison's Principles of Internal Medicine, 12th ed. New York, McGraw-Hill Book Company, 1991.

Knoebel, S. B., et al. Guidelines for ambulatory electrocardiography. J Am Coll Cardiol 13:249–58, 1989.

Kopp, D. E., and D. J. Wilber. Palpitations and arrhythmias: Separating the benign from the dangerous. Postgrad Med 91:241–51, 1992.

Levitt, M. A. Palpitations. In G. C. Hamilton, A. B. Sanders, G. R. Strange, and A. T. Trott (eds.). Emergency Medicine: An Approach To Clinical Problem Solving. Philadelphia, W.B. Saunders Company, 1991.

Linzer, M., et. al. Incremental diagnostic yield of loop electrocardiographic recorders in unexplained syncope. Am J Cardiol 66:214, 1990.

CHAPTER 38

HYPERTENSION

Alan K. Halperin, M.D.

H$_x$ A 52-year-old male firefighter comes in for a routine health maintenance examination. He feels well and has no major medical problems. Upon examination, his blood pressure in his left arm is 158/104 mm Hg and is unchanged after he has been sitting quietly for 5 minutes. The rest of his physical examination is normal.

Questions

1. How is the diagnosis of hypertension confirmed, and how is it classified?
2. What evaluation is necessary?
3. What life-style modifications lower blood pressure, and can they prevent the development of hypertension?
4. What pharmacologic agents are used to treat hypertension, and how would you select the most appropriate choice?
5. What are the long-term consequences of inadequately treated hypertension?

During the past 20 years, there has been remarkable progress in the detection, treatment, and control of hypertension. This has significantly contributed to the decline in the morbidity and mortality associated with coronary heart disease and stroke.

It is estimated that 50 million Americans (approximately 20% of the adult population of the United States) have hypertension, which is defined as a systolic blood pressure (SBP) greater than 140 mm Hg and/or a diastolic blood pressure (DBP) greater than 90 mm Hg. The prevalence of hypertension increases with age, in African Americans, in those with a family history of hypertension, and in those from lower socioeconomic groups. Hypertension is a major risk factor for coronary heart disease, congestive heart failure, stroke, and renal disease. Increased SBP and DBP both are strong predictors of morbidity and mortality. These relationships are continuous, graded, strong, independent, and epidemiologically significant.

CLINICAL PRESENTATION

Most people with hypertension are asymptomatic. Symptoms sometimes attributed to hypertension such as headache, epistaxis, and dizziness are equally present in the normotensive population. Occasionally, patients with hypertension can present with end organ damage, such as stroke, myocardial infarction, and renal failure.

PATHOPHYSIOLOGY

The mean arterial pressure is the product of cardiac output and systemic vascular resistance (SVR). Each of these elements is determined by an extremely complex interaction of many factors. The underlying abnormality in patients with essential or primary hypertension is unknown. However, the hallmark of established hypertension is increased SVR. SVR is both functional and structural and can result from a number of different pathways, including (1) increased sympathetic nervous system activity and catecholamines, (2) activation of the renin-angiotensin-aldosterone system, and (3) alterations of the permeability of cell membranes to cations such as sodium and calcium. Some of these factors are undoubtedly hereditary, since normotensive males have a 2.5 times greater relative risk of developing hypertension if they have one first-degree relative with hypertension. Although the initiating factors are not known, vascular hypertrophy is an inevitable result. Many of the pressor substances mentioned above are also growth factors that promote vascular hypertrophy. Hypertensive individuals may have an exaggerated response to both pressor and growth factor changes. The etiology and pathophysiology of many secondary causes of hypertension, such as renovascular hypertension, pheochromocytoma, and hyperaldosteronism, involve elaboration of excess pressor hormones.

DIFFERENTIAL DIAGNOSIS

In most people, blood pressure is labile, and the higher the pressure the greater the lability. Because of this lability, at least three readings are required for the diagnosis of hypertension unless the blood pressure is

TABLE 38–1. Classification System for Hypertension in Adults		
Category	SBP (mm Hg)	DBP (mm Hg)
Normal	< 130	< 85
High normal	130–139	85–89
Hypertension		
Stage 1 (mild)	140–159	90–99
Stage 2 (moderate)	160–179	100–109
Stage 3 (severe)	180–209	110–119
Stage 4 (very severe)	> 210	> 120

extremely elevated (e.g., > 200/120 mm Hg). Blood pressure measurements should be obtained after the patient has rested 5 minutes, is seated, and has on a properly sized cuff (the cuff should nearly encircle the arm). Blood pressure can be elevated in the office setting ("white coat" hypertension) but normal in other locations. Therefore, it is recommended that blood pressure measurements be obtained in the office, home, and other settings with inexpensive recording devices or automatic, portable, ambulatory recording devices. Treatment decisions should be based on all measurements. Table 38–1 provides a classification of blood pressure for adults.

The majority of hypertensive patients have stage 1 hypertension. Usually both SBP and DBP are elevated. When only the SBP is elevated, it is termed isolated systolic hypertension.

EVALUATION

The purpose of the evaluation is to (1) screen for secondary causes of hypertension, (2) determine whether target organ damage is present, (3) detect other cardiovascular risk factors, and (4) develop a treatment plan.

History

The following points should be stressed: the duration of hypertension; previous treatment and response; presence of a family history of hypertension, premature coronary heart disease, stroke, diabetes, or hyperlipidemia; patient history of target organ damage such as coronary heart disease, congestive heart failure, cerebrovascular disease, or renal disease; other risk factors such as diabetes and hyperlipidemia; habits such as physical activity and tobacco use; dietary assessment of salt and fat ingestion and alcohol use; use of competing substances such as nonsteroidal antiinflammatory drugs, oral contraceptives, decongestants or cold remedies, appetite suppressants, corticosteroids, cyclosporine, or erythropoietin; and psychosocial or socioeconomic factors that might influence blood pressure control.

In addition, patients should be questioned about the presence of secondary causes of hypertension (Table 38–2). Less than 5% of cases of hypertension are due to secondary causes; however, it is important to identify

---

Dx   **Hypertension**

- Three BP measurements over one to several weeks with mean SBP > 140 mm Hg and/or mean DBP > 90 mm Hg.
- One BP measurement > 210/120.

these causes because they are potentially curable and, if corrected, can obviate the need for lifelong medication. Most patients with hypertension have no symptoms. Symptoms often attributed to hypertension such as headache, epistaxis, and dizziness are equally common in hypertensive and normotensive persons.

Physical Examination

The physical examination emphasizes the vascular system and includes the following: verification of the blood pressure in both arms and legs if coarctation of the aorta is suspected; measurement of height and weight; funduscopic examination for arteriolar narrowing, arteriovenous nicking, hemorrhages, exudates, and papilledema (indicating the severity and duration of hypertension); examination of the carotid pulses for bruits (suggesting generalized arteriosclerosis); examination of the thyroid; examination of the heart for rate, size, murmurs, and extra sounds such as S_3 or S_4 gallops (suggesting congestive heart failure); examination of the abdomen for bruits (suggesting renovascular hypertension), enlarged kidneys (suggesting polycystic kidney disease), and aneurysms; examination of the extremities for pulses and edema; and a neurologic assessment.

Additional Evaluation

A small number of laboratory tests should be performed at the initial assessment including CBC, glucose, potassium, urinalysis, creatinine, lipids (cholesterol, high-density lipoprotein, triglyceride) and electrocardiogram. These tests serve as a baseline, detect other cardiac risk factors, and screen for secondary causes. Additional tests may be useful in selected patients if secondary causes are suspected (see Table 38–2). The most common causes of secondary hypertension are chronic renal disease and renovascular hypertension. Rarer causes of secondary hypertension are Cushing's disease, hypothyroidism, hyperparathyroidism, acromegaly, sleep apnea, and carcinoid.

TABLE 38–2. Evaluation of Secondary Causes of Hypertension

Condition	Screening Tests	Additional Tests
Chronic renal failure	Urinalysis, creatinine, renal sonography	Renogram, renal biopsy
Renovascular disease	Renal bruits, plasma renin 1 hour before and 1 hour after captopril, duplex scan	Captopril renogram, renal arteriogram
Coarctation of aorta	Blood pressure in legs lower than in arms	Chest x-ray, aortogram
Primary aldosteronism	Decreased plasma potassium and renin, weakness	Urinary potassium, serum aldosterone, adrenal CT scan
Pheochromocytoma	Variable BP, tachycardia, sweating	Urinary metanephrine, urine or plasma catechols, adrenal CT scan

MANAGEMENT

The goal of therapy is to reduce the morbidity and mortality associated with hypertension. Numerous studies have demonstrated lower morbidity and mortality from coronary events, congestive heart failure, stroke, renal failure, and progression of hypertension for treated patients. Treatment is beneficial for all ages, and both systolic and diastolic hypertension should be treated aggressively. In general, the blood pressure should be lowered to less than 140/90 mm Hg.

General Treatment

Life-style modifications have been shown to lower blood pressure and may reduce the need for costly medications with their associated side effects. Useful measures include weight reduction (if > 110% of ideal body weight), regular aerobic physical activity, reduction of dietary sodium to 2–3 g/d, and moderate intake of alcohol (less than two drinks per day). These measures should be stressed in all hypertensive individuals and should be tried for at least 3 months in those with mild hypertension before starting pharmacologic therapy. Other less proven modalities include increased intake of potassium, calcium, and magnesium and relaxation and biofeedback therapy. Physicians and other health care professionals can effectively promote life-style modifications. Patients should be referred for more intensive counseling or self-help groups when indicated.

Specific Treatment

The decision to initiate pharmacologic therapy should be based on the severity of the blood pressure, the presence of target organ damage, and other cardiovascular risk factors. The greater the number of risk factors, the more important it is to adequately control the blood pressure. In general, drugs should be started in low doses and adjustments in dosage made after 3 to 4 weeks of therapy, unless the hypertension is severe. If the blood pressure is not controlled, the dose of medication can be increased, the drug can be stopped and one from another class started, or a drug from another class can be added. Many authorities recommend that a diuretic be added if one drug from another class does not control the blood pressure. Diuretics should be a part of every regimen if more than two drugs are required. Once the blood pressure is controlled (< 130/85 mm Hg) for longer than 6 months, it may be possible to reduce the dose or number of drugs while monitoring the blood pressure. This is termed step-down therapy. Table 38–3 provides a list of drugs commonly used to treat hypertension and their most frequent adverse effects.

Factors involved in the initial selection of the most appropriate drug include efficacy in reducing morbidity and mortality, cost, metabolic effects, effects on quality of life, drug interactions, and associated diseases. The most effective and best tolerated drugs are the diuret-

TABLE 38–3.   Antihypertensive Medications

Drug	Adverse Effects
Thiazide diuretics	Decreased potassium, sodium, magnesium; increased uric acid, glucose, calcium, cholesterol, triglycerides; sexual dysfunction
β-Blocker	Bronchospasm, exacerbation of peripheral vascular disease, congestive heart failure (CHF), masking of hypoglycemia, increased triglycerides and decreased HDL, reduced exercise tolerance, sexual dysfunction
$α_1$-Blockers	Orthostatic hypotension, dizziness, syncope, weakness
ACE inhibitor	Cough, rash, dysgeusia, increased potassium, renal insufficiency
Calcium antagonists	Headache, dizziness, edema (dihydropyridines), constipation, atrioventricular block, bradycardia (verapamil); may exacerbate CHF
Central $α_2$-agonists	Sedation, fatigue, dry mouth, rebound hypertension
Peripheral adrenergic antagonists	Orthostatic hypotension, sedation, depression
Direct vasodilators	Edema, tachycardia, positive antinuclear antibodies (hydralazine), hypertrichosis (minoxidil)

ics, β-blockers, ACE inhibitors, and calcium antagonists. Diuretics and β-blockers in low doses are generally preferred because they are the only drugs that have been shown to decrease mortality in patients with hypertension and because they cost less than the other drugs do. Certain demographic groups respond differently to the various classes of antihypertensive agents. African American patients often respond well to diuretics and calcium antagonists but poorly to β-blockers or ACE inhibitors. Treatment of diabetic patients with ACE inhibitors may help preserve renal function. For patients with hyperlipidemia, calcium antagonists or ACE inhibitors are good choices because they do not adversely affect lipids, unlike diuretics and β-blockers. However, β-blockers have been shown to have cardioprotective properties when used following myocardial infarction. β-Blockers should not be used in patients with bronchospastic diseases or congestive heart failure. On the other hand, ACE inhibitors may benefit those with congestive heart failure. Because they have expanded plasma volumes, patients with advanced renal insufficiency (creatinine > 2.5 mg/dL) should be treated with loop diuretics.

Hypertensive Emergencies

In hypertensive emergencies, it is important to lower blood pressure rapidly to prevent target organ damage. Examples include hypertensive encephalopathy, acute pulmonary edema, dissecting aortic aneurysm, eclampsia, and myocardial infarction. In other conditions such as accelerated hypertension or severe hypertension, blood pressure can be lowered more gradually, within 2 to 3 days.

PATIENT AND FAMILY EDUCATION

Because of the complications of longstanding and untreated hypertension, it is imperative that patients adhere to both life-style modifications and pharmacologic therapy. Patient education programs stressing information about hypertension and its complications, family support, and adjustment of therapy to meet the needs of the patient have all been shown to improve blood pressure control and decrease hypertension-related morbidity and mortality. Other strategies for improving adherence include simplifying the regimen, encouraging self-monitoring of blood pressure, minimizing the cost of therapy, encouraging discussion about the side effects of medication, giving positive feedback for life-style modifications and blood pressure control, and arranging regular office visits.

NATURAL HISTORY/PROGNOSIS

Generally, the higher the blood pressure is and the longer it remains elevated, the greater the morbidity and mortality. Hypertension and its subsequent complications represent important preventable diseases. Related aspects of prevention include maintaining ideal body weight, reducing sodium intake and alcohol consumption, and exercising regularly. Those who develop hypertension as adults tend to have higher blood pressures even as children. Hypertension usually becomes established between 30 and 50 years of age. Complications usually occur 20 or more years after recognition. Complications of hypertension include coronary heart disease, left ventricular hypertrophy, congestive heart failure, arrhythmias, peripheral vascular disease, abdominal aortic aneurysms, aortic dissection, cerebrovascular disease, and renal failure. If hypertension is recognized and treated early, the risk of complications is greatly reduced.

Research Questions

1. Which blood pressure measurements (office, home, work) should be used to guide therapy?
2. How can patients be persuaded to adhere to life-style modifications and drug therapy?
3. How frequently should stable hypertensive individuals be evaluated?

Case Resolution

The patient's medical history revealed long-standing hypertension on both sides of his family. Screening laboratory tests were normal, and he was given the diagnosis of essential hypertension. After a trial of a low-sodium diet and exercise, he was still hypertensive and a thiazide diuretic was started and proved effective in managing his hypertension.

Selected Readings

Joint National Committee on Detection, Evaluation, and Treatment of High Blood Pressure Fifth Report (JNC V). Arch Intern Med 153:154–83, 1993.

Kaplan, N. M. *Clinical Hypertension*, 5th ed. Baltimore, Williams & Wilkins, 1990.

National High Blood Pressure Education Program Working Group Report on Primary Prevention of Hypertension. Arch Intern Med 153:186–208, 1993.

Stamler, J, R. Stamler, and J. D. Neaton. Blood pressure, systolic and diastolic, and cardiovascular risks. Arch Intern Med 153:598–614, 1993.

CHAPTER 39

MURMURS AND VALVULAR HEART DISEASE

Veena Raizada, M.D.

H$_x$1 A 60-year-old male insurance company executive presents for his routine health maintenance check. He has no cardiac symptoms, specifically denying chest pain, shortness of breath, pedal edema, dizziness, syncope or easy fatigability. His blood pressure is 120/82 mm Hg, the carotid pulse is noted to rise slowly with a decreased pulse volume, and the jugular venous pressure is not elevated. The heart sounds are normal, and no click is audible. A harsh crescendo-decrescendo systolic murmur is audible in the right second intercostal space and radiates to both carotid arteries. The murmur begins with the first heart sound and ends before the second heart sound, peaking late in systole. In addition, a short, blowing, early diastolic decrescendo murmur is audible at the mid and lower left sternal border. The chest is clear, and the liver is not enlarged. His electrocardiogram reveals left bundle branch block.

H$_x$2 A 25-year-old Hispanic female farm worker presents with a 1-week history of an irregular heartbeat and exertional shortness of breath. On examination, she is dyspneic at rest, the cardiac apical impulse is irregular, and a rumbling diastolic murmur preceded by an opening snap is heard at the apex. S$_1$ is loud, and rales are heard at both lung bases. The liver is not enlarged, and there is no pedal edema.

QUESTIONS

1. How is an innocent murmur differentiated from an organic murmur?
2. What bedside maneuvers can assist in the diagnosis of murmurs?
3. What additional diagnostic studies can assist in the diagnosis of murmurs?
4. When is surgery indicated in the management of valvular heart disease?

A major responsibility of the primary care physician in the outpatient setting is to establish whether a murmur found on routine physical examination is "innocent" or due to organic heart disease.

The four most significant valvular abnormalities in adults are aortic stenosis, aortic regurgitation, mitral stenosis, and mitral regurgitation. Aortic stenosis (AS) and mitral regurgitation (MR) generate systolic murmurs, whereas aortic regurgitation (AR) and mitral stenosis (MS) generate diastolic murmurs.

PATHOPHYSIOLOGY

In **aortic stenosis**, the aortic valve orifice is narrow, resulting in obstruction of blood flow from the left ventricle to the aorta during systole. As a result, left ventricular pressure is elevated and left ventricular hypertrophy without cavity enlargement occurs. The size of the normal aortic valve orifice is 2 to 3 cm^2; when the orifice is smaller than one third of the normal size (i.e., ≤ 0.8 cm^2), symptoms of fatigability, dyspnea, angina, or syncope usually appear. Patients with aortic stenosis are at risk for sudden death. The true incidence of sudden death in asymptomatic AS patients is uncertain but may be as high as 4%. In young and middle-aged patients, half of the surgical cases of AS are caused by calcification of a congenital bicuspid aortic valve. In contrast, in patients 70 years of age or older, half of the cases are caused by degenerative calcification of the aortic valve. Rheumatic fever is an uncommon cause of isolated AS; the rheumatic aortic valve is regurgitant as well as stenotic and is usually associated with mitral valve disease. Aging, hypertension, diabetes mellitus and severe hypercholesterolemia seem to promote degenerative calcification. Other causes of calcific AS include Paget's disease of bone, end-stage renal disease, and rheumatoid arthritis.

Mitral regurgitation is characterized by an incompetent mitral valve that allows retrograde ejection of blood into the left atrium. In chronic MR, both the left atrium and the left ventricle are markedly enlarged. In the United States, nonrheumatic causes of isolated chronic MR (e.g., myxomatous valvular disease or other connective tissue disorders, isolated rupture of chordae tendineae, infective endocarditis, mitral annular calcification in the elderly, or papillary muscle dysfunction due to coronary artery disease) account for 45%–95% of cases. Before its decline in the United States and other developed countries, rheumatic fever was the major cause of chronic MR. Rheumatic fever still accounts for the majority of cases of chronic MR in developing countries. Bacterial endocarditis, acute myocardial infarction, and malfunction of a prosthesis are the common causes of acute MR.

In **mitral stenosis**, the mitral valve orifice is narrow, resulting in obstruction of blood flow from the left atrium to the left ventricle during diastole. The normal area of the mitral valve orifice is 4 to 6 cm^2. The reduced valve area results in an abnormal diastolic gradient across the mitral valve and subsequent elevation of the left atrial and pulmonary venous pressures. When the mitral valve orifice is minimally or moderately decreased (2 cm^2), left atrial pressure is only mildly or moderately elevated and the patient is usually asymptomatic. With more severe reduction in the orifice (≤ 1 cm^2), left atrial pressure becomes significantly elevated, causing pulmonary venous congestion and shortness of breath. Over a period of years, the obstruction can lead to the development of pulmonary hypertension, right ventricular hypertrophy, tricuspid regurgitation, and right heart failure. Conditions associated with increased cardiac output and mitral flow (e.g., fever, pregnancy, physical exertion, and emotional upset) can acutely elevate the left atrial and pulmonary venous pressures, resulting in pulmonary edema. Mitral stenosis is nearly always due to rheumatic fever; however, systemic conditions such as rheumatoid arthritis, systemic lupus erythematosus (SLE), mitral valve calcification, malignant carcinoid syndrome, and amyloidosis can lead to MS. There is also a rare congenital form.

Aortic regurgitation is due to incompetence of the aortic valve with blood regurgitating from the aorta into the left ventricle during diastole. Chronic AR gradually increases left ventricular diastolic volume because the left ventricle receives blood from both the left atrium and the systemic circulation; over a period of time, this leads to progressively severe left ventricular cavity dilatation in addition to hypertrophy. Rheumatic fever is a common cause of chronic AR. Progressive AR can also result from a bicuspid aortic valve, a myxomatous valve, aortic root dilatation in Marfan's syndrome, an aneurysm of the ascending aorta, and syphilitic aortitis. The two most common causes of acute AR are infective endocarditis and aortic dissection.

DIFFERENTIAL DIAGNOSIS

Causes of systolic and diastolic murmurs are presented in Table 39–1.

EVALUATION

History

Patients with valvular heart disease may be asymptomatic or may present with symptoms of variable severity. The most common symptoms associated with valvular heart disease include exertional dyspnea, orthopnea, paroxysmal nocturnal dyspnea, edema, hemoptysis, palpitations, syncope, and easy fatigability.

Symptoms associated with AS include easy fatigability, dyspnea, angina, and syncope; sudden cardiac death in previously asymptomatic patients may also occur but is uncommon.

Most patients with MS are asymptomatic at rest but complain of dyspnea with physical activity. Acute pulmonary edema may be the first symptom of MS and can be precipitated by pregnancy, new-onset atrial fibrillation, or a febrile illness due to infection. Hemoptysis stemming from bronchial venous bleeding is fairly common. In a small proportion of patients with severe MS, no significant symptoms are present despite severe pulmonary hypertension. Some patients with advanced MS learn to restrict their physical activity over the years and may be unaware of the full extent of their physical disability and underlying cardiac disease.

Patients with severe MR and AR may remain asymptomatic for many years. Development of symptoms (e.g., shortness of breath, palpitations) in these patients may occur gradually or follow an acute event such as bacterial endocarditis or myocardial infarction. Acute pulmonary edema in previously asymptomatic patients is usually due to new-onset atrial fibrillation with a rapid ventricular rate, ruptured chordae tendineae, or bacterial endocarditis.

TABLE 39–1.   Classification of Common Murmurs

Innocent Murmurs

Systolic
   In children and young adults
   In the elderly
   Hyperdynamic states
Continuous
   Venous hum
   Mammary souffle

Pathologic Murmurs

Systolic
   Aortic stenosis
   Hypertrophic subvalvular obstruction
   Mitral regurgitation
   Tricuspid regurgitation
   Pulmonic stenosis
   Atrial septal defect
   Ventricular septal defect
Diastolic
   Mitral stenosis
   Tricuspid stenosis
   Aortic regurgitation
   Pulmonic regurgitation
Continuous
   Patent ductus arteriosus

TABLE 39–2. Responses of Cardiac Murmurs to Bedside Physiologic Maneuvers

Valvular Lesion	Shape of the Murmur	Maneuver			
		Valsalva	Handgrip	Erect Posture	Squatting
Systolic murmurs	S₁ EC S₂				
Valvular aortic stenosis		↓	↓	↓	↑
Mitral regurgitation		↓	↑	↓	↑
Diastolic murmurs	OS				
Mitral stenosis		↓	↑	↓	↑
Aortic regurgitation		↓	↑	↑	↑

↑ Increase in intensity. ↓ Decrease in intensity. S₁, first heart sound; S₂, second heart sound; EC, ejection click; OS, opening snap.

Physical Examination

All valvular lesions have classical auscultatory findings. Dynamic auscultation, i.e., evaluation of murmurs by using physiologic and pharmacologic maneuvers to alter circulatory dynamics, is of great value in the differentiation of valvular lesions (Table 39–2).

A diastolic murmur nearly always represents underlying valvular pathology. A systolic murmur, on the other hand, can be either innocent or due to valvular disease. Innocent murmurs are a common finding in normal children, with a prevalence as high as 60%. Most innocent murmurs are soft and systolic in timing, with their graphic configuration resembling the ejection murmurs; these murmurs are typically attenuated by rapid standing from a lying position. A short systolic murmur is usually heard to the left of the sternal border during pregnancy and in patients with anemia or thyrotoxicosis (pulmonic scratch murmur). Adults with hypertension or diabetes mellitus (and older patients without these conditions) often have a systolic murmur at the base of the heart that mimics mild aortic stenosis. However, this murmur is due to the turbulence of blood flow around an aortic valve that has degenerative changes without any narrowing of the valve orifice (so-called aortic sclerosis).

A systolic murmur is present in both AS and MR. The systolic murmur of aortic stenosis is midsystolic and is a crescendo-decrescendo ejection murmur. A late-peaking systolic murmur, a faint or inaudible A₂, and an S₄ are generally associated with more severe aortic stenosis. The murmur is loudest at the right second intercostal space and radiates to the carotid arteries and the rest of the precordium (especially the left sternal border and apex). It is important to remember that in patients with severe AS and advanced left ventricular dysfunction, the murmur may be very soft when the cardiac output is low. Conversely, a loud murmur may be associated with trivial AS. The loudness of the murmur is related to the cardiac output and the systolic turbulence surrounding the valve rather than to the severity of the AS. The classic murmur of MR is holosystolic and is best heard at the apex with radiation to the left axilla and back. An S₃, when present, is indicative of moderate to severe MR.

A diastolic murmur is present in both MS and AR. The classic diastolic murmur of MS is a low-frequency, mid-diastolic rumble localized to the apex. It is best heard with the bell of the stethoscope with the patient lying on the left side, and it can be further enhanced by light exercise such as sit-ups, a brief walk in the clinic area, or a few vigorous coughs. Other findings in MS include a loud S₁ and an opening snap.

In contrast to the situation in MS, the diastolic murmur of AR is usually best heard along the left parasternal border, at the apex, and in the second right intercostal space. The murmur is early diastolic in timing, is high pitched, and is best heard with the diaphragm of the stethoscope with the patient in the sitting position and leaning forward with the breath held in expiration. The murmur increases with sudden squatting, isometric handgrip, or any maneuver that increases afterload; sudden squatting often makes an inaudible murmur audible. Massive acute AR from severe damage to the valve (i.e., due to acute bacterial endocarditis or a severe intravalvular leak of a prosthesis) is usually associated with a faint diastolic murmur. An apical mid-diastolic rumble, known as an Austin-Flint murmur, may also be audible in AR. This is not due to mitral stenosis but is related to partial closure of the septal mitral leaflet during diastole by the aortic regurgitant stream.

Additional Evaluation

Dynamic Auscultation

A variety of maneuvers can be used to alter circulatory dynamics, resulting in changes in the characteristics of several specific cardiac murmurs. Table 39–2 summarizes these maneuvers and the resultant changes in murmur intensity and timing. Response of the auscultatory findings in hypertrophic obstructive cardiomyopathy (HCM) and mitral valve prolapse (MVP) deserve special attention. The systolic murmur of HCM is louder with assumption of erect posture and with the Valsalva maneuver and is attenuated by handgrip and squatting. The systolic click and murmur of MVP occur earlier in systole with erect posture and Valsalva and later with handgrip and squatting. In certain valvular conditions, cardiologists might use the vasodilator amyl nitrite as well. In response to amyl nitrite, (1) the systolic murmurs of aortic stenosis and hypertrophic obstructive cardiomyopathy are augmented, whereas the murmur of mitral regurgitation is diminished, and (2) the diastolic murmur of mitral stenosis is enhanced, whereas the murmur of aortic regurgitation is diminished.

Noninvasive and Invasive Tests

Noninvasive tests such as echo-Doppler studies, electrocardiogram (ECG), and chest x-ray are of great value in assessing valvular lesions and their hemodynamic consequences. Echo-Doppler examination is of particular value, since it provides direct visualization of cardiac structures and aids in determining the pathology of the lesion. Cardiac chamber size and wall thickness, ventricular function, and the severity of valvular lesions (particularly AS and MS) can be reliably assessed. In contrast to cardiac catheterization, these noninvasive tests can be used to follow patients over time. Information from echo-Doppler examination is usually sufficient to plan management, including the timing and nature of surgery. In the great majority of valvular patients, cardiac catheterization is performed before valve surgery only to evaluate for possible concomitant coronary artery disease.

In AS, the ECG is helpful in documenting the presence of left ventricular hypertrophy (LVH) with strain, a pattern seen in approximately 85% of patients with severe stenosis. Approximately 5% of patients with calcific AS manifest various forms and degrees of atrioventricular or intraventricular conduction block. The heart size on chest x-ray may be entirely normal, even in severe AS. Echo-Doppler studies allow quantitation of the left ventricular-aortic systolic pressure gradient as well as the aortic valve area, which correlate with measurements obtained by left heart catheterization.

The ECG is generally not very helpful in assessing the severity of AR or MR. In AR, a left axis shift and LVH are generally seen on the ECG, whereas left atrial enlargement is commonly seen in MR. Echocardiography, however, can provide valuable information about both the etiology and severity of AR and MR. Echo-Doppler and radionuclide (MUGA) examinations permit quantitative evaluation of left ventricular ejection fraction and both end-systolic and end-diastolic volumes. These measurements can be of great help in planning the timing of valvular surgery. Transesophageal echo (TEE) can be employed with confidence in detecting complications of aortic and mitral valvular endocarditis, including acute AR and MR and abscesses. In acute aortic dissection, TEE helps determine the extent of dissection and the degree of associated AR.

In MS, the ECG—in addition to detecting left atrial enlargement in 90% of patients—can provide clues regarding pulmonary artery pressure. The presence of right ventricular hypertrophy (RVH) on ECG usually indicates a pulmonary artery systolic pressure between 70 and 100 mm Hg. The chest x-ray is of immense value in demonstrating interstitial edema due to pulmonary venous hypertension; however, left atrial size, right heart changes, and pulmonary artery pressures are better evaluated by echo-Doppler examination. In addition, this study reliably evaluates the mitral valve area, the pliability and degree of calcification of the mitral valve, and pulmonary artery pressures. The echo-Doppler examination in MS provides sufficiently reliable information to allow for the planning of surgical intervention (valve replacement, commissurotomy, or balloon valvuloplasty) without cardiac catheterization.

MANAGEMENT

Asymptomatic patients with AS should be advised to watch for the development of cardiac symptoms. In patients with an aortic valve area < 0.8 cm^2 and with cardiac symptoms due to AS, aortic valve replacement is indicated; in asymptomatic patients with a tight aortic valve, surgery is indicated in the presence of left ventricular dysfunction and left ventricular enlargement. In patients with severe aortic stenosis, including those in their 70s and 80s, aortic valve replacement results in substantial clinical and hemodynamic improvement, with a 5-year actuarial survival of 85%. In contrast to the case for AR, left ventricular performance usually returns to normal in AS. In selected patients with severely depressed left ventricular function and frank left heart failure, aortic valve replacement may be lifesaving despite its overall high rate of surgical mortality.

Patients with MS who have symptoms and severe disease (i.e., valve area < 1 cm^2) should undergo mitral valve surgery (balloon valvuloplasty, mitral commis-surotomy, or valve replacement). Marked symptomatic improvement has been shown to occur in > 80% of these patients, and the 10-year survival rate is > 80%.

In MR, patients should be considered for valve replacement when symptoms develop or when there is evidence of left ventricular dysfunction, i.e., an ejection fraction (EF) ≤ 50%–55% as demonstrated on echocardiography or radionuclide ventriculography. In most patients with MR, symptoms improve after surgery. Postoperatively, pulmonary hypertension, left ventricular size and mass, and left atrial size are also reduced. However, patients with marked left ventricular dysfunction usually remain symptomatic. Preoperative hemodynamic predictors of a favorable surgical outcome are an EF > 70% and an end-systolic volume index < 50 mL/m^2. An EF of < 55%, an end-systolic volume index > 70 mL/m^2, and a mean pulmonary artery pressure > 20 mm Hg predict an unfavorable postoperative course.

Patients with AR should have aortic valve replacement when they have symptoms or evidence of left ventricular dysfunction on noninvasive or invasive testing. Patients with normal left ventricular systolic function preoperatively remain asymptomatic after aortic valve replacement; those with decreased EF and only a brief duration (< 1 year) of left ventricular dysfunction have a favorable postoperative outcome. Patients with a severely depressed preoperative EF are likely to develop irreversible left ventricular dysfunction and are at a high risk of dying of congestive heart failure.

It is important to remember that all patients with valvular disease require prophylactic antibiotics before and after selected procedures that have been associated with a significant incidence of transient bacteremia (e.g., dental work, cystoscopy). Although conclusive evidence is lacking, such prophylaxis is believed to decrease the risk of these patients developing subacute bacterial endocarditis (SBE). Rheumatic valvular lesions, both mitral and aortic, are commonly involved in endocarditis. Associated diabetes mellitus causes patients with degenerative valvular disease to be more susceptible to endocarditis.

PATIENT AND FAMILY EDUCATION

Patients and families should be instructed about (1) the need to see the physician every 3–6 months, (2) the importance of calling the physician promptly if cardiovascular symptoms develop, and (3) the necessity for SBE antibiotic prophylaxis (see above).

NATURAL HISTORY/PROGNOSIS

All chronic valvular lesions are progressive but tend to be tolerated without symptoms for many years. Once symptoms develop, survival is shortened.

In AS, the development of symptoms presages a significant reduction in life expectancy. For patients not treated surgically, survival averages approximately 5–7 years after the onset of angina, 3–5 years after the onset of syncope, and 2 years after the onset of shortness of breath and heart failure.

In MS, atrial fibrillation develops in at least 50% of patients. Systemic arterial embolism occurs in 10%–20% of patients. The prognosis for MS depends upon the stage of the disease and the severity of the symptoms. The 10-year survival rate in asymptomatic patients exceeds 60%, but survival decreases progressively as symptoms become more severe.

Both chronic MR and AR are tolerated for a long time before left ventricular failure develops. The status of left ventricular function is an important determinant of long-term prognosis and survival in patients with these lesions. For moderately symptomatic patients with chronic MR, the 5-year survival is 50% and the 10-year survival is 20%; for severely symptomatic patients, the 5-year survival is approximately 40% and the 10-year survival is 15%. Atrial fibrillation occurs in 10%–20% of patients and may be complicated by systemic arterial emboli. Up to 95% of asymptomatic patients with mild to moderate AR will survive for 10 years. However, survival is shortened once symptoms arise. Severe AR has 5- and 10-year survivals of approximately 75% and 50%, respectively. After the onset of angina, however, the 5-year survival is approximately 50%; after the development of heart failure, survival is usually less than 2 years.

Research Question

1. How can better noninvasive techniques to measure left ventricular function be developed?

Case Resolutions

The first patient's echocardiogram demonstrated a moderately calcified aortic valve with moderate aortic stenosis. A follow-up echocardiogram in 6 months was advised.

The second patient's echocardiogram documented severe mitral stenosis. She underwent mitral commissurotomy and has been asymptomatic since her surgery.

Selected Readings

Braunwald, E. *Heart Disease,* 4th ed. Philadelphia, W.B. Saunders Company, 1992, pp. 13, 43, 1007.

Eagle, K. A., et al. *The Practice of Cardiology,* 2nd ed. Boston, Little, Brown & Co., 1988, pp. 655–764.

Giuliani, E. R., V. Fuster, B. J. Gersh, et al. *Cardiology: Fundamentals and Practice,* 2nd ed. St. Louis, Mosby–Year Book, 1991, p. 1505.

Kulick, D. L., and S. H. Rahimtoola. Selection of patients for cardiac valve replacement. *In* E. Braunwald (ed.). *Heart Disease Update,* 3rd ed. Philadelphia, W.B. Saunders Company, 1990, pp. 257–72.

Osborn, L. A., and M. H. Crawford. Mitral regurgitation. *In* A. S. Kapoor and B. N. Singh (eds.). *Prognosis and Risk Assessment in Cardiovascular Disease.* New York, Churchill Livingstone, 1993, p. 251.

Schlant, R. C., and R. W. Alexander. *The Heart,* 8th ed. New York, McGraw-Hill, Inc., 1994, p. 1391.

CONGESTIVE HEART FAILURE

Michael H. Crawford, M.D.

H$_x$ A 64-year-old male city manager presents because of two episodes of paroxysmal nocturnal dyspnea in the last week. The patient was in good health until 2 years ago when he suffered an anterior myocardial infarction complicated by congestive heart failure. Cardiac catheterization at that time showed a complete occlusion of the proximal left anterior descending coronary artery with a large area of anteroseptal akinesia, resulting in an overall left ventricular ejection fraction of 35%. The other coronary arteries were without lesions, and he had no mitral regurgitation. The patient was placed on captopril (25 mg twice a day) and aspirin (81 mg/d) and left the hospital asymptomatic. He continued to do well in a cardiac rehabilitation program until about 2 weeks ago when he suffered an exacerbation of degenerative joint disease and was placed on two 325-mg aspirin tablets every 4 hours. He noted some swelling of the ankles after a few days of this treatment and subsequently noted increased dyspnea on exertion. Finally, he experienced two episodes of paroxysmal nocturnal dyspnea, which occasioned his return visit. He denies chest pain, cough, dietary changes, or any other changes in his medications. On the physical examination, blood pressure was 110/70 mm Hg, pulse was 90/min and regular, and there was 1+ pitting edema of the ankles. His lungs showed fine bibasilar rales. The jugular veins were distended with a right atrial pressure of 12 cm H$_2$O. His cardiac examination revealed an S$_3$.

Questions

1. Why did this patient's heart failure recur?
2. What additional studies would you obtain?
3. How would you treat this patient?

Heart failure is a major public health problem in the United States. Three to four million people experience heart failure each year and there are approximately 400,000 new cases annually, resulting in more than 11 million outpatient visits per year. Heart failure is the most common diagnosis in hospitalized patients greater than 65 years of age; estimated health care costs related to heart failure totaled almost 9 billion dollars in 1990.

CLINICAL PRESENTATION

Heart failure occurs when the cardiac output decreases below what is necessary for adequate tissue perfusion. Typical symptoms include shortness of breath, orthopnea, paroxysmal nocturnal dyspnea, and lower extremity edema.

PATHOPHYSIOLOGY

The first event in the sequence of events leading to heart failure is usually some form of myocardial damage that reduces the stroke volume of the left ventricle (Fig. 40–1). One early compensatory mechanism for this fall in stroke volume (SV) is an increase in adrenergic tone in the body. This results in an increase in heart rate (HR), a response that tends to keep the cardiac output (CO) in the normal range (CO = SV × HR). In addition, increased adrenergic tone causes peripheral vasoconstriction and increased systemic vascular resistance (SVR), thus serving to keep the blood pressure (BP) in the normal range (BP = SV × SVR). If these mechanisms are insufficient to compensate for the reduction in stroke volume, organ hypoperfusion results. Reduced renal perfusion results in increased secretion of renin, which catalyzes the conversion of angiotensin I in the plasma to angiotensin II. Angiotensin II is a potent vasoconstrictor and contributes to peripheral vasoconstriction. In addition, it stimulates the release of aldosterone from the adrenal glands, resulting in salt and water retention.

Salt and water retention and constriction of the venous beds by heightened adrenergic tone result in an increased preload to the heart that can enhance stroke volume via the Frank-Starling mechanism. This compensatory mechanism, however, is of limited usefulness in the severely damaged myocardium, and the resultant left ventricular dilation increases afterload. The increased sympathetic tone and angiotensin II production result in marked vasoconstriction, which also contributes to an increase in afterload and further depression of left ventricular function. As left ventricular function decreases, the increased preload ends up in the lungs as pulmonary edema. Thus, the very mechanisms the body employs to compensate for myocardial damage eventually result in further *depression* of myocardial function. A vicious circle ensues that, if not broken by medical intervention, will eventually lead to the death of the patient, either through hemodynamic collapse or the induction of lethal arrhythmias.

It is not surprising, therefore, that edema, tachycardia, and a third heart sound (due to increased left ventricular filling) are some of the first signs of early congestive heart failure. As heart function decreases in relationship to the available preload, the left ventricle cannot accommodate the increased venous return that results from assuming the supine posture (i.e., since no further augmentation of stroke volume is possible). Fluid accumulates in the lungs, and the patient experiences paroxysmal nocturnal dyspnea within a few hours

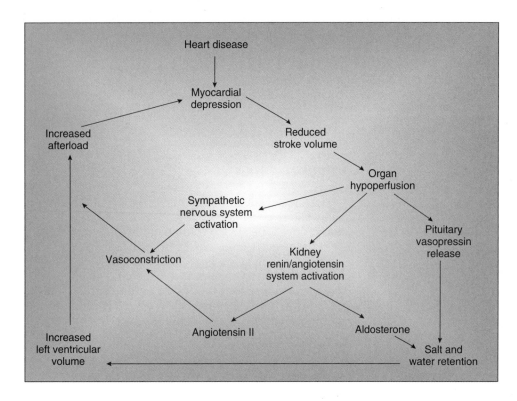

FIGURE 40–1. *Pathophysiologic schema of compensatory responses to myocardial depression that lead ultimately to further myocardial depression and a vicious circle unless treatment intervenes.*

after lying down at night. As the mismatch between ventricular performance and preload worsens, the patient cannot assume the supine position for even a few minutes without becoming dyspneic (a symptom referred to as orthopnea).

DIFFERENTIAL DIAGNOSIS

In every patient who presents with heart failure, it is imperative to ascertain (1) the etiology of the left ventricular dysfunction and (2) the reason for cardiac decompensation at that time.

Causes of decreased left ventricular function (and subsequent heart failure) are listed in Table 40–1. Patients with reduced left ventricular performance may be marginally compensated under ideal conditions, but any change in homeostasis can lead to an exacerbation of heart failure (Table 40–2). A frequent problem is increased salt and water retention due to dietary indiscretion, often seen at times of cultural celebration when increased food intake is common. Certain medications (e.g., corticosteroids, NSAIDs) can also lead to increased salt and water retention. It is thus imperative to determine the cause of the lack of homeostasis.

D_x Congestive Heart Failure

- Dyspnea, orthopnea, paroxysmal nocturnal dyspnea.
- S_3, increased jugular venous pressure, rales.
- Lower extremity edema.

EVALUATION

History

The diagnosis of congestive heart failure can usually be made from the history and physical examination. The most specific historical features are dyspnea on exertion, paroxysmal nocturnal dyspnea, and orthopnea. Helpful (but less specific) complaints such as fatigue, edema, and decreased appetite should also be sought.

Physical Examination

Common physical findings include tachycardia; cool, clammy skin; jugular venous distention; pulmonary rales; an enlarged heart; a third heart sound; tender hepatomegaly; and edema. There may be evidence of specific cardiac abnormalities, such as murmurs due to valvular heart disease or findings suggestive of an apical

---

TABLE 40–1. Causes of Heart Failure

Myocardial damage
  Ischemia*
  Infarction*
  Myocarditis
  Dilated cardiomyopathy*
  Restrictive cardiac disease (e.g., amyloidosis)
  Toxins (e.g., Adriamycin)
Valvular heart disease*
Congenital heart disease
Constrictive pericarditis
Hypertrophic cardiomyopathy (diastolic dysfunction)*

*Most common causes.

TABLE 40–2. Causes of Cardiac Decompensation in Patients with Reduced Left Ventricular Performance

Common Causes

Ischemia
Infarction
Dietary indiscretion
Failure to take medication
Arrhythmias (e.g., atrial fibrillation)
Systemic hypertension
Myocardial depressants (e.g., calcium blockers or β-blockers)
Infection (e.g., pneumonia)

Less Common Causes

Thyrotoxicosis
Hypothyroidism
Iatrogenic fluid overload
Myocarditis
Worsening valvular function
Drugs that retain salt and water (e.g., corticosteroids, NSAIDs)
Pulmonary embolus

aneurysm (e.g., displaced apical impulse) or congenital heart disease (e.g., cyanosis).

Additional Evaluation

If the exact nature of the problem is not clear from the history and physical examination, a cardiac evaluation should be performed as soon as possible (Table 40–3). Every patient with an exacerbation of heart failure should have an electrocardiogram (ECG) performed to ascertain if myocardial ischemia or infarction underlies the symptomatology. Since many patients with coronary artery disease have silent episodes of ischemia or infarction, a lack of chest pain history does not exclude this possibility. A chest x-ray is helpful, especially if pulmonary pathology is suspected. A chest x-ray can reveal pulmonary venous congestion, enlargement of the heart, and occasionally specific abnormalities of the cardiac chambers or great vessels that point to a particular diagnosis.

The most useful test for ascertaining the presence or absence of cardiac disease is the echocardiogram, which allows anatomic visualization of all cardiac structures and permits an assessment of their performance.

TABLE 40–3. Evaluation of Heart Failure

Usually Indicated Tests

Electrocardiogram (ECG)
Chest x-ray
Echocardiogram

Sometimes Indicated Tests

Creatine kinase (CK), electrolytes, Mg, blood urea nitrogen (BUN), creatinine
Drug blood levels
Blood cultures
Ambulatory ECG monitoring
Electrophysiologic testing
Cardiac catheterization
Thyroid-stimulating hormone (TSH)
Arterial blood gases (ABG)
Ventilation/perfusion (V/Q) lung scan

Other testing depends on the clinical situation. If anemia or infection is suspected, a CBC may be useful. If endocarditis is suspected, blood cultures are needed, and consideration should be given to performing transesophageal echocardiography (which is more sensitive for detecting cardiac vegetations than transthoracic echocardiography). A suspicion of myocardial infarction requires a creative kinase–MB measurement. Drug levels in the blood should be assessed if drug toxicity (e.g., digoxin) is suspected. Finally, if metabolic derangements are suspected, a glucose or thyroid-stimulating hormone level may be useful.

MANAGEMENT

The most important aspect of the treatment of heart failure is to remove any precipitating cause (Box 40–1). For example, NSAID use should be avoided, since these agents can lead to salt and water retention. If this is not possible, an alternative is to treat the patient with an NSAID during arthritis flares but to initiate diuretic therapy simultaneously to compensate for the salt- and water-retaining properties of the NSAID.

Coexisting infections should be promptly treated. Patients with heart failure should also be encouraged to have a flu shot every fall as well as periodic (i.e., every 6 years) vaccination against pneumococcal pneumonia, and they should have top priority in these preventive programs.

If a precipitating cause cannot be found or remedied, increased medical treatment should be attempted. Many patients respond to an increase in diuretic (e.g., furosemide) therapy, even when a specific cause for increased salt and water retention is not apparent. However, once the furosemide dose exceeds 160 mg/d, there is little hope that a further increase will result in additional diuresis. In such cases, it is often useful to add metolazone to augment diuresis by blocking the entire loop of Henle. Profound diuresis often results that should be maintained for only a few days. The patient must be watched carefully during this time for evidence of overdiuresis, including hypotension, impaired organ perfusion, and hypochloremic alkalosis. Rarely, patients will need to be on daily metolazone in addition to daily furosemide. Switching to another loop diuretic (e.g., bumetanide) occasionally can be helpful.

Recent data support the value of digoxin treatment in patients with systolic dysfunction of the left ventricle complicated by heart failure. Comparison studies with angiotensin converting enzyme (ACE) inhibitors have

BOX 40–1. Management of Heart Failure

Remove precipitating causes (e.g., ischemia, arrhythmias)
Give inotropic support (e.g., digoxin)
Provide diuresis (e.g., furosemide)
Administer vasodilators (ACE inhibitors preferred)
Restrict salt and water intake
Prescribe bed rest followed by progressive ambulation

shown that digoxin can play a beneficial role, especially in patients with moderate or severe symptoms of heart failure.

Considerable data now demonstrate that ACE inhibitors are indicated in almost all patients with congestive heart failure, including asymptomatic postmyocardial infarction patients with low ejection fractions (< 35%). Interestingly, trials performed to date suggest that larger rather than smaller doses should be used for maximal benefit (e.g., captopril, 150 mg/d, or enalapril, 20 mg/d). When increasing the ACE inhibitor dose, care must be taken not to produce hypotension and further compromise of organ perfusion. ACE inhibitors often take several weeks to reach their full therapeutic effect in patients with heart failure. Thus, dosage increments should be made slowly, allowing adequate time for the patient to adjust to the new dose.

For patients who cannot take ACE inhibitors or do not seem to respond to them, the combination of hydralazine and isosorbide dinitrate has been shown to be effective in clinical trials. Nitrates also can be beneficial either alone or in combination with ACE inhibitor therapy, especially in patients with ischemic heart disease who also have angina pectoris.

PATIENT AND FAMILY EDUCATION

Patients with congestive heart failure do better if they adhere to a low sodium diet, preferably 4 g/d or less. It is preferable for the entire family to follow this diet rather than to prepare special meals for the patient. Thus, education of the patient's family, especially the meal preparers, is very important. If the patient has ischemic heart disease, consideration should be given also to a low-fat diet (i.e., < 30% of total caloric intake). Patients with congestive heart failure often take several medications, and it is important that the patient and close family members understand the actions of these medications as well as potential adverse effects.

Continued physical activity is important for the heart failure patient, although a period of physical rest is necessary when the patient is in a state of decompensation. Once patients have reached the compensated state, they should begin regular exercise in modest fashion. The heart failure patient experiences considerable peripheral muscle atrophy and metabolic downregulation. This situation can be improved by regular physical activity. The patient should avoid strenuous or competitive activity, however, since it may be intolerable and might incite dangerous ventricular arrhythmias. If feasible, a structured rehabilitation program in which the patient can be carefully monitored is ideal, especially during the initiation phase of the exercise program.

Follow-up visits for encouragement purposes are quite important, since heart failure is often associated with depression. In addition, the key medications used in the heart failure regimen need to be monitored for possible side effects, including hypokalemia, digoxin toxicity, or decreasing renal function. Usually, heart failure patients are seen three to six times a year depending on their disease severity.

NATURAL HISTORY/PROGNOSIS

Although the etiology of heart failure influences the prognosis, the general rule is that the lower the left ventricular systolic performance (ejection fraction), the higher the mortality. The mortality curve is exponential in that, once the ejection fraction falls below 35%, mortality rises dramatically. When the patient's ejection fraction falls below 20% and no reversible component is apparent, the patient becomes a potential candidate for cardiac transplantation. Usually patients are considered for transplantation if (1) their life expectancy is less than 12 months without transplantation; (2) there is no severe, irreversible pulmonary hypertension; and (3) other debilitating diseases that would limit life are not present. However, donor hearts are scarce, and patients frequently die awaiting transplantation. Consequently, a great deal of attention is now being focused on how heart failure, as well as asymptomatic left ventricular dysfunction, can be prevented.

Research Questions

1. Should all patients with heart failure receive digoxin therapy?
2. How can painful arthritis best be managed in heart failure patients?

Case Resolution

This case represents an example of exacerbation of heart failure in a patient with known left ventricular dysfunction who was previously well compensated. The patient responded quickly to stopping aspirin and beginning oral furosemide. Over time, his captopril dose was increased and the furosemide dose lowered. This heart failure regimen allowed the occasional use of NSAIDs for arthritis flares.

Selected Readings

Cohn, J. N., G. Johnson, S. Ziesche, et al. A comparison of enalapril with hydralazine-isosorbide dinitrate in the treatment of chronic congestive heart failure. N Engl J Med 325:300–10, 1991.

Konstam, M. A., M. F. Rousseau, M. W. Kronenberg, et al. Effects of the angiotensin converting enzyme inhibitor enalapril on the long-term progression of left ventricular dysfunction in patients with heart failure. Circulation 86:431–38, 1992.

Pfeffer, M. A., E. Braunwald, L. A. Moye, et al. Effect of captopril on mortality and morbidity in patients with left ventricular dysfunction after myocardial infarction. N Engl J Med 327:669–77, 1992.

SOLVD Investigators. Effect of enalapril on mortality and the development of heart failure in asymptomatic patients with reduced left ventricular ejection fractions. N Engl J Med 327:685–91, 1992.

SOLVD Investigators. Effect of enalapril on survival in patients with reduced left ventricular ejection fractions and congestive heart failure. N Engl J Med 325:293–302, 1991.

ARTERIAL INSUFFICIENCY OF THE LEGS

Mark Langsfeld, M.D., Eric S. Weinstein, M.D., and Robert D. DeFrang, M.D.

H$_x$ A 62-year-old male hotel clerk presents with increasing pain in his right calf associated with walking. He describes the pain as cramping, and states that he has had it for several years, but now it bothers him when he walks 15 m (50 ft) to his mailbox. His medical history is pertinent for hypertension diagnosed 10 years ago. He has cut down to smoking three cigarettes a day but has a greater than 50 pack-year history. Six weeks ago his wife trimmed his toenails, and since that time he has had a shallow ulcer at the tip of his right great toe. On physical examination, his femoral pulses are strong bilaterally, but none of the distal pulses are palpable. The tip of his right great toe is bluish-black with a small uninfected ulcer present.

Questions

1. What are the diagnostic possibilities for a patient who presents with leg pain associated with ambulation?
2. What physical findings indicate arterial insufficiency as the main problem in this patient?
3. What signs and symptoms are associated with life-threatening ischemia in an extremity?

Lower extremity arterial insufficiency is a common problem particularly in an aging population. Its most typical manifestation is pain in the leg (most commonly in the calf) that occurs with ambulation. Advanced ischemia is manifested by pain in the foot that occurs at rest or evidence of tissue loss such as gangrene or a nonhealing ulcer.

PATHOPHYSIOLOGY

Leg pain induced by ambulation, known as claudication, is most commonly associated with atherosclerosis. Atherosclerosis is a systemic, degenerative process involving the arterial system. There are well-known risk factors, and its etiology is likely multifactorial. Claudication is up to nine times more common in smokers than in nonsmokers.

The arterial system should not be viewed as a simple conduit for blood flow but as a complex organ with many cell-to-cell interactions. The most popular theory regarding the etiology of atherosclerosis involves an initial injury to the inner lining of the blood vessel, the endothelium. Endothelial injury, whether due to mechanical forces, immunologic mechanisms, or chemical abnormalities, is thought to be the initiating event

in plaque formation. Platelets appear to play a role, since platelet byproducts add to the abnormal cellular proliferation.

Hemodynamic forces also appear to be involved. Experimental models show that plaque formation does not occur in areas where blood flow is rapid and laminar. Rather, plaques tend to occur at arterial bifurcations, particularly in areas of low shear stress and low flow velocity.

Blood flow is governed by Poiseuille's law, which states that energy losses are inversely proportionate to the fourth power of the radius of the vessel. A small change in the diameter of the vessel therefore results in a large change in flow. In patients with claudication, flow is adequate through an arterial stenosis at rest. However, with exercise, there is greater demand for blood flow in the leg muscles. Peripheral resistance drops, producing an increase in flow velocity and a subsequent loss of kinetic energy and pressure drop across the stenosis. A hemodynamically insignificant stenosis at rest therefore becomes significant with exercise.

As a stenosis progresses, tissue hypoxia promotes collateralization of blood vessels. Flow through these collaterals is at greater resistance. Up to a certain point, improvement in walking distance with exercise in patients with intermittent claudication is due to collateralization; beyond that point, improved walking is likely due to metabolic adaptation of the muscle.

If the atherosclerotic process continues unabated, tissue hypoxia will progress to occur at rest. Rest pain always occurs in the foot, over the dorsum of the foot or toes. When that transpires, the limb is in jeopardy, particularly if subsequent tissue trauma occurs.

DIFFERENTIAL DIAGNOSIS

Orthopedic/Neurogenic Conditions

It is important to determine whether the onset of symptoms is related to trauma to the extremity. Direct bony or joint trauma will result in extremity pain aggravated by ambulation. Arthritic conditions or degenerative joint disease will also result in painful ambulation. However, all these conditions are associated with a variable onset of pain, including pain at rest.

The most common neurogenic condition confused with vascular claudication is a syndrome called pseudoclaudication. In this disorder, lumbar spinal stenosis or a herniated disk may cause pain whenever an increase in lumbar lordosis occurs, as with walking or standing.

Affected individuals must often sit or lie down to stop the pain, which usually takes 5 to 10 minutes or longer to subside.

A painful extremity due to neuritis in patients with diabetes is uncommon. Usually diabetes is associated with *painless* neuropathy in a stocking-and-glove distribution. However, diabetes is a significant risk factor for the development of lower extremity claudication, and a vascular etiology may be responsible for a painful extremity in a diabetic patient.

Venous Insufficiency

Superficial thrombophlebitis and deep vein thrombosis can cause a painful extremity but the discomfort is not typically worsened by ambulation. A condition occasionally associated with deep vein thrombosis, however, may lead to a painful sensation when a patient walks. This venous claudication results from functional iliofemoral venous obstruction. Obstructed or poorly recanalized veins cannot handle the increased venous outflow associated with exercise. Affected individuals will have other signs of chronic venous insufficiency, such as swelling or stasis dermatitis.

Arterial Insufficiency

The word claudication is derived from a Latin word meaning "to limp." Claudication occurs in the antigravity muscles of the lower extremity, i.e., hip and buttocks, anterior thigh, and calf muscles. The pain occurs after a fixed distance of walking, is repetitive and easily described by the patient, and is relieved after 1 to 2 minutes of standing still.

EVALUATION

History

A thorough history will distinguish the cause of leg pain in over 90% of patients. Since atherosclerosis is a systemic disease, a complete history involving multiple organ systems is necessary. The presence of the major risk factors for atherosclerosis (i.e., smoking, diabetes, hypercholesterolemia, family history of atherosclerosis, and hypertension) should be ascertained. Smoking and diabetes are the main risk factors associated with claudication. Careful questioning about cerebrovascular insufficiency (e.g., transient ischemic attacks, amaurosis fugax, previous stroke), coronary artery disease (e.g., chest pain, shortness of breath, myocardial infarction, arrhythmia), and renal insufficiency should be pursued.

The next crucial piece of history is determining the rapidity of onset of symptoms. The patient should be asked whether the claudication occurred suddenly one day, with no previous symptoms. This situation may indicate an acute event such as an embolism from the heart or from a proximal abdominal aortic aneurysm.

Gradual onset of claudication is more consistent with the progressive obliteration of lower extremity vessels and formation of collaterals. Claudication symptoms often plateau when progressive shortening of walking distance occurs, except when the patient continues to smoke.

Finally, the clinician must distinguish between claudication and the limb-threatened state. The latter may present with rest pain on recumbency, often awakening the patient at night. The patient may wake up and dangle the foot over the side of the bed or get up and walk around to relieve the pain. (This is entirely different from night cramps in calf muscles.) Nonhealing ulceration and rest pain are the final stages of arterial ischemia.

Physical Examination

Signs of vascular insufficiency should be sought throughout the body. A complete pulse examination should include evaluation of cervical, radial, ulnar, brachial, femoral, popliteal, dorsalis pedis, and posterior tibial pulses bilaterally. Some form of consistent grading of the pulses should be used. A pulse examination using a 2 in the denominator is adequate, with 0/2 meaning pulse absent, 1/2 diminished, 2/2 normal, and 3/2 bounding. The clinician should use the same pulse examination in all patients, since only extensive practice will yield accurate examinations. Up to 10% of normal patients may have an absent pedal pulse. Upper extremity blood pressures should be taken bilaterally.

Bruits, which signify turbulence and possible atherosclerotic narrowing, should be listened for with the diaphragm of a stethoscope. Cervical, supraclavicular, abdominal, flank, and groin areas should be examined bilaterally.

A routine cardiopulmonary examination should be performed. Aneurysms should be palpated for in the abdomen (at the level of the umbilicus) and in the popliteal fossae. Examination of the popliteal pulse is difficult for the inexperienced examiner. The fingers of both hands should meet behind the slightly flexed knee. The patient should be told to relax the leg in the examiner's hands, and careful but deep palpation should reveal the pulse.

The "six Ps" of acute arterial ischemia should be committed to memory: pain, paresthesia, paralysis, poikilothermy, pallor, and pulselessness. The signs of ischemia may not be as pronounced in the patient with chronic claudication. Examination of both extremities is necessary for comparison purposes. In critical ischemia, the affected extremity is usually cooler and pulseless and becomes pale upon elevation followed by dependent rubor with dangling. Evidence of ulceration or pregangrenous changes must be noted. Finally, a sensory examination, particularly in patients with diabetes, is done to note the presence of neuropathy or sensory deficits associated with ischemia.

Additional Evaluation

Whenever there is a question of extremity arterial insufficiency, Doppler testing should be routine. Doppler evaluation can help quantitate the degree of ischemia when pulses are absent. A hand-held continuous wave Doppler instrument is used to obtain the highest systolic blood pressure in each arm. The arterial Doppler signals are then localized over the dorsalis pedis and posterior tibial arteries in each foot. A blood pressure cuff is placed just above each ankle, and the pressure in each individual pedal vessel is recorded. The higher of the two ankle pressures is then placed over the highest brachial pressure, creating an ankle/brachial index (ABI). A normal ABI is > 0.9. Abnormal levels consistent with claudication are in the 0.6–0.9 range. Levels ≤ 0.5 are consistent with severe ischemia. Pressures may be spuriously elevated in patients with diabetes, whose vessels may become noncompressible owing to medial calcification. An ABI > 1.0 in feet without palpable pulses is likely due to this effect. In this event, toe pressures obtained in the noninvasive vascular laboratory (see below) can give objective information about the degree of arterial insufficiency. Doppler wave form patterns can also give important information about the degree of ischemia.

Arteriography has no role in the initial assessment of patients with arterial insufficiency. This study is not necessary in most cases to make a diagnosis, and should be obtained only as a preoperative study after the patient has been assessed by a vascular surgeon.

Noninvasive Vascular Laboratory Tests

In assessing a patient with lower extremity arterial insufficiency, an ABI is the study of first choice to indicate the overall level of foot perfusion. Occasionally, a patient with classic claudication symptoms and palpable pulses will need to have exercise treadmill testing. These patients often have aortoiliac disease that is not hemodynamically significant at rest, but with exercise, ankle pressures drop significantly. A drop in ankle pressure to 60 mm Hg or less on a treadmill test is consistent with significant claudication.

Transcutaneous oxygen measurement indirectly measures arterial flow by evaluating skin perfusion. This test is most often used in assessing the healing potential of an amputation level or the healing potential of an ulcer. Oxygen levels > 40 mm Hg are consistent with good healing, < 20 mm Hg have poor healing potential, and in the 20–40 mm Hg range have variable healing potential.

Noninvasive testing beyond the ABI and possibly exercise treadmill stress testing should be discussed with a vascular surgeon. Localization of the disease process to inflow (aortoiliac) disease versus outflow disease (femoral-popliteal-tibial disease) is most important. This can easily be done with segmental pressure testing or with duplex scanning. Most laboratories are equipped with the simpler segmental pressure testing equipment.

MANAGEMENT

The overall management scheme for a patient with intermittent claudication is presented in Box 41–1.

Modification of risk factors, especially abstaining from tobacco products, is critical. Searching for evidence of life-threatening cardiovascular disease is important. The patient should be started on a regular exercise regimen. Walking for 30 minutes three or four times a week is the minimum recommended exercise. Most patients who can stop smoking and commit to this type of exercise program will stabilize or improve.

Drug therapy is not a substitute for exercise, but concomitant use of a rheologic agent, such as pentoxifylline, may be helpful in extending ambulation distances for about 25% of patients. This drug enhances red blood cell deformability, thereby decreasing blood viscosity and improving oxygen delivery in the microcirculation. Other drugs are currently being investigated, including L-carnitine.

Conservative treatment will be unacceptable to some patients whose life-style is limited by their walking disability. Life-style modification is thus recommended. In those patients whose job is dependent upon their walking ability, or in those patients whose disease progresses to the point of limb threat, vascular surgery consultation is necessary.

Revascularization for lower extremity ischemia is complex. However, the clinician should be aware that graft patency rates in both diabetics and nondiabetics can achieve 80% at 5 years, with even higher limb salvage rates. Less invasive methods of revascularization, such as balloon angioplasty and stenting, are being utilized more frequently. Endovascular grafting via minimal arterial access is on the horizon. A patient with claudication who experiences a deterioration in symptoms or signs of progressive ischemia should be immediately referred for surgical evaluation.

Patients who present with arterial ischemia and foot infections must be handled carefully. Treatment of infection is best done with intravenous antibiotics and bed rest. Debridement of infected or necrotic tissue must be performed concomitantly with revascularization.

BOX 41–1. Management of Patient with Claudication

Establish diagnosis by history and physical examination.
Rule out acute ischemia or limb-threatened state (in consultation with vascular surgeon).
Perform baseline ABIs.
Counsel patient about modification of risk factors:
    Total abstinence from nicotine.
    Hypertension control.
    Fat intake modification.
    Strict control of diabetes.
Establish a regular exercise program for the patient:
    At least 30 minutes of walking three or four times a week.
Reassess the patient at 8 weeks.
If no improvement, consider pentoxifylline use (minimum of 8 weeks to assess efficacy).
If still no improvement (or patient is worse), encourage risk factor modification and exercise and obtain evaluation by vascular surgeon.
Follow-up every 6 months with general cardiovascular assessment and ABIs.

BOX 41–2. Recommendations to Patient/Family about Lower Extremity Ischemia

Perform meticulous daily foot care.
 Inspect feet daily for sores, ulcers, abrasions, etc.
 Wear properly fitting shoes.
 Do not walk barefoot.
 Inspect footwear for foreign objects.
 Do not soak feet.
 Trim toenails carefully.
Remove footwear at each visit to physician.
Recognize signs of increasing ischemia; e.g., increased pain, increased pallor or cyanosis, rest pain.
 Report to physician immediately with signs of increasing ischemia or evidence of infection.

PATIENT AND FAMILY EDUCATION

Recommendations to the patient with arterial insufficiency are summarized in Box 41–2. In general, patients should be taught to inspect their feet and toes daily. Any visit to a physician should cause the patient to remove footwear, i.e., to remind the physician to inspect the feet. The patient should wear properly fitting shoes and avoid barefoot walking. Avoidance of trauma to the feet is critical. Cutting of toenails, in particular, should be done carefully. If the patient is incapable of self-inspection and proper foot care, a family member should assume this role.

The patient should be taught about advancing signs of ischemia. Increased pain in an extremity, particularly the foot, should be reported promptly to the physician. Rest pain, evidence of pallor, cyanosis, and foot or toe ulceration are also indicative of advanced ischemia. Patients should be scheduled for regular follow-up visits. ABI testing should be performed at least every 6 months.

Counseling about smoking cessation may be the most critical component of patient education. Referral to a smoking cessation program can be helpful. Of utmost importance, however, is the concern and empathy shown by the physician. The physician must take the time to teach the patient about the association between arterial ischemia and cigarette smoking.

NATURAL HISTORY/PROGNOSIS

In general, claudication is a relatively benign disorder. However, it is a marker for systemic disease, and the life expectancy of patients with generalized atherosclerosis is 5–10 years less than that of the general population. In particular, life-threatening coronary artery disease may be present in as many as 30% of patients with lower extremity ischemia.

Natural history studies of patients with intermittent claudication are difficult to interpret, but it is generally accepted that the amputation rate after 5 years is approximately 5%–10%. Patients who refuse to modify their risk factors (e.g., by stopping tobacco use) will have a high incidence of disease progression. Diabetics also tend to have progression of disease. Overall, approximately 25% of patients who present with intermittent claudication will require surgical intervention. Follow-up by noninvasive studies is critical. Limb-threatening ischemia has a poor prognosis unless aggressively managed.

Research Questions

1. How might you predict which patients will have progressive atherosclerotic obstruction despite modification of risk factors?
2. Can pharmacologic agents be developed to arrest or reverse the atherosclerotic process?

Case Resolution

This patient had a nonhealing toe ulcer, consistent with severe arterial insufficiency. He continued to smoke several cigarettes daily and eventually developed a mild cellulitis extending from his affected toe to the dorsum of his foot. He was admitted to the hospital for bed rest and intravenous antibiotics. Since ABIs and toe pressures suggested that a great toe amputation would not heal, he underwent angiography. This study revealed a right superficial femoral artery occlusion and severe distal tibial arterial disease. He underwent a right femoral to posterior tibial artery bypass, using saphenous vein as a conduit, and a great toe amputation. The amputation site healed completely, and he was discharged home on one aspirin daily.

Selected Readings

Castronuevo, J. J., and D. P. Flanigan. Pseudoclaudication of neurospinal origin. Vasc Diag Ther 5:21–6, 1984.
Criado, E., F. Ramadan, B. A. Keagy, and G. Johnson. Intermittent claudication. Surg Gynecol Obstet 173:163–70, 1991.
Green, R. M., and J. McNamara. The effects of pentoxifylline on patients with intermittent claudication. J Vasc Surg 7:356–62, 1988.
Krupski, W. C., and J. H. Rapp. Smoking and atherosclerosis. Perspect Vasc Surg 1:103–34, 1988.
Lundgren, F., A. G. Dahllof, and K. Lundholm. Intermittent claudication: Surgical reconstruction or physical training? A prospective randomized trial of treatment efficacy. Ann Surg 209:346–55, 1989.
Strandness, D. E. Intermittent claudication. Cardiovasc Clin 3:53–63, 1971.

CHAPTER 42

LEG EDEMA

Bruce K. Shively, M.D.

H$_x$ A 65-year-old male retired chaplain complains that 4 months ago his shoes became difficult to remove at the end of the day because of ankle swelling. He denies any ankle or leg pain. He admits to shortness of breath when mowing his lawn. He has no other medical problems except hypertension, for which he takes diltiazem. When he was 42, he was hospitalized for "a blood clot in the lung." The physical examination reveals an obese, elderly man with normal vital signs and mild periorbital puffiness. His jugular venous pressure is estimated to be 12 mm Hg. The chest examination is normal. Cardiac examination reveals distant heart sounds and a II/VI murmur at the lower left sternal border that increases with inspiration. His abdomen is protuberant but without a fluid wave, and his liver span is 14 cm. Examination of his legs is unremarkable except for 2+ bilateral pitting edema limited to the ankles.

Questions

1. What other questions would you want to ask this patient?
2. What is meant by "2+ pitting"?
3. What does the elevation of jugular venous pressure imply about his heart?
4. Which laboratory tests would be helpful?

Leg edema is an abnormal increase in the interstitial fluid content of the subcutaneous tissues of the leg. Synonymous terms are dependent edema and peripheral edema. Leg edema is not to be confused with joint swelling (see Chapter 87) or pretibial myxedema, which is an abnormal thickening of the skin of the anterior lower leg and foot seen in hypothyroidism. Leg edema is not an indicator of a specific disease but rather a marker for either an increase in interstitial fluid content of the entire body or an obstruction to the normal flow of blood and lymph from the leg. The importance of leg edema as a sign in clinical medicine stems from its frequent association with major organ dysfunction and with several diseases that may be acutely life threatening.

PATHOPHYSIOLOGY

Edema is caused by an imbalance of factors affecting the distribution of extracellular fluid between the plasma compartment of blood and the interstitial compartment of tissues. The most important factors contributing to the accumulation of interstitial fluid are (1) increased hydrostatic pressure in capillaries, (2) reduced oncotic pressure in capillaries, and (3) increased capillary permeability. These factors were first identified by Starling in 1895. In addition, edema formation is prevented or reduced by lymphatic drainage of fluid from the interstitial space. The causes of leg edema can be categorized according to which of these factors initiates edema formation (Table 42–1). Certain diseases cause edema by altering more than one of the above factors.

Because of the force of gravity, generalized (total body) edema is prominently manifested as leg edema and, when the edema is mild, may be manifested as leg edema only. Clinically detectable leg edema does not appear until total body interstitial fluid volume has increased by several liters. Other signs of generalized edema that should be sought include periorbital puffiness and stethoscope indentation of the chest wall during auscultation.

DIFFERENTIAL DIAGNOSIS

Most cases of leg edema are caused by **increased capillary hydrostatic pressure,** due in turn to increased venous pressure. Increased venous pressure in the lower body is usually a result of either elevated right atrial pressure or obstruction in the venous system below the right atrium (with normal or low right atrial pressure). If the obstruction is in the inferior vena cava (above the iliac bifurcation of the venous system, approximately at the level of the umbilicus), leg edema is bilateral. If the obstruction is below the bifurcation, edema occurs on the side of the obstruction.

Severe or complete inferior vena caval obstruction occurs rarely but can be seen with malignancy (almost always renal cancer) or a hypercoagulable state (causing thrombosis). Leg edema in these cases is usually severe and refractory to therapy. Partial inferior vena caval obstruction may be caused by abdominal or pelvic masses, marked lymphadenopathy, ascites, pregnancy, and obesity. This leg edema usually is mild. Obstruction of the lymphatic system above its bifurcation produces bilateral leg edema indistinguishable from that due to venous obstruction. The term lymphedema describes this phenomenon. Lymphatic obstruction is almost always caused by lymphadenopathy.

Venous obstruction in the leg is the most important diagnostic possibility when a patient presents with unilateral leg edema. The cause is often thrombosis of the deep venous system in the leg, which carries a high risk of life-threatening pulmonary embolization. Other potential causes of unilateral edema due to venous obstruction are related to extrinsic compression of veins such as occurs with inguinal adenopathy or a

TABLE 42–1. Causes of Leg Edema by Mechanism

Mechanism	Subset	Disease/Syndrome	Usual Clinical Features
Increased capillary pressure	Inferior vena cava obstruction	Thrombosis, malignancy	Bilateral, severe (may be mild if partial obstruction)
	Deep venous obstruction in leg	Thrombosis, extrinsic compression	Unilateral, mild
	Reduced venous channels or venous valve incompetence	Coronary bypass grafting, stroke, varicosities	Unilateral or bilateral, mild
	Right atrial hypertension	Left ventricular dysfunction	Bilateral
		Pulmonary disease	Bilateral
		Valve disease	Bilateral
		Renal dysfunction	Bilateral, mild
Reduced lymphatic clearance	Lymphatic obstruction	Lymphadenopathy, filariasis	Unilateral or bilateral
Decreased capillary oncotic pressure (hypoalbuminemia)		Severe malnutrition; liver, renal, GI disease	Bilateral, mild or severe, generalized, poor prognosis
Increased capillary permeability		Calcium channel blockers	Bilateral, mild
		Idiopathic cyclic edema	Bilateral, mild, premenstrual female

tumor in the leg, and these causes may be complicated by deep venous thrombosis. Because of the importance of ruling out deep venous thrombosis, patients with recent onset of unilateral leg edema should almost always urgently undergo ultrasound duplex scanning of the leg. Unilateral leg edema may also result from lymphatic obstruction in the leg.

A unilateral increase in the hydrostatic pressure in the venous system without obstruction may occur when venous valves become incompetent such as in stroke (loss of venous tone), following vein removal for coronary bypass grafting, or after deep venous thrombosis. Otherwise healthy middle-aged and elderly patients may also develop bilateral edema when malfunction of the deep venous system is caused by reduced venous tone, valve incompetence, or decreased muscular activity. Leg edema from these causes is common and typically mild. Enlarged subcutaneous veins, called varicose veins, may be caused by increased pressure in the deep venous system and often are accompanied by leg edema.

Increased right atrial pressure is the initiating mechanism in many medically important cases of bilateral leg edema. Elevated right atrial pressure may be defined as > 8 mm Hg. Right atrial hypertension has many possible causes; some are common and easy to diagnose, while others are rare and difficult to prove. In the former category is right ventricular failure, almost always due to pulmonary hypertension, in turn usually caused by left atrial hypertension from left ventricular failure. By this mechanism, right atrial hypertension may result from left ventricular failure of any cause. However, right atrial hypertension may also occur from a variety of pulmonary diseases, and this possibility becomes more likely if the patient has no history of coronary or other heart disease or if the left ventricular ejection fraction is normal. A commonly used term for right heart failure due to pulmonary disease is cor pulmonale.

Uncommon causes of leg edema due to right atrial hypertension include those marked by accompanying left atrial hypertension without decreased left ventricular systolic function, such as mitral stenosis or regurgitation or constrictive and restrictive left ventricular

disease. Diseases in which right atrial hypertension is not accompanied by left atrial hypertension include tricuspid valve stenosis and regurgitation, in addition to severe pulmonary disease.

The many possible causes of right atrial hypertension—with one exception—are often accompanied by reduced cardiac output. This decrease in body perfusion is detected by the kidneys, in which a system of neurohumoral compensatory mechanisms is activated to restore cardiac output toward normal by expanding blood volume. The best understood components of this system are diagrammed in Fig. 42–1. Decreased cardiac output with consequent retention of Na^+ and H_2O may even play a role in other causes of edema not related to right atrial hypertension. For example, venous obstruction may reduce venous return to the heart, and loss of intravascular volume due to decreased oncotic pressure (see below) may limit cardiac output as well.

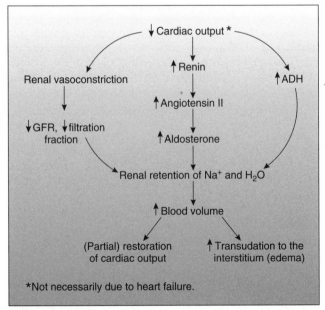

FIGURE 42–1. *Neurohumoral mechanisms promoting edema formation when cardiac output is low.* ADH, antidiuretic hormone; GFR, glomerular filtration rate.

The exceptional cause of leg edema due to right atrial hypertension that is not accompanied by reduced cardiac output is renal failure. Renal dysfunction resulting from many causes is associated with inability of the kidney to excrete the daily intake of Na^+ and H_2O; acute glomerulonephritis and the nephrotic syndrome are the renal diseases most associated with edema due to this mechanism. When renal failure is the underlying cause of leg edema, it is usually accompanied by elevated BUN and creatinine levels and an "active" (inflammatory) urinary sediment (one containing cellular casts and protein). Mild impairment of renal excretion of Na^+ and H_2O may also occur in renal disease without frank renal failure and as an adverse effect of certain drugs, especially NSAIDs and corticosteroids with mineralo-corticoid activity. These causes should be considered when approaching the patient with mild leg edema.

Decreased capillary oncotic pressure is usually the initiating mechanism of edema when the patient's albumin level is < 2.0 mg/dL and is likely to be a contributing factor with albumin levels ≤ 2.5 mg/dL. Because albumin accounts for approximately 65% of the total oncotic pressure of plasma, hypoalbuminemia alone may account for leg edema resulting from decreased oncotic pressure. Although this mechanism may produce leg edema of a nonspecific type (bilateral and worse in the evening), hypoalbuminemia should be suspected when the edema is generalized (i.e., apparent above the waist) and accompanied by severe underlying disease. Hypoalbuminemia results from either an impairment of synthesis due to malnutrition or severe liver insufficiency or severe losses that exceed the liver's synthetic capacity. Losses of this magnitude are usually due to the nephrotic syndrome with urinary protein > 3.5 g/d or rarely protein-losing intestinal disease. These diseases are always suggested by the patient's history or physical examination and carry a poor prognosis.

Leg edema due to **increased capillary permeability** is bilateral, mild, and usually unaccompanied by signs of generalized edema. The diagnosis is one of exclusion, since there is no specific test for capillary integrity. The patient's history is key because the cause will be either a drug or a poorly understood syndrome called idiopathic cyclic edema (see below). Calcium channel blockers (especially nifedipine) are the most frequent cause of leg edema by this mechanism; most drugs associated with leg edema act by increasing renal Na^+ and H_2O retention. Increased capillary permeability also plays a role in edema due to injury and inflammation. When edema is acute and accompanied by redness and tenderness, cellulitis or a burn (especially from hot water) should be considered. A history of other types of chemical or physical injury should be sought.

Idiopathic cyclic edema is a syndrome of abnormal diurnal fluctuations of total body Na^+ and H_2O resulting in leg edema most noticeable at the end of the day. The diagnosis should be considered only when the other causes of edema have been excluded. It is almost always seen in women, increases during the premenstrual period, and is probably due to hormonally mediated changes in capillary permeability.

EVALUATION

History

Leg edema usually is not painful and sometimes goes unnoticed by the patient. The physician should suspect leg edema when a patient mentions that shoes seem too small or are difficult to put on. Another frequent complaint is a feeling of tight or tender skin of the foot or leg. The patient may notice increased indentation of the skin over the ankle caused by ribbed socks. Edema may be noticed at any time of day but is most common in the evening, when gravity tends to distribute it to the lower extremity. When leg edema is painful, the physician must consider the possibility of accompanying cellulitis, a diagnosis requiring urgent treatment (see Chapter 115).

Physical Examination

Leg edema is most easily detected on physical examination by indentation of the skin over the ankle when the physician gently presses with one or two fingers. Indentation of the skin in this manner is called pitting. The depth and location of pitting are related to the degree of interstitial fluid accumulation. Pitting may be graded by measuring the depth of the indentation after pressure is held for approximately 10 seconds. Pitting may also be graded by its extent upward from the feet (e.g., "pitting to the mid-calf"). Physicians fre-

---

TABLE 42–2. Clinical Evaluation of Leg Edema

History

Duration and rate of progression of swelling
Diurmal variation (morning versus evening)
Organ system symptoms
　Heart: exertional dyspnea, orthopnea
　Lung: dyspnea, hemoptysis, smoking and other exposures
　Liver: fatigue, bleeding, abdominal distention
　Kidney: change in urinary habits, malaise
Other symptoms: abdominal/pelvic pain, leg pain, change in bowel habits
Prior deep venous thrombosis or pulmonary embolism

Physical Examination

Unilateral or bilateral edema
Severity (grade)
Generalized vs. localized
Brawny vs. pitting
Organ system signs
　Heart: jugular venous pressure and V waves, right ventricular lift and S_3, loud P_2, abnormal PMI murmurs of mitral stenosis or regurgitation
　Lung: abnormal breath sounds, rales, kyphosis
　Liver: jaundice, spider angiomata, palmar erythema, ascites
Other signs: abdominal/pelvic masses; inguinal adenopathy; leg tenderness, redness, or masses

Laboratory Tests

Blood: albumin, BUN/creatinine, liver enzymes, INR
Urinalysis: protein, microscopic examination, 24-hour collection for protein and creatinine excretion
Chest x-ray: heart size, pulmonary vascular congestion, other pulmonary parenchymal or vascular disease
Echocardiogram*: estimation of right atrial and pulmonary artery pressure; function of ventricles, valves
Pulmonary function tests: to assess for hypoxemia, restrictive or obstructive pattern
Leg duplex scan: to detect deep venous thrombosis

*ECG is not sufficiently specific to differentiate cardiac vs. noncardiac etiologies.

quently grade pitting on the ubiquitous scale of 1+ to 4+. Although there are no firmly standardized criteria for assignment of each rank, the following rules of thumb may be used. In general, 1+ leg edema is 1–3 mm of indentation of the skin limited to the ankle or below, 2+ is 4–10 mm also limited to the ankle or below, 3+ is a similar depth of pitting extending up to the knee, and 4+ leg edema is pitting extending above the knee.

When leg edema does not show pitting, it is called brawny (i.e., muscle-like) edema. Edema tends to become brawny when it is chronic, since the long-standing interference of normal metabolism within subcutaneous tissues by edema results in low-grade inflammation and fibrosis. The causes of brawny edema are the same as those of pitting edema (see Table 42–1).

Additional Evaluation

Leg edema in the outpatient is approached differently than in other settings because edema is more likely to be the presenting problem and less likely to be accompanied by major organ system failure (Table 42–2 and Fig. 42–2). In particular, malnutrition and severe liver, intestinal, and nonlymphatic malignant disease are unlikely to present with leg edema as the sole feature. In contrast, heart failure, renal dysfunction, and deep venous thrombosis warrant immediate consideration in the outpatient setting and must be excluded before

assigning a less readily confirmable diagnosis such as idiopathic cyclic edema. Symptoms and signs of cardiac disease should be sought, including orthopnea and paroxysmal nocturnal dyspnea by history and the presence of an S_3 and increased jugular venous pressure on the physical examination. Since lower extremity edema may be the only physical finding in renal disease, a BUN, creatinine, and urinalysis should be obtained. When the patient is at risk for heart disease or has no other explanation for edema, echocardiography may be indicated. Mild proteinuria is common in heart failure, and a 24-hour quantification of urinary protein excretion may be helpful in diagnosing the nephrotic syndrome.

If these studies are negative and a potentially responsible drug has been excluded, then venous obstruction or insufficiency should be considered. If the patient is obese or elderly or has a history suggestive of idiopathic edema, then symptomatic therapy should be given. If leg edema is refractory or progressive during therapy, further testing may be warranted.

Unilateral leg edema, in the absence of evidence of vein harvesting for coronary bypass grafting, cellulitis, or chemical and physical injury, should almost always prompt the exclusion of deep venous thrombosis with urgent ultrasound duplex scanning of the leg. If this study is inconclusive, venography may be indicated. A high-probability lung ventilation/perfusion scan can be substituted for venography in the absence of chronic

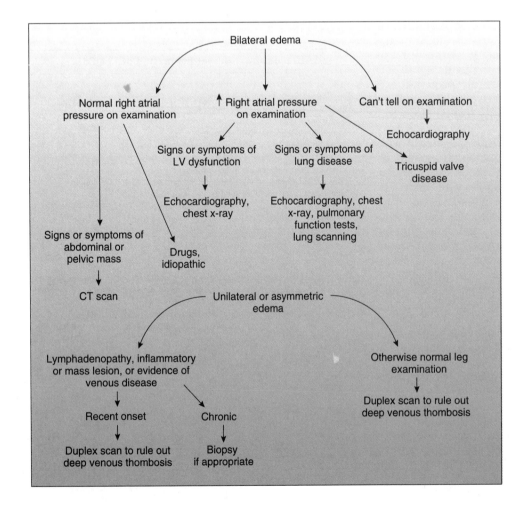

FIGURE 42–2. *Algorithm for evaluation of leg edema in outpatients.*

pulmonary disease or left ventricular failure. With negative duplex scanning (with or without lung scanning), a follow-up visit in a few days is advisable. This approach assumes that the leg has been carefully examined for inguinal adenopathy and mass lesions. A history of prior deep venous thrombosis should be sought because chronic venous insufficiency may result from venous scarring (called postphlebitic syndrome), and chronic cor pulmonale (and right atrial hypertension) may result from multiple prior pulmonary emboli.

MANAGEMENT

Patients with leg edema should be routinely counseled to avoid sitting with the knees bent (e.g., by propping up their legs on a stool or chair). If further measures are needed, some patients may be willing to attempt sleeping with their ankles elevated to above shoulder level on pillows. Support stockings worn during the day are helpful. Those that extend above the knee are especially effective but can be uncomfortable.

When leg edema complicates left heart failure, a moderate or severe degree of left ventricular dysfunction is strongly implied. After severe mitral valve stenosis is ruled out by echocardiography, treatment with an afterload-reducing regimen (either an angiotensin-converting enzyme [ACE] inhibitor or a combination of hydralazine and isosorbide dinitrate) is indicated. Elevation of the legs at night is likely to worsen orthopnea. Salt restriction should be attempted but often meets with limited success. A low daily dose of a diuretic is usually needed. Although in mild cases a thiazide diuretic may be sufficient, usually furosemide with potassium supplementation is given.

Diuretic therapy may be deleterious when leg edema is due to right atrial hypertension. If severe valve disease, cor pulmonale, or a low cardiac output state resulting from severe left ventricular dysfunction is present, diuretic therapy may precipitate cardiogenic shock owing to an excessive reduction in left ventricular filling pressure. In these settings, diuretic therapy is often used but should be initiated and titrated cautiously. To maintain adequate cardiac output, the patient may have to accept the persistence of mild edema.

Edema due to venous disease and drugs usually responds adequately to withdrawal of the drug or to a nonpharmacologic strategy. Low-dose diuretic therapy may be considered if these measures fail or if the patient has a compelling indication for continuation of the calcium channel antagonist, such as severe angina.

In idiopathic cyclic edema, nonpharmacologic treatment (such as salt restriction) should always be attempted initially. Diuretic therapy should be used with caution because for unknown reasons it may exacerbate the edema. ACE inhibitors and progesterone have been reported to be useful in some patients.

Research Questions

1. By what mechanism do calcium channel antagonists cause an increase in capillary permeability?
2. In patients with chronic edema, lymphatic channels return a larger volume of interstitial fluid per hour to the superior vena cava. How does this change come about?

Case Resolution

The patient was found to have increased pulmonary artery pressure on Doppler-echocardiography. A lung scan confirmed multiple prior pulmonary emboli. He was started on warfarin anticoagulation therapy. His physician plans to monitor his pulmonary artery pressure with follow-up Doppler-echocardiography, since increasing pulmonary artery pressure may warrant surgical removal of the emboli. A low dose of furosemide was prescribed for the patient's leg edema.

Selected Readings

Dzau, V. J., W. S. Colucci, and N. K. Hollenberg. Relation of renin-angiotensin-aldosterone system to clinical state in congestive heart failure. Circulation 63:645, 1981.

Gore, R. W., and P. F. McDonagh. Fluid exchange across single capillaries. Annu Rev Physiol 42:337, 1980.

Paller, M. S., and R. W. Schrier. Pathogenesis of sodium and water retention in edematous disorders. Am J Kidney Dis 2:241, 1982.

Staub, N. B., and A. E. Taylor (eds.). *Edema.* New York, Raven Press, 1984.

Streeten, D. H. P. Idiopathic edema: Pathogenesis, clinical features and treatment. Metabolism 27:353, 1978.

COMMON GASTROINTESTINAL PROBLEMS

C H A P T E R   4 3

ABDOMINAL PAIN

Melissa Martinez, M.D.

H$_x$ A 32-year-old female x-ray technologist has had cramping abdominal pain on and off for several months. The pain is associated with diarrhea (3–4 loose stools per day) and abdominal distention, mostly in the left lower quadrant and periumbilical areas. She denies fever, nausea, vomiting, melena, rectal bleeding, or abdominal trauma. She has a 15 pack-year history of cigarette smoking and had a cesarean section several years ago. She has had no major illnesses. She is a well-developed woman in moderate distress. She is afebrile, and her blood pressure is 110/80 mm Hg. The abdominal examination is unremarkable except for moderate left lower quadrant tenderness without guarding or rebound. The pelvic and rectal examinations are normal.

Questions

1. Does the nature of the patient's pain provide any clues to its origin?
2. What tests would you order?
3. How would your approach differ if the patient had guarding and rebound tenderness?

PATHOPHYSIOLOGY

The nature of abdominal pain is in part a result of the mechanism responsible for the pain. Table 43–1 presents some mechanisms of abdominal pain and provides examples of each. Distention or spasm of a hollow viscus causes a "visceral" type of pain originating from pain receptors located in the organs (viscera) of the abdomen. Visceral pain is poorly localized and often described as "dull." Vascular compromise, mucosal irritation, and organ capsule distention usually produce pain that is more visceral in nature. Conversely, peritoneal irritation causes a "parietal pain" that is sharp and well localized. Any given pain can have more than one mechanism. For example, as the appendix becomes inflamed, it produces a visceral type of pain. Later in the course of appendicitis, the adjacent peritoneum be-

comes involved and the pain becomes more parietal in nature.

DIFFERENTIAL DIAGNOSIS

The differential diagnosis of abdominal pain is extensive. Table 43–1 lists some of the more common causes of abdominal pain as well as descriptions of typical presentations. The nature of the pain, the clinical setting, and the associated symptoms can help narrow the differential. Certain presentations are considered "classic" for specific diseases. For example, appendicitis usually presents as pain in the right lower quadrant (McBurney's point) associated with fever and an elevated white blood cell count. However, not all patients will have a classic presentation of their illness. This is especially true of infants, the elderly, and debilitated patients.

EVALUATION

History

A first step is to question the patient about the nature of the pain, which may provide a clue to the mechanism. Another valuable piece of information is the location of the pain. Table 43–2 summarizes some of the more common causes of abdominal pain by location. It is important to remember that (1) abdominal pain can be referred from sites outside the abdomen and (2) the description of pain will vary from patient to patient. The presence or absence of associated symptoms provides additional key information. For example, the presence of jaundice in a patient with right upper quadrant pain points to a hepatobiliary process. Finally, some medical conditions predispose patients to a specific abdominal disorder. A patient with known atherosclerosis, for example, is at increased risk for ischemic bowel. Similarly, a patient who has had a prior appendectomy is at risk of developing small bowel obstruction secondary to adhesions. Table 43–3 summarizes issues to inquire about when taking a history.

TABLE 43-1. Mechanisms and Nature of Abdominal Pain

Pathology	Mechanism of Pain	Nature of Pain
Distention or Spasm of a Hollow Organ		
Obstruction of bowel	Distention and spasm of bowel.	"Colicky" (comes and goes in waves)
Biliary tract obstruction	Gallstone lodging in biliary tract.	Colicky or constant pain in right upper quadrant, epigastric area, or right infrascapular region
Urinary tract obstruction	Passage of renal stone, distention and spasm of the ureter.	Severe colicky pain in back, flank, groin or abdomen
Irritable bowel syndrome	May be related to "oversensitivity" to normal distention and peristalsis.	Chronic, intermittent, cramp-like pain associated with a sensation of abdominal distention or bloating
Gastroenteritis	Toxins, bacteria or parasites cause bowel spasm, distention, irritation, increased peristalsis.	Diffuse, cramping pain
Organ Capsule Distention or Inflammation		
Hepatitis	Pain is sensed by the organ capsule, not the insensitive parenchyma.	Dull ache in area of the organ
Pyelonephritis		
Peritoneal Irritation		
Peritonitis	Infection, blood, or other irritant to the peritoneum.	Sharp, well-localized pain, causing involuntary guarding and rebound tenderness
Vascular Compromise		
Mesenteric vessel ischemia	Thromboembolism, atherosclerosis, or vasospasm of the mesenteric vessels.	Acute, severe pain out of proportion to abdominal examination findings, preceded by recurrent, transient postprandial pain
Mucosal Irritation		
Peptic ulcer	Gastric contents cause irritation and ulceration of stomach and duodenal mucosa.	Burning pain in epigastric or right or left upper quadrant regions
Inflammatory bowel disease	Inflammation and narrowing of the intestine.	Cramping or burning pain, often in right or left lower quadrant
Referred Pain		
Referred pain	Exact mechanism unknown.	Various presentations
Systemic Diseases		
Sickle cell crisis	Unknown.	Varies, can mimic "acute abdomen"
"Strep" throat (especially in children)		
Diabetic ketoacidosis		
Abdominal Wall Pain		
Herpes zoster	Viral invasion of nerve root.	Severe burning pain before any lesions appear
Abdominal wall muscle strain	Stretching of abdominal wall muscles, can occur with vomiting or coughing.	Pain on movement of the abdomen, which can be mistaken for peritoneal pain
Psychogenic		
Psychosomatic pain	Indirect result of sexual abuse or other traumatic life events.	Chronic, associated with emotional stress, negative workup

Physical Examination

A complete examination with emphasis on the abdominal, rectal, pelvic, and genital regions is essential. It is especially important to search for signs of peritoneal irritation such as guarding and rebound tenderness as well as for the exact location of the pain.

TABLE 43-2. Abdominal Pain by Region

Location	Common Causes of Pain
Epigastric	Peptic ulcer, gastroesophageal reflux, pancreatitis, cholecystitis, bowel obstruction, pleurisy, myocardial infarction, early appendicitis, abdominal aortic aneurysm
Right upper quadrant	Hepatitis, cholecystitis, pancreatitis, appendicitis (if appendix is high), bowel obstruction, peptic ulcer, pleurisy
Left upper quadrant	Gastric ulcer, gastritis, pancreatitis, splenic abscess, pleurisy
Right lower quadrant	Appendicitis, pelvic inflammatory disease, bowel obstruction, ectopic pregnancy, inguinal hernia, inflammatory bowel disease
Left lower quadrant	Diverticulitis, bowel obstruction, pelvic inflammatory disease, ectopic pregnancy, inguinal hernia inflamatory bowel disease, irritable bowel syndrome
Periumbilical	Gastroenteritis, appendicitis (early), bowel obstruction

Additional Evaluation

A CBC may reveal an elevated white blood cell count (suggesting infection or inflammation) or a decreased hemoglobin level (consistent with blood loss). Electrolytes, liver function tests, serum amylase and lipase, arterial blood gases, and other tests can be ordered based on the most likely cause of the pain.

Plain films of the abdomen are insensitive and of limited value especially in the evaluation of chronic abdominal pain. Specific indications for ordering plain films include searching for free air under the diaphragm (a sign of perforation), dilated loops of bowel or air-fluid levels (a sign of ileus or obstruction), and radiopaque objects such as renal stones or gallstones. Abdominal or pelvic sonography, CT scans, and contrast studies such as barium enemas or upper gastrointestinal studies should be obtained only when a specific disease is suggested by the history and physical examination.

MANAGEMENT

The treatment of abdominal pain depends on its cause and is beyond the scope of this chapter.

TABLE 43-3. Information to Elicit During the History

Timing
Onset, duration
Frequency (if recurrent)
Relationship to associated symptoms

Severity
On a scale of 1 to 10

Locations
Region (see Table 43-2)
Diffuse versus localized
Radiation

Quality
Colicky, sharp, dull, burning, etc.

Palliative/Provocative Factors
(what makes it better/worse)
Movement
Positioning
Food
Medications

Associated Symptoms
Appetite
Jaundice
Heartburn
Dysphagia
Acid taste
Nausea
Vomiting
Diarrhea
Constipation
Flatus
Fever
Chills
Malaise
Dysuria
Frequency
Hematuria
Melena
Hematochezia

Clinical Setting
Age
Habits (smoking, alcohol, drug use)
Medications (including over-the-counter drugs)
Current and past medical problems
Prior abdominal surgery

Acute Abdomen

The term "acute abdomen" is used to describe abdominal pain of sudden onset requiring surgical intervention. The severity of the pain usually causes patients to seek medical care within a few hours after its onset. Patients with an acute abdomen should be hospitalized, made NPO (i.e., given nothing by mouth), and administered intravenous fluids until the workup and surgical consultation is completed. The workup should proceed as rapidly as possible, since emergent intervention may be required. Even with a careful and complete workup, the cause of acute abdominal pain is sometimes elusive. In these instances, "watchful waiting" with serial examinations may be helpful.

Chronic or Recurrent Abdominal Pain

No set time criterion distinguishes acute from chronic (or recurrent) abdominal pain, and it is sometimes difficult to differentiate the two. Chronic abdominal pain is usually less emergent than acute abdominal pain. Many causes of abdominal pain can cause both chronic and acute pain. For example, cholelithiasis can cause chronic intermittent pain until a stone obstructs and inflames the biliary tract with resultant acute pain.

Sometimes the cause of abdominal pain, especially chronic pain, is never determined. Such chronic pain may be a clue to an underlying problem such as depression, anxiety, or a history of sexual abuse. In the case of pain secondary to depression or other psychiatric causes, treatment may involve helping the patient gain insight into factors provoking the pain. This must be done carefully. Telling patients that the pain is "all in their head" or "not real" is not productive and impedes recovery.

PATIENT AND FAMILY EDUCATION

When abdominal pain is chronic and a functional problem is suspected, the physician should consider a meeting with the patient and the patient's family to help the physician better understand the psychosocial context and to discuss strategies to improve the patient's symptoms.

NATURAL HISTORY/PROGNOSIS

Many causes of severe acute abdominal pain have the potential to be fatal if untreated. Many causes of chronic abdominal pain can also produce significant morbidity and mortality if untreated.

Research Questions

1. Diabetic ketoacidosis sometimes presents with severe abdominal pain that can mimic an abdominal disorder such as appendicitis. What is the mechanism of this pain?
2. What is the mechanism of referred pain?
3. Why are elderly patients less likely to experience abdominal pain as a symptom of abdominal disease?

Case Resolution

On further questioning, the patient revealed that she had a great deal of stress in her life including a recent divorce, a new job, and conflicts with her youngest daughter. Flexible sigmoidoscopy showed no evidence of inflammatory bowel disease. A high-fiber diet and an antispasmodic were prescribed and resulted in dramatic symptomatic relief.

Selected Readings

Bender, J. S. Approach to the acute abdomen. Med Clin North Am 73:1413–22, 1989.
Birnbaumer, D. M., W. A. Woolery, and C. M. Wyte. Abdominal pain: Triaging the elderly. Patient Care 27(9):72–99, 1993.

Ganong, W. F. Cutaneous, deep, and visceral pain. *In* W. F. Ganong. *Review of Medical Physiology,* 16th ed. East Norwalk, Connecticut, Appleton & Lange, 1993, pp. 124–129.

Richter, M. J., and L. F. Butterly. Evaluation of abdominal pain. *In* A. H. Goroll, L. A. May, and A. G. Mulley (eds.). *Primary Care Medicine.* Philadelphia, J. B. Lippincott Company, 1987.

Silen, W. (ed.) *Cope's Early Diagnosis of the Acute Abdomen,* 18th ed. New York, Oxford University Press, 1991.

Soybel, D. The acute abdomen: Let the location and intensity of the pain guide your diagnosis. Mod Med 61:64–73, 1993.

C H A P T E R   4 4

NAUSEA AND VOMITING

Nona M. Girardi, M.D.

Hx   A 17-year-old female high school student is brought in by her concerned and anxious mother. The patient has been experiencing nausea and vomiting for a week. She is able to eat but her appetite is decreased. The nausea and vomiting are worse after a large meal. She feels tired but has no fever, chills, diarrhea, or abdominal pain. There is no noticeable weight loss. She has no history of recent travel. She ate a fast food burrito the day before her symptoms began. She is in good general health and takes an oral contraceptive, vitamins, diet pills, and an oral medication for acne.

Questions

1. What is your differential diagnosis?
2. What additional history do you want to obtain?
3. What would you focus on during the physical examination?

Nausea and vomiting are frequently caused by infections that result in a self-limited acute gastroenteritis. However, nausea and vomiting may be signs of more serious disease of the gastrointestinal (GI) tract or other organ systems.

PATHOPHYSIOLOGY

Nausea and vomiting often occur together. Alterations in the motility of the stomach and small intestine can cause nausea. Severe nausea is often accompanied by increased parasympathetic activity manifested by pallor, diaphoresis, salivation, and other vasovagal signs such as hypotension and bradycardia.

Vomiting is a reflex response involving visceral and somatic components that are integrated in the vomiting center and the chemoreceptor trigger zone (CTZ) of the medulla oblongata. The vomiting reflex begins with stimulation of receptor sites in the mucosa of the upper GI tract, the labyrinthine apparatus (inner ear), higher cortical centers (e.g., emesis can occur in response to emotional stimuli), or the CTZ (dopamine receptors), which is stimulated by specific mediators in the blood. Afferent nerves then carry the impulses to the vomiting center. Efferent pathways, including phrenic nerves to the diaphragm, spinal nerves to the abdominal musculature, and visceral efferent nerves to the stomach and esophagus, carry these impulses to the effector muscles. This causes relaxation of the gastric fundus and the gastroesophageal sphincter, contraction of the gastric pylorus, and reverse peristalsis in the esophagus. The glottis closes, preventing aspiration and increasing intrathoracic pressure, and the diaphragm and abdominal wall muscles contract, causing a sudden increase in intraabdominal pressure, which forces the stomach contents out through the mouth.

DIFFERENTIAL DIAGNOSIS

Although disease in the gastrointestinal system is frequently the cause, nausea and vomiting can also result from a myriad of other disorders (Table 44–1).

EVALUATION

History

The patient should be asked about the timing, frequency, and duration of the nausea and vomiting. Morning vomiting occurs in early pregnancy, uremia, and alcoholic gastritis. Vomiting occurs shortly after eating in pylorospasm, gastritis, and some psychogenic disorders. Vomiting 4–6 hours after eating, with food still undigested, suggests gastric retention (as in diabetic gastric atony or pyloric obstruction).

Bile is commonly present when there is prolonged vomiting due to any cause. Regurgitation occurs without nausea and without muscular contraction of the diaphragm or abdominal wall and may be due to esophageal stricture, esophageal diverticula, or gastroesophageal sphincter incompetence (especially when associated with a hiatal hernia). Projectile vomiting without nausea can occur with central nervous system

TABLE 44–1. Differential Diagnosis of Nausea and Vomiting

Common Causes

Acute GI infections, "food poisoning" (secondary to bacterial toxin)
Acute systemic infections with fever (especially in children)
Pregnancy (morning sickness, hyperemesis gravidarum)
Adverse effects of drugs and chemicals (which may cause gastric irritation or stimulate chemoreceptor trigger zone)
   Antibiotics, especially erythromycin and metronidazole
   Opiates
   Estrogen
   Ipecac (used to induce vomiting)
   Digitalis
   Chemotherapy
   Theophylline
Motion sickness

Less Common Causes

Acute abdomen
   Intestinal obstruction
   Inflammation of peritoneum or viscus (peritonitis, appendicitis, cholecystitis)
Other GI disorders
   Gastritis (including alcoholic)
   Peptic ulcer
   Radiation sickness
   Aerophagia
   Food intolerance (e.g., "allergy," celiac sprue [gluten enteropathy], lactase deficiency, fatty foods)
   Diabetic gastric atony
Cardiac disorders
   Acute myocardial infarction
   Congestive heart failure (nausea and vomiting are due to hepatic congestion)
Endocrine disorders
   Diabetic ketoacidosis
   Adrenal insufficiency
Hepatitis (especially viral)
Uremia
Psychogenic causes
   Transient, secondary to emotional upset
   Bulimia nervosa (chronic, induced vomiting)
CNS disorders
   Increased intracranial pressure (secondary to inflammation, acute hydrocephalus, neoplasm)
   Migraine headache
   Meningitis
   Disorders of the labyrinthine apparatus (acute labyrinthitis, Ménière's disease)
   Altitude sickness

(CNS) lesions. Feculent or putrid odor (due to bacterial overgrowth) occurs in lower intestinal obstruction or gastrocolic fistula. Blood in the vomitus usually indicates bleeding from the esophagus, stomach, or duodenum but occasionally is due to swallowed blood (e.g., from epistaxis.)

Associated symptoms should be assessed. Anorexia is common and therefore of little diagnostic value. Fever suggests an infectious etiology. Diarrhea often occurs in gastroenteritis. While the pain of peptic ulcer is frequently temporarily relieved by vomiting, pain steadily worsens in an acute abdomen. Vertigo and tinnitus suggest Ménière's disease, while headache and other neurologic symptoms suggest other CNS causes.

The patient should be asked about possible exposures, including medications, toxins, and contaminated food or water.

A past medical history of diabetes mellitus, heart disease, or renal insufficiency raises the possibility that a complication related to one of these is causing the nausea and vomiting. Past history of abdominal surgery may rule out certain causes (e.g., if the appendix or gallbladder has been removed), but it increases the patient's risk of adhesions and intestinal obstruction.

Physical Examination

The patient's general condition should be assessed. Is there evidence of dehydration (dry mucous membranes, orthostatic hypotension) or of weight loss? Icterus suggests hepatitis or cholestasis.

The abdomen should be carefully examined. Distention suggests (1) ileus; (2) obstruction; or (3) ascites, which can be further evaluated by assessing the patient for shifting dullness. On auscultation, the absence of bowel sounds suggests an ileus; high-pitched, tinkling bowel sounds occur with obstruction; and hyperactive bowel sounds often occur with acute gastroenteritis. Epigastric tenderness is common in gastritis and peptic ulcer disease. Tenderness with guarding (muscular rigidity) and rebound tenderness occur with peritoneal or visceral inflammation. These signs can occur in the right upper quadrant in acute cholecystitis, and in the right lower quadrant in acute appendicitis. The presence of organomegaly or masses should be assessed by palpation. For example, enlargement and tenderness of the liver can occur in hepatitis or right-sided congestive heart failure.

A neurologic, cardiovascular, or pelvic examination may be indicated by the history.

Additional Evaluation

Laboratory and radiologic studies are often not needed. For example, a 1- to 2-day history of nausea and vomiting in an otherwise healthy patient with a normal physical examination suggests acute gastroenteritis. Further evaluation is indicated only if the symptoms do not resolve.

If the patient seems more seriously ill, if nausea and vomiting are persistent, or if the clinical presentation is

TABLE 44–2. Some Useful Tests in Selected Cases of Nausea and Vomiting

Test	Useful in Diagnosis of
Abdominal x-rays (flat and upright)	Obstruction or ileus
Upper GI series or endoscopy	Gastritis, peptic ulcer
Abdominal ultrasound	Cholelithiasis
ECG	Myocardial infarction
Urinalysis	Dehydration (increased specific gravity), infection (pyelonephritis)
β-hCG level (urine or serum)	Pregnancy
Liver function tests	Hepatitis or cholestasis
BUN, creatinine	Renal failure, dehydration
Glucose	Diabetic gastroparesis, diabetic ketoacidosis
Electrolytes	Diabetic ketoacidosis, electrolyte imbalance or dehydration due to prolonged nausea and vomiting
WBC	Appendicitis or other acute infection
Drug levels	Digitalis toxicity, theophylline toxicity

TABLE 44–3.   Medications for Control of Nausea and Vomiting

Classification	Example	Presumed Site/ Mechanism	Use	Adverse Effects
Anticholinergic (antimuscarinic)	Scopolamine	Labyrinth receptors, chemoreceptor trigger zone, vomiting center	Motion sickness	Dry mouth, drowsiness, blurred vision; rarely, CNS effects
Antihistamine	Dimenhydrinate, promethazine, hydroxyzine, meclizine	Labyrinth efferents/CNS depressant	Motion sickness, drug-induced, postoperative, during labor	Usually less than scopolamine; drowsiness, dry mouth, blurred vision, headache; paradoxical CNS stimulation (especially in children)
Antidopaminergic (phenothiazine derivatives)	Prochlorperazine	Chemoreceptor trigger zone	Toxins (metabolic, microbial), cytotoxic drugs, radiation, postoperative	Extrapyramidal reactions (especially in children and psychiatric inpatients)
Antidopaminergic and cholinergic	Metoclopramide	Chemoreceptor trigger zone/Stimulates upper GI motility, increases lower esophageal sphincter pressure	Diabetic gastroparesis, postoperative	Restlessness, drowsiness, fatigue; extrapyramidal reactions, especially in children
Tetrahydrocannabinoids	Dronabinol	Unknown	Cancer chemotherapy	CNS effects: depersonalization, dysphoria

more complicated, further evaluation should be pursued based on the diagnosis or complication suspected (Table 44–2).

MANAGEMENT

Management is directed at treating the underlying cause.

If there are no signs of severe underlying pathology, nausea and vomiting can often be managed by simple changes in diet. Adequate fluid and electrolyte intake is necessary to avoid dehydration. This can usually be done orally, with clear liquids taken in small amounts at frequent intervals. In mild cases without diarrhea, water, juices, and broth often work as well as oral rehydration solutions. If nausea and vomiting are prolonged or severe, if significant dehydration has already occurred, or if intraabdominal or other pathology make the oral route unsafe, intravenous hydration and correction of electrolyte imbalance may be necessary.

Nausea and vomiting due to food intolerance resolve with elimination of offending foods from the diet.

Nausea and vomiting in pregnancy often respond to changes in diet, e.g., eating smaller meals, separating liquids from dry foods, and avoiding foods with strong odors. These symptoms often resolve spontaneously after the first trimester.

Nausea and vomiting resulting from medication use can often be relieved by decreasing the dose, changing the timing of dosing (many drugs are better tolerated when taken with meals; oral contraceptives are often better tolerated at bedtime), or changing the preparation (e.g., enteric-coated erythromycin).

Medications that provide symptomatic relief are sometimes useful for patient comfort or to prevent complications. However, they can cause adverse reactions, especially in children, and their safety in pregnancy has not been well established. Many of these medications have combined anticholinergic, antihistaminic, and CNS depressant activity, but the exact mechanism of their antiemetic activity often is unclear (Table 44–3).

PATIENT AND FAMILY EDUCATION

In acute gastroenteritis or in pregnancy, the patient and family should be reassured that nausea and vomiting are usually self-limited and can be managed by the dietary changes mentioned above. Medication is usually unnecessary. They should be alerted to the importance of maintaining adequate hydration (and in small infants and pregnant women, adequate nutrition) and to the signs of dehydration.

NATURAL HISTORY/PROGNOSIS

Recurrent emesis can cause complications including Mallory-Weiss syndrome (hematemesis resulting from a tear at the cardioesophageal junction), dehydration, metabolic alkalosis (owing to loss of hydrochloric acid), hypokalemia (owing to loss of gastric secretions), and aspiration pneumonia (in patients with CNS depression).

Bulimia nervosa, a disorder characterized by binge eating alternating with purging (often by self-induced vomiting), can lead to any of these complications and, if unrecognized or untreated, can be fatal. Successful treatment may require comanagement with a psychiatrist or psychologist.

Research Questions

1. Why does seeing or smelling something disgusting, or feeling very nervous, make people "sick to the stomach"? Does this serve any adaptive function?

2. What causes "morning sickness" in pregnancy, and why is its severity variable?

Case Resolution

Further questioning revealed that the patient's oral acne medication was erythromycin, which she had started taking a week ago. Her physical examination was entirely normal, except for her mild acne. The oral erythromycin was stopped, and her nausea and vomiting resolved completely by the next day.

Selected Readings

Ganong, W. F. *Review of Medical Physiology,* 16th ed. Norwalk, Connecticut, Appleton & Lange, 1993.
Gilman, A. G., et al. (eds.). *Goodman and Gilman's The Pharmacological Basis of Therapeutics,* 8th ed. New York, Pergamon, 1990.
Kousen, M. Treatment of nausea and vomiting in pregnancy. Am Fam Physician 48(7):1279–84, 1993.
McEvoy, G. K. (ed.). AHFS Drug Information. Bethesda, American Society of Hospital Pharmacists, 1995.
Wilson, J. D., et al. (eds.). *Harrison's Principles of Internal Medicine,* 13th ed. New York, McGraw-Hill, Inc., 1994.

CHAPTER 45

DYSPHAGIA AND ODYNOPHAGIA

Howard K. Gogel, M.D.

H$_x$ The patient is a 46-year-old male architect who has had difficulty swallowing for years, but his symptoms have progressed over the last 6 months. Food and drink "hang up" in his chest. After a short while, they usually go through, but sometimes he regurgitates. It makes no difference what he eats or drinks; solids and liquids are equally difficult. Some days he has little trouble, and other days he is miserable. He has lost 4.5 kg (10 lb) over the last 4 months. He has had minimal heartburn but no chest pain. He occasionally awakens at night with a dry cough. When he belches, the odor is foul. The physical examination is normal.

Questions

1. If the dysphagia occurred with solid food only, would the differential diagnosis be altered?
2. Is there a relationship between his dysphagia and his cough?
3. Does the presence or absence of a history of heartburn help in the differential diagnosis?
4. What diagnostic tests would be most helpful?

Dysphagia

PATHOPHYSIOLOGY

Although much is known about the control and regulation of swallowing, the level of understanding has not reached a point that allows for specific pathophysiologically based therapies of the various swallowing disorders. It seems likely that many "diseases" such as achalasia are really syndromes (much like

anemia) and are caused by several pathologic mechanisms.

Dysphagia is the symptom resulting from the failure to move a food bolus from the mouth to the stomach. There is a sense of something caught or stuck, but pain is unusual. The earliest sensation of dysphagia is that of delayed passage of a food bolus. When dysphagia is severe, regurgitation is common. There are two chief pathophysiologic mechanisms: neuromuscular disorders (motility disorders) and anatomic obstruction of an otherwise normal swallowing mechanism (Table 45–1).

DIFFERENTIAL DIAGNOSIS

Neuromuscular failure in the pharynx results in the inability to organize a bolus of food for delivery to the upper esophageal sphincter. Liquids are more difficult

---

TABLE 45–1.   Causes of Dysphagia

Neuromuscular	
Primary esophageal disease	
Achalasia	
Chagas' disease	
Other motor disorders	
Secondary (Table 45–2)	
Anatomic	
Benign	
Peptic strictures	
Rings and webs	
Caustic scars	
Cancer	
Primary esophageal	
Extrinsic compression	

TABLE 45–2.   Systemic Illness Causing Dysphagia

Collagen Vascular Disease

Scleroderma
Systemic lupus erythematosus
Mixed connective tissue disease
Polymyositis and dermatomyositis
Rheumatoid arthritis
Sjögren's syndrome

Neuromuscular Disease

Myotonic dystrophy
Myasthenia gravis
Multiple sclerosis
Parkinson's disease
Chronic idiopathic intestinal pseudo-obstruction
Diabetes mellitus
Botulism
Amyotrophic lateral sclerosis

Endocrine Disease

Severe hypothyroidism
Diabetes mellitus

Amyloidosis

to organize than solids. This is called **transfer dysphagia** or **oropharyngeal dysphagia** and is commonly accompanied by aspiration, cough, or nasal speech tone. Transfer dysphagia is often the result of a cerebrovascular accident or systemic neuromuscular disease. A pharyngeal motor disorder can also result from failure of the cricopharyngeal muscle to relax appropriately (so-called **cricopharyngeal achalasia**). This is often associated with Zenker's diverticulum (an outpouching of the esophageal wall just above the cricopharyngeus muscle). Zenker's diverticulum is probably a secondary phenomenon.

Neuromuscular disorders of peristalsis in the esophageal body can occur with primary esophageal disease (Chagas' disease, achalasia) or with esophageal involvement in systemic disease (Table 45–2). The pharynx and proximal third of the esophagus are made up of striated muscle and are subject to striated muscle disorders (e.g., myasthenia gravis, polymyositis). The distal third of the esophagus is subject to smooth muscle disorders (e.g., scleroderma).

Anatomic distortion of the pharynx, with associated motility disorders, can occur with head and neck tumors. Anatomic esophageal obstruction is most often due to benign strictures (caused by persistent, severe acid reflux), tumors, or rings. Achalasia-like disorders can develop in patients with carcinoma of the esophagogastric junction (secondary achalasia) as well as in certain patients with benign obstruction.

EVALUATION

History

Patients with neuromuscular dysphagia have as much or more trouble with liquids as with solids (Table 45–3). Symptoms often vary from day to day and can be made worse by extremes of temperature of food and drink. Patients with anatomic narrowing have the most trouble with chunky solids and breads. Their degree of dysphagia is more predictable from one meal to the next. If the anatomic narrowing is progressive, dysphagia for

soft solids and then liquids develops. Symptom progression can be subtle in disorders with a long natural history. Many patients will make an unconscious alteration in diet to lessen dysphagia. Progression is inevitable with esophageal cancer and common with peptic strictures. Schatzki's ring (a thin, uninflamed narrowing at the squamocolumnar junction) most often causes intermittent dysphagia for solids only. A history of symptoms of systemic diseases associated with dysphagia can also be helpful (see Table 45–2).

Pain is usually not associated with dysphagia. Pain occurs in 2%–5% of patients with achalasia and only late in esophageal cancer. Esophageal spasm can cause chest pain and dysphagia may accompany this pain, but isolated dysphagia is rarely the major complaint.

The sensation of something being persistently present in the throat or esophagus independent of swallowing is called "globus." Whereas dysphagia is nearly always caused by a definable organic illness, globus is often functional. A careful ENT examination should be done in patients with globus to avoid misdiagnosing those with definable organic pathology.

Acute total dysphagia is usually due to an esophageal foreign body or food bolus impaction. Mild pain is frequent, but severe pain should lead to the consideration of associated esophageal perforation.

Physical Examination

Weight loss is a nonspecific and late finding. A pathologic supraclavicular node may indicate advanced esophageal cancer. Halitosis may accompany esophageal stasis, particularly in achalasia. Signs of systemic or neuromuscular diseases capable of causing esophageal dysfunction may be present (see Table 45–2).

Additional Evaluation

An anatomic study of the esophagus is the first test to perform. Some controversy remains regarding the best anatomic study—endoscopy or barium swallow. Endoscopy is a reasonable first choice because ultimately the evaluation frequently includes it. Lesions seen radiographically often require biopsy or endoscopic treatment. A barium swallow is an excellent choice for patients with contraindications to endoscopy. When done carefully, considerable information regarding esophageal motor function can be obtained. Follow-

TABLE 45–3.   Dysphagia for Solids versus Liquids

Dysphagia for Solids

Progressive
   Cancer
   Peptic stricture
Intermittent
   Esophageal ring

Dysphagia for Liquids

Progressive
   Achalasia
Intermittent
   Motor disorders

ing a barium study, a standard size barium tablet or barium-coated marshmallow can be used to detect subtle abnormalities in patients with solid-food dysphagia. After the anatomy is defined, an esophageal motility study can be performed.

MANAGEMENT AND PROGNOSIS

Transfer dysphagia is best managed by speech therapists who have an interest in rehabilitating patients with this particular disability. These patients do better with a semisoft diet than with liquids. Patients who fail rehabilitation require gastrostomy feeding. Cricopharyngeal discoordination is treated by surgical division of the muscle. This procedure should be considered only in highly selected patients because aspiration risk is greatly increased in patients without upper esophageal sphincter function. Before surgery is considered, peristalsis and lower esophageal sphincter function must be proved adequate. Achalasia is treated by decreasing lower esophageal sphincter pressure. Current modalities (in order of increasing effectiveness and completeness of lower esophageal sphincter destruction) are drugs, dilation, and surgery. Unfortunately, the risk increases with increasing effectiveness.

Dilation of peptic strictures provides rapid, effective relief from dysphagia. Dilation does not, however, address underlying acid reflux, and peptic strictures often recur. Adequate control of acid reflux with lifestyle modification, inhibition of acid production, promotility agents, or surgery is necessary (see Chapter 51). Dysphagia caused by cancer can be improved by dilation, radiotherapy, or laser ablation. Where possible, surgical resection of the neoplastic stricture provides the best palliation, but cure is infrequent.

Acute total dysphagia due to food impaction may occur because of a mild stricture or ring. Secondary esophageal spasm can interfere with spontaneous resolution. Treatment with intravenous glucagon or atropine is often successful and obviates the need for urgent endoscopic therapy. A barium study should not be done because it interferes with endoscopy. After clearance of the obstruction, patients should be referred for elective endoscopy to evaluate the underlying cause.

PATIENT AND FAMILY EDUCATION

Many people consider heartburn normal. Persistent heartburn should be considered significant and sought out when taking a review of symptoms. Smoking and alcohol intake are the only potentially modifiable risk factors for the deadliest cause of dysphagia—esophageal cancer. Smoking also makes reflux more difficult to manage.

Odynophagia

PATHOPHYSIOLOGY

Odynophagia means pain on swallowing. It is caused by a number of unrelated disorders, which are characterized by inflammation extending deeply into the

---

TABLE 45–4.   Causes of Odynophagia

Chemical Burns
Caustic ingestion
Pill esophagitis
Sclerotherapy

Infection
Fungal
Viral

Perforation
Foreign body
Boerhaave's syndrome
Trauma
Instrumental perforation
Surgical injury

Cancer

Inflammation
Severe peptic esophagitis
Radiation esophagitis

---

esophageal wall (Table 45–4). Secondary esophageal spasm may contribute to the pain.

DIFFERENTIAL DIAGNOSIS

Odynophagia may result from chemical burns, infections, or perforation.

Chemical burns are most frequently caused by ingestion of prescribed pills. Most cases of pill esophagitis occur in patients with a normal esophagus. Pills usually hang up at the impression of the aortic arch or just above the lower esophageal sphincter, where a localized chemical burn occurs. In these patients, the location of the burn will vary. Pathologic conditions predisposing to pill ulcers include left atrial enlargement, esophageal motility disorders, and esophageal strictures.

Pills most likely to cause this trouble are antibiotics (especially tetracycline), potassium chloride, iron, quinidine, and nonsteroidal antiinflammatory drugs. Large, round, lightweight pills (as compared to small, oval, heavy pills), gelatin capsules, and sustained-release products are especially troublesome.

A chemical burn may also result from **sclerotherapy** for esophageal varices, as a natural consequence of effective treatment. Mild odynophagia is frequent and often persists for several days. Severe odynophagia can be a sign of perforation or a deep ulcer.

Infectious esophagitis should be considered in immunocompromised patients with odynophagia (Table 45–5). In immunocompetent individuals with no history compatible with other causes of odynophagia, infections must also be considered. Esophageal infections are most commonly caused by *Candida,* herpesvirus, or cytomegalovirus (CMV).

Colonization of the oropharynx and esophagus with *Candida* is common and can occur with imbalances in bacterial ecology, with failure of the clearance function of the swallowing mechanism, and with immune dysfunction. Infection can be asymptomatic. **Candida esophagitis** may be isolated or part of systemic infection as suggested by fever and other symptoms. Infection is accompanied by tissue invasion and the development of hyphal forms.

**TABLE 45–5. Predisposing Factors
to Infectious Esophagitis**

Profound Immunosuppression

AIDS
Leukemia
Lymphoma
Posttransplantation
Chemotherapy

Mild to Moderate Immunosuppression

Diabetes
Hypoparathyroidism
Adrenal insufficiency
Malnutrition
Advanced age
Hypochlorhydria
Broad-spectrum antibiotics
Corticosteroid administration
Chronic mucocutaneous candidiasis

Esophageal Stasis

Achalasia
Scleroderma
Anatomic obstruction

In comparison with fungal esophagitis, **viral esophagitis** is more often confined to immunosuppressed hosts. The clinical presentation and evaluation are otherwise similar. Herpetic lesions of the mouth or nose are helpful in suggesting a diagnosis. CMV esophagitis is more often part of systemic infection than are herpes or candidal infections.

Odynophagia may also result from foreign bodies, particularly if they are sharp and lodged in the esophageal wall. **Perforation** may ensue and is usually painful. Other causes of perforation are also likely to cause odynophagia (see Table 45–4).

EVALUATION

Pill esophagitis is easy to suspect from a careful history. Nonspecific ulceration detected by barium swallow or endoscopy combined with a favorable clinical course confirm the diagnosis.

For odynophagia in immunosuppressed patients, endoscopy with directed brushings and biopsy is usually required to direct treatment. Thrush in AIDS patients will predict *Candida* esophagitis in about three quarters of these patients with esophageal symptoms. A double-contrast barium swallow can be highly suggestive of infection and may even indicate a specific infectious agent. Radiocontrast studies are particularly useful in patients with bleeding disorders, possible strictures, or perforations.

MANAGEMENT

Treatment of pill esophagitis consists of withholding the offending pills or substituting a liquid preparation.

H_2-receptor antagonists, omeprazole, or antacids may promote healing. Pill esophagitis can be prevented by taking pills in the upright position with sufficient water.

For immunocompetent patients with infection localized to the esophagus, topical therapy for ***Candida esophagitis*** usually is adequate. Tablets of amphotericin B or clotrimazole (to be sucked) or nystatin suspension generally are effective. Patients with immune suppression usually require systemic therapy. Fluconazole or ketoconazole can be given orally, and fluconazole or amphotericin B can be given intravenously. Ketoconazole is poorly absorbed in patients with hypochlorhydria.

Foreign bodies can be removed endoscopically, but if perforation is present, surgical repair is required.

Research Questions

1. Why do only some patients with reflux develop strictures?
2. Why do many patients with peptic strictures have minimal preexisting heartburn?

Case Resolution

The patient had achalasia. The variability of the symptoms and the significant difficulty with liquids strongly suggested a motility disorder. His barium swallow showed poor motility and a "bird beak" appearance of the distal esophagus. Aperistalsis and poor lower esophageal sphincter relaxation at manometry confirmed the diagnosis. Endoscopy successfully ruled out secondary achalasia. The patient's dysphagia was relieved with dilation of the lower esophageal sphincter with a 35-mm balloon.

Selected Readings

Castell D. O., and M. W. Donner. Evaluation of dysphagia: A careful history is crucial. Dysphagia 2:65–71, 1987.

Castell, D. O., J. E. Richter, and C. B. Dalton (eds.). *Esophageal Motility Testing.* New York, Elsevier, 1987.

Diamant, N. E. Physiology of the esophagus. *In* M. H. Sleisenger and J. S. Fordtran (eds.). *Gastrointestinal Disease,* 5th ed. Philadelphia, W.B. Saunders Company, 1993, pp. 319–30.

Edwards, D. A. Discriminate information in the diagnosis of dysphagia. J R Coll Physicians Lond 9:257–63, 1975.

Richter, J. E. Heartburn, dysphagia, odynophagia and other esophageal symptoms. *In* M. H. Sleisenger and J. S. Fordtran (eds.). *Gastrointestinal Disease,* 5th ed. Philadelphia, W.B. Saunders Company, 1993.

DIARRHEA

Daniel J. Derksen, M.D.

H$_x$ A 20-year-old male college student complains of a 4-day bout of diarrhea with four to six episodes of watery stools per day. The diarrhea is preceded by severe abdominal cramping. The student has not been feverish, and he has not noticed any blood in his stool. Lacking interest in eating solid foods, he has limited his intake to liquids for the last few days. The student has recently returned from Mexico, where he spent the last 3 months teaching English in an orphanage. He says that in addition to boiling his water for 20 minutes, he thoroughly washed all fruits and vegetables in clean water before eating them. After returning to the United States, he went fishing for 3 days in a wilderness area in New Mexico. There he used water purification tablets.

Questions

1. What are the possible causes of this patient's diarrhea?
2. Does the time spent in Mexico or the recent fishing trip make certain causes of diarrhea more likely than others?

Diarrhea is an increase in the frequency, volume, or fluid content of stools. In the United States, where dietary fiber intake is low, the daily stool usually weighs less than 200 g. Diarrhea can be defined as a stool volume greater than 200 g/d or a frequency of three or more bowel movements per day. In a primary care practice, acute episodes of diarrhea are common. Worldwide, there are one billion cases of diarrhea involving children each year and diarrhea is the leading cause of death of children under 5 years of age; over 4 million deaths occur each year. In the United States from 1979 through 1987, 28,500 persons, primarily elderly individuals, died of diarrhea.

PATHOPHYSIOLOGY

Figure 46–1 illustrates normal daily fluid movement in the digestive tract. Diarrhea can result from damage to the lining of the intestine, absorption problems, abnormal motility, or the presence of osmotically active solutes in the gut. It is useful to think of diarrhea as acute or chronic (> 3 weeks' duration), infectious or noninfectious, and secretory or osmotic. Table 46–1 summarizes the types and mechanisms of diarrhea.

DIFFERENTIAL DIAGNOSIS

Table 46–2 lists the causes of diarrhea. Viruses account for about 70% of infectious causes, with rotavirus being the most common viral agent. Other infectious causes of acute diarrhea are bacteria and protozoa. Noninfectious causes of acute diarrhea include excessive fruit ingestion, laxative abuse, and disruption of the normal gut flora by certain antibiotics.

EVALUATION

History

The evaluation of the cause of a patient's diarrhea begins with a thorough history (Table 46–3). As always, a comprehensive review of systems may elicit information that the patient does not think is important but that illuminates the correct diagnosis. Information about recent travel is particularly important. Acute diarrhea in patients who have traveled to endemic areas will suggest specific viral, bacterial, or protozoal causes.

Physical Examination

The next step in the evaluation of diarrhea is the focused physical examination. Vital signs, including blood pressure, pulse, weight, and temperature, should be measured. The skin and sclerae should be examined for evidence of jaundice, and the thyroid gland should be checked for signs of tenderness, nodules, or increased size. The abdomen should be inspected for evidence of surgical scars, localized swelling, or ascites. Auscultation of the abdomen should precede palpation and often reveals hyperactive bowel sounds in acute diarrhea. Palpation is performed to assess liver size, determine whether the spleen or kidneys are palpable, and locate any areas of tenderness. Percussion can be used to determine the size of the liver or spleen. The rectal vault should be examined for evidence of cancer or polyps.

Additional Evaluation

The stool on the examination glove should be tested for the presence of occult blood, and a smear can be stained with methylene blue to check for sheets of polymorphonuclear cells (PMNs, or "polys"). If none are present on the smear, cultures are usually not helpful. Laboratory evaluation can also include a Gram stain to look for PMNs or eosinophils, culture of the stool (for *Shigella, Salmonella, Campylobacter, Yersinia*), and examination of a stool smear for ova and parasites *(Entamoeba histolytica, Giardia lamblia, Cryptosporidium)*. One serum enzyme-linked immunosorbent assay (ELISA) can be used to determine the presence of *G. lamblia* and another to screen for the presence of the human immu-

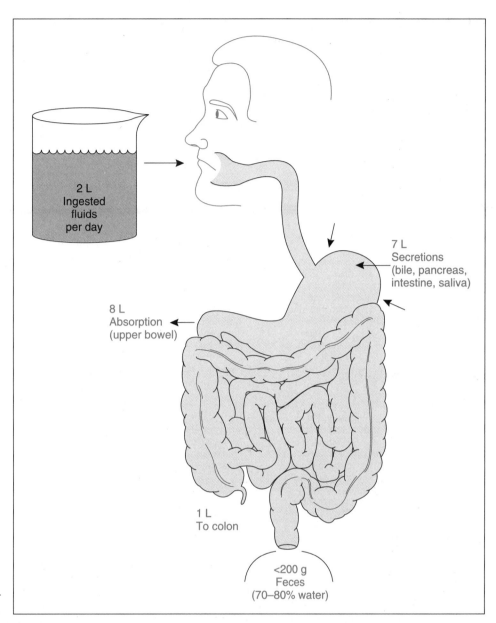

FIGURE 46–1. *Fluid movement in the digestive tract of a healthy 70-kg person.*

2 L
Ingested
fluids
per day

7 L
Secretions
(bile, pancreas,
intestine, saliva)

8 L
Absorption
(upper bowel)

1 L
To colon

<200 g
Feces
(70–80% water)

nodeficiency virus (HIV). Liver function tests should be checked if the patient has jaundice or liver tenderness. Also, flexible sigmoidoscopy should be considered in patients whose presentation is compatible with inflammatory bowel disease; in patients older than 50 years, colonscopy may be necessary to rule out a colonic neoplasm. Table 46–4 summarizes this list.

MANAGEMENT

In general, treatment of acute diarrhea involves hydration, symptomatic relief, and patient reassurance. Identification of the cause of diarrhea helps determine whether additional treatment is necessary. Replacement of fluids and electrolytes may be necessary. Diarrhea in young, otherwise healthy patients is usually due to infectious causes. Antibiotic therapy often is not necessary for acute cases of bacterial diarrhea. The need for antibiotics depends on the causative organism and the clinical situation. For example, antibiotics may prolong the carrier state in *Salmonella* infections. Thus, most *Salmonella* infections do not require treatment unless bacteremia ensues. However, *Shigella*-caused diarrhea is usually treated with trimethoprim-sulfamethoxazole. Symptomatic relief of diarrhea can sometimes be obtained with opiate-containing medications (e.g., Lomotil, Imodium), but such treatment may prolong the illness or lead to toxic megacolon in the occasional patient who has invasive bacterial infection.

Chronic or recurrent diarrhea that is due to inflammatory bowel disease (e.g., ulcerative colitis, Crohn's disease), irritable bowel syndrome, diverticulitis, malabsorption (e.g., lactase deficiency), pancreatic insufficiency (e.g., chronic pancreatitis, cystic fibrosis), or endocrine disorders (e.g., diabetes, hyperthyroidism) often resolves with treatment of the underlying problem.

PATIENT AND FAMILY EDUCATION

Hydration is the most important principle in testing a patient with acute diarrhea. This can usually be accomplished by oral hydration. Many infectious causes of diarrhea can be avoided by careful hygiene. Fecal contamination of water or food supplies can be reduced or eliminated by chlorination of the water supply, filtration systems, and institution of simple hygienic measures such as thorough hand washing after bowel movements. Traveler's diarrhea, which is often due to enterotoxigenic *Escherichia coli*, can be prevented by the use of bismuth subsalicylate (Pepto-Bismol).

TABLE 46–1.   Types of Diarrhea

Type of Diarrhea	Mechanism	Examples
Osmotic	Increased amount of poorly absorbed solutes in lumen resulting in increased retention of intraluminal water	Laxative abuse, undigested disaccharides (as from diet beverages), lactase deficiency
Secretory	Increased active ion secretion, abnormal secretion of water and electrolytes into intestinal lumen	Cholera, invasive *E. coli*, gastrinoma
Increased transit time or malabsorption	Decreased contact of food with lumen surface with decreased ability of mucosa to absorb food	Postsurgical (short bowel syndrome), diverticulosis, celiac sprue
Medication-induced	Disruption of normal balance of bacterial flora	Antibiotics (amoxicillin, tetracycline)
Inflammatory bowel disease	Inflammation of mucosal lining of lumen	Crohn's disease, ulcerative colitis

TABLE 46–2.   Causes of Diarrhea

More Common Causes	Less Common Causes
Irritable bowel syndrome	Infectious agents
Dietary factors	Viruses
Lactase deficiency	Coronavirus
Excess fruit intake	Adenovirus
Laxative abuse	Hepatitis (A, B, C)
Infectious agents	Bacteria
Viruses	*Campylobacter jejuni*
Rotavirus	*Yersinia enterocolitica*
Norwalk-like viruses	*Clostridium* species
Bacteria	*Vibrio* species
E. coli	Parasites
S. aureus	*Entamoeba histolytica*
Shigella species	*Cryptosporidium*
Salmonella species	Secretory conditions
Parasites	Gastrinoma
G. lamblia	Malabsorption
AIDS	Celiac sprue
Opportunistic agents	Postsurgery
Cytomegalovirus	Diverticulitis
Cryptosporidium	Endocrine disorders
Isospora	Hyperthyroidism
Gay bowel syndrome	Diabetes mellitus

TABLE 46–3.   Important History to Obtain from Patients with Diarrhea

Stool Characteristics
Frequency
Volume
Fluidity
Color (e.g., black or tarry, bloody)
Presence of steatorrhea or fecal incontinence
Other History
Dietary history
Recent travel
Source of drinking water
Medication use
Medical history
Surgical history
Sexual practices (e.g., anal intercourse, frequency of anal intercourse, number and sex of partners)
Social history (e.g., living situation)
Family history (e.g., inflammatory bowel disease, colon cancer)
Dimensions of the Problem
Associated symptoms (e.g., abdominal pain, fever, vomiting)
Exacerbating or alleviating factors

TABLE 46–4.   Laboratory Assessment for Diarrhea

Stool
  Occult blood
  Stool smear (methylene blue or Gram stain)
  Stool culture *(Shigella, Salmonella, Campylobacter, Yersinia)*
  Ova and parasites
  Clostridium difficile toxin
  Rotavirus assay
CBC
Electrolytes, BUN, creatinine
HIV
Flexible sigmoidoscopy or colonoscopy

NATURAL HISTORY/PROGNOSIS

Acute cases of virus-related diarrhea are self-limited and resolve spontaneously over a period of several days. Diarrhea caused by bacteria may also resolve spontaneously. However, some bacterial and many parasitic causes of diarrhea require antimicrobial intervention. With appropriate treatment, recovery is relatively quick, although loose stools can persist for days to weeks. Patients with chronic diarrhea may respond to specific therapy, or diarrheal exacerbations may be reduced in frequency or duration by appropriate medical regimens (e.g., the use of corticosteroids and sulfasalazine in patients with ulcerative colitis).

Research Questions

1. Can vaccines be developed that might reduce the frequency of infectious causes of diarrhea?
2. What is the cost-benefit analysis of the common treatments for diarrhea?

Selected Readings

Binder, H. J. Pathophysiology of acute diarrhea. Am J Med 88(suppl 6A):2S–4S, 1990.

Braude, A. J., C. E. Davis, and J. Fierer (eds.). *Infectious Diseases and Medical Microbiology,* 2nd ed. Philadelphia, W.B. Saunders Company, 1986.

Bruckstein, A. H. Acute diarrhea. Am Fam Physician 38:217–28, 1988.

Johnson, P. C., and C. D. Ericsson. Acute diarrhea in developed countries: A rationale for self-treatment. Am J Med 88(suppl 6A):5S–9S, 1990.

Lew, J. F., R. I. Glass, R. E. Gangarosa, et al: Diarrheal deaths in the United States, 1979 through 1987: A special problem for the elderly. JAMA 265:3280–4, 1991.

Research priorities for diarrheal disease vaccines: Memorandum from a WHO meeting. Bull WHO 69:667–76. 1991.

CHAPTER 47

CONSTIPATION

Toby B. Palley, M.D.

H$_x$ A 72-year-old widow complains of constipation for 3 weeks. She reports having a bowel movement about every 3–4 days. She feels bloated and uncomfortable. She denies blood in the stools, weight loss, abdominal pain, or fecal incontinence. She denies a history of constipation. Of note, she sustained a compression fracture of T10 a month earlier for which she was hospitalized for 5 days for pain control. While in the hospital, she was discovered to be hypertensive and was started on a calcium channel blocker. She was discharged home on the calcium channel blocker and acetaminophen with codeine for pain. Since her discharge, she has been in considerable pain, particularly when getting up. She also states that it hurts her back to strain at stool. The physical examination is normal except for tenderness at T10. The abdomen is soft, nontender, and without masses. The rectal examination shows normal tone, no masses, and a small amount of hard brown stool. The stool is negative for occult blood. CBC, electrolytes, and thyroid function test results are normal.

Questions

1. What factors might be contributing to the patient's constipation? How?
2. What other questions might you want to ask the patient?
3. Does this patient require further testing or evaluation?

Constipation is the most commonly experienced gastrointestinal disorder in the United States. More than 2.5 million people consult a physician every year because of constipation. Hundreds of millions of dollars are spent annually on prescription and over-the-counter laxatives.

Constipation is a symptom, not a disease. Normal stool frequency is between three stools per day and three stools per week. Some authors define fewer than three stools per week as constipation. Patients also refer to the inability to expel stool and very hard stools as constipation.

PATHOPHYSIOLOGY

The function of the colon is to absorb water and electrolytes and to transport fecal material to the sigmoid colon for eventual elimination. Three types of colonic muscular activity are involved in normal colonic motility: retrograde motion (back toward the cecum), segmenting motion (chopping and mixing), and mass movements (propelling fecal matter forward). If retrograde or segmenting motion is increased, transit can be slowed and more water absorbed.

Mechanical obstruction caused by strictures or tumors can cause constipation by preventing normal passage of stool through the colon.

Innervation of the colon and rectum is via the intrinsic myenteric plexus and the extrinsic autonomic nervous system, both sympathetic and parasympathetic. Therefore, drugs and neurologic disorders that affect the autonomic nervous system can cause constipation by disrupting the normal innervation and reflexes of the colon. Various hormones and peptides such as vasoactive intestinal peptides and enkephalins also affect colonic motility.

TABLE 47-1. Medications Commonly
Associated with Constipation

Aluminum-containing antacids
Antidepressants (especially tricyclics)
Antipsychotics and anticholinergics
Antiparkinsonian drugs
Antihistamines
Opiates
Seizure medications (e.g., phenobarbital, phenytoin, carbamazepine)
Antihypertensives (e.g., calcium channel blockers, clonidine, ganglionic blockers)
Iron preparations
Sympathomimetics (e.g., pseudoephedrine, phenylpropanolamine, terbutaline)
Bismuth-containing products
Nonsteroidal anti-inflammatory drugs (NSAIDs)

DIFFERENTIAL DIAGNOSIS

Most constipation is caused by poor dietary habits, decreased activity, poor bowel habits, irritable bowel syndrome, or medications with constipating properties (Table 47-1). Less commonly, constipation is related to systemic, neurologic, musculoskeletal, or collagen vascular disease or to mechanical obstruction secondary to tumors, strictures, or intussusception (Table 47-2). The etiology is often multifactorial.

The lack of adequate amounts or proper type of dietary fiber can lead to constipation. Dietary fiber has been shown to increase stool weight, increase stool water content, and decrease colonic transit time.

Inadequate fluid intake can cause constipation by producing dry, hard, small stools that are difficult to pass. Sedentary life-style and inactivity may contribute to constipation.

Since the voluntary process of defecation can be promoted by assuming a squatting position, which increases the intraabdominal pressure, poor positioning on the commode can impede defecation. The time of greatest motility and mass movements is postprandial, particularly following breakfast. Failure to take time for defecation when the urge strikes can lead to loss of rectal sensitivity and reflexes.

EVALUATION

History

First, patients should be asked what they mean by constipation. Next, dietary habits, fiber intake, fluid intake, and exercise habits should be explored. Questions regarding toilet habits should include timing, adequacy of time allowed, and whether the urge is often suppressed. Patients should be asked about stool frequency, consistency, size, and shape. Inquiry should be made about the presence of blood in the stool and pain with defecation. The duration of constipation must also be determined. A medication history, including both over-the-counter and prescribed medications, should be obtained.

Constipation present for many years is more likely to be due to a functional motility disorder, whereas constipation of recent onset, especially if associated with blood, pain, or weight loss, is suspicious for carcinoma. A long history of intermittent constipation and diarrhea, cramping, and bloating is consistent with irritable bowel syndrome. Constipation that develops in infancy suggests Hirschsprung's disease, a congenital absence of the myenteric plexus.

A detailed review of systems may suggest endocrine, neurologic, or other systemic disorders contributing to constipation.

Physical Examination

The patient's general condition should be noted. A complete physical examination should be carried out with special attention to the abdominal and rectal examination. The abdomen should be carefully examined for bowel sounds, masses, tenderness, surgical scars, and organomegaly. The anorectal examination is performed to detect the presence of hemorrhoids, fissures, rectal and anal masses, and anorectal tone. The stool should be tested for the presence of occult blood. In women, a vaginal examination should be performed to evaluate for rectocele and masses.

TABLE 47-2. Causes of Constipation

Common Causes	*Less Common Causes*	*Rare Causes*
Low-fiber diet, inadequate fluid intake	Endocrine disorders (e.g., diabetes, hypothyroidism, hyperparathyroidism)	Myelomeningocele
Poor toilet habits		Hirschsprung's disease
Prescription and nonprescription medications	Neurologic disorders (e.g., multiple sclerosis, Parkinson's disease, autonomic neuropathy, dementia, cerebrovascular accident, spinal cord injury)	Chagas' disease
Irritable bowel syndrome		Intestinal pseudo-obstruction
Inactivity, generalized muscle weakness		Cauda equina tumors
Chronic laxative use or abuse	Mechanical obstruction (e.g., neoplasm, stricture, external compression)	Pheochromocytoma
Pregnancy	Psychosis or depression	Porphyria
	Electrolyte disorders	Heavy metal poisoning
	Anorectal disorders (e.g., fissures, hemorrhoids, abscess, rectocele, rectal prolapse, tumors)	Pudendal and splanchnic nerve injuries
	Other systemic disorders (e.g., scleroderma, uremia)	
	Decreased rectal tone and sensation (due to surgery, childbirth, excessive straining)	

TABLE 47–3. Agents Used to Treat Constipation

Type (and Examples)	Use	Comment
Bulking agents (psyllium preparations, e.g., Metamucil; methylcellulose preparations, e.g., Citrucel)	Regular use in chronic constipation and irritable bowel syndrome.	May contain sugar or sodium. May cause flatulence or bloating. Slow onset of action. Adequate fluid intake required.
Hyperosmolar preparations (lactulose, sorbitol)	Acute constipation. Preferred agent for intermittent use in chronic constipation.	Nonabsorbable sugars. Lactulose is expensive, may cause flatulence, bloating, and diarrhea.
Stool softeners (docusate sodium, e.g., Colace, Surfak)	Frequently used for prevention of constipation and chronic constipation. Probably ineffective for prevention.	Possible hepatotoxicity when combined with irritant laxatives.
Lubricants (mineral oil)	Intermittent use in chronic constipation.	Risk of lipoid pneumonia if aspirated.
Saline laxatives (magnesium hydroxide, sodium phosphate)	Intermittent use in chronic constipation. Bowel preparation.	Can cause electrolyte disorders and dehydration.
Stimulant/irritative laxatives (cascara, senna, bisacodyl, phenolphthalein)	Occasional use in acute constipation. Should not be used in chronic constipation. Bowel preparation.	Can lead to cathartic colon and dependence. May injure the myenteric plexus. Can cause dehydration, electrolyte disorders.
Local agents (enemas, suppositories)	Bowel preparation. Impaction. Occasionally used to stimulate rectal reflexes in neurologic disorders.	May damage rectal mucosa and inhibit reflexes. Dependence can develop.

Additional Evaluation

In a young and otherwise healthy person, constipation related to a low-fiber diet can be treated with a trial of dietary and life-style modification. If such interventions relieve the constipation, then further investigation is unnecessary.

The presence of (1) occult blood in the stool, (2) weight loss, (3) anemia, (4) severe straining at stool, or (5) a sensation of rectal fullness mandates a more thorough evaluation. The work-up may include anoscopy, flexible sigmoidoscopy, barium enema, or colonoscopy. In rare instances of severe chronic constipation, further studies may include (1) colonic transit times and anorectal manometry to evaluate the function of the internal and external anal sphincter, (2) rectal biopsy, and (3) electromyography.

MANAGEMENT

Many patients respond to simple education. Most often, the treatment of constipation consists of bowel retraining, dietary interventions, and life-style changes. The patient is encouraged to eat a high-fiber breakfast followed by mild exercise. The patient must then allow adequate time to sit on the toilet; i.e., at least 10 minutes. If no bowel movement occurs, the patient should try again after the next meal. Proper positioning on the commode is important to generate adequate intraabdominal pressure. This process of retraining may take many months, and the patient may need considerable positive reinforcement during that time.

Patients should be encouraged to increase their intake of dietary fiber to 20–30 g/d. The best dietary fiber source is bran and whole-grain cereals. Fruits and vegetables are also important sources of fiber. Dietary fiber can be supplemented with bulking agents if necessary.

Hydration is important in the prevention of constipation, and patients may need to drink up to eight glasses of water daily.

Some patients become overly concerned and even obsessed with bowel function. They may require psychological evaluation.

Electrolyte disorders and hypothyroidism are causes of constipation that are usually easily correctable. Identified anatomic or mechanical causes of constipation also need to be addressed.

All laxative use should be stopped. Constipating medications should be withdrawn or replaced by nonconstipating medications whenever possible.

Patients who have abused laxatives for a long time or who have systemic diseases affecting colonic motility (e.g., diabetes mellitus, multiple sclerosis, scleroderma) often do not fully respond to the above measures and may require intermittent laxative use.

Pharmacologic Agents

Agents used to treat constipation are listed in Table 47–3. Nearly all these agents are available without prescription.

Bulk agents are the only products recommended for chronic use in constipation. Bulk agents include such commercially available sources of fiber as natural psyllium or synthetic methylcellulose. They should be added to the diet gradually because, if introduced too rapidly, they can cause flatulence, bloating, and abdominal discomfort. The patient should be told that such agents act slowly and that it may take several weeks to see an effect.

The remainder of the agents listed should not be used in chronic constipation except in special circumstances.

Complications

Fecal impaction can occur in the elderly, debilitated patient. Decreased mobility, decreased bowel motility, and decreased fluid intake are contributing factors. Enemas and manual disimpaction may be necessary.

Toxic megacolon can present with abdominal distention. It can occur in elderly, debilitated patients or in depressed or psychotic patients, or it can be the result of autonomic dysfunction or anticholinergic medications. The colon is massively dilated and at risk for perforation. Cathartics and bulk agents should be avoided. The patient should be hospitalized and observed closely, while decompression is carried out with gentle enemas. Toxic megacolon due to ulcerative colitis requires aggressive management of the underlying disease.

NATURAL HISTORY/PROGNOSIS

Patients with chronic constipation who undergo bowel retraining will have a good outcome. Patients with a long history of laxative abuse or with systemic diseases affecting bowel motility often require the intermittent use of laxatives. They may never fully regain "normal" bowel function, but substantial improvement in symptoms and quality of life can usually be attained.

Research Questions

1. How might hormones and vasoactive peptides be used in development of treatments for constipation?
2. How does the epidemiology of constipation relate to the epidemiology of colon cancer in the United States? What are some possible mechanisms connecting the two?

Case Resolution

The patient had been given two medications known to cause constipation: codeine and a calcium channel blocker. In addition, she had decreased her activity and fluid intake. Her antihypertensive medication was changed to an angiotensin-converting enzyme (ACE) inhibitor. The codeine was discontinued, and she was told to use acetaminophen for mild pain and ibuprofen for more severe pain. The patient's constipation resolved quickly, and no further treatment was required.

Selected Readings

Castle, S. C. Constipation: Endemic in the elderly? Med Clin North Am 73:1497–1509, 1989.

Chopra, S., and R. May (eds.). *Pathophysiology of Gastrointestinal Diseases.* Boston, Little, Brown & Co., 1989, pp. 247–59.

Donatelle, E. P. Constipation: Pathophysiology and treatment. Am Fam Physician 42:1335–42, 1990.

Falk, G. W. Constipation. *In* E. Achkar, R. G. Farmer, and B. Fleshler (eds.). *Clinical Gastroenterology,* 2nd ed. Philadelphia, Lea & Febiger, 1992.

Graham, D. Y., S. E. Moser, and M. K. Estes. The effect of bran on bowel function in constipation. Am J Gastroenterol 77:599–603, 1982.

Holdstock, D. J., J. J. Misiewicz, T. Smith, and N. Rowlands. Propulsion (mass movements) in the human colon and its relationship to meals and somatic activity. Gut 11:91–9, 1970.

Keeling, W. F., and B. J. Marin. Gastrointestinal transit during mild exercise. J Appl Physiol 63(3):978–81, 1987.

Sonnenberg, A., and T. Koch. Physician visits in the United States for constipation: 1958-1986. Dig Dis Sci 34:606–11, 1989.

Wald, A. Disorders of defecation and fecal continence. Cleve Clin J Med 56:491–501, 1989.

CHAPTER 48

UPPER GASTROINTESTINAL BLEEDING

Howard K. Gogel, M.D.

H$_x$ The patient is a vigorous 66-year-old male waiter with a 20-year history of mild indigestion. He presented to his physician's office with melena and weakness but no pain. He has a 20 pack-year history of cigarette smoking. He began taking aspirin 2 weeks previously for back pain. Supine blood pressure was normal, and the physical examination was unremarkable except for the presence of melanotic stool on the rectal examination. A spun hematocrit was 41%. He was referred to a hospital x-ray department for an upper gastrointestinal series. As he swallowed the barium, he became hypotensive and slumped to the floor. He was taken to the emergency room and resuscitation was begun. He was transfused with normal saline and packed red blood cells and transferred to the intensive care unit. The hypotension resolved, but endoscopy was delayed because of the barium in the stomach. After initial stabilization, he vomited blood and had a second but briefer episode of hypotension. Oliguria was noted despite replenishment of intravascular volume.

Questions

1. What is the paramount clinical priority in upper gastrointestinal bleeding?
2. What are the risk factors for upper gastrointestinal bleeding?
3. What is the role of upper gastrointestinal x-rays in the management of acute upper gastrointestinal bleeding?

Upper gastrointestinal (GI) bleeding results in over 250,000 hospital admissions per year in the United States, or about 100 episodes/100,000 population. Acute care costs alone amount to more than 1 billion dollars annually, and approximately 15% of intensive care beds are utilized for patients with this diagnosis. Whereas many other clinical syndromes require initial close attention to differential diagnosis, acute upper GI bleeding requires that initial attention be directed to resuscitation and monitoring. The differential diagnosis should be addressed only after the patient's safety has been assured.

PATHOPHYSIOLOGY

The reader is referred to other texts for a discussion of the pathophysiology of hypovolemic and hemorrhagic shock. Upper GI bleeding is a syndrome that presents with hematemesis, melena, and/or bright red blood per rectum, with or without nonspecific signs of hypovolemia and shock. Upper GI bleeding may be the underlying problem when patients present with angina, syncope, dyspnea, seizures, or confusion. Hematemesis is caused by blood loss of ≥ 500 mL. Melena results from a blood loss of at least 200 mL. The overall mortality due to upper GI bleeding may be as high as 10%. Hospitalization is almost always necessary. Bleeding stops spontaneously in 80% of patients, but rebleeding is not uncommon, and all patients require careful management.

INITIAL EVALUATION AND MANAGEMENT

The first priority is resuscitation, which is similar to that for any type of hemorrhagic shock. Adequate resuscitation is the key to avoiding preventable deaths and complications. A minimum of two 18-gauge intravenous catheters should be inserted, and isotonic saline should be given until blood is available and needed. The initial hematocrit should not be used to make transfusion decisions, since the hematocrit merely reflects the percentage of circulating blood volume composed of red cells. It is not uncommon for a patient to present with hemorrhagic shock and a normal hematocrit. The hematocrit accurately reflects blood loss only after equilibration between extra- and intravascular fluid spaces

has occurred. After fluid resuscitation, the hematocrit reflects blood loss more accurately. Clinical signs of hypovolemia (vital signs, urine output) are key. If edematous states, drugs, cardiac disease, or mental status make these signs hard to interpret, a central venous line or Swan-Ganz catheter should be placed. Anticoagulation should be reversed, since bleeding usually is riskier than thrombosis. The major exception is in patients with artificial heart valves.

Most deaths and complications occur as a result of underlying nongastrointestinal disease exacerbation rather than exsanguination. Indeed, the rapidity of blood loss and the presence of underlying disease are the two most important prognostic factors.

History

The specific bleeding lesion usually has little impact on the body's ability to cope with the rigors of hemorrhagic shock, endoscopy, and surgery. A single preexisting major organ system failure increases mortality by 10% or more. Thus, clinical history taking should be aimed at identifying serious underlying diseases, predicting the need for monitoring and urgent endoscopy, and assessing the risk of surgery. The clinical history does, however, yield tantalizing clues to the source of bleeding (Table 48–1).

TABLE 48–1. Relationship Between Medical History and Etiology of Bleeding

Medical History	Etiology of Bleeding
Previous hemorrhage	Recurrence at the same site
Pain patterns	Duodenal ulcer, gastric ulcer, esophagitis
Bleeding diathesis	Diffuse gastric mucosal hemorrhage
Retching	Mallory-Weiss tear
Abdominal trauma	Hemobilia, Budd-Chiari syndrome with esophageal varices
Liver disease	Gastritis, esophageal varices
Recurrent bleeding with negative evaluations	Arteriovenous malformations, ectopic gastric mucosa, small bowel lesions
Multiple trauma, burns, sepsis, respiratory failure, etc.	Gastric erosions
Anorexia, weight loss	Gastric cancer, gastric ulcer
Recurrent nose bleeds	Hereditary hemorrhagic telangiectasia
Dysphagia	Esophagitis, esophageal ulcer, esophageal cancer
Aspirin, alcohol, NSAIDs, corticosteroids	Gastritis, gastric ulcer
Previous aortic graft, "herald bleed"	Aortoduodenal fistula
Biliary colic, jaundice	Hemobilia
Renal failure	Gastritis
Head trauma	Cushing's ulcer
Pancreatitis, pancreatic cancer	Gastric varices, splenic artery aneurysms, esophageal varices
Myeloid metaplasia	Esophageal varices
Immunosuppression	Gastritis, candidal esophagitis
Tetracycline, potassium tablets	Esophageal ulcer
Polycystic kidneys	Congenital hepatic fibrosis with esophageal varices
Contraceptive steroids	Budd-Chiari syndrome with esophageal varices
Polycythemia	Peptic ulcer
Leukemia	Leukemic infiltrate

Reproduced, with permission, from H. K Gogel and D. Tandberg. Emergency management of upper gastrointestinal hemorrhage. Am J Emerg Med 4:152, 1986.

TABLE 48–2. Relationship Between Physical Examination Results and Etiology of Bleeding

Physical Examination Results	Etiology of Bleeding
Arteriovenous malformations on skin and mucous membranes	Hereditary hemorrhagic telangiectasia
Blue skin nevi	Angiomas
Acanthosis nigricans	Gastric cancer
Retinal angioid streaks	Pseudoxanthoma elasticum
Hyperextensible joints	Ehlers-Danlos syndrome
Bleeding from gums	Scurvy, leukemia, thrombocytopenia
Stigmata of chronic liver disease	Esophageal varices
Body cast	Esophagitis
Scleroderma, mixed connective tissue disease	Esophagitis
Surgical abdominal scar	Recurrent ulcer after gastric surgery
Supraclavicular adenopathy	Esophageal cancer, gastric cancer
Isolated splenomegaly	Gastric varices
Pulsatile mass	Aortoduodenal fistula
Thrush	Monilial esophagitis

Reproduced, with permission, from H. K. Gogel and D. Tandberg. Emergency management of upper gastrointestinal hemorrhage. Am J Emerg Med 4:153, 1986.

Patients with a history of abdominal aortic aneurysm repair should be admitted for close observation. Patients with Dacron aortic grafts can develop a fistula between the aorta and the small bowel. Torrential bleeding can occur through the fistula. A clinically mild bleeding episode (the so-called herald bleed) may be the harbinger of exsanguination.

Physical Examination

Similarly, the physical examination should be focused on detecting underlying disease that could compromise the bleeding patient. Physical findings can also act as clues to the bleeding site (Table 48–2).

Additional Evaluation

Useful points regarding laboratory interpretation are listed in Table 48–3. The initial clinical evaluation must include confirmation of an upper GI source of blood loss. When a patient presents with melena, a gastric tube should be passed to determine the region of bleeding. The oral route of passage is preferred in patients with nasal abnormalities or bleeding disorders in order to avoid confounding nose bleeds. Bleeding duodenal lesions may deliver all of their blood downstream; therefore, the gastric aspirate is considered negative only if it contains bile but no blood. The gastric aspirate should not be tested for occult blood because the result is often misleading. Patients presenting with bright red blood per rectum from the upper GI tract have lost enough blood to cause a marked decrease in intestinal transit time. They are usually hemodynamically unstable. Conversely, a patient with bright red blood per rectum and normal vital signs will nearly always be bleeding from the colon or rectum. A gastric tube should be passed in any case. Rarely, patients with upper GI bleeding and bright red blood per rectum will be stable.

Gastric aspirate findings are 79% sensitive and 53% specific for determining whether bleeding is ongoing. When both stool and gastric aspirate are red, the mortality rate is 30%. As a rule, the BUN and BUN/creatinine ratio will be elevated more often in patients with upper GI bleeding than in patients with lower GI bleeding. Unfortunately, these trends are not accurate enough to apply with confidence to the individual patient.

Patients presenting with melena that cleared more than 72 hours previously can be evaluated as outpatients, provided they are hemodynamically stable, have no severe underlying disease, and the hemoglobin is > 9 g/dL.

After resuscitation, an effort to define a bleeding source should be made. In general, patients with upper GI bleeding should have an endoscopic diagnosis. The most likely responsible lesions are listed in Table 48–4. In addition to being diagnostic, endoscopy provides a vehicle for delivering treatment. Moreover, the appearance of a lesion may allow for prognosis and prediction of rebleeding. Most importantly, endoscopic therapy has now been shown to improve outcome in actively bleeding patients. Barium studies should almost never be used in the acute setting because they interfere with endoscopy, surgery, and arteriography.

Nonspecific therapy for upper GI bleeding is generally not helpful. Omeprazole, H_2-receptor blockers, antacids, and all varieties of gastric lavage do not stop active bleeding. However, there is a trend toward improved overall outcome with H_2-receptor blockers. Intravenous vasopressin can slow the rate of bleeding from esophageal varices and is useful in temporizing while more definitive therapy is being arranged. Because clearing the stomach aids endoscopy, lavage should be performed in anticipation of this procedure. Despite the general success of endoscopy, surgical consultation should be sought early in the clinical course. When support, observation, and endoscopic

TABLE 48–3. Laboratory Tests in Upper Gastrointestinal Hemorrhage

Test	Rationale
Chest radiograph	Evaluate for concomitant aspiration and pneumonia.
Electrocardiogram	Check for myocardial ischemia precipitated by hypovolemia.
Urinalysis	Assess degree of hydration with specific gravity.
Electrolytes	Rule out hypokalemia, hyponatremia, and accompanying hypovolemia.
Prothrombin time (PT), partial thromboplastin time (PTT)	Use to guide the consideration of fresh-frozen plasma therapy and to assess for the presence of vitamin K deficiency, liver dysfunction, or consumptive coagulopathy.
Platelet count	Use to determine the need for platelet transfusion and to evaluate for marrow suppression or platelet consumption.
Kidney, ureter, and bladder (KUB) x-ray	Evaluate for the (rare) presence of obstruction and signs of ischemia.
AST, bilirubin, alkaline phosphatase, albumin	Check for abnormalities reflecting acute liver injury or decreased synthetic function.

Modified, with permission, from H. K Gogel and D. Tandberg. Emergency management of upper gastrointestinal hemorrhage. Am J Emerg Med 4:154, 1986.

TABLE 48–4. Relative Frequencies of Bleeding Sites

Diagnosis	Weighted Average (%)
Esophagitis	5
Esophageal ulcer	2
Esophageal varices	10
Mallory-Weiss tear	5
Gastritis	13
Gastric ulcer	16
Stomal ulcer	2
Duodenal ulcer	29
Neoplasm	3
Duodenitis	5
Unusual or undetermined diagnosis	10

therapy are unsuccessful, consideration should be given to surgical intervention before transfusion of more than six units of red blood cells.

SPECIFIC MANAGEMENT

For management purposes, there are three classes of lesions: (1) diffuse mucosal disease (esophagitis, gastritis, and duodenitis); (2) focal penetrating disease (esophageal, gastric, and duodenal ulcers and Mallory-Weiss tears); and (3) portal hypertensive bleeding (esophageal varices, gastric varices, and gastritis). Diffuse lesions are not amenable to endoscopic therapy. Surgical treatment, when required, involves wide resections of the involved mucosal surface. Fortunately, the bleeding is usually from capillaries and usually stops spontaneously. Bleeding from ulcers is more often arterial. Endoscopic hemostasis is effective about 85% of the time. Surgery is nearly always effective but is riskier. Endoscopic therapy consists of local injection (alcohol or epinephrine) or thermal cautery (heater probe or bipolar electrode).

For Mallory-Weiss tears, the prognosis is excellent and the need for surgery is unusual. For active or recurrent bleeding, endoscopic injection therapy or bipolar cautery can be employed. Patients should be treated with antiemetics to avoid recurrent retching. (The cause of the retching should also be clarified.) Rebleeding is unusual.

Patients with esophagitis also rarely require surgery. The bed should be placed in the reverse Trendelenburg position and antisecretory drugs administered. Gastritis is best managed by removing its causes: alcohol, NSAIDs, sepsis, hypovolemia, and hypoxia. H_2-receptor blockers and antacids should be used to neutralize gastric acid. Duodenitis usually resolves rapidly with medical therapy only, and early discharge can be planned.

Although the rate of variceal hemorrhage is slowed by vasopressin, overall mortality is not improved with this drug, and it should be considered a temporizing measure only. The safety of this dangerous drug may be improved by the simultaneous intravenous infusion of nitroglycerin. Early endoscopy with endoscopic injection sclerotherapy or rubber band ligation is indicated. Propranolol may help prevent variceal bleeding but should not be used in the acute setting because it interferes with normal hemodynamic responses to bleeding. Gastric varices can also be treated endoscopically, but this is technically more difficult and rebleeding is more frequent. A second attempt at endoscopic treatment for rebleeding is reasonable, but failure of endoscopic management should lead quickly to decompression of the portal system. Decompression can be accomplished by a radiologist (via transjugular intrahepatic portosystemic shunt [TIPS]) or by a surgeon. Since portal hypertensive gastritis is not amenable to endoscopic therapy, decompression is required in this case in the unusual circumstance of persistent bleeding.

PREVENTION

Many causes of upper GI bleeding have identifiable risk factors. Smoking unquestionably increases the risk of duodenal ulceration and inhibits healing. Acutely, alcohol inhibits mucosal defenses, which may lead to gastritis, gastric ulcers, or the worsening of preexisting lesions. Vomiting associated with alcohol intake can lead to a Mallory-Weiss tear. Chronically, alcohol causes liver disease and inhibits platelet production. Severe liver disease can lead to both coagulopathy and portal hypertension. Hypersplenism associated with portal hypertension decreases the platelet count. Discussions with patients and families about the dangers of smoking and drinking are warranted. Referral to treatment programs should occur when possible.

Medications play a major role in upper GI bleeding. Aspirin increases the risk of gastric ulceration and, via membrane acetylation, causes platelet dysfunction that persists for the life of the exposed platelet. Other NSAIDs also damage the gastric mucosa, but their deleterious effects on platelets are reversible. Corticosteroids may contribute to the risk of gastric ulcers but usually only with prolonged use of high doses. In cases in which NSAIDs cannot be discontinued and there is a history of upper GI disease or bleeding, prophylaxis with misoprostol or an H_2-receptor blocker is recommended.

It is unwise to treat a patient with portal hypertension with NSAIDs. Drug combinations such as warfarin and NSAIDs should also be avoided.

Gastritis, gastric ulcers, duodenitis, and duodenal ulcers are all associated with *Helicobacter pylori* infection. Recurrence rates for duodenal ulcers are proved to be reduced with treatment for *Helicobacter pylori*. Bleeding from portal hypertensive lesions can be reduced by propranolol administration, by the cessation of alcohol intake, or by liver transplantation.

Research Questions

1. What clinical findings will best predict which patients will benefit from urgent endoscopic hemostatic treatments?
2. Which specific endoscopic techniques are most effective?

Case Resolution

Vigorous gastric lavage was undertaken to cleanse most of the barium and blood from the patient's stomach. Endoscopy was performed, and an actively bleeding duodenal ulcer was successfully cauterized. The patient's recuperation, although complete, was delayed by gradual resolution of acute renal failure, presumably caused by prolonged hypotension.

Selected Readings

Cowley, R. A., and B. F. Trump (eds.). *Pathophysiology of Shock, Anoxia and Ischemia.* Baltimore, Williams & Wilkins, 1982.

Friedman, L. S. (ed.). Gastrointestinal bleeding. Gastroenterol Clin North Am 22(4):1, 1993 [entire issue].

Gogel, H. K., and D. Tandberg. Emergency management of upper gastrointestinal hemorrhage. Am J Emerg Med 4:150–89, 1986.

Peterson, W. L., and L. Laine. Gastrointestinal bleeding. *In* M. H. Sleisenger and J. S. Fordtran (eds.). *Gastrointestinal Disease,* 5th ed. Philadelphia, W.B. Saunders Company, 1993.

CHAPTER 49

LOWER GASTROINTESTINAL BLEEDING

David V. Gonzales, M.D.

H*x* A 63-year-old male chemical engineer, mildly overweight but otherwise without significant medical history, presents with a complaint of three episodes of bright red blood per rectum over a 2-week period. The patient denies any pain with defecation, abdominal pain, or weight loss. He also denies taking any medicines, and his family history is remarkable only for diabetes. The physical examination is unremarkable except for mild obesity. A rectal examination reveals a few small lesions around the anus consistent with hemorrhoids.

Questions

1. What are the most common causes of rectal bleeding in this patient's age group?
2. What tests would you order? How would the results affect subsequent evaluation?

Rectal bleeding is a common office complaint. Clinically, lower gastrointestinal (GI) bleeding can be defined as any blood loss from the GI tract below the ligament of Treitz whether noted by the patient or detected by chemical reaction tests. Severity can range from asymptomatic blood loss manifested as a positive occult blood test to massive hemorrhage resulting in death within minutes. The most common cause is bleeding from hemorrhoids.

PATHOPHYSIOLOGY

The pathophysiology of lower GI bleeding is straightforward, since the capillaries of the lower GI tract are separated from the intestinal lumen by a single layer of cells. Disruption of this lining results in blood loss.

Normal healthy people lose microscopic amounts of blood from their GI tract every day. Most authorities agree that a normal rate of GI blood loss is less than 1 mL/d. (These studies utilize the fecal occult bleeding test, which detects the peroxidase-like activity of hemoglobin. A small amount of stool is applied to the impregnated surface of the sample window. A few drops of developer are applied, and a positive test is manifested by a blue color. This test is sensitive enough to detect blood loss of 1 mL/d but requires greater than 20 mL/d to be reliably positive.) If the amount of blood lost exceeds the body's ability to replace the loss, anemia (as evidenced by a lower than normal hemoglobin or hematocrit) occurs. The severity of the anemia depends on the volume and rate of blood loss over time.

DIFFERENTIAL DIAGNOSIS

The differential diagnosis of lower GI bleeding is long but can be remembered more easily if diagnoses are grouped by prevalence according to age (Table 49–1).

Bleeding from diverticular disease (see Chapter 52) is common in older adults. In industrialized countries, diverticulosis is present in 50% of those over 50 years of age, with a similar prevalence in both sexes. Diverticula occur mostly in the sigmoid colon, which consequently is the most common bleeding site. Bleeding can be severe or life threatening. This diagnosis may be difficult to make, sometimes requiring resection of the bleeding segment of colon. Most diverticula, however, do not bleed.

Angiodysplasia (also called vascular ectasias and arteriovenous malformations [AVMs]) is a common vascular lesion of the GI tract. Vascular ectasias are abnormal dilatations of vascular structures, either

**TABLE 49–1. Causes of Lower GI Bleeding
(Most Common Listed First)**

Age < 10 Years

Meckel's diverticulum
Bleeding diathesis
Infectious diarrhea
Necrotizing enterocolitis
Anorectal trauma

Age 10–50 Years

Hemorrhoids
Anal fissures
Inflammatory bowel disease
Angiodysplasia
Meckel's diverticulum
Colonic or rectal polyps
Colonic or rectal cancer
Infectious diarrhea

Age > 50 Years

Hemorrhoids
Diverticular disease
Angiodysplasia
Colonic and rectal polyps
Colonic and rectal cancers
Colonic ischemia
Inflammatory bowel disease
Infectious diarrhea

congenital or acquired. The most common type of angiodysplasia occurs in patients older than age 60 years. Like diverticula, asymptomatic angiodysplasia is commonly found in autopsy series. These are usually multiple, located in the cecum and right colon, and less than 5 mm in size. If bleeding occurs, it can range from low-grade bleeding to massive hemorrhage.

Neoplasia includes premalignant and malignant growths. The most common premalignant growths are polyps, which can be precursors of cancer and are difficult to distinguish from cancer without a biopsy. Neoplasia, both benign and malignant, is a common cause of lower GI bleeding. Bleeding, both gross and occult, has been described as a "warning sign" of colon cancer; however, a significant number of cancers do not bleed until the lesion is well advanced. This inconsistent propensity of GI cancers to bleed has been the subject of much study, and the use of the fecal occult blood test in the early detection of colon cancer is controversial. Polyps and cancers share the same characteristics with regard to race and sex of affected individuals; the distribution of cancers within the colon is illustrated in Figure 49–1. The prevalence of polyps increases with age. Almost half of patients attaining age 80 years will have polyps; an estimated 11% of the U.S. population is believed to have polyps. Most authorities believe that the majority of colon cancers arise from adenomatous polyps, the most common type of polyp.

Inflammatory bowel disease (see Chapter 53) can cause lower GI bleeding of variable severity.

Diseases of the anus are a common cause of rectal bleeding. Hemorrhoids and anal fissures are discussed in Chapter 60.

Meckel's diverticulum is a common developmental anomaly of the small intestine and is an occasional cause of bleeding. The majority of Meckel's diverticula are asymptomatic. Most patients with complications are less than 10 years of age, but bleeding can occur at any age. The most common presentation is rectal bleeding with bright red or maroon stools.

Colonic ischemia can present as rectal bleeding. Usually these patients experience a sudden onset of crampy abdominal pain. Colonic ischemia affects people over age 50 years, and the mortality rate can be as high as 70%–80%. The incidence has increased over the past 40 years, probably because of the aging population. Diagnosis can be difficult to make, but colonic ischemia occurs more frequently in high-risk patients: those with congestive heart failure, recent myocardial infarction, hypovolemia, or sepsis or those who are taking splanchnic vasoconstrictor drugs. The splenic flexure and descending and sigmoid colon are most commonly

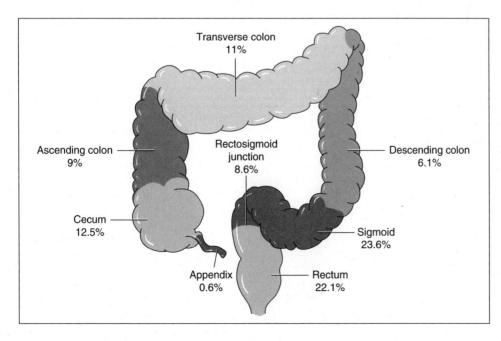

FIGURE 49–1. *Frequency of distribution of colon cancer by anatomic segment. Data from D. Shottenfeld and J. Fraumeni, Jr. (eds.).* Cancer Epidemiology and Prevention. *Philadelphia, W.B. Saunders Co., 1982.*

affected. If bowel infarction occurs, stricture, segmental colitis, gangrene, or perforation can result.

Bleeding is a common manifestation of infectious diarrhea, especially if the diarrhea is due to invasive strains of bacteria such as *Shigella, Campylobacter, Salmonella,* and invasive *Escherichia coli.* A stool guaiac test should be performed routinely in the evaluation of diarrhea (see Chapter 46).

EVALUATION

History

The age of the patient will help establish the differential diagnosis (see Table 49–1). Prior and coexisting diseases can help identify the most likely diagnoses. In elderly patients with a history of congestive heart failure or hypovolemia who present with abdominal pain and rectal bleeding, ischemia of the colon should be considered. How a patient presents is helpful. For example, a 25-year-old who presents with painless rectal bleeding while straining with a bowel movement is far more likely to have hemorrhoids than cancer, while a 70-year-old presenting in shock with massive rectal bleeding will most likely have diverticulosis or angiodysplasia.

Physical Examination

Vital signs (including orthostatic assessment) are important to check in any case of rectal bleeding, since hypotension and tachycardia can be signs of significant blood loss. The abdominal examination should include inspection, auscultation, percussion, and palpation. Palpation should be performed last, since it may be painful for the patient. Is the patient guarding a region of the abdomen? Are bowel sounds or bruits present? Is the liver or spleen enlarged? Is the abdomen rigid, or is rebound tenderness present? Are masses palpable? A rectal examination can serve many purposes, including searching for rectal masses and obtaining stool to test for the presence of blood. Proctoscopy, which does not require preparation, is useful in the examination of the anus and a portion of the rectum, areas where hemorrhoids, fissures, and proctitis might be found.

Additional Evaluation

A CBC can help document the presence or absence of anemia; in addition, a decreased mean corpuscular volume (MCV) suggests iron deficiency (such as might be found in chronic blood loss).

Commonly, more invasive procedures are required to localize the site of bleeding, an issue key to appropriate management (Table 49–2). Flexible sigmoidoscopy and colonoscopy have revolutionized the evaluation of lower GI bleeding. After appropriate preparation of the colon, lesions can be directly visualized and (in many cases) treated during the same procedure. Flexible sigmoidoscopy can be learned easily by primary care providers, while colonoscopy usually requires the skill of a gastroenterologist or surgeon.

The most common radiologic studies used in the evaluation of lower GI bleeding include a barium enema and angiography. The former is indicated primarily to detect colonic polyps and cancers, and the latter is useful to find the source of brisk (> 0.5 mL/min) bleeding.

In cases in which a bleeding source cannot be identified by the procedures described above, nuclear medicine studies, such as a radioisotope-labeled RBC scan, may be helpful. However, a significantly rapid bleed (> 0.1 mL/min) is required to pinpoint the location of the bleed.

MANAGEMENT

Management, including decisions about inpatient versus outpatient evaluation, depends on the severity of the lower GI bleed. The initial care of a patient with rectal bleeding consists of three steps: (1) **Fluid resuscitation** with IV fluids or transfusions is paramount if the patient presents with shock or other evidence of significant hypovolemia. (2) **Locating the source** is the next step, using any of the methods described above. (3) **Stopping the bleeding** should also be attempted, the exact method depending on the severity and source of the bleed. For severe bleeds, vasopressin (a vasoconstrictor), has been used with some success. Colonoscopy can be used, in conjunction with cauterization or polypectomy, to stop bleeding from angiodysplasia,

---

TABLE 49–2. Tests and Procedures Used in Diagnosis of Lower GI Bleeding

Method	Indication	Advantage	Disadvantage
CBC	Evaluation of anemia	Quick, inexpensive	Nonspecific
Flexible sigmoidoscopy	Evaluation of lower GI bleeding	Easy preparation, relatively inexpensive, can be performed by primary care provider	Limited to first 60 cm of colon
Barium enema	Evaluation of colon	Can be ordered by primary care provider, relatively inexpensive	Poor view of rectum
Colonoscopy	Evaluation of colon	Best sensitivity/specificity	Requires GI specialist, extensive colon preparation; greater patient discomfort; expensive
Radioisotope-labeled RBC scan	Identification of bleeding site	Sometimes only means to identify bleeding site	Requires brisk bleed; expensive
Mesenteric angiography	Localization of arterial bleeding	Identifies arterial bleeding	Invasive; requires brisk bleed; very expensive

diverticula, or polyps. When bleeding is massive or recurrent, the patient probably will require surgery.

Minor bleeds are treated according to the underlying diagnosis. For example, small polyps can be excised completely by colonoscopy. Hemorrhoids are usually treated conservatively with stool softeners and an increase of fiber in the diet. Inflammatory bowel disease is usually treated with antiinflammatory drugs.

PATIENT AND FAMILY EDUCATION

Some causes of lower GI bleeding may be preventable. Hemorrhoids have been called a "disease of the Western world" because of the typical Western diet, which is low in fiber and high in refined sugars, and the typical defecation posture. Consuming a diet high in fiber content and developing good bowel habits may help prevent hemorrhoids. Similar measures may also help prevent colon cancer and diverticulosis. In addition to changes in diet, aspirin, aspirin-related drugs, and certain vitamins (e.g, antioxidants such as vitamins A and E) may also decrease the incidence of colon cancers.

NATURAL HISTORY/PROGNOSIS

Colorectal cancer is a leading cause of death in the United States. Associated risk factors include family history, inflammatory bowel disease, and possibly a low-fiber/high-fat diet. Prognosis is determined by the stage of cancer at the time of diagnosis. Five-year survival rates can be as high as 85% for locally invasive cancer and as low as 6% for metastatic cancer.

Bleeding from diverticula can be severe and is usually worse than bleeding from angiodysplasia. In 75% of cases, diverticular bleeding will stop spontaneously. Approximately 20% of patients will eventually rebleed and will require partial colectomy. The prognosis is related to the age of the patient but is generally good because of improved surgical techniques.

Patients with bleeding due to angiodysplasia will usually have recurrent low-grade hemorrhages. In 15%, massive hemorrhage will occur, but even in these cases bleeding will stop in 90%. The prognosis is generally good once the lesion is identified and treated, often with cauterization via the colonoscope.

Bleeding resulting from acute mesenteric ischemia has a highly variable prognosis. Generally, half of patients with acute mesenteric ischemia will have "reversible" changes and recover uneventfully, while the other half will develop "irreversible" changes resulting in chronic colitis, gangrene, or obstruction.

Research Questions

1. How can fecal occult blood testing be made more sensitive and specific?
2. What dietary changes can patients make to lower their chances of developing colon cancer?

Case Resolution

The patient underwent flexible sigmoidoscopy the following week. Two 1-cm polyps were seen in the sigmoid colon, with the remainder of the examination being normal. The patient was referred to a gastroenterologist, who excised the polyps via colonoscopy. The pathology report noted focal areas of adenocarcinoma with clear margins. The patient opted to have a partial colectomy performed, and repeat yearly colonoscopic examinations have subsequently been normal.

Selected Readings

Boley, S., L. Brandt, and M. Frank. Severe lower intestinal bleeding: Diagnosis and treatment. Clin Gastroenterol 10(1):65–91, 1981.

Braunwald, E. (ed.). *Harrison's Principles of Internal Medicine,* 12th ed. New York, McGraw-Hill Book Company, 1991.

Fenoglio-Preiser, C., and R. Hutler. Colorectal polyps. CA 35(6):322–59, 1985.

Kelley, W. N. (ed.). *Textbook of Internal Medicine,* 2nd ed. Philadelphia, J. B. Lippincott Company, 1991.

Richert-Boe, K., and L. Humphrey. Screening for cancer of the lung and colon. Arch Intern Med 152:2398–404, 1992.

Stein, J. (ed.). *Internal Medicine,* 4th ed. St. Louis, Missouri, Mosby–Year Book, 1994.

PEPTIC ULCER DISEASE

Denis M. McCarthy, M.D., M.Sc.*

H_x A 45-year-old male rancher complains of midepigastric pain of increasing severity over the past 4 weeks, accompanied by tenderness 2.5 cm (1 in.) to the right of the midline. The pain occurs 2–3 hours after he eats and often awakens him around 1–2 AM. It is relieved by milk, food, or antacids but returns after a few hours. The pain does not radiate and is unrelated to exercise, breathing, posture, swallowing, defecation, or micturition. The patient is often hungry and snacks frequently, including on retiring, although he avoids coffee and cola drinks. He denies nausea and vomiting. He reports a 25-year history of similar pain, usually occurring in winter and usually relieved by over-the-counter antacids or cimetidine. Last October, he experienced a bout of pneumonia and was treated with amoxicillin for 2 weeks; this winter, he did not experience his usual pain spell. He has a 30 pack-year history of cigarette smoking, drinks moderately, and has never used aspirin or drugs other than cimetidine. On physical examination, there is tenderness in the epigastrium to the right of the midline but no rebound tenderness.

H_x A 76-year-old female who has had arthritis for 20 years is brought to the emergency room by her daughter, who noticed that her mother was pale and weak and had "jet-black, sticky stools that looked like tar" for 2 days. The patient has no pain but on questioning admits to occasional nausea, a poor appetite, and 5-kg (11-lb) weight loss since her doctor prescribed indomethacin 2 months ago for her joint pain. She does not smoke or drink and has never had an ulcer.

Questions

1. What do you think is causing the first patient's symptoms?
2. Why is he awakened from sleep?
3. Why was he pain-free last winter?
4. In the case of the second patient, why has she bled without warning symptoms?
5. What is the best drug with which to treat her arthritis?
6. Does she have to stop taking indomethacin?

A peptic ulcer is an area of loss of the surface mucosa of the gut > 5 mm in diameter and deep enough to reach or penetrate the muscularis mucosa, occurring in a site exposed to peptic juice (acid and pepsin). The area has usually been damaged initially by a factor such as infection or medication. Peptic ulcers occur commonly in the stomach or duodenum and only rarely in other sites. Peptic ulcer disease (PUD) refers to the lifelong tendency to develop recurrent episodes of ulcers or ulcer

complications (e.g., hemorrhage or perforation). Over a lifetime of ulcer disease, about 30% of patients suffer from bleeding and 10% to 15% from perforation; approximately 2% die as a result of ulcer-related complications. Mortality from PUD has not changed since 1930, but patients are now dying two to three decades later, principally in their 70s. PUD is a 20th century disease that reached a peak prevalence in the mid-1950s, when it affected approximately 10% of the U. S. population. The total direct and indirect costs of diagnosing and testing PUD currently exceed 3 billion dollars annually. Until recently, PUD appeared to be incurable.

PATHOPHYSIOLOGY

PUD has many causes; only the two principal causes are discussed here: *Helicobacter pylori* infection and use of aspirin or other NSAIDs. In the presence of generally normal amounts of peptic juice (acid and pepsin), mucosal injury induced by infection or drugs leads to formation of an ulcer, which, when deep enough to inflame the serosa, causes pain, bleeding, or perforation. Via mechanisms that are not understood, other factors (e.g., smoking, psychological stress, depression, and probably the use of caffeine-containing beverages) appear to exacerbate ulcer disease in some individuals; however, in the absence of *H. pylori* infection or NSAID-related injury, peptic ulcers are rare. *H. pylori* antral gastritis is found in approximately 95% of patients with duodenal ulcer (DU) and in about 70% of patients with gastric ulcer (GU). Only one of six patients with *H. pylori* gastritis develop ulcers, so *H. pylori* must interact with other factors if ulcerogenesis is to occur. Principal among these is gastric acid secretion. At present, many ulcers are healed by suppressing or neutralizing gastric acid; however, this practice is rapidly changing to treating first with antiinfective drugs except in those patients using aspirin or other NSAIDs where the primary aim is to discontinue use of these drugs.

Duodenal Ulcer

DIFFERENTIAL DIAGNOSIS

Other causes of similar pain include gastric ulcer and gastric cancer; gallbladder, biliary, and pancreatic disease; nonulcer dyspepsia; and mesenteric ischemia. Many ulcer patients are asymptomatic, and atypical symptom presentations are not uncommon.

* This chapter is in the public domain.

EVALUATION

Nocturnal pain; alleviation of symptoms by food, antacids, and H$_2$-blockers; winter exacerbations; and tenderness 2.5 cm to the right of the midline are highly suggestive of DU. Weight is typically maintained or increased. When patients lack such features, the physician should consider other diagnoses.

Definitive diagnosis is made by means of endoscopy (i.e., esophagogastroduodenoscopy [EGD]) as well as biopsies of any lesion seen and of the gastric antrum and fundus for evidence of *H. pylori* gastritis. Because endoscopy is not easily performed by generalists and is expensive, most physicians begin with an upper GI x-ray series, with a double-contrast barium meal study using air and barium being more sensitive and specific than a single-contrast study (Table 50–1). Endoscopy is not necessary when a DU crater is obvious on x-ray or when symptoms similar to those experienced previously recur within 1 year after a definitive diagnosis of DU is made. However, endoscopy may be needed when (1) x-rays are negative; (2) a scarred duodenal cap, profuse gastric secretions, prominent folds, active bleeding, or localized spasm makes it hard to interpret the x-ray with confidence; (3) symptoms persist despite therapy; or (4) surgery is being considered. As the cost of endoscopy falls, its use may increase still further.

In patients who are *H. pylori*-negative and who have a family history of ulcers or kidney stones, fasting serum gastrin and serum calcium levels should be measured to exclude underlying hypersecretory disorders (e.g., Zollinger-Ellison syndrome or hyperparathyroidism).

MANAGEMENT

The standard approach is to administer an H$_2$-antagonist (e.g., cimetidine, ranitidine, famotidine, or nizatidine) once per day on retiring (or half the daily dose twice daily) for 8 weeks. Low or moderate doses of aluminum-containing antacids are probably similarly

effective but have not been well studied in the United States. The newer proton pump-inhibiting drugs such as omeprazole or lansoprazole heal 90% of ulcers in 4 weeks. Long-term maintenance therapy with half-doses of the H$_2$-antagonists will keep most ulcers healed for as long as the drug is taken, but many ulcers relapse when treatment is discontinued. In patients who have *H. pylori* gastritis, eradication of the infection almost totally abolishes ulcer recurrences, even in heavy smokers. However, no single drug therapy achieves eradication, and a variety of two-, three-, and four-drug treatment regimens, while effective in the majority of cases, are rendered difficult by the generally high incidence of adverse effects, poor compliance, and the high cost of some regimens. In PUD patients infected with *H. pylori*, eradication of infection has become first-line therapy. In noninfected patients, traditional antisecretory therapy should be initiated.

Whatever the treatment, relief of symptoms occurs fairly rapidly (i.e., within days) but is a poor guide to healing, which takes months. For this reason, a full 8 weeks of H$_2$-antagonist therapy is recommended by some, even for those who have received antibiotic therapy. Surgery is reserved for complications such as perforation, pyloric channel obstruction, or uncontrollable hemorrhage. Lesser hemorrhages cease in 90% of cases with either medical therapy or a combination of medical therapy and transendoscopic electrocautery.

NATURAL HISTORY/PROGNOSIS

Mortality from PUD is increased in those with major hemorrhage who are over age 60 years or who have serious disease affecting other organ systems.

Gastric Ulcer

DIFFERENTIAL DIAGNOSIS

Benign GU must be differentiated from (1) ulcerating malignant tumors of the stomach (e.g., carcinomas, lymphomas, or sarcomas) and (2) other causes of benign ulcers such as infections. The pain of GU may sometimes resemble the pain of gallbladder, pancreatic, or colonic disease. Relief of symptoms by antacids does not significantly help in distinguishing between GU and other gastrointestinal disorders, since these drugs can also alleviate symptoms in esophagitis, gastric cancer, duodenal ulcer, duodenitis, and pancreatic or biliary disease.

EVALUATION

While GU often causes pain that comes on soon after eating and is relieved by vomiting, the pain is less stereotypical than that of DU; it may radiate to the right, to the left, or posteriorly, and is often described as dull. GU is uncommon below age 40 unless the patient is taking aspirin or another NSAID. More than 85% of gastric ulcers occur in patients over 40 years of age,

TABLE 50–1. Comparative Features of Esophagogastroduodenoscopy (EGD) and Double-Contrast Barium Meal (DCBM)

Double-contrast Barium Meal	*Esophagogastroduodenoscopy*
Provides sensitivity of 54% and specificity of 91%	Provides sensitivity of 92% and specificity of 100%
Is less expensive, quickly and widely available, and safe	Is more expensive
Detects extrinsic lesions and dysmotility better	Allows direct visualization, tissue biopsy, and luminal sampling
Forms a permanent record	Detects superficial lesions
Is poorly tolerated in immobile, elderly patients	Distinguishes active ulcers from old scars
	Is reliable in postgastrectomy patients
	Is well tolerated in immobile, elderly patients

Data from Colin-Jones, D. G. Endoscopy or radiology for upper gastrointestinal symptoms? Lancet 1:1022–3, 1986; and Dooley, C. P., et al. Double-contrast barium meal and upper gastrointestinal endoscopy: A comparative study. Ann Intern Med 101:538–45, 1984.

65%–70% in *H. pylori*-infected patients and 30%–35% in uninfected patients, most of whom are taking aspirin or another NSAID. Only a minority develop ulcer complications; in two thirds of those who do, both risk factors are present.

EGD is required in the evaluation of GU. Unlike duodenal ulcers, which are never malignant, there is a 2%–5% chance of malignancy in GU. For this reason, a biopsy of the ulcer is needed in most patients with GU to exclude cancer; in addition, biopsies of the antrum are taken to search for the presence of *H. pylori*.

MANAGEMENT

If *H. pylori* is present, eradication with antiinfective agents should be attempted. This may be combined with H$_2$-antagonist or acid-suppressive therapy similar to that used in the management of *H. pylori*-related DU except that it should continue for 12 weeks. The efficacy of antiinfective therapy alone is currently under assessment. If aspirin or another NSAID was being used, it should be discontinued if possible and a nonulcerogenic drug such as acetaminophen substituted. If necessary, aspirin or other NSAIDs can be continued (in combination with acid-suppressive drugs), and in most cases, ulcers will heal satisfactorily although healing may be delayed. Antiulcer therapy should be continued for as long as aspirin or other NSAIDs are prescribed. However, in patients hospitalized because of bleeding, aspirin or other NSAIDs should be stopped until the ulcer is healed. The prostaglandin E$_1$ analog misoprostol may also be used to prevent the development of GU or DU in aspirin or NSAID users, but it is not clear whether it reduces PUD complications in such patients. Surgery is reserved for complications and should generally be used minimally or avoided in NSAID users, since postoperative bile reflux increases the injurious effects of NSAIDs.

NATURAL HISTORY/PROGNOSIS

When GU is complicated by hemorrhage or perforation, mortality is 30%–50% in those older than 75 years of age.

Research Questions

1. How does *H. pylori* infection lead to peptic ulcer disease?
2. Why does prognosis deteriorate with age?
3. What is the relationship between stress and ulcerogenesis?
4. How do NSAIDs cause ulcers?

Case Resolutions

1. An upper GI series documented the presence of a duodenal ulcer. The patient was treated with triple drug therapy (tetracycline, metronidazole, and bismuth subsalicylate) for 2 weeks and started on cimetidine, and his symptoms resolved after several days. Cimetidine was continued for an 8-week course. Eight months later, he had a recurrence of upper abdominal pain to the right of the midline, which also responded to an 8-week course of cimetidine.

2. EGD demonstrated a 1.5-cm gastric ulcer. Biopsies proved negative for malignancy as well as for *H. pylori*. The patient's hemoglobin level in the emergency room was 7.2 g, and she was transfused with 2 units of packed cells. Indomethacin was discontinued, and a 12-week course of cimetidine was begun. She is currently feeling well, with no gastrointestinal complaints, and acetaminophen seems to provide adequate control of her chronic joint discomfort.

Selected Readings

Feldman, M., P. N. Maton, R. W. McCallum, and D. M. McCarthy. Treating ulcers and reflux. Patient Care 26(13):53–76, 1992.

Hawkey, C. J., and R. P. Walt. Prostaglandins for peptic ulcer: A promise unfulfilled. Lancet 2:1084–7, 1986.

McCarthy, D. M. Acid peptic disease in the elderly. Clin Geriatr 7(2):231–53, 1991.

McCarthy, D. M. NSAID-induced gastrointestinal damage: A critical review of prophylaxis and therapy. J Clin Gastroenterol 12(suppl 2):S13–S20, 1989.

Soll, A. H. Pathogenesis of peptic ulcer and implications for therapy. N Engl J Med 322:909–16, 1990.

Zakim, D., and A. J. Dannenberg. *Peptic Ulcer Disease and Other Related Disorders.* West Point, Pennsylvania, Academic Research Associates, Merck, 1991.

CHAPTER 51

GASTROESOPHAGEAL REFLUX

Denis M. McCarthy, M.D., M.Sc.*

H$_x$ An obese 40-year-old male surveyor reports a 2-week history of solid food "sticking in his throat" when he eats.

There is no pain, and the sensation goes away after a few minutes. For many years, he has suffered from "heartburn,"

---

* This chapter is in the public domain.

especially when he lies down. It is relieved by antacids or antiulcer drugs. His symptoms are mild unless he "parties a lot." He has a 20 pack-year history of cigarette smoking and drinks "moderately" (one to two 6-packs of beer) on weekends. He sometimes experiences "acid" in his mouth and for 6 months has noted a morning cough and hoarseness. In addition, on several occasions he has awakened "coughing and choking." His weight has remained stable, and the physical examination is normal except for obesity. Several doctors have told him he has a "hiatus hernia."

Questions

1. What causes heartburn?
2. Is hiatus hernia a disease?
3. How might the patient's physique or life-style affect his heartburn?
4. How might the current sense of "food sticking" be related to his heartburn or hiatus hernia?

Gastroesophageal reflux disease (GERD) is primarily a motility disorder in which noxious gastric or duodenal contents are refluxed into the esophagus. Contact with the mucosa for a prolonged period results in inflammation and injury, with the subsequent development of "heartburn," a burning retrosternal sensation. Clearance of the refluxed material and restoration of intraluminal pH to 4.0 or greater are also impaired. Chief among the irritants causing pain is acid; neutralization of acid or suppression of its secretion usually affords rapid relief. However, some patients have pain and inflammation even in the absence of acid. Heartburn is common in the general population, occurring daily in 7%, weekly in 14%, monthly in 15%, and in 36% at some time or other in their lives. However, not all episodes of heartburn are related to GERD.

CLINICAL PRESENTATION

Most often GERD presents with heartburn (retrosternal pain or discomfort), with the discomfort being worse after a large meal, especially if the patient slouches or lies down. Pain occurring shortly after retiring is common.

PATHOPHYSIOLOGY

Acid, pepsin, and certain chemicals of duodenal origin (lysolecithin, pancreatic enzymes, etc.) can injure and inflame the stratified squamous epithelium of the esophagus, leading to friability, erosions, ulcers, strictures, metaplastic and dysplastic changes in the epithelium (Barrett's esophagus), and eventually, in a small percentage of cases, adenocarcinoma. Regurgitation of gastric contents into the pharynx, larynx, bronchi, etc., can lead to pharyngitis, laryngitis, hoarseness, aspiration into the lungs, and occasionally asphyxia or aspiration pneumonia. Chronic low-grade bleeding is common, and GERD is the most common cause of iron-deficiency anemia in the elderly. Alcohol, aspirin and other NSAIDs, and many other drugs may exacer-

bate GERD and cause progression to stricture. Similarly, hiatus hernia (HH) may predispose the patient to GERD, although many patients with HH have no reflux and many with GERD have no HH.

DIFFERENTIAL DIAGNOSIS

Occasionally, the pain of GERD is atypical and must be differentiated from other causes of chest pain, including myocardial ischemia (myocardial infarction or angina), pericarditis, costochondritis, referred pain (e.g., cervical spondylosis), or even functional pain (e.g., esophageal spasm). Occasionally, patients with angina are treated with medications (e.g., calcium channel blockers, nitrates) that can affect esophageal muscle and lead to heartburn. Thus, the two pain conditions (angina and GERD) often coexist, giving rise to a mixture of symptoms. GERD can also coexist with peptic ulcer disease (see Chapter 50), which should be suspected when epigastric pain or tenderness is present, or with gallbladder disease (see Chapter 59), which causes pain in the right subcostal area. Dysphagia is discussed in Chapter 45.

EVALUATION

In most cases, a good history is sufficient to make the diagnosis, following which the patient can be treated empirically. However, if the chest pain is atypical, it might be prudent to obtain an electrocardiogram and an exercise stress test, especially in patients with cardiac risk factors. More importantly, patients with anemia, weight loss, dysphagia, or odynophagia should have full evaluations prior to any therapy.

Even when the decision is made to treat empirically, it is usually wise to perform a barium swallow and upper GI series, especially in patients over age 40 or in those with severe or prolonged symptoms. This enables the physician to *exclude* the presence of (1) complications indicative of severe GERD (e.g., mucosal abnormalities, ulcers, or strictures); (2) anatomic abnormalities (e.g., webs, hernias, or extrinsic compression); (3) gastric lesions in the area of the fundus; and (4) motility disorders. Failure to respond to treatment within 7 days should lead to cessation of empiric therapy.

When more precise assessment of heartburn is necessary, the best test is upper gastrointestinal endoscopy with biopsy. Biopsy may reveal esophagitis even when no changes are evident to the endoscopist. In a minority of cases, quantitation of reflux is desirable; this is accomplished by means of 24-hour intraesophageal pH monitoring. Radioisotopic scintiscanning should also be considered in patients with alkaline reflux. This

---

| D_x | **Gastroesophageal Reflux** |

- Retrosternal pain or discomfort.
- Pain typically worse after a large meal, especially after a period of recumbency.

technique is unaffected by pH and is more sensitive than x-ray in showing reflux of gastric or duodenal contents into the esophagus.

MANAGEMENT

General Approach

GERD is common and varies considerably in severity. Normal individuals may have occasional transient heartburn following dietary indiscretions, especially when followed by slouching or recumbency. This situation is especially common in the elderly, most of whom self-medicate with antacids and do not consult a doctor.

It is hard to define when "heartburn" becomes a disease. Certainly, the presence of histologic abnormalities on esophageal mucosal biopsy constitutes GERD, although in some patients with microscopic inflammation, symptoms may be trivial or absent. In other patients, symptoms are severe even though there are normal findings on endoscopy and biopsy. In those with mild GERD, symptom relief is the goal of treatment, but in more severe or persistent disease, the maintenance of a healed mucosa and the prevention of complications are also major objectives. On the whole, severity of symptoms is a poor guide to treatment, except insofar as persistent symptoms indicate inadequate therapy and respiratory symptoms indicate the presence of serious reflux disease.

Specific Treatment

Stage 1

The principal aim is to modify life-style by (1) dieting (returning body weight to normal in obese patients); (2) eating frequent, small meals, with the main meal in the middle of the day and no meal for 4 hours prior to bedtime; (3) avoiding prebedtime snacks; (4) stopping smoking; (5) consuming no more than one or two alcohol-containing drinks per day; (6) avoiding tight belts or garments; (7) elevating the head of the bed 15–20 cm (6–8 in), using blocks or bricks but not extra pillows; and (8) avoiding foods that bring on heartburn or are known to reduce lower esophageal sphincter pressure (e.g., coffee and caffeinated beverages, chocolate, peppermints, oils, fats, tomatoes, and citrus fruits). These measures should be stressed in all patients, regardless of disease severity, and sometimes must be continued until some other factor (e.g., obesity, pregnancy, tense ascites, an ovarian cyst, or the use of a plaster spica) can be eliminated or corrected. These life-style modifications, alone or combined with antacids or agents that increase salivation (e.g., lozenges, nuts, or chewing gum), may be all that is needed to control symptoms. However, in many patients, additional measures are required.

Stage 2

The mainstay of therapy for moderately severe GERD is H_2-antagonist drugs. Other drugs used in stage 2 patients include antacids, sucralfate, sodium alginate, and so-called prokinetic drugs such as bethanecol or cisapride. In most cases, combination therapy should be avoided, especially in the elderly. H_2-antagonist therapy, in combination with the life-style modifications described in stage 1, will ameliorate even moderately severe disease in 66%–75% of cases when properly used. H_2-blockers must be given at least twice daily with meals, and cimetidine works marginally better when given as one 400-mg tablet four times a day. Alternatives to cimetidine include ranitidine, famotidine, and nizatidine. The efficacy of all these drugs is dose dependent. Overall, based on cost, potency, duration of action, and relief of symptoms, famotidine (20 mg) given twice a day is probably the best drug for use in stage 2 management. Therapy should be continued for 8–12 weeks, and adequate healing may take 16–20 weeks, occurring long after symptoms have been controlled. The longer the time needed to control symptoms or heal the mucosa, the more likely it is that the patient will require long-term therapy. Long-term therapy has not been approved by the U. S. Food and Drug Administration (FDA) but is widely employed in practice, since many patients demand continued therapy rather than making the recommended life-style modifications. Failure to respond to regular doses of H_2-antagonists should lead to referral to a gastroenterologist for further investigation and assessment.

Stage 3

Occasional patients with severe disease (< 5% of all those with GERD and < 20% of those seeking medical care) do not respond to H_2-antagonists in moderate dosage; treatment with higher doses or combination therapy is usually not cost effective. Many of these patients have extensive or circumferential mucosal erosions, ulcers, strictures, or Barrett's epithelium with dysplastic changes, or they have symptoms that persist or progress despite months of high-dose H_2-antagonist therapy. Such patients should be treated by a gastroenterologist with a proton pump–inhibitor drug such as omeprazole or lansoprazole.

Stage 4

A minority of patients who have intractable disease or GERD-related complications not amenable to medical or endoscopic therapy are candidates for antireflux surgery (e.g., Nissen or Belsey procedures). Some of these procedures can now be successfully performed using laparoscopic techniques. Since delayed gastric emptying and the presence of duodenal contents in gastric juice exacerbate the esophageal inflammatory response to reflux, operations such as vagotomy and gastric "drainage" procedures should be avoided, and any ulcers present in the esophagus, stomach, or duodenum should be managed medically.

NATURAL HISTORY/PROGNOSIS

Most mild GERD symptoms clear up within a few weeks after initiation of therapy but may recur episodically for long or short periods, usually following failure to comply with stage 1 measures. If GERD occurs in the setting of aspirin or other NSAID use, the prognosis is excellent if the drugs can be discontinued but is otherwise uncertain; of those who end up with esophageal strictures, over one third are long-term users of aspirin or other NSAIDs. These drugs are particularly dangerous in patients with dysmotility.

Moderate disease responds over months, with both symptom relief and healing; many patients can be gradually weaned from all drugs, as long as they adhere to stage 1 therapy. In severe disease, symptoms respond rapidly in most cases to omeprazole. However, mucosal healing may require 8–24 weeks of therapy, and when the drug is stopped, both symptoms and erosive injury recur rapidly in > 80% of cases. Long-term management often requires the aid of a specialist, and decisions related to long-term medical or surgical care must be based on careful assessment of the pathogenetic factors involved. About 5% of chronic cases require surgery. The apparently rising incidence of adenocarcinoma of the esophagus, especially in white middle-class males, is being blamed by some authors on the widespread use of medical therapy in suboptimal dosages, adequate to relieve symptoms but not adequate to suppress the chronic inflammation that leads to cancer. New methods of localizing and classifying these tumors may also be contributing to the apparent increase.

Research Questions

1. How does the esophagus restore luminal pH to 7.0 after an episode of reflux?
2. What gastric factors are involved in the genesis of GERD?

Case Resolution

The patient underwent esophagogastroduodenoscopy (EGD), which demonstrated esophagitis and a mild esophageal stricture. Biopsies showed chronic inflammatory changes with no evidence of dysplasia or malignancy. The patient was placed on omeprazole and was also advised to lose weight, quit smoking, and reduce his use of alcohol.

Selected Readings

Baldi, F., et al. Oesophageal function before, during, and after healing of erosive esophagitis. Gut 29(2):157–60, 1988.

Castell, D. O. Ambulatory monitoring in esophageal disease. Viewpoints on Dig Dis 21(1):1–4, 1989.

Castell, D. O., and E. G. Hewson. Current medical therapy of gastroesophageal reflux disease. Practical Gastroenterol 12:11–22, 1988.

Frank, W. O., J. Wetherington, R. H. Palmer, and M. D. Young. Cimetidine: Effective therapy for reflux esophagitis. Gastroenterol 96:A156, 1989.

Harvey, R. F., N. Hadley, and T. R. Gill. Effects of sleeping with a bed-head raised and of ranitidine in patients with severe peptic oesophagitis. Lancet 2:1200–3, 1987.

Johnson, L. F. Gastroesophageal reflux, esophagitis, and pH monitoring. Curr Opin Gastroenterol 5:529–37, 1989.

Nebel, O. T., M. F. Fornes, and D. O. Castell. Symptomatic gastroesophageal reflux: Incidence and precipitating factors. Am J Dig Dis 21:953–6, 1976.

Richter, J. E., and D. O. Castell. Gastroesophageal reflux: Pathogenesis, diagnosis and therapy. Ann Intern Med 97:93–103, 1982.

Sandmark, S., et al. Omeprazole or ranitidine in the treatment of reflux esophagitis. Scand J Gastroenterol 23:625–32, 1988.

Tytgat, G. N. J. Drug therapy of reflux oesophagitis: An update. Scand J Gastroenterol 24(suppl 168):38–49, 1989.

CHAPTER 52

DIVERTICULAR DISEASE

M. Mazen Jamal, M.D.

H$_x$ A 72-year-old male retired industrial designer presents with lower abdominal cramping pain that he has had for the past 24 hours. He has felt warm, but his temperature was not taken. His appetite is poor, he feels bloated, and he has been unable to expel gas or stool. His usual bowel pattern over the past year has alternated between constipation and diarrhea. A barium enema study done a year ago showed colonic diverticulosis involving the sigmoid colon. Physical findings include the following: temperature 38.3° C (101° F), pulse 108/min, blood pressure 145/88 mm Hg, mild abdominal distention with diffuse tympanitic percussion and infrequent bowel sounds, moderate tenderness in the left lower quadrant with a palpable sausage-like mass, and guarding without rebound tenderness. Rectal examination reveals tenderness with mass effect.

Questions

1. What would be your differential diagnosis?
2. What diagnostic studies would you order?
3. How would you manage this patient?

Diverticula are acquired herniations of mucosa through the muscular wall of the colon. Diverticulosis is asymptomatic diverticular disease in the large bowel, and diverticulitis is the presence of associated inflammation. Diverticular disease is common in industrialized countries and infrequent in less well-developed countries. The prevalence of the disease in the United States is 33%–50% of the population over 50 years of age and greater than 50% in those over 80 years of age.

PATHOPHYSIOLOGY

Diverticulosis is an acquired condition. The herniation of the mucosa through the muscular layer of the colon is a function of two factors: (1) the strength of the bowel wall and (2) the pressure differential between the lumen of the colon and the peritoneal cavity.

The etiology of colonic diverticulosis is multifactorial: the roles of colonic muscle changes, abnormal intraluminal pressure, motor dysfunction, and dietary fiber in the pathogenesis of diverticulosis are likely interrelated but remain to be elucidated.

Colonic diverticula are pseudodiverticular in that they consist of mucosa and serosa with no muscular coat. They may be single or exist in a series of saccular protrusions from the colonic lumen. Most (94%) of patients with diverticulosis have diverticula in the sigmoid colon. The distribution of diverticula is as follows: 65% are limited to the sigmoid colon, 25% are located in the sigmoid as well as another segment of the colon, 7% are dispersed over the entire colon, and 4% are limited to a segment proximal to the sigmoid colon. Most patients with sigmoid diverticula have thickening of the circular muscle layer with luminal narrowing. The cause of this muscular thickening is unknown, but the characteristic decreased diameter of the colon creates a situation that may result in high intraluminal pressure with no compensatory increase in wall strength.

DIFFERENTIAL DIAGNOSIS

Generally, any disease causing abnormal intestinal motility, abdominal inflammation, or rectal bleeding must be considered (Table 52–1). **Irritable bowel syndrome** with abdominal pain and altered bowel habits may be indistinguishable from diverticulosis. **Crohn's colitis,** like diverticulitis, is associated with fistula formation, obstruction, and abscess formation.

TABLE 52–1. Differential Diagnosis of Diverticular Disease

Irritable bowel syndrome
Colon cancer
Appendicitis
Inflammatory bowel disease (Crohn's colitis, ulcerative colitis)
Upper GI bleeding with rapid blood loss
Vascular ectasia
Colitis (ischemic, radiation-induced, infectious)

TABLE 52–2. Complications of Diverticulosis

Acute diverticulitis with localized peritonitis
Abscess formation
Perforation with local or generalized peritonitis
Fistula formation (colovesical or colovaginal)
Stricture/obstruction
Hemorrhage

Appendicitis may be indistinguishable from right-sided diverticulitis but is more common in younger patients. **Colonic carcinoma** and diverticular disease are both common in elderly patients. Both may cause luminal obstruction and rectal bleeding, but carcinoma rarely causes massive hemorrhage. **Angiodysplasia, upper GI hemorrhage with rapid blood loss, Meckel's diverticulum,** and **colitis** (ischemic, radiation-induced, and infectious) should also be considered.

EVALUATION

History

About 70% of patients with diverticulosis have **asymptomatic diverticular disease** as an incidental finding at endoscopy, barium enema, or surgery. Probably less than one fourth of those actually develop related symptoms. Patients with **symptomatic diverticular disease** experience intermittent colicky abdominal pain in the lower or central abdomen associated with flatulence, distention, and altered bowel habits. Complications of diverticulosis are listed in Table 52–2.

Acute diverticulitis occurs in 10%–25% of patients with diverticulosis and begins with microperforation of the bowel wall and peridiverticulitis. The occurrence of diverticulitis increases in incidence with the duration of the preexisting diverticulosis and is associated with the patient's age. Diverticulitis is more common in individuals with higher numbers of diverticula. The site of inflammation and perforation is almost always the sigmoid colon. Patients experience constant pain localized to the left iliac fossa, which lasts for several days and is associated with fever, nausea, vomiting, and distention. A small portion of patients develop a **diverticular abscess.**

The patient with **free perforation** presents with diffuse peritonitis. Large bowel **obstruction** is secondary to a fibrous diverticular **stricture** or occlusion of the lumen due to an acute infection. **Fistula formation** is a common complication in patients with diverticulitis. The most frequent site of fistula formation is between the colon and the bladder. Patients with colovesical fistulas experience pneumaturia and have recurrent urinary tract infections. Fistulas associated with the uterus and vagina cause a feculent vaginal discharge.

Painless **rectal bleeding** has been reported in 47% of patients, but bleeding is usually minor and stops spontaneously. Diverticulosis is the most common cause of massive lower intestinal bleeding, but only 5% of patients experience massive bleeding. It is highly unusual for both diverticulitis and bleeding to be present in the same patient. Whereas 95% of diverticula are found in the sigmoid, 70% of diverticular bleeding occurs on the right side.

Physical Examination

Physical findings in diverticulosis are limited to mild tenderness, usually located in the left iliac fossa. In diverticulitis, fever and tenderness over the involved colonic segment are common; often a tender fullness or discrete mass can be appreciated. Rectal examination often reveals tenderness and possible mass effect. Patients with perforation often have signs of peritonitis, including decreased bowel sounds and rebound tenderness.

Additional Evaluation

Laboratory studies are not particularly useful in defining the diagnosis. Leukocytosis is seen in less than 50% of patients, even when complicated diverticulitis is seen. Urinalysis may demonstrate pyuria or hematuria (or both).

Plain abdominal x-rays usually are normal. However, patients with diverticulitis may have a localized ileus, evidence of colonic obstruction, or extracolonic air in an abscess. When the clinical diagnosis is reasonably secure, additional radiologic testing is of no benefit.

Contrast radiology is reserved for patients in whom the diagnosis is in doubt and is not indicated in early stages of acute diverticulitis. Frequently, barium studies are done to rule out concomitant lesions such as neoplasms. Diverticula appear as barium-filled globular protrusions from the external surface of the colon. The radiologic features of diverticulitis include displacement or narrowing of the bowel, an altered mucosal pattern (sawtoothing), a soft tissue mass, gas lucencies, or an air fluid level. Computed tomography (CT) is the initial procedure of choice in the evaluation of complicated cases of diverticulitis because it provides a more accurate estimate of the degree of the inflammation and precisely locates abscesses. CT should be performed when (1) there is uncertainty about the diagnosis of diverticulitis during the acute attack, (2) there is clinical suspicion that an abscess or fistula is present, (3) the patient is immunocompromised and the clinical evaluation is not a reliable indicator of the patient's condition, or (4) the patient fails to respond to medical treatment.

Selective mesenteric angiography is occasionally used in those patients with massive hemorrhage from diverticulosis.

Lower gastrointestinal endoscopy is used to assess the large bowel for coexisting disease rather than for the diagnosis of diverticular disease. Sigmoidoscopy is seldom indicated during the acute phase of diverticular disease.

MANAGEMENT

There is support in the literature for the treatment of symptomatic diverticulosis with high-fiber diets and bulk-forming agents. This treatment results in a reduction in associated abdominal symptoms.

Medical treatment for diverticulitis involves bowel rest, intravenous fluids, and broad-spectrum parenteral antibiotics (Table 52–3). Nasogastric suction is used only in the presence of vomiting or when there is evidence of colonic obstruction. The antibiotic regimen should cover the major colonic anaerobes (e.g., *Bacteroides fragilis*), gram-negative bacilli (e.g., *Escherichia coli*), and gram-positive coliforms (e.g., *Streptococcus faecalis*).

In most patients, symptoms respond promptly (within 2–4 days). The antibiotic course should be maintained for 7 to 10 days. Dietary intake is permitted when the patient has subjectively and objectively improved. If a favorable response is not forthcoming within 3–4 days following the initiation of therapy, a CT scan should be done to exclude secondary complications (abscess, fistula, or obstruction).

Surgical management is indicated in 15%–30% of patients with diverticulitis. The surgical indications are free perforation with fecal peritonitis, suppurative peritonitis secondary to ruptured abscess, abdominal or pelvic abscess, fistula, obstruction, recurrent diverticulitis, inability to exclude carcinoma, and massive hemorrhage.

PATIENT EDUCATION

Patients with diverticula should be advised to eat a high-fiber diet, since epidemiologic studies show that the development of diverticulosis may result from a fiber-deficient diet. Dietary fiber speeds the progress of food passing through the digestive tract and promotes regular bowel movements. The increased ease of stool passage keeps the intestinal muscles in good shape and prevents stool sitting dormant in the colon for long periods of time. Fiber is the structural part of fruits, vegetables, and grains. The daily recommended consumption of fiber is 25–35 g.

NATURAL HISTORY/PROGNOSIS

The majority of patients with colonic diverticula have an uncomplicated course. However, 10%–25% develop diverticulitis and its sequelae. Massive hemorrhage occurs in approximately 5% of patients. Spontaneous cessation of bleeding occurs in approximately 80% and recurrence of bleeding occurs in approximately 20% of patients.

TABLE 52–3.   Treatment of Diverticular Disease

Clinical Presentation	Treatment
Uncomplicated	High-fiber diet, bulk laxative, antispasmodic
Diverticulitis	Fluid support, broad-spectrum antibiotic
Abscess	Percutaneous drainage
Perforation	Laparotomy with resection, peritoneal lavage, antibiotics, delayed anastomosis
Fistula	Resection with primary anastomosis
Hemorrhage	Resuscitation, colectomy if life threatening
Obstruction	Resection with delayed anastomosis

Research Questions

1. Is abdominal pain in diverticulosis secondary to the presence of diverticula, or is it related to colonic dysmotility?
2. Does colonic ischemia play a role in the development of diverticular stricture?

Case Resolution

The patient was admitted to the hospital. His CBC revealed a white blood cell count of 14,000/mm³ with 68% neutrophils and 16% band forms. Plain abdominal x-rays were nondiagnostic. A flexible sigmoidoscopic examination was attempted, but the instrument could not be passed into the spastic rectosigmoid region. An abdominal and pelvic CT examination revealed evidence of colonic diverticular disease and thickening of the sigmoid colon wall. The patient responded to conservative management that included intravenous antibiotics, intravenous fluids, and no oral intake. The patient became afebrile within 48 hours.

A liquid diet was introduced and tolerated on the sixth hospital day, and the patient was discharged on day 10. The final diagnosis was acute diverticulitis.

Selected Readings

Albright, A., and C. Hines. Diverticula of the alimentary tract. *In* R. E. Rakel (ed.). *Current Therapy, 1993: Latest Approved Methods of Treatment for the Practicing Physician.* Philadelphia, W.B. Saunders Company, 1993.

Almy, T. P., and D. A. Howell. Diverticular disease of the colon. N Engl J Med 302:324–31, 1980.

Cheskin, L. J., M. Bohlman, and M. M. Schuster. Diverticular disease in the elderly. Gastroenterol Clin North Am 19:391–403, 1990.

Floch, M. H. Update on diverticulitis: Diagnostic and therapeutic options. J Crit Ill 8:43–55, 1993.

Hughes, L. E. Complications of diverticular disease: Inflammation, obstruction and bleeding. Clin Gastroenterol 4:147–70, 1975.

Mendeloff, A. I. Thoughts on the epidemiology of diverticular disease. Clin Gastroenterol 15:855–77, 1986.

Naitove, A., and R. E. Smith. Diverticular disease of the colon. *In* M. H. Sleisenger and J. S. Fordtran (eds.). *Gastrointestinal Disease,* 5th ed. Philadelphia, W.B. Saunders Company, 1993.

CHAPTER   53

INFLAMMATORY BOWEL DISEASE

Sanjeev Arora, M.D.

H$_x$ A 26-year-old female dental student presents with a history of rectal bleeding, diarrhea, and lower abdominal cramping of 3 months' duration. She reports having eight to ten loose stools each day and is usually awakened two or three times each night by the need to have a bowel movement. She describes moderate urgency and tenesmus prior to each stool and crampy lower abdominal and suprapubic pain that typically abates after each bowel movement. The stools are liquid and are mixed with mucus and blood. Her symptoms have been gradually worsening, and she has lost 4.5 kg (10 lb). She describes occasional joint pains but no joint swelling. The physical examination is normal except for the presence of a small amount of blood on the glove when a digital rectal examination is performed.

Questions

1. What are the possible causes of this symptom complex?
2. Could this be irritable bowel syndrome or hemorrhoidal bleeding?
3. What tests will rapidly indicate the diagnosis and allow effective treatment to be started that same day?

The term chronic idiopathic inflammatory bowel disease (IBD) is a diagnosis that comprises two major illnesses: ulcerative colitis and Crohn's disease. Though both are characterized by gastrointestinal (and a variety of extraintestinal) complaints, there are significant differences between them.

More than 250,000 people in the United States have inflammatory bowel disease. Although IBD can occur in any age group, its peak incidence is in young adults aged 15–35 years. The cause of ulcerative colitis and Crohn's disease is unknown, and major research efforts have focused on infectious and immunologic hypotheses.

Ulcerative colitis and Crohn's disease are more common in whites than in African Americans or Asian Americans, and some studies indicate a three- to six-fold greater prevalence in Jews compared to non-Jews. There is a clear genetic predisposition, with 10%–25% of patients having a first-degree relative with IBD.

PATHOPHYSIOLOGY

Ulcerative colitis is characterized by diffuse mucosal inflammation that is limited to the colon. It *always* involves the rectum and may extend proximally to a variable degree; in addition, the disease usually extends from the rectum in a noninterrupted fashion. The three major classes of ulcerative colitis are (1) **proctitis**—mucosal inflammation involving the rectum only; (2) **left-sided colitis**—mucosal inflammation up to the level of the splenic flexure; and (3) **pancolitis**—involvement of the entire colon.

Crohn's disease is characterized by transmural inflammation involving all layers of the intestinal wall. It may affect any part of the gastrointestinal tract from the mouth to the anus. In addition, the disease can be patchy, with areas of normal mucosa interspersed between diseased areas. The three major classes of Crohn's disease are (1) **regional ileitis**—inflammation of the small bowel alone (35% of cases); (2) **ileocolic Crohn's disease**—involvement of both the ileum and the colon (45% of cases); and (3) **colonic Crohn's disease,** which involves the colon alone (20% of cases).

Other areas of the gastrointestinal tract such as the esophagus, stomach, and duodenum are involved less frequently. A disabling complication of Crohn's disease is the development of fistulas that can be enteroenteric (connecting two loops of bowel), enterovesical (connecting bowel and bladder), and enterovaginal (connecting bowel and vagina).

Both ulcerative colitis and Crohn's disease can be associated with a wide array of extraintestinal manifestations (Table 53–1).

DIFFERENTIAL DIAGNOSIS

The differential diagnosis of abdominal pain is reviewed in Chapter 43, while that of diarrhea and of rectal bleeding is addressed in Chapters 46 and 49, respectively. The symptom complex of diarrhea, rectal bleeding, and crampy lower abdominal pain typically seen in ulcerative colitis (and colonic or ileocolonic Crohn's disease) can also be caused by a number of other disease processes, including infectious colitis and ischemic colitis (Table 53–2).

It is important to exclude infectious agents as the cause of this symptom complex, since treatment with corticosteroids (commonly used in IBD) may have deleterious consequences in infectious states.

TABLE 53–1. Extraintestinal Manifestations of Inflammatory Bowel Disease

Associated With Disease Activity of Colitis
Peripheral arthropathy
Erythema nodosum
Anterior uveitis/episcleritis
Aphthous ulcers in the mouth
Pyoderma gangrenosum
Not Associated With Disease Activity of Colitis
Primary sclerosing cholangitis
Sacroiliitis
Ankylosing spondylitis

TABLE 53–2. Differential Diagnosis of Inflammatory Bowel Disease

Diagnosis	Clinical Features	Histologic/ Culture/ Radiologic Features
Ulcerative colitis	Diarrhea, rectal bleeding	Acute inflammatory infiltrate, goblet cells depleted, crypt distortions and abscesses, negative cultures, rectum always involved
Crohn's disease	Abdominal pain, diarrhea, weight loss, perianal disease	Transmural inflammation, granulomas, focal involvement, skip areas, rectal sparing
Infectious colitis	Acute onset, history of exposure	Positive cultures for *Salmonella, Shigella, Campylobacter, Escherichia coli* 0:157
Pseudomembranous colitis	History of antibiotic exposure	*C. difficile* toxin in stool, discrete ulcers with normal intervening mucosa
Microscopic/ collagenous colitis	Watery diarrhea, female predominance	Macroscopically normal mucosa on colonoscopy; chronic inflammatory infiltrate, intraepithelial lymphocytes, thick subepithelial collagen layer on biopsy
Ischemic colitis	Elderly, atherosclerotic disease, sudden onset, rectal bleeding, abdominal pain	Segmental distribution, rectal sparing; "thumbprinting" (submucosal edema) on x-ray

EVALUATION

History

Most patients with **ulcerative colitis** present with rectal bleeding, tenesmus, lower abdominal cramping, and diarrhea. Fever and weight loss are additional clinical features in some patients. Severe abdominal pain is relatively infrequent because of the mucosal nature of the disease. Extraintestinal symptoms occur in a significant percentage of ulcerative colitis patients and include arthritis, skin lesions, eye involvement, and hepatobiliary dysfunction (see Table 53–1).

Patients with symptoms of diarrhea, rectal bleeding, and lower abdominal cramping should be asked about recent travel (amebic colitis, giardiasis) as well as recent exposure to unrefrigerated food or inadequately cooked meat (infectious colitis). Recent antibiotic use suggests the diagnosis of *Clostridium difficile* colitis.

Sudden onset of these symptoms in an elderly patient should alert the clinician to the possibility of ischemic colitis. A history of congestive heart failure, atherosclerotic vascular disease, cardiac arrhythmias, digoxin therapy, a hypercoagulable state, or recent aortography predisposes the patient to the development of colonic ischemia.

In addition to abdominal pain, symptoms frequently seen in patients with **Crohn's disease** include diarrhea, nausea, vomiting, fever, and generalized fatigability. Patients with regional ileitis or ileocolitis, in fact, can present with right lower quadrant pain (sometimes associated with rebound tenderness) and are often initially diagnosed as having appendicitis. Though rectal bleeding can occur, it is much less common than in ulcerative colitis, a reflection of both the patchy nature of the mucosal inflammation in Crohn's disease as well as the relative lack of rectal involvement. Symptoms such as severe abdominal pain and vomiting are often secondary to intestinal obstruction due to inflammation or fibrosis.

Because of the transmural nature of the disease, strictures in the intestine are common. In addition, as many as one-third of patients develop fistulas, sinus tracts (connections between the bowel and the skin), or abscesses. The extraintestinal manifestations of Crohn's disease are similar to those of ulcerative colitis.

Other diagnoses to consider in female patients are tubo-ovarian abnormalities, pelvic inflammatory disease, and ectopic pregnancy; taking a careful sexual and menstrual history is therefore mandatory. A recent history of vaginal discharge or vaginal bleeding provides important clues. A history of pain that is most severe during menstrual periods suggests endometriosis.

Onset of symptoms soon after travel to endemic areas suggests the diagnosis of amebic colitis. In developing countries, a common cause of right lower quadrant pain and tenderness is ileocecal tuberculosis. Patients with a sudden onset of pain who can precisely define the time of onset may have a variant of acute appendicitis or appendiceal abscess. A prior history of abdominal operations may point to partial obstruction secondary to adhesions. A careful history should be taken to evaluate risk factors for AIDS, since ileitis caused by cytomegalovirus infection or *Mycobacterium avium* complex can also mimic the clinical features of Crohn's disease. It is important to exclude infectious agents as the cause of this symptom complex, since treatment with corticosteroids (occasionally used for IBD) may have deleterious consequences in infectious states.

Physical Examination

Patients with ulcerative colitis often have a normal physical examination except for the presence of blood on the gloved examining finger when a digital rectal examination is performed. The presence of joint swelling, erythema nodosum (painful tender nodules on the anterior aspect of the legs), or aphthous ulcers should be noted. Some patients may have back pain, diminished range of motion of the spine, or spinal deformity due to ankylosing spondylitis.

Patients with severe ulcerative colitis who are hospitalized should be examined frequently for the development of tachycardia, hypoactive bowel sounds, and abdominal distention. These findings may indicate the onset of toxic megacolon, a dreaded complication of ulcerative colitis that often requires emergency surgery. Development of severe abdominal tenderness (not a typical feature of ulcerative colitis) and loss of liver dullness on percussion suggest the presence of a complication such as perforation.

Patients with suspected Crohn's disease will often have tenderness in the right lower quadrant. Distinctive features on examination include the presence of perianal or other enterocutaneous fistulas or perianal abscesses. The finding of abdominal distention in association with nausea and vomiting suggests intestinal obstruction secondary to inflammation or stricture formation. Severe rebound tenderness and development of hypoactive bowel sounds are not typical features of uncomplicated Crohn's disease, and their presence suggests a complication such as perforation or an alternative diagnosis such as appendicitis or appendiceal abscess.

Additional Evaluation

When patients present with diarrhea, lower abdominal cramping, and rectal bleeding, a stool specimen should be tested for fecal leukocytes, pathogenic bacteria, ova and parasites, and *C. difficile* toxin. If these tests exclude infection, flexible sigmoidoscopy should be performed. The presence of erythema, friability, exudate, and superficial ulcerations—as well as loss of the normal vascular pattern—is suggestive of ulcerative colitis. In ulcerative colitis, these findings always involve the rectum and extend upward to a variable extent. The inflammation is confluent, and no "skip areas" are seen.

In patients with ulcerative proctitis, rectal biopsies reveal an acute inflammatory infiltrate, crypt distortion, and abscesses. Goblet cell depletion is also seen. If the patient's symptoms are moderate or severe, no further testing need be performed and treatment can be started immediately. After symptoms improve, colonoscopy should be performed to evaluate the extent and severity of disease. A complete blood count and sedimentation rate should also be done at presentation. Anemia, leukocytosis, and an elevated sedimentation rate are signs of severe inflammation. In patients with severe diarrhea, serum electrolytes and renal function should also be monitored.

When Crohn's disease is suspected, an upper gastrointestinal series with small bowel follow-through is the procedure of choice. The most common site of disease is the terminal ileum, which typically demonstrates ulceration, narrowing, or nodularity. There can also be thickening of the bowel wall. In patients with long-standing disease, one can see marked luminal narrowing with a radiologic "string sign" (the marked narrowing causes the barium in the lumen to resemble a string). Fistulous tracts can be seen connecting adjacent loops of bowel or connecting the intestine with the bladder or vagina. Patients often have mild anemia and an elevated sedimentation rate. In patients with extensive Crohn's disease, a nutritional evaluation should also be performed. Patients with Crohn's disease can develop deficiencies of both fat- and water-soluble vitamins.

MANAGEMENT

For many years, **sulfasalazine** has been the mainstay of treatment for patients with ulcerative colitis and has also been widely used for management of patients with Crohn's disease. Sulfasalazine is a combination of an antibiotic, sulfapyridine, and an antiinflammatory drug, 5-aminosalicylic acid (5-ASA). Studies suggest that the 5-ASA portion of sulfasalazine is the active ingredient and that sulfapyridine acts as a carrier molecule, preventing the absorption of 5-ASA in the proximal small intestine.

Sulfasalazine is highly effective in inducing remission in mild to moderate ulcerative colitis in a dose-dependent fashion. In addition, it is effective for maintenance of remission once the disease is symptomatically and endoscopically quiescent.

Multicenter studies performed in both the United States and Europe have found sulfasalazine to be effective in the treatment of Crohn's colitis and Crohn's ileocolitis. In contrast, there has been no demonstrable efficacy in Crohn's ileitis. Experienced clinicians, however, continue to use sulfasalazine for Crohn's ileitis in the belief that it helps some patients. Similarly, although sulfasalazine has not been shown to be effective in maintaining remission in Crohn's disease, many experienced gastroenterologists advise life-long sulfasalazine therapy for patients with Crohn's disease.

The use of sulfasalazine is associated with a high frequency of side effects. Dose-related intolerance usually occurs in association with a high level of sulfapyridine in the blood, as is often seen in slow hepatic acetylators of sulfapyridine. Common complaints in these individuals include nausea, malaise, and headache. In addition, sulfasalazine is a gastric irritant; however, symptoms of epigastric burning and dyspepsia can be lessened by using an enteric-coated preparation. Sulfasalazine use is also associated with a high incidence of allergic reactions, usually a skin rash or fever. Hematologic side effects, including hemolysis, macrocytic anemia, and neutropenia, are also seen. Use of sulfasalazine can cause abnormal sperm morphology or motility and may be a direct cause of infertility in young males taking this medication. This side effect is completely reversible after discontinuation of the medicine for a few weeks.

While sulfapyridine accounts for the majority of adverse effects, the 5-ASA moiety of sulfasalazine is responsible for its therapeutic efficacy. Therefore, pharmaceutical companies have attempted to develop ways of delivering 5-ASA to the colon without having to administer another drug concomitantly. Several forms of oral 5-ASA (also known as mesalamine) are currently available. Delayed-release forms of mesalamine include Pentasa; Asacol (the release of which is pH-dependent); and olsalazine (Dipentum), in which 5-ASA is conjugated with another 5-ASA molecule.

Topical 5-ASA agents are commercially available for treatment of proctitis and left-sided ulcerative colitis. These drugs are effective and have a favorable side effect profile. In several large studies, 5-ASA enemas induced remission in as many as 90% of patients with distal colitis. These trials proved that 5-ASA enemas, used at bedtime daily for 6 weeks, are more effective than hydrocortisone enemas. Many patients appear to benefit from a maintenance regimen of a 5-ASA enema given every 2–3 nights. For patients with very limited proctitis (< 15 cm), a 5-ASA suppository administered 2 to 3 times daily is probably the treatment of choice.

Corticosteroids have long been used in the treatment of patients with IBD, but long-term daily use is associated with an unacceptable number of severe side effects, thus making it an inappropriate choice for chronic management of IBD. Even low doses should generally not be used for more than 1 year. It has been suggested that long-term therapy with corticosteroids may *increase* the overall mortality of patients with IBD. In patients with Crohn's disease not controlled by other modalities, 5–10 mg of prednisone on alternate days may help control disease activity and minimize side effects.

Topical corticosteroids in the form of hydrocortisone enemas are effective for treatment of distal colitis. Long-term use is associated with the same side effects seen with systemic corticosteroids.

Antibiotics have long been used by experienced clinicians for treatment of Crohn's disease. Metronidazole is useful in the management of Crohn's colitis, perianal abscesses, perianal fistulas, and rectovaginal fistulas.

Immunosuppressive agents such as azathioprine and 6-mercaptopurine are indicated for management of refractory Crohn's disease that is unresponsive to sulfasalazine, corticosteroids, or antibiotics. They are a useful addition when the patient is corticosteroid-dependent and attempts to taper prednisone have resulted in reactivation of the disease. In this setting, 6-mercaptopurine and azathioprine have a corticosteroid-sparing effect. These drugs are also efficacious for treatment of perianal disease and refractory fistulas and for maintenance of remission in patients with Crohn's disease.

PATIENT AND FAMILY EDUCATION

Key issues in patient education involve (1) the chronic/recurrent nature of IBD, (2) the need for compliance with prescribed medications, (3) an awareness of medication side effects, (4) the need to call the physician promptly if flare-ups occur, and (5) the risk of malignancy in patients with long-standing ulcerative colitis and the need for periodic colonoscopic surveillance.

The Crohn's and Colitis Foundation of America is an active patient support group that plays a major role in patient education. It also funds research and informs its membership about advances in treatment. Patients should be encouraged to join this organization.

NATURAL HISTORY/PROGNOSIS

Patients with ulcerative colitis or Crohn's disease have recurrent relapses and remissions throughout their lives.

Patients with ulcerative proctitis have symptoms that are a nuisance but are easily managed. With proctitis alone, there is no risk of life-threatening complications or future development of malignancy. Patients with diffuse colitis have a more debilitating illness, but modern therapy is successful and there is no excess mortality over that of the general population.

A total proctocolectomy cures ulcerative colitis. This operative procedure is generally recommended only (1) for patients with disease unresponsive to medical therapy and (2) in long-standing disease to prevent the development of malignancy.

Patients with Crohn's disease have a higher mortality rate than that of either the general population or patients with ulcerative colitis. This excess mortality is probably due to the need for multiple surgical resections in some patients and the inability of surgery to cure the disease. Extensive small bowel involvement leading to nutritional compromise is probably an additional factor contributing to increased mortality.

Research Questions

1. Is there an infectious agent that triggers the onset of Crohn's disease in genetically susceptible patients? Will identification of such an agent lead to a cure?

2. Why do some patients with ulcerative colitis develop only proctitis while others have involvement of the entire colon?

Case Resolution

The patient's workup, including stool studies looking for parasites and pathogenic bacteria, was negative for infectious colitis. On flexible sigmoidoscopy, however, she was found to have left-sided ulcerative colitis. She was started on sulfasalazine and 5-ASA enemas and currently reports marked improvement in her symptoms.

Selected Readings

Bernstein, L. H., M. S. Frank, L. J. Brandt, and S. J. Boley. Healing of perineal Crohn's disease with metronidazole. Gastroenterology 79:357–65, 1980.

Danielsson, A., G. Hellers, E. Lyrenas, et al. A controlled randomized trial of budesonide versus prednisone retention enemas in active distal ulcerative colitis. Scand J Gastroenterol 22:987–92, 1987.

Korelitz, B. I, and D. H. Present. Favorable effect of 6-mercaptopurine on fistulas of Crohn's disease. Dig Dis Sci 30:58–64, 1985.

Mulder, C. J., G. N. Tytgat, I. T. Weterman, et al. Double-blind comparison of slow-release 5-aminosalicylic acid and sulfasalazine in remission maintenance in ulcerative colitis. Gastroenterology 95:1449–53, 1988.

Peppercorn, M. D. Advances in drug therapy for inflammatory bowel disease. Ann Intern Med 112:50, 1990.

Present, D. H., B. I. Korelitz, N. Wisch, et al. Treatment of Crohn's disease with 6-mercaptopurine: A long-term, randomized, double-blind study. N Engl J Med 302:981–7, 1980.

Present, D. H., et al. 6-Mercaptopurine in the management of inflammatory bowel disease: Short- and long-term toxicity. Ann Intern Med 111:641, 1989.

Rao, S. S., P. A. Cann, and C. D. Holdworth. Clinical experiences of the tolerance of mesalazine and olsalazine in patients intolerant of sulfasalazine. Scand J Gastroenterol 22:322–6, 1987.

Rhodes, J., D. Bainton, P. Beck, and H. Campbell. Controlled trial of azathioprine in Crohn's disease. Lancet 2:1273–6, 1971.

Ursing, B., T. Alm, F. Barany, et al. A comparative study of metronidazole and sulfasalazine for active Crohn's disease: The cooperative Crohn's disease study in Sweden. Gastroenterology 83:550–62, 1982.

CHAPTER 54

IRRITABLE BOWEL SYNDROME

Carol Y. Nishikubo, M.D.

Hx A 25-year-old female business school student presents to the student health clinic with a 4-month history of abdominal pain and diarrhea. She describes the pain as crampy, worse in her lower abdomen, and improved after passing a diarrheal stool. Her bowel movements are loose, occasionally contain mucus, and occur up to five times a day. She denies any fever, chills, nausea, vomiting, blood in the stool, or melena; she has no tenesmus or fecal incontinence. Her only medication is an oral contraceptive, which she has taken for 8 years. She does not smoke and states that she drinks one or two beers on the weekends. She denies any recent travel and is involved in a monogamous relationship with her male partner of 3 years. The physical examination is normal, including the abdominal examination, and her stool is negative for occult blood.

The irritable bowel syndrome (IBS) is estimated to be present in up to 15% of the population worldwide, although not all people with symptoms seek medical attention. It is classified as a functional bowel disorder rather than a structural problem because its symptoms cannot be attributed to a structural cause. IBS is more common in women in Western countries, although in some Asian cultures male predominance is the rule.

CLINICAL PRESENTATION

Irritable bowel syndrome is a symptom complex usually appearing in young adulthood. Patients usually have abdominal pain and either diarrhea or constipation (an individual patient will generally have either one or the other), and relapses tend to be of the same type. Symptoms are typically worse in times of physical or emotional stress, and patients can sometimes identify foods that provoke exacerbations of their illness (e.g., caffeine, fatty foods, and lactose).

Until the mid-1970s, IBS was mainly a diagnosis of exclusion; however, there is now a set of defining criteria, which were established by Manning. Symptoms must be present for at least 3 months. Abdominal discomfort is characteristically relieved by the passage of stool or is associated with a change in the frequency or character of the stool. In order to diagnose IBS in a given individual, at least three of the following features should be present at least 25% of the time: altered stool frequency, altered stool character, altered stool passage (straining or urgency, feeling of incomplete evacuation), mucus in the stool, and bloating or abdominal distention.

PATHOPHYSIOLOGY

Several mechanisms have been proposed to explain the observed symptoms of IBS.

Motility Dysfunction

An abnormal amplitude or frequency of small bowel contractions has been observed in patients with IBS. Studies have demonstrated abdominal pain mimicking a given patient's symptoms in response to high-amplitude pressure contractions of the small bowel. Other studies have shown an increased number of colonic contractions and decreased total gut transit time in patients with diarrhea-predominant IBS; the converse is observed in constipation-predominant cases.

Abnormal Pain Perception

Patients with IBS have been shown to be more sensitive to balloon distention at several sites along the small and large intestine when compared to normal controls.

Dietary Irritants

Lactase deficiency is manifested by symptoms similar to those of IBS. Other (as yet unidentified) dietary substances may play an analogous role, since some patients can relate increased symptoms to the ingestion of specific substances such as fats, caffeine, or alcohol.

Psychological Factors

For many years, the irritable bowel syndrome was regarded as mainly a psychological disorder. IBS patients were thought to be more anxious and to have more psychiatric disorders than did the non-IBS population. The relationship of the symptoms to stress, at least in some IBS patients, reinforced this belief. However, studies comparing people with IBS to those with lactase deficiency showed no increased incidence of anxiety in the IBS group, raising the question of whether the symptoms themselves might be causing the psychiatric features of IBS.

DIFFERENTIAL DIAGNOSIS

The clinical manifestations of **lactase deficiency** are similar to those seen in patients with IBS. **Infectious diarrhea** may be due to a parasitic infection (e.g., *Giardia, Entamoeba histolytica,* or *Cryptosporidium*). Tuberculosis and fungal infections may cause a chronic diarrhea. Since IBS is more common in the United States in women, **pelvic and gynecologic** causes of abdominal pain and bloating, such as endometriosis or pelvic inflammatory disease, should be considered. Women with a history of **sexual abuse** as children will sometimes present with nonspecific abdominal or pelvic pain as adults. Abuse of certain **drugs**, such as laxatives and antacids, can cause the clinical picture of IBS. This is especially important to consider in young women, in whom eating disorders are common. **Inflammatory bowel disease** sometimes causes abdominal pain, bloating, and diarrhea. The presence of blood in the stool, however, as is often seen in inflammatory bowel disease, cannot be attributed to IBS and always warrants further workup. **Hypothyroidism** and **hyperthyroidism** may

---

Dx Irritable Bowel Syndrome

- Abdominal discomfort relieved by passage of stool or associated with diarrhea, constipation, or mucus in stool.
- Onset of symptoms in young adulthood.
- No blood in stool.
- Symptoms present for at least 3 months.

result in disturbances in stool frequency and therefore should be considered in the differential. **Porphyria** is an unusual cause of abdominal pain but may be a consideration, especially with a suggestive family history.

EVALUATION

History

The history is the most important diagnostic tool in identifying patients with IBS. In addition to the classic manifestations, there may be improvement or relief of symptoms with passage of stool and exacerbation of symptoms with stress or certain types of foods. A history of fever, blood in the stool, tenesmus, or epigastric pain is not typical and should prompt consideration of other disorders. Medication, travel, and sexual histories are helpful in distinguishing IBS from other disorders.

Physical Examination

Patients with IBS will typically have a normal physical examination, other than possible abdominal distention. Any abnormalities beyond that should steer the clinician away from the diagnosis of irritable bowel syndrome.

Additional Evaluation

Laboratory tests that can be helpful in making a diagnosis include serum electrolytes, a CBC, and an erythrocyte sedimentation rate (the latter two to check for evidence of infection or inflammation). Stool should be sent for parasitic examination and for laxative screen if indicated. A flexible sigmoidoscopy is useful in excluding structural abnormalities or inflammation. Some authors recommend a lactose tolerance test or a trial of a lactose-free diet to exclude lactase deficiency.

MANAGEMENT

Treatment of patients with IBS can be initiated with a stepped-care approach, depending on the severity of symptoms. **Patient education** is the most important aspect of management (see below).

If patients identify dietary factors that exacerbate symptoms, institution of a **diet** that restricts these products may be beneficial. Common substances that have been identified by patients as exacerbating their disease are caffeine, fatty foods, alcohol, and lactose. Encouraging the patient to make dietary changes to relieve specific symptoms may be helpful, for instance, recommending a high-fiber diet for patients with constipation-predominant disease.

Pharmacologic therapy is directed at the predominant symptom. Abdominal pain can be treated with antispasmodics such as anticholinergic drugs (e.g., dicyclomine). For unremitting pain, antidepressants such as amitriptyline or trazodone are effective although these drugs may worsen constipation. The use of opioids is controversial and is not currently standard

practice. Cholestyramine and loperamide have been used effectively for the control of diarrheal symptoms, and fiber or cisapride are used for constipation. Other drugs currently under investigation include calcium channel blockers and serotonin antagonists.

Behavioral treatments are more successful in diarrhea-predominant IBS as compared with constipation-predominant cases. Group therapy is less effective than individual therapy. Relaxation training, biofeedback, and, in some studies, hypnosis have all been shown to improve symptoms in some people.

PATIENT EDUCATION

Patients often can learn to control their symptoms once they have an understanding of the disease process. They should understand that there is no cure for IBS and that the disease is chronic; however, they need to be reassured that symptoms can be controlled with both medical and psychological interventions. Since patients are often concerned that there is a more serious underlying problem (e.g., infection, cancer), these concerns should be addressed explicitly. Patients also should understand that any change in symptoms warrants a new evaluation.

NATURAL HISTORY/PROGNOSIS

There is no cure for irritable bowel syndrome, and treatment provides symptom relief only. IBS *per se* does not decrease life expectancy. Patients with IBS are, nevertheless, often subjected to extensive workups (including in some cases abdominal surgery), which can cause significant morbidity and mortality.

Research Questions

1. What is the exact mechanism of symptom production in patients with the irritable bowel syndrome?
2. Will more effective pharmaceutical treatments become available in the near future, and if so, by what mechanism of action will they be effective?

Case Resolution

The patient continued to have symptoms of diarrhea and abdominal pain despite patient education and dieting modification. She chose, however, not to treat her symptoms with medication and continues to be intermittently symptomatic.

Selected Readings

Blanchard, E. B., et al. Two controlled evaluations of multicomponent psychological treatment of irritable bowel syndrome. Behav Res Ther 30(2):175–89, 1992.

Camilleri, M., and C. M. Prather. The irritable bowel syndrome: Mechanisms and a practical approach to management. Ann Intern Med 116:1001–8, 1992.

Christensen, J. Pathophysiology of the irritable bowel syndrome. Lancet 340:1444–6, 1992.

Drossman, D. A., and W. G. Thompson. The irritable bowel syndrome: Review and a graduated multicomponent treatment approach. Ann Intern Med 116:1009–16, 1992.

Friedman, G. (ed.). The irritable bowel syndrome: Realities and trends. Gastroenterol Clin North Am 20(2), 1991 [entire issue].

Guthrie, E., et al. A controlled trial of psychological treatment for the irritable bowel syndrome. Gastroenterology 100:450–7, 1991.

Lynn, R. B., and L. S. Friedman. Irritable bowel syndrome. N Engl J Med 329:1940–5, 1993.

Talley, N, J., et al. Diagnostic value of the Manning criteria in irritable bowel syndrome. Gut 31:77–81, 1990.

Weber, F. H., and R. W. McCallum. Clinical approaches to irritable bowel syndrome. Lancet 340:1447–51, 1992.

C H A P T E R   5 5

ACUTE PANCREATITIS

Michael W. Gavin, M.D.

H$_x$ A 36-year-old female aerobics instructor presents with a 1-day history of acute, unrelenting, mid-epigastric pain radiating to the back. Persistent nausea and vomiting are associated with the pain. The woman recalls having occasional episodes of mid-epigastric pain several hours after meals during the preceding weeks. These self-limited episodes were less intense and lasted for only several hours. She reports no dyspepsia, hematemesis, melena, or change in bowel habits. When asked about medication use, the woman says that, in addition to oral contraceptives, she takes ibuprofen on occasion for headaches. Her last menstrual period was 2 weeks ago. She rarely uses alcohol. Her pulse is 100/min, but there is no postural hypotension or fever. Abdominal examination reveals marked tenderness in the mid-epigastrium, with quiet bowel sounds. The remainder of the patient's examination is unremarkable.

Questions

1. What is the differential diagnosis of this patient's abdominal pain?
2. What tests would help confirm the most likely diagnosis?
3. How might her medications be related to her pain?

Pancreatitis may be classified as acute or chronic based on morphologic considerations. Clinical manifestations are diverse, ranging from mild abdominal pain to an acute abdomen with shock.

In acute pancreatitis, no long-term morphologic or functional abnormalities follow the attack.

CLINICAL PRESENTATION

Acute pancreatitis is marked by acute abdominal pain, which may be severe. The pain is epigastric and can radiate to the midback. It tends to be constant (not colicky) in nature. Nausea and vomiting occur, and fever may also be present.

PATHOPHYSIOLOGY

In nearly 80% of cases of acute pancreatitis (Table 55–1), either gallstone disease (biliary pancreatitis) or

---

TABLE 55–1.   Etiology of Acute Pancreatitis

Alcohol Use
Obstruction
Choledocholithiasis
Ampullary or pancreatic tumors
Medications
Azathioprine/6-mercaptopurine
Dideoxyinosine (DDI)
Valproic acid
Thiazide diuretics
Pentamidine
Estrogens
Tetracycline
L-Asparaginase
Methyldopa
Metronidazole
Cimetidine
Nitrofurantoin
Furosemide
Sulfonamide
Sulindac
Sulfasalazine
Metabolic Causes
Hypertriglyceridemia
Hypercalcemia
Miscellaneous Causes
Postoperative (e.g., cardiac bypass)
Infections (e.g., ascariasis, mycoplasmal, viral)
Vasculitis (e.g., systemic lupus erythematosus)
Trauma
Familial
Idiopathic

TABLE 55–2.   Complications of Acute Pancreatitis

Local

Pseudocyst—sterile or infected
Phlegmon—sterile necrosis or infected (abscess)
Gastrointestinal hemorrhage
   Gastric varices due to splenic vein thrombosis
   Hemorrhagic pancreatitis due to autodigestion of pancreatic blood vessels
Pancreatic ascites due to disrupted pancreatic ducts

Systemic

Pulmonary—atelectasis, pleural effusion, adult respiratory distress syndrome (ARDS)
Renal—azotemia
Hematologic—coagulopathy
Metabolic—hypocalcemia, hyperglycemia, hypoalbuminemia
Neurologic—altered sensorium, psychosis
Cardiovascular—hypotension, pericardial effusion

---

alcohol abuse (alcoholic pancreatitis; see Chapter 56) is implicated. Hypertriglyceridemia, medications, trauma, and other rare causes account for approximately 10% of cases; the remaining 10% are considered idiopathic.

The mechanism by which these causal factors trigger the events that lead to pancreatitis is not well understood. The acinar cells of the pancreas synthesize and secrete a multitude of digestive enzymes—trypsin, chymotrypsin, amylase, lipase, phospholipase, and others. Pancreatitis is believed to result from injury to the pancreas by these digestive enzymes. The inappropriate activation of trypsin from trypsinogen (the inactive precursor) is thought to initiate the process that leads to autodigestion of the pancreatic gland. Release of these potent cytolytic enzymes has both local and systemic effects (Table 55–2).

Gallstones or other obstructions are believed to transiently obstruct the distal pancreatic duct, resulting in increased pressure in the pancreatic duct. Continued secretion of pancreatic enzymes leads to extravasation of the enzymes into the gland parenchyma, with subsequent intra-acinar activation of the zymogens. The clinical improvement seen in severe biliary pancreatitis following emergent endoscopic sphincterotomy (cutting the ampulla and sphincter), which allows stone removal and decompression of the pancreatic ductal system, supports this theoretical mechanism.

Direct toxic effects on the pancreas may result from **medication and alcohol use** (see Table 55–1). Dideoxyinosine (DDI) and azathioprine/6-mercaptopurine are known to have the highest frequency of drug-associated acute pancreatitis. Marked hypertriglyceridemia (triglycerides usually >1000 mg/dL) may cause pancreatitis from the effects of excessive fatty acids on the acinar cells.

D_x   Acute Pancreatitis

- Moderate to severe epigastric pain radiating to the back.
- Elevated levels of serum amylase, lipase, or both.

DIFFERENTIAL DIAGNOSIS

Because of the wide spectrum of clinical manifestations seen in acute pancreatitis, **gastroduodenal ulcer** (e.g., penetration of a posterior ulcer into the gland), **perforated viscus, cholangitis** (infection from obstruction of the biliary system), and **intestinal obstruction** should be considered. Cholangitis and acute pancreatitis may coexist in the setting of choledocholithiasis (common bile duct stones). In patients with underlying valvular heart disease or in the elderly, **mesenteric ischemia** should be considered. A **ruptured ectopic pregnancy,** usually presenting with acute abdominal pain and shock, is of grave importance in a female of reproductive age. Elevated serum amylase and lipase levels are used to define acute pancreatitis in patients with acute abdominal pain, but a perforated viscus, bowel obstruction, mesenteric ischemia, and ruptured ectopic pregnancy all can cause increases in these enzyme concentrations (Table 55–3). Amylase is filtered by the kidneys, and therefore chronic renal failure can also be associated with hyperamylasemia.

It should be noted that pancreatic carcinoma may initially present as acute pancreatitis.

EVALUATION

History

The patient should be asked about the nature of the abdominal pain and the presence of associated symptoms. Risk factors for acute pancreatitis, e.g., alcohol use, a history of gallstones, medication use, should be sought (see Table 55–1).

Physical Examination

In mild cases, physical findings may be limited to tachycardia with epigastric tenderness. In severe cases, hypotension, marked tachycardia, and fever may be evident. Diffuse abdominal tenderness with peritoneal signs (an "acute abdomen") may be present, and bowel sounds may be decreased or absent.

TABLE 55–3.   Conditions Associated with Hyperamylasemia

Pancreatic

Pancreatitis, acute or chronic
Pancreatic pseudocyst, ascites, or abscess
Pancreatic cancer
Pancreatic trauma
Post-endoscopic retrograde cholangiopancreatography (ERCP)

Abdominal

Perforated viscus
Mesenteric infarction
Intestinal obstruction
Ruptured ectopic pregnancy
Ovarian cysts/tumors

Renal Failure

Miscellaneous

Salivary gland origin
Diabetic ketoacidosis
Macroamylasemia

Jaundice, usually resulting from obstruction of the common bile duct, may be seen. The obstruction can be either intrinsic (e.g., choledocholithiasis) or extrinsic (e.g., pancreatic cancer). Flank or periumbilical ecchymosis (Turner's or Cullen's signs, respectively) can be seen with hemorrhagic pancreatitis.

Additional Evaluation

Laboratory Tests

Measurement of serum amylase and lipase should be performed. Although not specific for pancreatitis, hyperamylasemia supports the diagnosis of suspected pancreatitis. In pancreatitis, the serum amylase level usually peaks several hours after onset and declines in the next 3–5 days. The magnitude of the elevation has no prognostic significance. Other conditions associated with hyperamylasemia (see Table 55–3) may have a similar clinical presentation to acute pancreatitis.

Although an increased serum lipase is more specific for pancreatitis than is an elevated amylase, high lipase levels are also seen with other acute abdominal conditions. Serum lipase usually declines more slowly than does serum amylase.

Leukocytosis, hyperglycemia, hypocalcemia, and elevation of serum transaminases have prognostic significance in acute pancreatitis. These laboratory findings are included in Ranson's criteria (Table 55–4).

Fasting serum triglyceride and serum calcium measurements should be obtained in those patients with no evidence of biliary disease or alcohol use, i.e., to search for a possible metabolic etiology pancreatitis.

Imaging Studies

Plain abdominal radiographs should be obtained on presentation to help exclude nonpancreatic disease such as small bowel obstruction or a perforated viscus. Abdominal ultrasound is helpful in screening for possible associated cholelithiasis and biliary obstruction. Evaluation of the pancreas itself is often limited, however, because of excessive bowel gas. A CT scan of the abdomen is often preferred for diagnosis in acutely ill patients and in detection of possible complicating processes, such as an abscess or pseudocyst.

MANAGEMENT

The management of patients with acute pancreatitis has three components: use of supportive measures, identification of etiologic factors, and observation for complications.

Supportive measures include (1) administering intravenous hydration with careful attention to fluid and electrolyte status, (2) withholding oral feedings to avoid pancreatic stimulation until abdominal pain resolves (usually also associated with a declining serum amylase), (3) prescribing parenteral analgesics (e.g., meperidine) to control pain, and (4) using nasogastric suctioning when nausea and vomiting are present.

Etiologic factors for acute pancreatitis should be identified. If evidence of a possible biliary cause or cholangitis exists, endoscopic retrograde cholangiopancreatography (ERCP) should be performed early in the clinical course. In severely ill patients with a retained common bile duct stone, endoscopic sphincterotomy with clearance of the duct may improve their condition, often lowering morbidity and mortality.

Patients with the presumed diagnosis of acute pancreatitis should be hospitalized and carefully observed during the first 24–48 hours. If aggressive nonoperative treatment does not lead to improvement, a CT scan of the abdomen should be performed to confirm pancreatic inflammation.

Close observation for associated complications is necessary. Findings of persistent fever, abdominal tenderness, or clinical deterioration should alert the physician to the possibility of a septic complication such as infected pseudocyst or abscess. Surgical drainage is indicated when evidence of an infected pseudocyst or abscess exists.

The complications of acute pancreatitis can be considered either local or systemic (see Table 55–2). **Local complications** result from the acute inflammatory process, which may lead to tissue necrosis and ductal disruption with resulting fluid collections and extravasation. Superimposed bacterial infection of either the pancreatic phlegmon (inflammatory, necrotic parenchyma) or pseudocyst (collection of fluid within or around the gland) is an important cause of death in acute pancreatitis. The management of both the pancreatic phlegmon and pseudocyst is generally nonsurgical unless infection develops, in which case surgical drainage is always required. Some practitioners advocate the drainage of a sterile pseudocyst if it is larger than 6 cm and persists for more than 6 weeks.

Systemic complications can be diverse (see Table 55–2). Pulmonary manifestations range from atelectasis to acute respiratory distress syndrome (ARDS) requiring mechanical ventilation. Acute tubular necrosis, which is usually attributable to shock and hypovolemia, may lead to renal insufficiency.

TABLE 55–4. Ranson's Prognostic Signs of Pancreatitis

At Admission
Age > 55 years
WBC > 16,000/mm³
Blood glucose > 200 mg/dL
Serum LDH > 350 U/L
Serum AST > 250 U/L

During Initial 48 Hours
Hematocrit decrease > 10%
BUN rise > 5 mg/dL
Serum calcium < 8 mg/dL
Arterial PO_2 < 60 mm Hg
Base deficit > 4 meq/L
Fluid sequestration > 6 L

Mortality
1%–10%	< 3 positive Ranson's signs
10%–40%	3–5 positive Ranson's signs
50%	≥ 6 positive Ranson's signs

PATIENT EDUCATION

If alcohol or a medication is the presumed etiologic agent, instruction regarding discontinuation of the offending agent is obviously important.

NATURAL HISTORY/PROGNOSIS

With general supportive measures alone, the majority of acute pancreatitis cases resolve within 3–10 days. To predict those patients at risk for a more complicated course, Ranson and coworkers defined a variety of clinical and biochemical features identifiable on admission and at 48 hours (see Table 55–4). Five positive signs are associated with a 40% mortality.

Research Questions

1. What role does the lipolytic enzyme phospholipase A have in the development of the acute respiratory distress syndrome associated with acute pancreatitis?
2. Would prophylactic antibiotic therapy be helpful in decreasing the rate of infectious complications associated with severe pancreatitis?

Case Resolution

Laboratory studies revealed marked serum hyperamylasemia and a serum alkaline phosphatase twice the normal level. Ultrasonography of the right upper quadrant demonstrated cholelithiasis and a dilated common bile duct. Biliary pancreatitis was therefore suspected, and endoscopic retrograde cholangiopancreatography (ERCP) demonstrated choledocholithiasis. Endoscopic sphincterotomy was performed, and two common bile duct stones were removed. Supportive therapy (including intravenous hydration and bowel rest) was initiated with resolution of symptoms within 72 hours. An elective laparoscopic cholecystectomy was performed 2 weeks following discharge.

Selected Readings

Fan, S., E. C. S. Lai, F. P. T. Mok, et al. Early treatment of acute biliary pancreatitis by endoscopic papillotomy. N Engl J Med 328:228–32, 1992.

Lee, S. P., J. F. Nicholls, and H. Z. Park. Biliary sludge as a cause of acute pancreatitis. N Engl J Med 326:589–93, 1992.

Marshall, J. B. Acute pancreatitis: A review with an emphasis on new developments. Arch Intern Med 153:1185–98, 1993.

Ranson, J. H. C. Etiological and prognostic factors in human acute pancreatitis: A review. Am J Gastroenterol 77:633–8, 1982.

Steinberg, W., and S. Tenner. Acute pancreatitis. N Engl J Med 330:1196–1210, 1994.

CHAPTER 56

CHRONIC PANCREATITIS

Michael W. Gavin, M.D.

Hx A 44-year-old male chef with a long history of alcohol abuse and chronic abdominal pain attributed to chronic pancreatitis presents with a 6-month history of progressive diarrhea. The stools, which are usually postprandial, are loose, bulky, and foul-smelling. The man has experienced a 4.5-kg (10-lb) weight loss in 3 months. He says that alcohol seems to make his persistent epigastric pain worse, and he has decreased his alcohol use to 3–6 beers a day. The physical examination is notable for a cachectic-appearing male. The abdomen is mildly tender in the mid-epigastrium with normal bowel sounds.

Questions

1. What simple test might confirm the diagnosis of chronic pancreatitis?
2. What is the likely cause of this man's diarrhea? What tests would verify the clinical impression?
3. What endocrine abnormality is commonly associated with long-standing chronic pancreatitis?

Chronic pancreatitis may be defined from a morphologic or clinical perspective. Pancreatic inflammation and sclerosis with resultant destruction of exocrine tissue are the morphologic hallmarks. Clinically, chronic pancreatitis is characterized by persistent or recurrent abdominal pain that is sometimes associated with pancreatic exocrine or endocrine insufficiency, which is manifested by steatorrhea, diabetes mellitus, and weight loss.

CLINICAL PRESENTATION

The most prominent presenting symptom is usually persistent, boring, epigastric pain. Patients may present with an acute flare (i.e., with symptoms typical of acute pancreatitis), but over time they usually develop continuous pain. Chronic pancreatitis is painless in less than 15% of patients, usually those who have an idiopathic cause.

Diarrhea results from pancreatic exocrine insufficiency, which causes malabsorption (or more exactly, maldigestion) related to the inadequate amount of digestive enzymes secreted.

Weight loss, the third of the three most common presenting symptoms, results from malabsorption and anorexia. Food ingestion often exacerbates pain.

Diabetes mellitus due to pancreatic endocrine insufficiency occurs in 30% of patients with chronic pancreatitis. However, 70% of patients with advanced alcoholic pancreatitis with pancreatic calcifications develop diabetes mellitus.

PATHOPHYSIOLOGY

The pathophysiologic basis of chronic pancreatitis is not well understood. Chronic alcoholism is the main cause of chronic pancreatitis in Western countries. Based on morphologic findings, two different types of chronic pancreatitis have been identified. The most common form is **chronic calcifying pancreatitis** (CCP). The formation of protein plugs and calculi (pancreatic lithogenesis) in the pancreatic ducts leads to atrophy of the involved acinar and ductal epithelium. Resultant morphologic findings are chronic patchy inflammation and progressive fibrosis of the exocrine parenchyma. Multiple strictures and segmental dilatations of the pancreatic ductal system, associated with intraductal calculi and protein plugs, characterize chronic calcifying pancreatitis.

The less common form of chronic pancreatitis, **chronic obstructive pancreatitis,** is associated with obstruction of the main pancreatic duct by tumors, strictures from previous trauma, congenital abnormalities, or papillary stenosis. In contrast to chronic calcifying pancreatitis, fibrosis is uniform (not patchy), intraductal calculi and protein plugs are rarely seen, and on correction of the obstruction, the lesion may be partially reversible.

Tropical pancreatitis occurs in children and young adults in Africa and Asia. Although the etiology is not well understood, malnutrition appears to play a role in its pathogenesis. Other less common causes of chronic pancreatitis are presented in Table 56–1.

Dx Chronic Pancreatitis

- Pain, malabsorption, and weight loss often present.
- Chronic pancreatic inflammation and scarring.
- Pancreatic calcifications on x-ray (40% of patients).

TABLE 56–1. Etiology of Chronic Pancreatitis

Alcohol
Idiopathic
Malnutrition
Familial
Congenital abnormalities
Trauma
Hypertriglyceridemia
Hyperparathyroidism

DIFFERENTIAL DIAGNOSIS

The clinical presentation of both chronic pancreatitis and pancreatic cancer may be similar, and the two diseases may coexist. Chronic pancreatitis has recently been shown to be a risk factor for pancreatic carcinoma.

On a CT scan, pancreatitis may occasionally appear as an inflammatory mass. Imaging studies (e.g., CT), endoscopic pancreatography with brush biopsies, CT-directed needle biopsies, and measurement of serum tumor markers (e.g., CA-19-9) may all be nondiagnostic in the evaluation of a pancreatic mass. Surgery sometimes is required to differentiate between pancreatic cancer and chronic pancreatitis in difficult cases.

Pancreas divisum, the absence of fusion of the dorsal and ventral pancreatic ducts, is the most common congenital abnormality of the pancreas. However, it rarely represents a true obstructive lesion leading to pancreatitis.

EVALUATION

History

The history should focus on clarifying the nature and duration of the epigastric pain, on eliciting risk factors for chronic pancreatitis, and on defining the severity of malabsorption or weight loss. Pain is nearly always constant (with occasional exacerbations). It may radiate to the midback. The physician should take a careful alcohol history, since excessive alcohol use is the major risk factor. Any diarrhea should be quantified as to volume, frequency, and consistency. Weight loss should be documented by obtaining a history of previous weights and by ascertaining the rapidity of weight loss.

Physical Examination

The typical patient with chronic pancreatitis has mild mid-epigastric tenderness. In an acute flare, physical findings are similar to those seen in acute pancreatitis (see Chapter 55).

Additional Evaluation
Imaging Studies

Plain abdominal radiographs may demonstrate calcifications of the pancreas in 40% of patients, which is a pathognomonic finding. Ultrasound of the abdomen may demonstrate pancreatic calcifications, a dilated pancreatic duct, or a pseudocyst. A satisfactory examination by sonography is often precluded by overlying intestinal gas. CT of the abdomen is more sensitive in detecting the above findings. In addition, CT may help distinguish pancreatic carcinoma from chronic pancreatitis.

Endoscopic retrograde cholangiopancreatography (ERCP) is the most sensitive method for studying the pancreatic ductal system. In rare instances, this examination may be normal in the early stages of chronic pancreatitis. Early pancreatographic changes are seen only in the side branches, followed by severe changes in the pancreatic duct involving multiple strictures and dilatations forming the so-called chain of lakes.

When considering the diagnosis of chronic pancreatitis in a patient with compatible clinical manifestations, a plain film of the abdomen should be performed initially. If no calcifications are seen, a CT scan of the abdomen should follow. ERCP should be reserved for those patients whose initial studies are negative.

Laboratory Tests

Unlike the situation in acute pancreatitis, serum pancreatic enzymes (amylase, lipase) may be normal in chronic pancreatitis, even in the setting of an acute flare. The secretin or secretin-cholecystokinin (CCK) stimulation test is considered the "gold standard" in the diagnosis of exocrine insufficiency in chronic pancreatitis. Following duodenal intubation, collection of pancreatic secretions is performed after intravenous injection of secretin, CCK, or both. Bicarbonate output is then measured from the collected pancreatic fluid. A secretin or secretin-CCK stimulation test should be performed (if available) when ERCP is nondiagnostic.

Because ERCP requires some expertise to perform, indirect tests of pancreatic function often are used. The bentiromide test involves oral administration of bentiromide. Chymotrypsin secreted by the exocrine pancreas is required to cleave bentiromide into *para*-aminobenzoic acid (PABA), which is absorbed and measured by urine analysis. Although the sensitivity of this test is only 50% in early disease, it is as high as 100% in severe disease.

MANAGEMENT

Therapeutic measures in chronic pancreatitis are directed toward (1) pain control, (2) pancreatic exocrine insufficiency (diarrhea with steatorrhea), and (3) pancreatic endocrine insufficiency (diabetes mellitus).

In an acute flare, such supportive measures as restriction of oral intake, intravenous hydration, and administration of appropriate parenteral analgesics for 3 to 10 days are usually necessary. In alcoholic chronic pancreatitis, abstinence from alcohol decreases the frequency and severity of acute attacks. Irreversible exocrine destruction usually has occurred by initial presentation, however, and may progress despite abstinence from alcohol.

Patients with persistent or chronic abdominal pain should be given a 1-month trial of pancreatic enzyme therapy. This is most effective in idiopathic chronic pancreatitis but occasionally may be helpful in alcoholic chronic pancreatitis. The proposed therapeutic effect involves inhibition of pancreatic secretion ("resting the pancreas"). The nonenteric-coated pancrelipase preparations (four tablets four times a day) should be used initially, since they are less expensive than enteric-coated or high-potency preparations.

If medical management of chronic pancreatitis does not result in pain relief, other causes of epigastric pain (e.g., peptic ulcer disease) should be considered. With marked pancreatic ductal dilatation caused by fibrotic strictures, surgical drainage of the duct may be helpful (e.g., longitudinal pancreaticojejunostomy).

Celiac ganglionectomy achieved by the injection of anesthetic and ablative agents into the celiac ganglion plays a limited role in the management of pain in chronic pancreatitis. Pain relief lasting up to 6 months is seen in approximately 50% of patients.

Because diarrhea in chronic pancreatitis results from maldigestion, pancreatic enzyme replacement for this complication is essential. Two factors are important to consider. First, 28,000 U of lipase is required for each meal. Some commercial preparations contain as little as 4000 U/tablet, so up to eight tablets per meal may be necessary. Second, gastric acid may inactivate pancreatic enzymes. Therefore, if a nonenteric-coated preparation is used, sodium bicarbonate or an H_2-receptor antagonist (e.g., cimetidine) should be added to prevent acid inactivation if diarrhea does not abate with supplements alone. Restriction of dietary fat (< 80 g/d) may be helpful.

In the treatment of diabetes mellitus caused by chronic pancreatitis, the physician should be aware of the increased risk of hypoglycemia with insulin therapy. This is attributable both to impaired glucagon secretion and erratic carbohydrate absorption.

PATIENT AND FAMILY EDUCATION

Three educational issues should be emphasized. First, the pain of chronic pancreatitis usually lasts 5–10 years and then generally diminishes. Second, complications of pancreatic exocrine and endocrine insufficiency (malabsorption and hyperglycemia) develop approximately 10 years after the onset of chronic pancreatitis. Third, abstinence from alcohol does not halt the course of chronic pancreatitis but does lessen the frequency and duration of acutely painful flares.

TABLE 56–2.   Complications of Chronic Pancreatitis

Chronic pain
Diarrhea due to maldigestion
Hyperglycemia
Pancreatic pseudocyst
Pancreatic abscess
Pancreatic ascites
Common bile duct obstruction
Duodenal obstruction
Splenic vein thrombosis

NATURAL HISTORY/PROGNOSIS

Complications of chronic pancreatitis are listed in Table 56–2.

Mortality in chronic pancreatitis is not clearly defined, although 50% mortality at 20 years has been reported.

Research Questions

1. What is the cause of tropical pancreatitis?
2. What therapeutic role might dissolution therapy for pancreatic stones have in chronic calcifying pancreatitis?

Case Resolution

A plain film of the abdomen in this patient revealed multiple calcifications across the epigastrium. The physician suspected malabsorption as the cause of the diarrhea. A 72-hour stool collection for fat was abnormal. A bentiromide test also was abnormal, supporting the diagnosis of malabsorption caused by chronic calcifying pancreatitis with exocrine insufficiency. The patient was placed on pancreatic enzyme supplementation, with subsequent resolution of the diarrhea and eventual weight gain.

Selected Readings

Dutta, S. K. Chronic pancreatitis: Exocrine and endocrine insufficiency. *In* J. P. Kassirer. *Current Therapy in Internal Medicine,* 3rd ed. St. Louis, Mosby–Year Book, 1990.

Karanjia, N. D., and H. H. Reber. The cure and management of the pain of chronic pancreatitis. Gastroenterol Clin North Am 19:895–904, 1990.

Sarles, H., J. P. Bernard, and L. Gullo. Pathogenesis of chronic pancreatitis. Gut 31:629–32, 1990.

Toskes, P. P. Medical therapy of chronic pancreatitis. Semin Gastrointest Dis 3:188–193, 1991.

CHAPTER 57

JAUNDICE AND LIVER FUNCTION ABNORMALITIES

Dana Fotieo, M.D., and Marc Masotti, M.D.

Hx A 64-year-old male machinist was found to have a cecal mass 8 months ago while undergoing a workup for iron deficiency anemia. Biopsy of the mass revealed adenocarcinoma, and the patient underwent a partial colectomy. He subsequently refused further treatment and was lost to follow-up until he presented to the emergency room with complaints of weakness, increasing abdominal girth, and yellow discoloration of his skin. He was an elderly appearing man in no acute distress. He was not oriented to time or place upon questioning. He was afebrile and markedly jaundiced with scleral icterus. The rest of the physical examination was remarkable for the presence of shifting dullness and a fluid wave, a liver span of 18 cm (8 in), 2+ to 3+ pitting edema of the lower extremities, and asterixis. There was no gynecomastia, testicular atrophy, palmar erythema, or spider angiomas. The laboratory examination showed a mild normochromic/normocytic anemia and mild thrombocytopenia. Coagulation studies revealed a prothrombin time (PT) of 17.9 seconds with an INR of 2.3 and an activated partial thromboplastin time (PTT) of 68 seconds. Electrolytes were within normal limits. Liver function tests showed an aspartate aminotransferase (AST, SGOT) of 110 U/L, an alanine aminotransferase (ALT, SGPT) of 103 U/L, an alkaline phosphatase of 1295 U/L, a γ-glutamyltranspeptidase (GGT) of 5292 U/L, a total bilirubin of 13.2 mg/dL with a direct fraction of 12.5 mg/dL, a lactic dehydrogenase (LDH) of 1583 U/L, a total protein of 5.6 g/dL, and an albumin of 2.5 g/dL.

Questions

1. What are the possible causes of the patient's laboratory abnormalities?
2. What is the predominant pattern of the abnormalities?
3. How would you approach making the diagnosis?

The problem of how to evaluate a patient with abnormal liver function tests (LFTs) arises in all field of medicine. Because the appearance of jaundice is so dramatic and frightening, patients usually seek medical attention promptly. Some patients with abnormal LFTs, however, are asymptomatic. It is up to the clinician to determine the significance of the laboratory abnormalities and to investigate the underlying cause.

PATHOPHYSIOLOGY

In some ways, the term liver function tests is a misnomer. These tests are usually ordered as part of laboratory chemistry profiles and can provide some information regarding separate hepatic parameters, such as hepatocellular damage, cholestasis, biosynthetic function, and detoxification/excretion. Appropriate interpretation of abnormal LFTs requires an understanding of what specific information can be obtained from a particular assay.

The transaminases (AST and ALT) are good indicators of hepatocyte damage due to a variety of causes. AST is present in the mitochondria and cytoplasm of hepatocytes but also is found in other tissues such as skeletal muscle, heart, and brain. ALT is located primarily in hepatocyte cytoplasm and is found to a lesser extent in extrahepatic tissues, thereby making it more specific for liver damage. Both enzymes will be elevated in most hepatic diseases although levels below 300 U/L are nonspecific. LDH is another enzyme liberated from damaged hepatocytes but is much less specific than the transaminases owing to its widespread distribution in extrahepatic tissues. Cellular necrosis and lysis secondary to any cause will result in release of these three enzymes.

Cholestasis is assessed through levels of alkaline phosphatase, GGT, and to a lesser extent 5'-nucleotidase. Alkaline phosphatase and 5'-nucleotidase are found in biliary canalicular membranes; GGT is in biliary epithelium as well as extrahepatic tissues, making it less specific. When there is cholestasis, GGT and alkaline phosphatase levels usually rise in parallel. In this instance, GGT elevation is a very sensitive marker for biliary tract disease. Moreover, because GGT levels can be increased by inducers of the microsomal enzyme system, GGT will often be elevated out of proportion to other liver enzymes in certain conditions (e.g., alcoholic liver disease). Isolated alkaline phosphatase elevations are usually due to other illnesses (e.g., bone disease). Mild to moderate increases of alkaline phosphatase (up to 3 times normal) are nonspecific and can be seen in almost any type of liver disease. The most striking elevations (> 3 times normal) occur with mechanical obstruction of the biliary system, e.g., with obstructing tumor, stricture, or stone impaction. 5'-Nucleotidase is nonspecific although generally associated with hepatobiliary disease. Its main use is to help confirm the hepatic origin of an elevated alkaline phosphatase; however, it does not correlate as well with alkaline phosphatase elevation as GGT does.

Measurement of serum proteins and certain coagulation factors (factors I, II, V, VII, IX, and X) provide information about the liver's synthetic capability. Owing to the long half-life of albumin, decreases in its serum concentration reflect subacute or chronic illness. Given the short half-life of the clotting factors—up to 5 days for factor I—prolongation of the PT will be seen prior to a decrease in the serum albumin as a marker for significant liver injury.

Finally, serum bilirubin can be considered a test of the liver's detoxifying capability and excretory function.

Bilirubin is primarily derived from catabolism of senescent red blood cells by the reticuloendothelial system. This initial bilirubin is unconjugated, is not water soluble, and is measured as the indirect fraction. This unconjugated portion is bound to albumin, then transported to the liver where is it taken up by the hepatocyte, conjugated with glucuronic acid, and excreted by the hepatocyte into the biliary system. The conjugated, water-soluble fraction is measured as the direct fraction of bilirubin and is the fraction found in the urine in patients with hyperbilirubinemia. Disorders of bilirubin metabolism can occur at each of the above steps and can be considered in terms of the following mechanisms: (1) increased production of bilirubin, (2) decreased uptake of bilirubin by the hepatocyte, (3) decreased conjugation of bilirubin, and (4) decreased excretion of bilirubin. It should be remembered that jaundice (icterus) usually will not be clinically evident until the serum bilirubin level exceeds 2–2.5 mg/dL.

DIFFERENTIAL DIAGNOSIS

The differential diagnosis of abnormal liver function tests is too extensive to be covered completely in this chapter. The most common causes—hepatocellular and cholestatic—are discussed briefly below.

Transaminase elevations < 300 are nonspecific; the most striking elevations (> 1000) occur in acute viral hepatitis, toxin- or drug-induced hepatitis, and ischemic liver injury. Cholestatic patterns of elevation usually have mild transaminase elevations and a predominance of alkaline phosphatase, GGT, 5'-nucleotidase, and bilirubin elevations. Cholestasis can be intra- or extrahepatic, acute or chronic. Extrahepatic causes are considered obstructive and include stones, strictures of the biliary tree, and tumors of the pancreas or bile ducts. Intrahepatic causes are nonobstructive and numerous (Table 57–1). Commonly used drugs that can result in cholestasis are listed in Table 57–2. Other causes of hyperbilirubinemia are given in Table 57–3.

EVALUATION

The first step is confirmation of the laboratory abnormality. Subsequently, a careful history and physical examination are undertaken.

TABLE 57–1. Common Causes of Intrahepatic Cholestasis

Acute	Chronic	Recurrent
Drugs (Table 57–2)	Chronic hepatitis	Dubin-Johnson
Alcohol	Hodgkin's disease	syndrome
Viral infection	Primary biliary cirrhosis	Rotor's syndrome
Toxic exposure	Sclerosing cholangitis	Pregnancy
Paraquat	Amyloidosis	
Rapeseed oil	Sarcoidosis	
Total parenteral nutrition	Congestive heart failure	
Postoperative	Drugs (Table 57–2)	
Sepsis		

TABLE 57–2. Commonly Used Drugs That Can Cause Cholestasis

Antibiotics
   Erythromycin
   Trimethoprim/sulfamethoxazole
   Amoxicillin/clavulanic acid
   Nitrofurantoin
   Griseofulvin
Analgesics
   Propoxyphene
   Sulindac
   Diflunisal
Allopurinol
Warfarin
Steroids (contraceptive and anabolic)
Phenytoin
Thiazide diuretics
Phenothiazines
Tricyclic antidepressants
Haloperidol
Parenteral gold
Oral hypoglycemics (chlorpropamide, tolbutamide)

TABLE 57–4. Symptoms and Signs of Liver Disease and Their Significance

Symptom/Sign	Significance
Fever	Nonspecific but might indicate hepatitis, chole-
Nausea/vomiting	cystitis, spontaneous bacterial peritonitis
Weight loss	Nonspecific but might indicate malignancy or
Anorexia	hepatitis
Fatigue	
Increased abdominal girth	Ascites from portal hypertension or hypoal-
	buminemia
Jaundice	Biliary obstruction
Clay-colored stools	
Dark urine	
Gastrointestinal bleeding	May indicate portal hypertension
Right upper quadrant pain	Hepatitis, cholecystitis, hepatocellular carci-
	noma, abscess
Pruritus	Biliary obstruction
Confusion	Encephalopathy secondary to liver failure or
	portal hypertension
Easy bruising	Splenomegaly secondary to portal hypertension
	with platelet sequestration, or coagulopathy
	secondary to decreased synthesis of clotting
	factors

History

Patients with abnormal LFTs or jaundice should be asked about their symptoms (Table 57–4). Another key aspect of the history is to determine risk factors for liver disease. Patients should be asked about past or present intravenous drug use, alcohol use, sexual practices, blood transfusions, and occupational exposures (e.g., vinyl chloride). A detailed medication history including over-the-counter drugs (e.g., acetaminophen) and herbal remedies is important because of the hepatotoxicity of many drugs. A family history should be obtained, since some liver diseases are inherited (e.g., α_1-antitrypsin deficiency and Wilson's disease).

Physical Examination

The physical examination is useful in determining the cause and chronicity of abnormal LFTs. Fever may be present in acute hepatitis, cholecystitis, and spontaneous bacterial peritonitis. Certain physical signs, such as

TABLE 57–3. Etiology of Hyperbilirubinemia

Increased production
   Hemolysis
   Ineffective erythropoiesis
Decreased uptake
   Drugs (flavaspidic acid)
   Gilbert's syndrome (variant)
Decreased conjugation
   Gilbert's syndrome
   Crigler-Najjar syndrome types I and II
   Drug inhibition of glucuronyl transferase
   Hypothyroidism
Decreased excretion
   Dubin-Johnson syndrome
   Rotor's syndrome
   Benign familial recurrent cholestasis
   Pregnancy
   Drug-induced cholestasis
   Extrahepatic obstruction (stone, stricture, mass)

spider angiomas, palmar erythema, gynecomastia, testicular atrophy, loss of body hair, and asterixis, are suggestive of end-stage liver disease (cirrhosis). If portal hypertension is present, the examiner might note splenic enlargement, ascites, or a caput medusae. The liver should be percussed and palpated to assess size, tenderness, and nodularity. A rectal examination is helpful to identify hemorrhoids (which can be a sign of portal hypertension) and evaluate for occult blood. The presence of jaundice (of either skin or sclera) is suggestive of severe liver disease or biliary obstruction. Finally, signs of hepatic encephalopathy such as decreased mental status and asterixis can occur in cirrhosis or fulminant hepatic failure.

Additional Evaluation

Although LFTs do not identify the cause of a particular liver disease, repeated laboratory panels can be used to assess the degree of hepatic damage, suggest possible underlying causes, and follow the progression of liver disease. For example, increases in transaminases suggest acute hepatitis. In general, patients with alcoholic hepatitis have levels < 300 U/L. Furthermore, an AST/ALT ratio of 2 is consistent with alcohol-induced hepatitis. More marked elevations suggest a viral or a toxin-mediated hepatitis.

Biliary obstruction is evaluated by alkaline phosphatase, GGT, and bilirubin. Direct hyperbilirubinemia typically is associated with hepatobiliary disease (e.g, gallstones, pancreatic tumor), whereas elevation of indirect bilirubin can occur with hemolysis, decreased hepatic uptake, and impaired conjugation (e.g., Gilbert's syndrome).

Tests of synthetic function such as albumin and PT can help determine chronicity of disease. Because of its long serum half-life, albumin may be normal in acute disease states. Albumin also can be affected by protein malnutrition, protein-losing states such as nephrotic syndrome, acute stress (e.g., sepsis), and other factors. Patients may have a prolonged PT secondary to decreased synthetic function, vitamin K deficiency, or disseminated intravascular coagulation. A trial of vitamin K can help distinguish hepatocellular disease from impaired vitamin K absorption. If liver synthetic function is adequate, the PT should improve by approximately 30% in 24 hours.

Further diagnostic workup depends on the pattern of LFT abnormalities and the physician's clinical suspicion. Serology can play an important role in evaluating increased LFTs. For example, an isolated elevation of transaminases might prompt the clinician to order a viral hepatitis panel. If biliary obstruction is suspected, a right upper quadrant ultrasound can be useful in looking for gallstones, intra- and extrahepatic duct dilatation, and masses. A CT scan might help define a mass (e.g., cyst, tumor, abscess) in addition to identifying calcified gallstones and biliary dilatation.

More invasive procedures such as endoscopic retrograde cholangiopancreatography (ERCP) can be helpful in diagnosing pancreatic cancer and obstructive jaundice. At times, a percutaneous liver biopsy is necessary to confirm a diagnosis suggested by laboratory findings or to evaluate persistent, unexplained LFT abnormalities.

MANAGEMENT AND PROGNOSIS

Management and prognosis depend on the cause. See Chapters 58 and 59, respectively, for a discussion of hepatitis and gallstones.

Research Questions

1. Are there better markers of liver synthetic function than albumin and PT?
2. Why is GGT elevated in acute alcohol ingestion and alcoholic liver disease?

Case Resolution

The patient was admitted to the hospital and found by CT scan to have lesions in his liver suggestive of metastatic carcinoma. The striking elevations of GGT, alkaline phosphatase, and bilirubin with only mild transaminase elevations were consistent with cholestasis. Prolongation of the PT and low albumin were evidence of synthetic dysfunction. Although the CT scan and clinical history were most suggestive of metastatic colon cancer, a guided liver biopsy was required for confirmation of this diagnosis. The biopsy confirmed metastatic adenocarcinoma. He declined further treatment and subsequently died several weeks later.

Selected Readings

Gordon, S. Jaundice and cholestasis. Postgrad Med 90(4):65–71, 1991.

Laker, M. F. Liver function tests. Br Med J 301:250–1, 1990.

McKenna, J. P., M. Moskovitz, and J. L. Cox. Abnormal liver function tests in asymptomatic patients. Am Fam Physician 39(3):117–26, 1989.

Tygstrup, N. Assessment of liver function: Principles and practice. J Gastroenterol Hepatol 5:1468–82, 1990.

Zimmerman, H. J., and K. W. Deschner. Differential diagnosis of jaundice. Hosp Pract 22(5):99–122, 1987.

CHAPTER 58

HEPATITIS

Glenn C. Robinson, M.D.

H$_x$ A 37-year-old female telephone operator presents with a 1-week history of malaise and fatigue. She complains of nausea, diminished appetite, and aching discomfort in her upper abdomen. She has had low-grade fever without chills for 3 days. Thinking she had "the same flu bug" from which her two young children in daycare had recovered 3 weeks earlier, she did not plan to seek medical attention. However, when her urine turned "cola-colored" and she lost her taste for cigarettes, she decided to see the doctor. Her past medical history is remarkable for two uncomplicated pregnancies and a third requiring a blood transfusion. She has had a tubal ligation. She takes no prescription medications but uses acetaminophen for headaches and takes vitamins. She has a 5 pack-year history of cigarette smoking and drinks alcohol only rarely. Physical examination reveals a tired-appearing but well-nourished woman with mild scleral icterus. Her vital signs are normal. Her skin is cool and clammy. The liver edge is tender with an 11-cm span; the spleen is not palpable. The remainder of the examination is normal.

Questions

1. What elements of her medical history are important? What else would you like to know concerning her medical history?
2. What diagnostic evaluation would you initiate at this point? Can the patient be evaluated as an outpatient, or must she be hospitalized?

The term "acute hepatitis" implies a process that takes place over the course of days to months in which the liver suffers an injury due to a wide variety of agents and pathophysiologic mechanisms. Generally, in acute hepatitis, symptoms, physical signs, and laboratory abnormalities have been present for fewer than 6 months.

Acute hepatitis is a common clinical problem worldwide. Hepatotropic viruses are by far the leading cause of hepatitis. Many cases are subclinical in children and adolescents; thus, the true incidence of acute viral hepatitis is difficult to measure. Drug- and toxin-related injury (e.g., ethanol abuse) is the next most common cause.

Viral hepatitis is a significant public health problem in less well-developed countries because of poor sanitation and suspect water supplies. Hepatitis A virus (HAV) is nonetheless responsible for 25% of overt hepatitis cases in industrialized nations. Hepatitis B virus (HBV) is harbored by an estimated 300 million carriers worldwide with prevalence rates as high as 15% in China, Southeast Asia, and sub-Saharan Africa. In areas of endemic HBV, intrafamilial spread and perinatal maternal-fetal infection are important vectors of transmission. Globally, hepatocellular carcinoma is the most common cancer of solid organs. Approximately 80% of hepatocellular carcinomas are related to chronic HBV or hepatitis C (HCV) infection. Hepatitis E virus (HEV) is responsible for 60% of sporadic cases of acute hepatitis in India. Because of its increasing prevalence in India, HEV will likely surpass HBV as the world's most common cause of hepatitis.

PATHOPHYSIOLOGY

Hepatic injury can occur via a variety of mechanisms and involve all cellular components of the liver acinus (Table 58–1). Hepatotropic viruses appear to cause injury either by direct cytopathic action (e.g., HCV) or by hepatocyte infection and immune-mediated injury (e.g., HBV). In 5% to 10% of icteric HAV cases, there is predominantly bile ductular and canalicular involvement resulting in prolonged cholestasis. Hepatitis D (HDV) is an incomplete virus and, in order for hepatitis to occur, the infected person must already be a carrier of hepatitis B surface antigen (HBsAg) (superinfection) or be simultaneously infected by HBV (coinfection).

Drug use can cause myriad histopathologic abnormalities in the liver (Table 58–2). Ethanol and acetaminophen, for example, can damage hepatocytes by the local generation of toxic metabolites, which damage cellular and subcellular structures. Ischemia (e.g., in hypotension or congestive heart failure) causes hypoxic injury to hepatocytes. In sepsis, hepatic injury is probably related to several factors including direct parenchymal invasion by the bacterial organism, hypoxia, malnutrition, and circulating endotoxins. Hepatocyte injury in autoimmune chronic active hepatitis (AICAH) may be caused by abnormal cell-mediated immune regulation that allows cytotoxic lymphocytes to attack specific hepatocyte membrane antigens. The hepatic manifestations of Wilson's disease are caused by hepatocyte defects resulting in impaired copper excretion into bile. α_1-Antitrypsin deficiency is associated with impaired synthesis and secretion of a protease inhibitor.

TABLE 58–1. Some Causes of Acute Hepatic Injury

Infectious	Noninfectious
Viral	*Drugs (Table 58–2)**
Hepatitis A*	*Toxins*
Hepatitis B*	*Amanita phalloides*
Hepatitis C*	Ethanol*
Hepatitis D	Herbs *(Senecio, Crotalaria)*
Hepatitis E	Carbon tetrachloride
Cytomegalovirus*	*Autoimmune Chronic Active Hepatitis*
Epstein-Barr virus*	*Metabolic Disorders*
Herpesvirus	Wilson's disease
Varicella zoster virus	α_1-Antitrypsin deficiency
Varicella	*Vascular Disorders*
Rubella	Ischemia (hypotension, shock)*
Yellow fever virus	Congestive heart failure*
Nonviral	Budd-Chiari syndrome
Bacterial abscess*	Veno-occlusive disease
Amebic abscess	*Pregnancy*
Syphilis	Acute fatty liver
Lyme disease	HELLP syndrome
Weil's syndrome (leptospirosis)	

*Common in North America.

TABLE 58–2. Some Common Drugs That Cause Liver Disease

Hepatocellular Injury/Inflammation/ or Necrosis	*Granulomatous Hepatitis*
Acetaminophen (overdose or in alcoholics)	Allopurinol
	Captopril
Aspirin (high dose)	Carbamazepine
Isoniazid	Hydralazine
Ketoconazole	Procainamide
Methyldopa	Quinidine
Nitrofurantoin	*Cholestasis*
NSAIDs (especially diclofenac, sulindac)	Anabolic steroids
Phenytoin	Azathioprine
Sulfonamides	Chlorpromazine
Fatty Liver	Erythromycin
Amiodarone	Estrogens
Corticosteroids	Nifedipine
Ethanol	Oral contraceptives
Gold	
Tetracycline	
Valproic acid	
Vitamin A (high dose)	

DIFFERENTIAL DIAGNOSIS

In the United States, viruses are the most common cause of hepatitis (Table 58–3) with HAV being the most common, followed by HBV and then HCV. Epstein-Barr virus (EBV) and cytomegalovirus (CMV), which both cause infectious mononucleosis syndromes, can also cause overt hepatitis. In patients with human immunodeficiency virus (HIV) or with an organ transplant, CMV is a common cause of often very severe hepatitis. Other infectious agents only rarely cause hepatitis in immunocompetent patients (see Table 58–1).

AICAH should be considered in young to middle-aged women with hepatitis. AICAH also affects men, albeit less frequently. Pregnant women in the last trimester may develop two distinct acute hepatitis-like syndromes: HELLP (hemolysis, elevated liver enzymes, low platelets) syndrome or AFLP (acute fatty liver of pregnancy). Although of uncertain etiology, both are associated with preeclampsia. It is important to remember, however, that viral hepatitis is the most common cause of hepatitis in pregnancy.

Finally, hepatitis can be caused by vascular and metabolic disease. In the elderly especially, ischemic hepatopathy may be a consequence of any severe cardiorespiratory or septic illness resulting in systemic hypotension or hypoxemia. Wilson's disease and α_1-antitrypsin deficiency are autosomal recessive diseases. They generally present with chronic liver test abnormalities or cirrhosis, but Wilson's disease may rarely manifest as an acute or even fulminant hepatitis.

With serum liver chemistries readily available, the detection of acute hepatocellular injury, cholestasis, or jaundice is rarely a diagnostic challenge. The symptoms of hepatitis in the anicteric phase may mimic those of infectious mononucleosis, viral gastroenteritis, appendicitis, meningitis, or cholecystitis. In the patient with acute jaundice, excluding extrahepatic biliary obstruction with or without cholangitis is important. Extrahepatic obstruction can occur either from benign disease (e.g., common duct stones) or malignancy (e.g., pancreatic carcinoma). Bacterial cholangitis with gram-negative sepsis often presents with Charcot's triad of fever, right upper quadrant pain, and jaundice. Recognizing and treating this condition early is critical because of its high mortality rate. Identifying patients with drug- or toxin-induced hepatitis with jaundice (e.g., due to ingestion of acetaminophen, isoniazid, or *Amanita phalloides* mushrooms) is also of great importance, since these patients have a higher mortality rate (> 10%) than do those with viral hepatitis.

EVALUATION

History

The symptoms of hepatitis are protean and often vague. Malaise, fatigue, anorexia, dysgeusia, fever, ar-

TABLE 58–3.   Comparative Features of the Hepatitis Viruses

Feature	A	B	C	D	E
Clinical presentation					
Onset	Abrupt	Insidious	Insidious	Insidious	Abrupt
Incubation period					
Range (days)	15–50	28–160	15–160	28–140	?
Mean (days)	30	70	50	?	40
Fever	Common	Uncommon	Uncommon	Uncommon	Common
Jaundice	Uncommon	More common	Uncommon	Common	Common
Laboratory data					
Duration of enzyme elevation	Short, 3–19 days	Prolonged, 35–200 days	Prolonged, like B	Prolonged, like B	Short, like A
Viral nucleic acid	RNA	DNA	DNA	DNA	RNA
Transmission					
Oral	Yes	Possibly	Uncertain	No	Yes
Percutaneous	Rare	Yes	Yes	Yes	No
Sexual	Yes	Yes	Yes	Yes	Uncertain
Perinatal	No	Yes	Rare	No	Uncertain
Outcome					
Severity	Mild	Mild to severe	Intermediate	Severe	Mild, severe in pregnancy
Mortality	< 1%	1%	< 1%	3%	< 1%, 20% in pregnancy
Chronic hepatitis (risk)	No	Yes (10%)	Yes (40%–90%)	Yes Superinfection: 70% Coinfection: 10%	No
Chronic carrier	No	Yes	Yes	Yes	No
Epidemiology					
Endemic areas	Worldwide	China, Southeast Asia, sub-Saharan Africa	Worldwide	Mediterranean, Middle East, North Africa	Southeast Asia (particularly India), Africa
Found in North America	Yes	Yes	Yes	Unusual (except intravenous drug users, hemophiliacs)	No

thralgias, nausea, and epigastric or right upper quadrant pain are often present in varied combinations. The prodrome of anorexia and nausea typically lasts from several days to several weeks and is followed by upper abdominal discomfort and a loss of taste for cigarettes and alcohol. Dark urine, light-colored stools, jaundice, and pruritus are due to impaired bile excretion but may be absent, especially initially. By the time icteric symptoms arise, constitutional symptoms are on the wane. Pruritus generally occurs only in prolonged cholestasis. Fever, if present, usually subsides before the onset of jaundice in hepatitis A–E. Persistence of fever suggests CMV, EBV, herpesvirus type 1, alcohol, or drugs as the cause. Sore throat and tender lymph nodes suggest a mononucleosis syndrome. Transient macular rashes can occur with all viral forms; however, if accompanied by fever and eosinophilia, a drug-induced hypersensitivity reaction should be suspected.

Medication history, exposures, social habits, and occupational history are important to elicit in detail. All medications taken during the 2 months prior to presentation should be noted. One must always inquire about use of nonprescription medications and remedies such as acetaminophen, aspirin, megadose vitamins (particularly vitamin A), herbal preparations, and, for bodybuilders, anabolic steroids. Women should be asked about oral contraceptive use. Every patient should be questioned regarding past exposure to blood products (red cells, plasma, factor concentrates), intravenous drug use (particularly needle sharing), tattoos, unsafe sexual practices (multiple sexual partners, prostitution), foreign travel (particularly to Southeast Asia), shellfish ingestion (HAV), wild mushroom ingestion, children in daycare (a reservoir for HAV), and exposure to jaundiced persons. Careful questioning about the amount of alcohol ingested and the duration of alcohol use is important. Recent operations and anesthetic exposures should be noted.

Physical Examination

Physical findings are often subtle and nonspecific. Jaundice occurs when the total serum bilirubin exceeds 2–3 mg/dL. Most patients with viral hepatitis have palpable hepatomegaly. Splenomegaly is found in 25% of acute viral cases and in 90% of EBV-related hepatitis. Exudative pharyngitis and cervical lymphadenopathy also suggest EBV. Clues to significant cardiovascular disease such as elevated jugular venous pressure, cardiomegaly, acrocyanosis, S_3, and pulmonary rales might suggest an ischemic or congestive hepatopathy.

The findings of spider angiomas, palmar erythema, digital clubbing, leukonychia (whitish nails), ascites, gynecomastia, and superficial abdominal collateral veins, although nonspecific, suggest chronic liver disease and cirrhosis. Patients with acute alcoholic hepatitis, however, generally have chronic liver disease and exhibit many of these findings. In men, finding both Dupuytren's contractures and testicular atrophy may help differentiate alcoholic from nonalcoholic cirrhosis.

Particular attention should be paid to the neurologic evaluation of any patient with severe hepatitis. Altered sensorium, drowsiness, asterixis, changes in muscle tone, and repeated vomiting suggest fulminant hepatic failure with portosystemic encephalopathy and portend a poor prognosis.

Additional Evaluation

Evaluation of serum liver enzymes and viral serologic markers is recommended for all patients with hepatitis. Aminotransferases (AST, ALT) are typically elevated dramatically and peak 1–2 weeks after symptom onset in viral hepatitis. ALT, which is liver-specific, is usually > 400 but may reach levels of 3000–4000 in hepatitis A–E. Drugs and other viruses cause increases of 2–15 times normal. Ischemic injury causes a dramatic and rapid rise and fall of aminotransferases in a time course of 2–4 days. In alcoholic hepatitis, the AST:ALT ratio is usually > 2 with the peak AST < 300-400. Peak aminotransferase levels do not correlate with clinical outcome in acute hepatitis.

Alkaline phosphatase is elevated less markedly (2 to 3 times normal). More significant elevations can be seen in HAV with prolonged cholestasis. In this instance, γ-glutamyltransferase (GGT) and bilirubin are also elevated. Total bilirubin rarely exceeds 10 mg/dL in acute viral hepatitis but may be elevated to 20–25 mg/dL in severe alcoholic hepatitis. The level of bilirubin elevation correlates well with prognosis in alcoholic but not in viral hepatitis. In all cases, cholestasis generally occurs after the AST and ALT peak.

The prothrombin time (PT) is an insensitive measure of most types of hepatocellular injury, since severe damage is required before PT prolongation occurs. The PT, however, is a sensitive indicator of hepatic dysfunction in ischemic or congestive hepatopathy. In viral hepatitis, a significant prolongation of the PT that is unresponsive to parenteral vitamin K administration connotes severe hepatocellular injury.

Serologic testing for viral antigens and antibodies is essential. Serum should be tested for anti-HAV IgM, HB surface antigen, anti-HB core IgM, and anti-HCV. Intravenous drug users should also be tested for anti-HDV IgM. HCV and HDV antibodies may take from 4 weeks to 4 months to develop, thus potentially creating a role for measuring HDV DNA and HCV RNA in the acute diagnosis. Currently these tests are not available for routine use. In the patient seronegative for hepatitis A–D, one should consider evaluating for HEV (HEVAb), EBV (Monospot or heterophile Ab), CMV (rise in convalescent titers or presence of IgMAb), AICAH (ANA [antinuclear antibody] and ASMA [anti-smooth muscle antibody]), and Wilson's disease (ceruloplasmin, 24-hour urine copper).

Routine CBCs are occasionally helpful. A mild lymphocytosis (WBC rarely > 12,000) generally accompanies cases of viral hepatitis. Atypical lymphocytosis suggests EBV or CMV. Hemoglobin and hematocrit are often normal, but mild anemia due to hemolysis may occur in glucose-6-phosphate dehydrogenase (G6PD) deficiency or in Zieve's syndrome (hemolysis due to alcoholic hepatitis). Megaloblastic changes may signal impaired folate metabolism from alcoholism. Aplastic anemia and agranulocytosis are rare, often fatal, sequelae of viral hepatitis.

Radiologic evaluation is usually unnecessary. Occasionally, abdominal ultrasonography may be required to rule out portal hypertension, mass lesions of the liver, and intra- or extrahepatic biliary obstruction. Liver biopsy generally is not required in acute hepatitis and, because of the risk to the patient, should be considered only when (1) serology is negative, (2) no drugs or toxins can be implicated, and (3) the results will alter therapy.

MANAGEMENT

Most cases of acute viral hepatitis are mild to moderate in severity and require only supportive outpatient care. General recommendations include avoidance of vigorous physical activity until symptoms abate, adequate hydration, a trial of low-fat, high-carbohydrate diet if anorexia is a problem, judicious use of antiemetics if needed, and avoidance of potentially hepatotoxic agents (narcotics, sedatives, analgesics, ethanol). Corticosteroids have no role in the treatment of acute viral hepatitis and may, in fact, impair the normal host immune response to infection, thus increasing the risk of development of chronic hepatitis.

In the case of drug- or alcohol-induced illness, use of the offending agent should be ceased indefinitely. In all cases treated on an outpatient basis, the patient and the patient's liver chemistries should be evaluated twice weekly while the aminotransferases are rising, weekly when they plateau, and every 1–2 weeks thereafter until resolution. In HBV, it is helpful to check for disappearance of HBsAg.

Severe acute hepatitis as evidenced by a prolonged PT (INR > 1.4), bilirubin > 10 mg/dL, persistent nausea and vomiting with dehydration, or any evidence of fulminant hepatic failure (FHF) requires hospitalization and careful monitoring. Patients with FHF should be transferred to a medical center with a specialized liver unit and the ability to perform liver transplantation. Patients without fulminant disease require supportive therapy with (1) intravenous hydration, (2) parenteral vitamin K or fresh-frozen plasma if coagulopathy is present, (3) avoidance of psychoactive medications, and (4) monitoring for neurologic changes suggestive of deterioration.

Specific therapies are few but include high-dose corticosteroids in selected patients with severe alcoholic hepatitis, acyclovir for herpetic hepatitis, and acetylcysteine in acetaminophen toxicity. To date, no antiviral agents have been found to be helpful in acute viral hepatitis. Alpha interferon, an immune stimulating agent, is efficacious in chronic viral hepatitis; its role in the treatment of acute infection is being evaluated. Acute fatty liver of pregnancy and the HELLP syndrome are definitively treated by prompt termination of the pregnancy.

PATIENT AND FAMILY EDUCATION

Patients, their immediate family, and sexual partners require careful instruction as to the cause of the hepatitis, the mode of transmission, if any, and preventive measures to be taken to avoid further liver injury as well as spread of the disease. Passive immunization with gamma globulin is recommended for close household contacts of patients with HAV. Frequent hand washing and good personal hygiene will help prevent further transmission. Those with HBV or HCV should not donate blood products. Patients persistently positive for HBsAg or HBeAg should be instructed to follow safe sex precautions. Recombinant HBV vaccine and HBV immune globulin (HBIG) should be administered to sexual partners. Close household contacts of HBsAg carriers should receive the HBV vaccine as well. Persons traveling to less well-developed countries with endemic HAV should receive gamma globulin prophylaxis prior to departure.

In general, those with HCV should follow the same precautions as those with HBV. Although the rate of sexual transmission of HCV is less well understood than that of HBV, safe sex measures seem prudent. For all patients with viral hepatitis, alcohol intake should be discouraged for 6 months. Patients should not share eating utensils, razors, and toothbrushes while still infectious. Those patients with HBV, HCV, and HDV who develop chronic hepatitis will need regular follow-up, consideration of antiviral therapy, and surveillance for hepatocellular carcinoma owing to the oncogenic potential of these viruses.

Patients with hepatitis stemming from alcohol or intravenous drug use require intensive substance abuse counseling by mental health professionals. If a specific medication, herbal preparation, or megadose vitamin is implicated, appropriate documentation should be made in the medical record and further use avoided. Rechallenging a patient with the suspected drug for diagnostic purposes is dangerous and is to be discouraged.

NATURAL HISTORY/PROGNOSIS

Prognosis and clinical course are dependent on the specific etiology. The mortality from acute viral hepatitis is, for all causes, less than 1%. Viral hepatitis tends to be milder in children and more severe in elderly patients and in those with multiple medical problems. In HBV and HDV, the more florid the acute illness, the lower the likelihood of chronic sequelae. Moreover, patients with HBV who suffer only mild icterus acutely, who have a relapsing episode, or who are immunocompromised are at a higher risk of developing chronic hepatitis. Provided that fulminant hepatitis does not ensue, the prognosis for complete recovery in drug- or toxin-mediated injury is excellent with discontinuation of exposure.

Many of the acute hepatitides can evolve into chronic hepatitis. Whereas approximately 10% of people with hepatitis B infection develop chronic hepatitis, more than half of those with hepatitis C develop chronic infection. Chronic hepatitis C generally is indolent, causing only a mild portal triaditis, but in perhaps 20% of uses it will cause more aggressive chronic active hepatitis, leading to cirrhosis. Current therapy for chronic hepatitis B or C is the immunomodulating agent alpha interferon.

Autoimmune chronic active hepatitis, by definition, is a chronic necroinflammatory process. Despite treatment with immunosuppressants such as corticosteroids and azathioprine, half of those with autoimmune hepatitis develop cirrhosis. If untreated, chronic hepatic iron and copper accumulation in hemochromatosis and Wilson's disease, respectively, leads to chronic hepatitis and cirrhosis. D-Penicillamine therapy in Wilson's disease and phlebotomy or iron chelation in hemochromatosis can halt progression and reverse the chronic inflammatory process if treatment is initiated before cirrhosis has developed.

Currently, there is no effective treatment for primary biliary cirrhosis or α_1-antitrypsin deficiency affecting the liver. Liver transplantation is often required.

Research Questions

1. What specific immunologic mechanisms contribute to acute liver injury? What can be done to modulate these responses without increasing the risk of chronic disease?

2. In an era of managed health care and scarcity of health resources, what will be the ultimate role of liver transplantation? Who should determine this role?

Case Resolution

The patient had significant elevation of aminotransferases, moderate hyperbilirubinemia, and viral serology remarkable for the presence of HAV IgM antibody. Two of her children also demonstrated HAV IgM antibody; her husband, their other child, and all the children and staff at the daycare center were given gamma globulin. Clinically and biochemically, the patient was back to normal in 3 weeks.

Selected Readings

Carey, W. D., et al. Viral hepatitis in the 1990s, Part III: Hepatitis C, hepatitis E, and other viruses. Cleve Clin J Med 59(6):595–601, 1992.

Hoofnagle, J. H. Therapy of acute and chronic viral hepatitis. Adv Intern Med 39:241–75, 1994.

Koff, R. S. Hepatitis B today: Clinical and diagnostic overview. Pediatr Infect Dis J 12(5):428–32, 1993.

Maddrey, W. C. Chronic hepatitis. Disease-a-Month 39(2):53–125, 1993.

Yarze, J. C., et al. Wilson's disease: Current status. Am J Med 92:643–54, 1992.

CHAPTER 59

GALLSTONES

Michael W. Gavin, M.D.

H$_x$ A previously healthy 39-year-old female records clerk presents to an outpatient clinic with a 12-hour history of both midepigastric and right upper quadrant pain. The pain, which is associated with nausea and vomiting, had awakened the patient at midnight. The woman complains of a recent "shaking chill." She recalls having had several similar episodes of epigastric pain, each lasting 3–4 hours, in the past several weeks. Antacids did not relieve the symptoms. The patient's only significant medical history is limited to her obstetric history—gravida 4, para 4. She takes oral contraceptives and an occasional acetaminophen tablet. The physical examination reveals a low-grade fever of 38.5° C (100.5° F). The sclerae are mildly icteric. On abdominal examination, marked right upper quadrant and epigastric tenderness is detectable on palpation.

Questions

1. What is the differential diagnosis of right upper quadrant pain?
2. What historical factors and physical findings support the diagnosis of biliary "colic" versus acute cholecystitis or acute cholangitis?
3. What are the patient's risk factors for the development of gallstones?

Approximately 20% of men and 35% of women in the United States will develop gallstones (cholelithiasis) during their lifetime. The majority of such individuals are asymptomatic, but up to one third become symptomatic. In the United States, 600,000 cholecystectomies are performed annually. Laparoscopic surgery and biliary endoscopy have been the most significant developments in the management of gallstones and their associated complications, although advances in the understanding of the pathogenesis of gallstones have also occurred.

CLINICAL PRESENTATION

Patients with symptomatic cholelithiasis may present with any of four clinical syndromes—biliary "colic," acute cholecystitis, cholangitis, or biliary pancreatitis. Right upper quadrant or midepigastric pain are commonly encountered, and the pain typically is not colicky but persistent. Chronic cholecystitis is a term often used to describe those patients who have had repeated episodes of biliary "colic" or acute cholecystitis.

PATHOPHYSIOLOGY

Gallstones may be classified as either cholesterol stones or pigment stones. In Western countries, 75% of gallstones are cholesterol stones, 20% are black pigment stones, and 5% are brown pigment stones.

Cholesterol Gallstones

Two main factors are involved in the formation of cholesterol gallstones—cholesterol supersaturation of bile and the potential role of the gallbladder in promoting nucleation (formation of cholesterol crystals).

In hepatocytes, cholesterol is solubilized with phospholipid, forming unilaminar vesicles. Upon secretion into the canaliculus, the vesicles may absorb bile salts, causing the formation of mixed micelles. When the vesicles become supersaturated with cholesterol, they fuse into multilaminar structures. Cholesterol crystals appear to originate from this process. Excessive hepatic secretion of cholesterol is the principal cause of cholesterol supersaturation of bile. Conditions associated with biliary cholesterol hypersecretion include rapid weight loss, obesity, heredity (e.g., Pima Indian descent), use of estrogen and oral contraceptives, and hypertriglyceridemia (Table 59–1).

TABLE 59–1. Risk Factors for Cholesterol Stone Formation

Cholesterol Hypersecretion in Bile

Obesity
Hypertriglyceridemia
Rapid weight loss
Estrogen therapy
Oral contraceptive use
Pima Indian descent

Gallbladder Hypomotility

Prolonged fasting (e.g., parenteral nutrition)
Pregnancy
Oral contraceptive use
Somatostatin analog (octreotide) therapy

TABLE 59–2. Characteristics of Pigment Stones

Characteristic	Black Pigment Stone	Brown Pigment Stone
Color	Black	Brown to orange
Consistency	Amorphous, powdery	Soft, laminated
Anatomic location	Gallbladder or ducts	Bile ducts
Geographic distribution	Europe, USA, and Asia	Mostly Asia
Disease association	Hemolysis, cirrhosis	Cholangitis, parasites
Bile culture	Usually sterile	Infected with *Escherichia coli*
Etiology	Increased excretion and hydrolysis of conjugated bilirubin to unconjugated bilirubin	Bacterial hydrolysis of conjugated to unconjugated bilirubin

The second factor in the formation of cholesterol gallstones is the gallbladder itself. Normally, contraction of the gallbladder may prevent cholelithiasis by expelling supersaturated bile and crystals. If hypomotility is present, however, the resulting stasis promotes the precipitation of crystals (i.e., nucleation). In addition, excessive secretion of mucin by the gallbladder acts to entrap crystals, thus promoting lithogenesis. This composite of cholesterol monohydrate crystals and calcium bilirubinate granules in thickened mucin is known as biliary sludge. Conditions associated with biliary sludge attributed to gallbladder hypomotility are pregnancy, prolonged total parenteral nutrition, rapid weight loss, and somatostatin analog (octreotide) therapy (see Table 59–1). In summary, the cumulative effects of cholesterol supersaturated bile in an aberrantly functioning gallbladder with excessive mucin production and stasis lead to the formation of cholesterol gallstones.

Pigment Gallstones

The pathogenesis of pigment gallstones depends on whether they are brown or black. Black pigment stones are associated with chronic hemolysis (e.g., cardiac valvular prosthesis) and cirrhosis. In these disorders, the secretion of bilirubin into the bile may increase tenfold. A complex of calcium and unconjugated bilirubin then forms, which leads to the formation of black pigment stones (Table 59–2).

Formation of brown pigment stones requires chronic anaerobic infection and hypomotility of the biliary system. Bacteria produce β-glucuronidase, which can cause deconjugation of bilirubin from glucuronide. The unconjugated bilirubin precipitates as calcium salts.

D_x Cholelithiasis

- Epigastric or right upper quadrant pain.
- More common in women, obese patients, and certain ethnic groups, e.g., Hispanics, Native Americans.

Brown pigment stones are commonly associated with parasitic infections of the biliary tree that are endemic to Asia (Table 59–2).

DIFFERENTIAL DIAGNOSIS

In the consideration of the cause of right upper quadrant or midepigastric pain, the discovery of gallstones does not preclude other causes of the patient's symptoms.

With migration of a gallstone into the common bile duct (choledocholithiasis), transient blockage of the ampulla may lead to acute cholangitis or biliary pancreatitis. Right upper quadrant pain, jaundice, and fever with chills (Charcot's triad) is the classic presentation for **acute cholangitis.** The presence of hypotension or confusion suggests sepsis and a worse outcome. Attributed to transient blockage of the pancreatic duct by a stone, **pancreatitis** may occur alone or be accompanied by cholangitis. A boring epigastric pain radiating to the back is usually present in pancreatitis. Biochemical and radiographic evaluations are usually required to confirm this diagnosis.

Peptic ulcer disease must be distinguished from biliary "colic." The pain associated with a duodenal ulcer often improves with eating and then becomes more severe approximately 1 hour postprandially. In addition, the nocturnal component of ulcer pain characteristically occurs between 2:00 and 3:00 AM, whereas biliary "colic" has been observed to awaken patients around midnight. Endoscopy or a barium study of the upper gastrointestinal tract may be necessary to distinguish between peptic ulcer disease and biliary "colic." **Renal colic** can present as right upper quadrant pain. However, the pain typically radiates toward the groin. A urinalysis will show red blood cells. **Colonic pain** may be distinguished from biliary pain by the paroxysmal cramping pattern associated with colonic distention. A barium enema should be performed if colicky pain is a predominant feature. Acute appendicitis due to a subhepatic appendix may present with right upper quadrant pain. A history of initial periumbilical pain moving to the right abdomen suggests possible appendiceal inflammation. Ultrasonography may help differentiate an inflammatory process of the gallbladder from appendicitis.

EVALUATION

History

Biliary "colic" is a persistent epigastric pain (*not* colicky) secondary to intermittent obstruction of the cystic duct, usually by a stone. A typical episode lasts several hours. Pain involving both the right upper quadrant and epigastrium that persists for more than 6 hours is consistent with acute cholecystitis. The epigastric pain is visceral, whereas the right upper quadrant pain is secondary to localized parietal irritation from the inflamed gallbladder. Right upper quadrant pain is not usually seen in biliary "colic" for this reason (i.e., absence of inflammation of the gallbladder).

The pain may also be referred to the right scapula. Nausea and vomiting may accompany the pain.

Physical Examination

Physical findings in biliary "colic" are usually limited to epigastric tenderness during an episode. With acute cholecystitis, right upper quadrant tenderness is often accompanied by low-grade fever. Murphy's sign is the sudden arrest of inspiration because of pain on palpation of the right upper quadrant.

In acute cholangitis, epigastric or right upper quadrant tenderness is present. Fever and icterus complete the classic Charcot's triad. In those patients who develop biliary pancreatitis in the setting of cholangitis, abdominal tenderness may be more severe and less localized.

Additional Evaluation
Laboratory Tests

In biliary "colic," all biochemical studies are usually normal. Leukocytosis with mild elevation of transaminases and bilirubin may be seen in acute cholecystitis. Acute cholangitis is marked by abnormally high bilirubin levels, usually 2–10 mg/dL depending on the degree and duration of obstruction. Alkaline phosphatase is elevated, usually twice normal, with transaminases ranging from normal to several times normal. Amylase and lipase are markedly elevated when concomitant biliary pancreatitis is present.

Imaging Studies

Plain films of the abdomen should be obtained in the evaluation of right upper quadrant pain. Although less than 20% of gallstones are radiopaque, plain films are helpful to exclude other causes of pain (e.g., bowel obstruction). The unusual finding of a calcified gallbladder wall (porcelain gallbladder) is an indication for cholecystectomy owing to the associated risk for gallbladder carcinoma.

Ultrasonography is the procedure of choice for evaluation of cholelithiasis. Gallstones are detectable beginning at a size of 1–2 mm. A thickened gallbladder wall and pericholecystic fluid are the characteristic findings in acute cholecystitis. Biliary sludge associated with acalculous cholecystis is seen as echogenic material, layering in the gallbladder. Dilatation of the common bile duct suggests possible obstruction, yet common duct stones may not be reliably seen (less than 40%) with ultrasound. CT scanning adds little to the evaluation of suspected gallstones.

Hepatobiliary scintigraphy, a nuclear study of the biliary system, may also be used in the diagnosis of acute cholecystitis and common bile duct obstruction. The radionucleotide, a technetium-labeled iminodiacetic acid derivative, is used to provide images of the common bile duct, gallbladder, and drainage into the small bowel, normally within 30 to 45 minutes. Nonvisualization of the gallbladder at 90 minutes is consistent with acute cholecystitis. Prolonged fasting (e.g., critically ill patients on parenteral nutrition) and nonfasting states can cause false-positive results.

The use of oral cholecystography (OCG) has greatly diminished since the emergence of ultrasonography and hepatobiliary scintigraphy. In rare cases in which oral gallstone dissolution is being considered, OCG can provide necessary information regarding patency of the cystic duct, stone size, and stone composition.

Endoscopic retrograde cholangiopancreatography (ERCP) is indicated in the evaluation and management of possible choledocholithiasis.

MANAGEMENT

Asymptomatic cholelithiasis generally requires no treatment.

Annually, approximately 1% to 2% of individuals with asymptomatic gallstones develop biliary symptoms. Prophylactic cholecystectomy should be performed if a "porcelain" (calcified) gallbladder, gallbladder polyp > 1 cm, or single gallstone > 3 cm is found because of the increased risk of gallbladder carcinoma in these situations.

For recurrent biliary "colic" or acute cholangitis, cholecystectomy is the "gold standard" of therapy. Because it is associated with decreased pain and a decreased postoperative recovery period, laparoscopic cholecystectomy (versus open cholecystectomy) is the most commonly employed technique. However, the risk of common bile duct injury is increased in laparoscopic cholecystectomy and may be related to the surgeon's experience and training. In those patients at markedly increased risk for surgery, medical therapy should be considered.

Dissolution of gallstones by both biochemical and mechanical methods is available. Oral dissolution therapy involves the use of ursodiol, a bile acid that has no significant adverse effects except occasional diarrhea. However, the gallstones must be cholesterol stones less than 1 cm in diameter and the gallbladder must be functioning for optimal results. After 6 months of therapy, 60% of patients will have achieved dissolution. Unfortunately, one half will have recurrent gallstones within 5 years.

Extracorporeal shock wave lithotripsy (ESWL) involves external application of sonic "shock waves" to the right upper quadrant overlying the gallbladder. It has limitations similar to those of oral dissolution therapy with regard to the selection criteria and high rate of recurrence of cholelithiasis. In addition, access to ESWL units is limited in the United States.

In the management of common bile duct stones and the resulting complication of cholangitis, ERCP has become important because it reduces the necessity of surgical common bile duct exploration and decreases the morbidity and mortality associated with acute cholangitis. When common bile duct stones are present, a sphincterotomy (cutting the papilla endoscopically) is performed to allow clearance of the obstructed duct. Decompression of the common bile duct results in resolution of the acute cholangitis episode. Laparoscopic cholecystectomy may then be performed in a nonemergent setting.

NATURAL HISTORY/PROGNOSIS

Up to 90% of complications related to cholelithiasis (including cholangitis and pancreatitis) are preceded by biliary "colic." The mortality associated with open cholecystectomy for symptomatic gallstones is low (0.05%) except in the high-risk patient. Perforation and gangrene of the gallbladder may occur in up to 10% of cases of acute cholecystitis. Fortunately, the majority of perforations are localized and are sealed by adjacent viscera and omentum. In free perforation, mortality is marked (30%).

Research Questions

1. Can a pharmacologic method be developed that can relax the sphincter of Oddi and thus allow drainage of biliary sludge obstructing the common bile duct?
2. Can the liver be pharmacologically induced to increase phospholipid biliary secretion and thereby dissolve gallstones?

Case Resolution

With clinical findings of fever, jaundice, and right upper quadrant pain (consistent with Charcot's triad), the patient was presumed to have acute cholangitis. Right upper quadrant ultrasound demonstrated multiple gallstones with a dilated common bile duct. The patient was hospitalized, placed on appropriate antibiotic coverage, and emergent ERCP was performed, with the cholangiogram demonstrating choledocholithiasis. Sphincterotomy was performed, with clearance of the common bile duct. Within 24 hours, all symptoms had resolved. The patient underwent elective laparoscopic cholecystectomy and was discharged on the third day of hospitalization.

Selected Readings

Carey, M. C. Pathogenesis of gallstones. Am J Surg 165:410–9, 1993.

Fai, E. C. S., et al. Endoscopic biliary drainage for severe acute cholangitis. N Engl J Med 326:1582–6, 1992.

Johnston, D. E., and M. M. Kaplan. Pathogenesis and treatment of gallstones. N Engl J Med 328:412–21, 1993.

Lee, S. P., and J. F. Nicholls. Nature and composition of biliary sludge. Gastroenterology 90:677–86, 1986.

NIH Consensus Conference. Gallstones and laparoscopic cholecystectomy. JAMA 269:1018–24, 1993.

Ostrow, J. D. The etiology of pigment gallstones. Hepatology 4:215–25, 1984.

CHAPTER 60

HEMORRHOIDS AND OTHER COMMON ANORECTAL DISORDERS

Elaine Marcus, M.D.

H$_x$ A 43-year-old female administrative assistant comes to the family health center complaining of a recent episode of rectal pain and bleeding with defecation. The blood was bright red and was present both on the wiping paper and in the bowl but was not mixed with the stool. The rectal pain was most severe with the passage of stool but sometimes persisted for hours after defecation. The bleeding occurred last week for 3–4 days and has now stopped. The pain has lessened but is still present with bowel movements. She gives a history of a similar but more severe episode of rectal pain and bleeding 1 year ago, which responded to dietary changes and sitz baths. A dietary inventory reveals the intake of a high-fat, low-fiber diet. The patient states that she has bowel movements every 2–3 days and that her stools are often hard and dry, requiring her to strain. The patient is moderately obese and appears comfortable. The physical examination is unremarkable except for the rectal examination, which reveals external skin tags at the anal verge. These are neither inflamed nor tender. A digital examination finds no masses, but there is moderate tenderness at the midline inferiorly. Stool in the vault is firm, brown, and negative for occult blood. Anoscopy reveals a healing fissure in the area of tenderness, with a fibrinous exudate at the base, but no bleeding or swelling. No internal hemorrhoids are noted.

Questions

1. What are possible causes of rectal pain and bleeding?
2. Of what relevance to this case is the history of constipation and hard stools?
3. What tests, if any, would you recommend?

CLINICAL PRESENTATION

Anorectal disorders are frequently responsible for a degree of patient discomfort far out of proportion to the severity of pathology present. Though these conditions are almost never life-threatening, they prompt a large number of visits to primary care doctors each year.

Common presenting complaints are rectal pain, bleeding, and itching.

PATHOPHYSIOLOGY

The anorectal canal represents the region of transition from gut to skin. On the mucosal surface, the pectinate line is the junction of columnar and cuboidal epithelium. Surrounding the epithelial components lie the hemorrhoidal "cushions." These are composed of the superior and inferior hemorrhoidal plexuses (which communicate with each other and contain a large number of arteriovenous connections) along with connective and elastic tissue. All these elements are encased in a double sleeve of muscle formed by the internal and external sphincter along with the levator ani (Fig. 60–1).

Hemorrhoids are categorized as either **internal** (occurring above the pectinate line) or **external** (occurring below it). Internal hemorrhoids can be further subdivided into first, second, third, and fourth degree, depending on the degree of prolapse and reducibility (Table 60–1). Since the rectal mucosa contains no pain fibers, internal hemorrhoids are painless unless they are severely prolapsed and have become ulcerated or infected. External hemorrhoids, however, are covered with sensitive anoderm (an extension of skin) and become exquisitely painful when thrombosis occurs. The thrombosed external hemorrhoids usually arise from the rupture of small hemorrhoidal veins with resultant hematoma formation and swelling. They are typically bluish in color, swollen, and tender.

It is currently felt that hemorrhoidal disease represents the swelling of the submucosal cushions in response to chronic increased intraabdominal pressure (due to constipation, straining at stool, pregnancy, or continuous heavy lifting). This swollen tissue then gets forced downward and becomes engorged. As the support structures are increasingly stretched, prolapse ensues.

Anal fissures are small tears in the mucosal surface of the anal canal, usually at the midline posteriorly. The pathophysiology of anal fissures is poorly understood, but they seem to be more common in persons with severe constipation or diarrhea. Fissures also occur in patients with Crohn's disease and heal poorly in these patients. Anal fissures are extremely painful and are frequently associated with rectal bleeding. Infection and abscess formation also occur. The pain is most intense with bowel movements and may persist for hours. Although most fissures heal spontaneously with conservative treatment, some do not. These lesions result in the development of hypertrophic skin at the base of the fissure, seen on external examination as a "sentinel pile."

Most **perirectal abscesses** result from infections of the anal crypt glands, with secondary infection of the

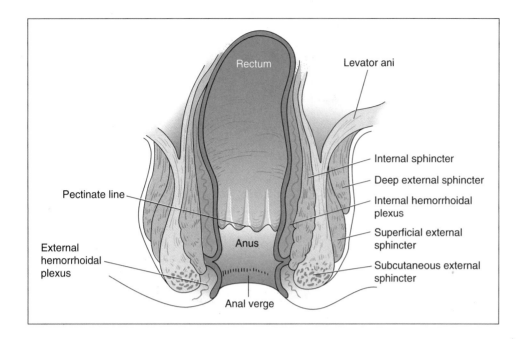

FIGURE 60–1. *Anatomy of the anus. (Reproduced, with permission, from D. A. Lieberman. Common anorectal disorders. Ann Intern Med 101:837–46, 1984.)*

intersphincteric space. The majority of these abscesses, if not treated, will result in rectal fistulas. **Rectal fistulas** are tracts from the mucosal surface of the anorectal canal to the skin surface in the perirectal area. These fistulas may also open into the vagina, the bladder, or other segments of the gastrointestinal tract. Their formation is frequently the result of a perirectal abscess, but fistulas may develop insidiously or as a manifestation of Crohn's disease. In the latter case, the tracts are usually complex, have more than one opening, and are extremely difficult to eradicate. The symptoms of a fistula include persistent or recurrent drainage or abscess in the perirectal area.

Infections of the anorectum (**proctitis**) result in rectal pain and tenesmus, with mucopurulent material visible on mucosal examination. Proctitis may result from inflammatory bowel disease or may have an infectious etiology. Infectious agents are frequently, but not always, sexually transmitted via unprotected anal intercourse (Table 60–2). Infections are especially aggressive and debilitating in patients infected with the human immunodeficiency virus (HIV).

Perirectal itching, or **pruritus ani,** is commonly associated with both too much and too little perianal hygiene. It may also be due to pinworm infestation or to other anorectal disorders associated with chronic mucus or stool seepage.

Neoplastic disease of the colon, most notably adenocarcinoma, may arise in the rectum, where it may present as rectal bleeding, a change in stool habits or stool caliber, weight loss, or intestinal obstruction. Squamous cell carcinoma is also encountered in the anorectum, most commonly in patients infected with HIV. This malignancy appears to be related to the transmission of oncogenic types of human papillomavirus via unprotected anal intercourse.

DIFFERENTIAL DIAGNOSIS

Most often a complete history and physical examination will serve to differentiate the various types of anorectal lesions. Patients will frequently complain of "hemorrhoids" when any one of a number of painful or bleeding rectal lesions is present. Systemic diseases (e.g., inflammatory bowel disease) can present first in the anorectum. Disease higher in the gastrointestinal tract, such as a peptic ulcer or colonic polyp, carcinoma, angiodysplasia, or diverticular disease may present with rectal bleeding.

TABLE 60–2. Causes of Proctitis

Infectious
Neisseria gonorrhoeae
Chlamydia trachomatis
Herpes simplex, types I and II
Cytomegalovirus (in patients with HIV)
Treponema pallidum
Lymphogranuloma venereum
Granuloma inguinale
Human papillomavirus (HPV)
Shigella
Campylobacter
Amebiasis
Noninfectious
Crohn's disease
Ulcerative colitis
Chemical irritation
Stool seepage
Poor hygiene

TABLE 60–1. Classification of Internal Hemorrhoids

Degree of Severity	Degree of Prolapse
First degree	Into anorectal canal but not through anus
Second degree	Through anus with defecation, reduces spontaneously
Third degree	Through anus, requires manual reduction
Fourth degree	Through anus, cannot be reduced

Anal Fissure

- Rectal bleeding and pain with defecation.
- Localized tenderness on digital rectal examination.
- Visible fissure in mucus membrane on anoscopy.

EVALUATION

History

Important historical information includes a description of bowel habits, concentrating on episodes of diarrhea, constipation, and straining at stool. A thorough sexual history should be taken, including questions about receptive anal intercourse or the insertion of foreign objects into the rectum. The severity and timing of pain and bleeding should be determined. The presence of swelling, drainage, and itching should be ascertained. Anal hygiene habits should be explored, along with a history of use of over-the-counter preparations for relief of symptoms. Previous similar episodes should be documented.

Physical Examination

The focused examination should begin with the patient lying on one side, with the knees drawn up to the chest. Alternatively, the male patient may stand and lean forward from the waist over an examining table. The perirectal skin is inspected for the presence of skin tags, sentinel piles, prolapsed internal hemorrhoids, induration, redness, abscess formation, rectal prolapse, excoriation, or bleeding. A gloved finger is inserted into the rectum to check for areas of tenderness, masses, and the presence of blood (either visible or occult).

Anoscopy should also be performed. This will reveal anal fissures, proctitis, rectal venereal warts, and internal hemorrhoids.

Since hemorrhoids are common, finding one does not guarantee that the source of rectal bleeding has been found. Colonoscopy (or a combination of flexible sigmoidoscopy and air-contrast barium enema) should be performed to rule out colorectal cancer or polyps, especially in patients over the age of 50 years.

Additional Evaluation

In the presence of large amounts of rectal bleeding, the hematocrit should be determined. Any stool in the vault and adherent to the glove on the examining finger should be tested for occult blood. In the case of proctitis suspected to be infectious, appropriate studies for bacterial, protozoan, and viral pathogens should be performed.

MANAGEMENT

Most patients with hemorrhoidal disease can be managed conservatively. Frequent sitz baths help alle-

viate pain and swelling. Attention should be given to measures that prevent straining during defecation such as using stool softeners and increasing the intake of dietary fiber.

Acutely thrombosed hemorrhoids can be evacuated through a small incision, affording relief of pain but resulting in several days of bloody drainage. Less painful thrombosed external hemorrhoids usually resolve over several days, leaving residual skin tags at the anal verge. Internal hemorrhoids that bleed chronically can be ligated or sclerosed by direct injection. Rubber band ligation is an office procedure. Since the rectal mucosa lacks pain fibers, the procedure is usually painless. Bacterial sepsis has been a rare complication, however. In the case of large, permanently prolapsed internal hemorrhoids, surgical excision may be required. This is an inpatient procedure with a prolonged recuperation period. Laser surgery can shorten the time to recovery.

Treatment of anal fissures is also directed at regulating bowel movements. Sitz baths and mild analgesics may be helpful during an acute episode. Surgical excision of fissures is rarely indicated and is frequently followed by recurrence.

A perirectal abscess requires surgical incision and drainage. In the case of deep abscesses extending into the ischiorectal space, general anesthesia is necessary. The majority of abscesses heal well. Recurrence, fistula formation, and cellulitis are the most common complications. Rectal fistulas with recurrent infection require surgical excision.

Treatment of infectious proctitis depends on the infectious agent. Proctitis as a manifestation of inflammatory bowel disease can be treated with topical corticosteroids in the form of enemas, foams, or suppositories. Topical 5-ASA in the form of enemas or suppositories is also useful in the treatment of ulcerative proctitis (see Chapter 53).

Pruritus ani is appropriately addressed by changes in anal hygiene. Keeping the area clean and dry, using gentle cleansing with water only, should be sufficient. Potentially sensitizing topical agents should be avoided. Pinworms may be treated with a single dose of mebendazole.

PATIENT AND FAMILY EDUCATION

Patient education is crucial to the successful treatment of most anorectal disorders. Regular bowel habits, promoted by a diet containing sufficient fiber and fluid, and regular physical activity are most important in preventing these disorders. The use of a latex condom during anal intercourse will prevent the spread of infectious agents (including HIV) via this route. The use of over-the-counter topical preparations should be discouraged, since many contain potentially sensitizing substances.

NATURAL HISTORY/PROGNOSIS

While symptoms of anorectal disorders can be annoying (or even alarming), they are usually due to self-limited conditions. Abnormalities of sphincter tone predispose some patients to these conditions, and aggravating factors (such as constipation, obesity, or other causes of increased intraabdominal pressure) should be avoided. Since patients may be reticent to discuss these potentially embarrassing problems, physicians should routinely include questions about bowel habits and anorectal symptoms in the review of systems.

Research Questions

1. What is the optimal workup (fiberoptic visualization with or without radiologic imaging studies) for patients with bright red rectal bleeding?
2. Why do some patients with mild constipation develop serious hemorrhoidal disease, while others with more severe constipation do not?

Case Resolution

The patient was advised to increase her dietary intake of fiber by making better food choices and using psyllium powder. She also was given docusate sodium as a stool softener. These measures, along with daily sitz baths, led to complete resolution of the patient's bleeding and discomfort in a week's time.

Selected Readings

Bassford, T. Treatment of common anorectal disorders. Am Fam Physician 45(4):1787–94, 1992.

Cocchiara, J. L. Hemorrhoids: A practical approach to an aggravating problem. Postgrad Med 89(1):149–52, 1991.

Hancock, B. D. Anal fissures and fistulas. Br Med J 304:904–7, 1992.

Jones, I. T., and V. W. Fazio. Anorectal diseases commonly encountered in clinical practice. *In* J. B. Kirschner and R. G. Shorter (eds.). *Diseases of the Colon, Rectum and Anal Canal.* Baltimore, Williams & Wilkins, 1988.

Lieberman D. A. Common anorectal disorders. Ann Intern Med 101:837–46, 1984.

McQuaid, K. R. Alimentary tract. *In* S. A. Schroeder, L. M. Tierney, Jr., et al. (eds.). *Current Medical Diagnosis and Treatment 1995.* Norwalk, Connecticut, Appleton & Lange, 1995.

Rex, D. K., R. A. Weddle, et al. Flexible sigmoidoscopy plus air contrast barium enema versus colonoscopy for suspected lower gastrointestinal bleeding. Gastroenterology 88:855–61, 1990.

Thomson, W. The nature of hemorrhoids. Br J Surg 67:542–52, 1975.

Vellacott, K. D., S. S. Amar, and J. D. Hardcastle. Comparison of rigid and flexible fiberoptic sigmoidoscopy with double contrast barium enema. Br J Surg 69:399–400, 1982.

COMMON GENITOURINARY PROBLEMS

CHAPTER 61

DYSURIA AND URINARY TRACT INFECTIONS

Lucy Fox, M.D.

H$_x$ A 28-year-old female paralegal reports a 2-day history of dysuria, urgency, and urinary frequency. She passes only scant amounts of strong-smelling urine, which is dark and occasionally blood-tinged. There is mild aching in the lower back but no fever, chills, diarrhea, nausea, vomiting, or vaginal discharge. She is sexually active with one steady partner and uses a diaphragm and spermicidal jelly. Her last menstrual period began 8 days ago and was normal. She denies a history of urinary tract infections (UTIs) but was given antibiotics for vaginitis at an urgent care clinic 2 years ago.

Questions

1. What diagnoses are you considering?
2. Would your perspective differ if this problem was recurrent?
3. If this patient were pregnant, how would you approach her diagnosis and management?

Dysuria, a complaint frequently addressed by the primary care physician, usually signifies a UTI. About 96% of UTIs occur in females, and the average woman has a 20% chance of developing an infection at least once in her lifetime. Most patient visits for UTIs are for uncomplicated cystitis, limited to the lower urinary tract and without signs of systemic illness. However, the primary care physician will also encounter challenging patients with complicated and recalcitrant infections.

PATHOPHYSIOLOGY

Most UTIs develop in an "ascending" fashion. Fecal organisms migrate to the perineum and vaginal mucosa and from there travel via the urethra into the bladder. In some cases, the infection ascends through the ureters to the collecting system. It is unusual for the urinary tract to be infected hematogenously, but this pattern does occur. Under normal conditions, nearly all organisms entering the urinary bladder are washed out with the next void. Those remaining must be adherent in order to be pathogenic.

Numerous virulence factors promoting infection have been identified. These can originate in either the organism or the host. Organism-derived factors (Table 61–1) are highlighted below. **Nonspecific adherence** involves hydrostatic and/or electrostatic interactions. **Specific adherence** is mediated by adhesins, also known as pili or fimbriae, which bind to receptors on epithelial cells or in epithelial mucus. Cell surface or capsular antigens, also known as K antigens, appear to enhance the resistance of *Escherichia coli* to phagocytosis. Their density is significantly greater on the surface of pyelonephritogenic strains. Certain somatic or O antigenic lipopolysaccharides (also known as endotoxins) are significant in *E. coli* infections and are believed to facilitate the inflammatory response, diminish ureteric peristalsis, and augment granulocyte activity. Resistance to serum-dependent bacteriolysis, mediated by both the classical and alternative complement pathways, is especially important in invasive infections and urosepsis. The association between hemolysin production and virulence in *E. coli* is well recognized.

Host factors (see Table 61–1) predisposing to infection may be systemic or local. Systemic factors include conditions such as malnutrition, diabetes mellitus, and

---

TABLE 61–1.   Organism- and Host-Related Factors in UTI

Organism-Derived Virulence Factors
Adherence (nonspecific or specific)
Cell surface antigens
Endotoxins
Serum resistance
Hemolysin

Host-Derived Defenses
Physical
   Flushing effect of micturition
   Cell exfoliation
Urinary
   Oligosaccharides
   Immunoglobulins (e.g., secretory IgA)
   Tamm-Horsfall proteins
Mucosal mucopolysaccharides (glycosaminoglycans)
Steric hindrance and bacterial interference
Phagocytosis (especially in upper tract infection)

TABLE 61–2.   Differential Diagnosis of Dysuria

Urinary Tract
Cystitis
  Infectious
  Interstitial/inflammatory
Pyelonephritis
Urethritis/obstruction
Prostatitis
Female Genital Tract
Vulvovaginitis
Cervicitis
Salpingitis (pelvic inflammatory disease, or PID)

immunodeficient states. Potential local factors are numerous; the most common include urinary stasis (pathologic or, in the case of pregnancy, physiologic), calculi, and the presence of catheters, stents, and other foreign bodies. Recent sexual intercourse increases the likelihood of developing a UTI. Oral contraceptive users are predisposed to UTIs because they tend to be sexually active. Women using diaphragms for contraception are at increased risk for UTIs owing to properties of the spermicidal agents used concomitantly.

DIFFERENTIAL DIAGNOSIS

A UTI generally is the cause of dysuria. However, dysuria (a symptom and not itself a disease) can signify the presence of numerous other conditions both within and extrinsic to the urinary tract (Table 61–2).

EVALUATION

History

The clinician should ask about general or nonspecific symptoms such as back and abdominal pain, fever, chills, rigors, nausea, vomiting, and diarrhea, all of which may accompany a UTI, especially pyelonephritis. The quality, intensity, and radiation of pain may suggest the presence of a stone. Direct questions regarding urinary patterns (frequency, urgency, nocturia, incontinence, quantity), the color and odor of the urine, the presence of obvious blood, and the passage of stones or gravel usually yield useful information. A sexual history in females is essential. How often is the patient having sexual intercourse? Does she habitually urinate following intercourse? What method of contraception is used? Has she recently begun using a diaphragm and spermicide? When was the last menstrual period?

A history of stones, UTI, prostatic hyperplasia, immunosuppression, and systemic diseases such as diabetes mellitus should be obtained. Recent urinary tract instrumentation, including indwelling or intermittent catheterization, is always significant.

Physical Examination

Although often unremarkable in uncomplicated lower tract infections, the physical examination should not be neglected. The presence of fever, hypotension, tachycardia, or tachypnea may signify a serious infection. The examination should focus on eliciting percussion tenderness over the costovertebral angles, suprapubic tenderness with palpation, bladder distention, and abdominal masses. Men should have a prostate examination. If a woman complains of vaginal discharge or has a history of pelvic inflammatory disease, a pelvic examination should be performed.

Additional Evaluation

The urinalysis, properly performed, is the single most important test. The patient should be instructed, and assisted if necessary, in the careful collection of a "clean-catch midstream" urine specimen. For a clean catch, retraction of the foreskin by uncircumcised males should be sufficient to prevent contamination by skin epithelium and periurethral bacteria. In females, the introitus must be cleansed thoroughly with water- or saline-soaked swabs. Antiseptic solutions should be avoided owing to their potential effect on culture results. The labia are held apart while the patient voids. Collection of a "midstream" specimen allows any urethral contaminants to be washed out initially. Catheterization is rarely justified, since the risk of infection is not insignificant. If it must be performed, strict aseptic technique should be employed.

The complete urinalysis includes both dipstick and microscopic examinations. A positive dipstick nitrite test, based on the conversion of nitrate to nitrite in the bladder, is an especially reliable marker for coliform infection. The dipstick leukocyte esterase (LCE) test is easy to perform and often serves as the basis for diagnosing UTIs. However, pyuria caused by nonbacterial inflammatory conditions may yield a falsely positive result. Although in many cases the microscopic examination does not add significantly to dipstick findings, it is a test worth performing in all cases of dysuria. Some clinicians prefer to centrifuge the urine, discard the supernatant, and then resuspend the sediment; others prefer to examine the unspun urine. In the latter case, the finding of either one organism per high power field or 10 leukocytes/mm^3 on a hemocytometer correlates strongly with infection. Whenever possible, the treating clinician should examine the freshly voided urine. This practice allows the diagnosis of UTI to be established immediately, often considerably before the laboratory urinalysis report becomes available.

Formerly, it was taught that $> 10^5$ colony-forming units (CFU) of bacteria per milliliter of voided urine constituted significant bacteriuria. However, the diagnostic criteria for UTIs (Table 61–3) have been liberalized.

Which patients require a urine culture? It is probably simpler to say that a healthy female who is neither diabetic nor pregnant, presenting with what appears to

TABLE 61–3.   Diagnostic Criteria for Bacteriuria

$> 10^2$ CFU/mm^3 (coliforms) or $> 10^5$ CFU/mm^3 (noncoliforms) in a symptomatic female
$> 10^3$ CFU/mm^3 in a symptomatic male
$> 10^5$ CFU/mm^3 on two occasions in asymptomatic individuals
$> 10^2$ CFU/mm^3 in a catheterized patient
Any growth on suprapubic catheterization in a symptomatic patient

be an uncomplicated first lower tract infection, can be managed without a culture. All others should have their urine cultured, but the results are not necessary to begin appropriate antimicrobial therapy.

Radiographic studies are not needed when the infection appears uncomplicated. When a stone is suspected, a plain abdominal film should be followed by an intravenous pyelogram (IVP) and, in some cases, tomograms. Although ultrasound can often demonstrate calculi, its sensitivity is lower than that of the IVU, and its delineation of urinary tract anatomy is less precise. However, in the presence of renal insufficiency or an allergy to iodinated contrast agents, ultrasound is clearly preferred.

Additional laboratory tests, such as a peripheral blood leukocyte count with differential, blood urea nitrogen, and serum creatinine, are usually obtained only when a complicated or systemic infection is suspected.

MANAGEMENT

Uncomplicated cases can be approached in several ways. Single-dose therapy has certain advantages (excellent compliance, lower cost, less chance of allergic reaction) and cures most cases of acute uncomplicated cystitis in healthy females. However, the frequency of relapse is higher with single-dose therapy (e.g, trimethoprim [TMP], trimethoprim-sulfamethoxazole [TMP-SMX], and nitrofurantoin) than with a 3-day regimen (e.g., TMP, TMP-SMX, nitrofurantoin, ciprofloxacin, and norfloxacin). Ampicillin and amoxicillin are associated with lower cure rates, regardless of the duration of therapy, probably owing to the high prevalence of resistant organisms. Oral cephalosporins are similarly not first-choice drugs, since they are associated with a high relapse rate and are relatively expensive. Recurrent infections should be treated with antibiotics for at least 7 days.

Selected individuals with acute pyelonephritis may be treated as outpatients, provided that there is no evidence of immunocompromise, the urinary tract anatomy is normal, associated systemic symptoms are absent, and intravenous rehydration is not indicated. Suggested regimens include 14 days of TMP-SMX, TMP, or ciprofloxacin. Some clinicians give an initial dose of IM or IV aminoglycoside or third-generation cephalosporin. Inpatients should be given parenteral antibiotics (TMP-SMX, a third-generation cephalosporin, or an aminoglycoside are reasonable initial choices) until they are afebrile/asymptomatic, at which time an oral agent can be chosen using culture and sensitivity data. A repeat urine culture should be obtained 2 weeks following completion of therapy.

Asymptomatic bacteriuria may actually be more prevalent than symptomatic infection, and the natural history of this condition as well as its appropriate management have been extensively investigated. In general, a patient's age and overall condition, as well as the presence or absence of structural/functional urinary tract abnormalities, should dictate the clinician's approach. The prevalence of asymptomatic bacteriuria in schoolgirls is 1%–2%, increasing by 1% with each decade thereafter. Some experts believe that children under 5

years of age or with abnormal urinary tract anatomy and/or function should receive antimicrobial therapy. In older children and healthy adults, treatment of asymptomatic bacteriuria does not appear to reduce morbidity, and in fact, the potential for adverse drug side effects and infection with resistant bacteria poses a greater problem.

Special Cases

Most UTIs are uncomplicated and can be managed in the ways outlined above, but certain special cases warrant mention.

Individuals with **diabetes mellitus** have a two- to fourfold increased incidence of UTI when compared with the general population. The immune response may be suboptimal, and diabetics with autonomic neuropathy may develop bladder dysfunction. Urine culture should be done in diabetic patients with dysuria. In some cases, the distinction between vulvovaginal candidiasis and fungal UTI is important. Perinephric abscess and emphysematous pyelonephritis should be sought using CT scanning or ultrasound when a diabetic patient appears seriously ill, particularly if appropriate drug therapy is ineffective.

In **pediatric patients**, up to 5% of girls and 1%–2% of boys will develop a UTI. Pathogens are similar to those infecting adults. Infants can present with nonspecific symptoms such as vomiting, diarrhea, and failure to thrive; up to 50% of these children have an abnormal urinary tract. Vesicoureteral reflux, neurogenic bladder, stones, and immune deficiency states must all be excluded. However, a voiding cystourethrogram should be deferred until the infection has fully resolved, since (1) the procedure itself can cause pyelonephritis and (2) transient reflux may occur during UTIs. Children under the age of 5 years are believed particularly vulnerable to renal scarring secondary to chronic reflux.

The **elderly** are prone to UTIs, both acute and chronic, because of urinary retention and catheterization. As males age, their risk increases as prostate disease develops. When elderly patients present with vague complaints such as lethargy and anorexia, the clinician must rule out UTI and particularly urosepsis. Treatment should continue for at least 10 days. Bacteriuria is prevalent in the elderly and often difficult to eradicate. Asymptomatic patients with colonized urinary tracts, while at risk for developing infection, do not benefit from expectant or prophylactic antibiotics.

During **pregnancy**, bacteriuria is detectable in 4%–10% of females. Left untreated, up to 60% will develop a UTI. Physiologic ureteral stasis and hydronephrosis place this group at risk for pyelonephritis, which increases perinatal mortality. Therefore, surveillance urinalyses must be performed frequently during pregnancy, and bacteriuria, even when asymptomatic, should be treated promptly.

PATIENT AND FAMILY EDUCATION

The need to finish an entire antibiotic prescription should be emphasized. Patients treated for pyelonephritis should be reminded to have their urine recultured 2 weeks after completing therapy. Those with recurrent infections need to recognize early warning signs; however, some diabetics with neuropathy can remain asymptomatic until urosepsis develops. High-risk diabetics with kidney transplants and recurrent UTIs should be taught to test their urine daily with LCE dipsticks. Sexually active females prone to UTI should avoid using the diaphragm for contraception and should urinate immediately after intercourse.

NATURAL HISTORY/PROGNOSIS

In healthy individuals with uncomplicated infections, the acute problem resolves rapidly and sequelae are extremely rare. Recurrences, while not uncommon, typically develop within 2 months of the initial infection and are confined to the lower tract. Women admitted to the hospital with acute pyelonephritis have a 23% recurrence rate at 6 months and 40% by 3 years, yet long-term renal damage is extremely unusual. The patient with frequently recurring infections, i.e., four or more in a year, may benefit from daily, thrice weekly, or postcoital prophylaxis using low-dose TMP-SMX, TMP, or nitrofurantoin. Patients using prophylaxis should be monitored at 3- to 4-month intervals for adverse drug reactions and breakthrough with resistant organisms.

Research Questions

1. How can the risk of symptomatic UTI be reduced in catheterized patients? (As the population ages, the use of indwelling catheters is likely to increase.)

2. Which bacteriuric individuals need further evaluation, and which invasive and radiologic tests are most useful and cost-effective?

Case Resolution

Urinalysis showed pyuria and bacteriuria. A 3-day course of TMP-SMX was prescribed, and the patient recovered rapidly and uneventfully.

Selected Readings

Johnson, J. R., and W. E. Stamm. Urinary tract infection in women: Diagnosis and treatment. Ann Intern Med 111:906–17, 1989.
Keys, T. F. Outpatient antibiotic therapy for urinary tract infections in women. Cleve Clin J Med 56:478–80, 1989.
Lipsky, B. A. Urinary tract infections in men: Epidemiology, pathophysiology, diagnosis, and treatment. Ann Intern Med 110:138–50, 1989.
Reid, G., and J. D. Sobel. Bacterial adherence in the pathogenesis of urinary tract infection: A review. Rev Infect Dis 9(3):470–87, 1987.
Stamm, W. E, and T. M. Hooton. Management of urinary tract infections in adults. N Engl J Med 329(18):1328–34, 1993.
Yoshikawa, T. T. Chronic urinary tract infections in elderly patients. Hosp Pract 65–76, June 15, 1993.
Zelikovic I. Urinary tract infections in children: An update. West J Med 157:554–61, 1992.

CHAPTER 62

HEMATURIA

Curtis O. Kapsner, M.D.

H$_x$ A 65-year-old male retired mail carrier presents to the urgent care clinic with a 1-day history of painless, gross hematuria. He has no history of diabetes mellitus, hypertension, or coronary artery disease. Physical examination showed a healthy-appearing man with a blood pressure of 145/78. Rectal examination revealed a symmetrically enlarged prostate without nodules. No other abnormalities were found. Renal function tests, liver function tests, clotting studies, and CBC were normal. Urinalysis showed 3+ blood and trace proteinuria on dipstick. Microscopic

examination revealed "too numerous to count" red blood cells (RBCs) per high-power field (hpf) without casts or other abnormalities. The red blood cells did not appear dysmorphic.

Questions

1. What are the most likely causes of hematuria in this setting?
2. What type of evaluation should be performed?

TABLE 62–1. Use of Dipstick and Microscopic Examinations in the Diagnosis of Hematuria

Positive Dipstick and Positive Microscopic Examination
Obvious diagnosis of hematuria
Positive Dipstick and Negative Microscopic Examination
1. Free hemoglobin in urine (from intravascular hemolysis or lysis of red cells in hypotonic urine)
2. Myoglobin in urine (from rhabdomyolysis)
Negative Dipstick and Positive Microscopic Examination
1. Objects mistaken for red cells (*Candida* spherules, calcium oxalate crystals, air bubbles, starch granules)
2. False-negative dipstick result caused by intake of large amounts of vitamin C

Normal persons can excrete up to 3 RBC/hpf on urinalysis. In menstruating women, red blood cells can enter the urine after it leaves the urethra, making determination of kidney or urinary tract disease difficult. This issue can be resolved by either repeating the urinalysis after the patient's menstrual period has ended or by obtaining the urine sample via bladder catheterization.

PATHOPHYSIOLOGY

The urine dipstick (an *ortho*-tolidine-impregnated paper strip) will give a positive (i.e., abnormal) result in the presence of 5 RBC/hpf on microscopic examination. The dipstick is not specific for red cells and will also turn positive in the presence of free hemoglobin or myoglobin. Usually the pattern is speckled in the presence of red cells and diffuse with free hemoglobin or myoglobin. Free hemoglobin can enter the urine in the presence of intravascular hemolysis, since some of the hemoglobin is filtered at the glomerulus. More commonly, red cells lyse in hypotonic urine after it is formed. Myoglobinuria occurs when rhabdomyolysis is present, and it can be screened for by measuring serum creatine phosphokinase (CPK) levels. Table 62–1 demonstrates the various combinations of dipstick and microscopic results possible. Often, a urinalysis that demonstrates hematuria shows additional abnormalities that suggest a cause of the hematuria. For example, the presence of hematuria with white blood cells and bacteria suggests

a urinary tract infection (UTI), while the presence of large amounts of protein suggests a glomerular etiology.

There are hundreds of potential causes of isolated hematuria; however, the major identifiable causes are relatively few and vary by age. In adults, the most common causes are prostate disease, nephrolithiasis, cancer (prostate, bladder, or kidney), and trauma. In children, glomerular disease, hypercalciuria, and perineal irritation or trauma are the most common etiologies.

DIFFERENTIAL DIAGNOSIS

Given the many causes of hematuria, it is useful to classify a particular patient as having glomerular hematuria; painless, gross hematuria in an older person; or flank pain with hematuria (Table 62–2).

The presence of three different laboratory abnormalities presenting concurrently with hematuria suggests a glomerular origin of the hematuria. (1) Nephrotic range proteinuria (> 3.5 g/24 h) is highly suggestive of glomerulonephritis. (2) The presence of red blood cell casts on urinalysis is indicative of glomerular disease. (3) Red cells that enter the urine via the glomerular capillary wall often are damaged and appear dysmorphic (with varying shapes, blebs, and buds), whereas red cells that enter the urine from other parts of the urinary tract tend to be normally shaped and uniform in size. This distinction is best appreciated using phase contrast microscopy but can be seen using standard light microscopy, especially if a supravital stain is employed.

Painless, gross hematuria in an older person is an ominous sign. Although some benign conditions (e.g., trauma, kidney stones) can cause gross hematuria, the most important consideration is malignancy. Prostate cancer, transitional cell cancer, and renal cell carcinoma are all more common in older age groups.

Flank pain with hematuria is commonly caused by the presence of a kidney stone in the upper collecting system of the involved kidney. However, there are a number of other causes. Trauma is usually suggested by the history. Pyelonephritis occasionally presents with hematuria being more predominant than pyuria. Adult

TABLE 62–2. Patient Classification by Presentation of Hematuria

	Glomerular Hematuria	Painless Gross Hematuria in an Older Person	Flank Pain with Hematuria
Etiology	1. Systemic diseases (SLE, SBE, Goodpasture's syndrome) 2. Primary renal diseases (PSGN, IgA nephropathy)	Renal cell, transitional cell, or prostate cancer	Kidney stone, trauma, pyelonephritis, PCKD, papillary necrosis (DM, sickle cell disease, analgesic nephropathy), renal infarction
Evaluation	1. Duration of hypertension or edema 2. Previous urinalyses and creatinine measurements 3. Physical examination—blood pressure, edema, rash, arthritis, pleural or pericardial rubs 4. Laboratory tests—BUN, creatinine, 24-hour urine collection for creatinine clearance and protein, ANA, ANCA, complement levels	1. Digital rectal examination 2. Platelet count, PT, PTT, PSA 3. IVP, ultrasound, or CT scan of abdomen 4. Cystoscopy	Depends on history; patients usually require an IVP

polycystic kidney disease (PCKD) can present with pain from bleeding into a cyst, with subsequent hematuria if the cyst ruptures into the collecting system. Papillary necrosis usually presents first with bleeding followed by pain if the necrosed papilla becomes lodged in the ureter, causing unilateral obstruction. Finally, acute renal infarction can cause immediate, severe pain and hematuria. Renal infarction has a variety of predisposing causes. Among them are acute thrombosis of the renal artery (which can occur in patients with atherosclerotic vascular disease who undergo angiographic or surgical manipulation of the renal artery or aorta) and embolism to the renal artery (which can occur in patients with cardiac disease such as arrhythmias or acute myocardial infarction).

EVALUATION

History

It is important to ask about symptoms of systemic diseases that can cause glomerulonephritis (GN), which often presents with edema and hypertension as well as hematuria. This group includes systemic lupus erythematosus (SLE) (skin rash, arthralgias, chest pain, neurologic symptoms); subacute bacterial endocarditis (SBE) (history of valvular abnormalities, dental or other procedures, IV drug abuse); and Goodpasture's syndrome (hemoptysis). The patient should be questioned about an antecedent upper respiratory tract infection. In poststreptococcal glomerulonephritis (PSGN), there is at least a 10-day latent period between the URI and renal involvement. IgA nephropathy is a more common cause of glomerular pathology and has a latent period of only a few days between the URI and renal involvement (which is often manifested as gross hematuria). To determine the duration of the renal involvement, it is useful to inquire about the duration of hypertension or edema and to review previous urinalyses or previous measurements of serum creatinine.

Physical Examination

It is important to measure the blood pressure and assess for the presence of edema. Skin rashes could be indicative of either SLE or IgA nephropathy. Serositis (suggestive of SLE) can manifest as joint effusions, pericardial rubs, or pleural rubs.

Additional Evaluation

Laboratory evaluation consists of BUN and serum creatinine measurements; a 24-hour urine collection for protein and creatinine clearance; and antinuclear antibody (ANA), antineutrophil cytoplasmic antibody (ANCA), and complement levels (low in SLE and PSGN). When the diagnosis is not apparent from this evaluation, a kidney biopsy may be required.

In an adult with painless, gross hematuria and a negative history and physical examination, a platelet count, partial thromboplastin time (PTT), and prothrombin time (PT) should be done to exclude a systemic bleeding disorder. Additionally, the patient requires tests to exclude renal cell, transitional cell, and prostate cancers. Renal cell carcinoma can be effectively excluded with an intravenous pyelogram, renal ultrasound, or CT scan of the abdomen. Transitional cell carcinoma can involve the renal pelvis, ureters, or bladder. Of the tests that exclude renal cell carcinoma, the only one that is sensitive for ureteral involvement is the intravenous pyelogram (IVP), so this is usually the preferred imaging procedure. In patients who are allergic to contrast media or who are at risk for contrast nephropathy, a retrograde ureterogram can be performed instead. Cystoscopic studies must be performed to exclude transitional cell involvement of the bladder. Finally, prostate cancer is excluded by the combination of digital rectal examination and prostate-specific antigen (PSA) measurement.

In patients presenting with flank pain, the cause is usually apparent from the history. Kidney stones, trauma, and pyelonephritis are usually obvious. Polycystic kidney disease is an autosomal dominant disorder and so the family history tends to be positive. Diabetes mellitus, analgesic nephropathy, and sickle cell disease are all risk factors for papillary necrosis. A history of arrhythmias or recent myocardial infarction suggests embolism and subsequent renal infarction. Other tests may be needed depending on the history; most of these patients ultimately require an IVP.

MANAGEMENT, PATIENT EDUCATION, AND PROGNOSIS

Except in cases of major trauma, hematuria rarely results in enough blood loss to be life-threatening. Thus, the initial approach to the patient consists of history taking, physical examination, and diagnostic evaluation aimed at determining the cause of the hematuria. Thereafter, management, patient education, and prognosis vary widely.

Research Question

1. What is the most reasonable (and cost-effective) approach to evaluating asymptomatic microscopic hematuria in the 40- to 50-year-old age group?

Case Resolution

Evaluation of this patient included an IVP, which showed a 2-cm by 3-cm mass. Subsequently, this mass was removed surgically, and pathologic examination indicated renal cell carcinoma. There was no evidence of metastasis.

Selected Readings

Rose, B. D. *Pathophysiology of Renal Disease,* 2nd ed., New York, McGraw-Hill Book Company, 1984, pp. 20, 53–56.
Sutton, J. M. Evaluation of hematuria in adults. JAMA 263:2475–80, 1990.

PROTEINURIA

Mark C. Saddler, M.D.

Hx A 46-year-old male pilot complains of ankle swelling that has lasted for the past 6 weeks. The man has had no shortness of breath but admits that his urine has been more "frothy" than usual lately. He has been taking ibuprofen daily for the last several years for recurrent lower back pain. Urinalysis shows 3+ protein, no blood, and occasional granular casts.

Questions

1. What are the possible causes of this patient's proteinuria?
2. What workup would be appropriate? Should a renal biopsy be performed?
3. What are possible complications of the proteinuria?

PATHOPHYSIOLOGY

The glomerulus normally provides a barrier to filtration of proteins as a result of both pore size and charge of the glomerular basement membrane. The presence of large amounts of protein in the urine, therefore, is usually a result of glomerular damage. Normal urinary protein excretion is less than 150 mg/d for an adult. Since the dipstick test for protein becomes positive at about 100 µg/mL, normal individuals may show "trace positive" tests for proteinuria. Excretion of more than 3.5 g/1.73 m^2/d is called "nephrotic range proteinuria" and, in the presence of edema and hypoproteinemia, defines the **nephrotic syndrome**. Individuals with nonglomerular forms of renal disease (e.g., interstitial nephritis, pyelonephritis, hypertension) frequently have a daily protein excretion of 150–1000 mg.

DIFFERENTIAL DIAGNOSIS

The causes of heavy proteinuria fall into two main groups: systemic diseases and primary glomerular diseases (Table 63–1). The latter are usually classified according to their histologic features. For example, "minimal change" disease is characterized by no visible changes on light microscopy and podocyte foot process fusion on electron microscopy; membranous nephropathy shows thickening of the glomerular and basement membrane; and proliferative glomerulonephritis features proliferation of cells within the glomerulus.

EVALUATION

Figure 63–1 shows a simple algorithm for the initial evaluation of a patient with proteinuria.

History

The aim of history taking is to determine the possible causes of the proteinuria and to assess the severity of the disease. Patients should be asked

TABLE 63–1. Causes of Proteinuria

Etiology	Comment
Systemic Diseases	
Diabetes	Most common cause of nephrotic syndrome in USA
Systemic lupus erythematosus	Several different pathologic types
Amyloidosis	
Infection	
Hepatitis B	Usually membranous pathology
Hepatitis C	Usually associated with cryoglobulinemia
Poststreptococcal	
Endocarditis	
HIV	Poor prognosis
Quartan malaria	
Syphilis	
Drugs	
NSAIDs	Proteinuria usually resolves when drug is stopped
Gold	
ᴅ-Penicillamine	
Multiple myeloma	
Neoplastic disease	
Lymphoma	Frequently minimal change pathology
Adenocarcinoma	Usually membranous pathology
Vasculitis, including Wegener's granulomatosis	Usually associated with upper or lower respiratory tract disease
Sickle cell disease	
Primary Glomerular Diseases	
Minimal change disease	Good prognosis, responds to glucocorticoids
Membranous nephropathy	Most frequent primary glomerular cause of nephrotic syndrome in USA
Membranoproliferative nephropathy	
Focal and segmental glomerulosclerosis	Poor prognosis, usually not responsive to treatment
Proliferative glomerulonephritis, including IgA nephropathy	IgA nephropathy more common in people with alcoholism and certain population groups (e.g., Japanese, Navajo), frequently presents with hematuria

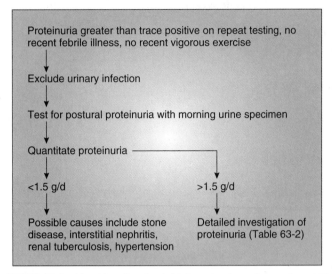

Proteinuria greater than trace positive on repeat testing, no recent febrile illness, no recent vigorous exercise

↓

Exclude urinary infection

↓

Test for postural proteinuria with morning urine specimen

↓

Quantitate proteinuria

<1.5 g/d   >1.5 g/d

↓   ↓

Possible causes include stone disease, interstitial nephritis, renal tuberculosis, hypertension

Detailed investigation of proteinuria (Table 63-2)

FIGURE 63–1. *Algorithm for the initial evaluation of a patient with proteinuria.*

whether ankle swelling or other evidence of volume overload has been present. A recent sore throat is suggestive of poststreptococcal glomerulonephritis. A complete drug history is important; nonsteroidal antiinflammatory drugs (NSAIDs), in particular, may give rise to a minimal change form of the nephrotic syndrome, which usually resolves on withdrawal of the drug. The family history also should be elicited because hereditary nephritis is a rare but important cause of the nephrotic syndrome and chronic renal failure. Where appropriate, the presence of risk factors for HIV should be determined. Any history of collagen vascular disease (especially systemic lupus erythematosus), diabetes, or myeloma is significant. Proteinuria is often a chronic condition, and the results of previous workups (especially previous renal biopsy) can help prevent duplication of expensive investigations.

Physical Examination

Evidence of edema or volume overload should be carefully sought. The optic fundi should be examined for evidence of diabetic retinopathy; pharyngeal inflammation and lymphadenopathy may suggest recent streptococcal infection. The presence of peripheral stigmata of endocarditis or lupus is also significant. Microscopic examination of the urine sediment helps distinguish proliferative glomerular lesions (which cause an "active" urine with numerous red cells and casts) from nonproliferative lesions (which cause an "inactive" urine, as in minimal change disease, membranous nephropathy, and sometimes focal segmental glomerulosclerosis).

Additional Evaluation

The urine should always be examined, and the presence of protein should be confirmed using the dipstick or sulfosalicylic acid (SSA) tests. The dipstick test, the most frequently used test for the detection of albumin in the urine, is simple, inexpensive, and quick.

However, it does not define the total *amount* of protein excreted. The urine protein *concentration* can be semiquantitatively determined using this test, from "1+" to "3+". It does not detect proteins other than albumin. In the SSA method, 2.5 mL of urine supernatant is mixed with 7.5 mL of 3% SSA. Turbidity indicates the presence of either albumin or any other protein. The most important situation in which nonalbumin proteinuria occurs is in multiple myeloma. Here immunoglobulin light chains (Bence Jones proteins) may spill into the urine, giving a positive result with SSA but a negative result with the dipstick.

Although the measurement of urine protein from a single specimen is valuable as a screening tool, protein excretion should also be measured quantitatively by a 24-hour urine collection. For the 24-hour urine collection, patients are instructed to empty the bladder at a specific time (usually in the morning on arising) and to discard this urine specimen. Every time they urinate subsequent to this for the next 24 hours, they collect the urine in a container. At the same time the next day, they again void, also into the container. The collection is then complete. In this way, they start and finish the test with an empty bladder. Alternatively, a urine protein/creatinine ratio can be performed on a single urine specimen. The protein (mg/dL) divided by the creatinine (mg/dL) normally is less than 0.2. Values greater than 3.5 are seen in the nephrotic syndrome.

Whenever urine is collected for evaluation of protein (or almost any other substance), the urine creatinine should also be measured. Since the excretion of creatinine is constant, measurement of urinary creatinine enables an assessment of the adequacy of the urine collection. Men usually excrete around 20–30 mg/kg and women 15–20 mg/kg of creatinine per day. If a urine collection contains only 5 mg/kg of creatinine for a given patient, urine collection is likely incomplete.

Before starting an extensive workup for proteinuria, exclusion of the syndrome of postural proteinuria may be worthwhile. In this disorder, which occurs in otherwise healthy asymptomatic individuals, urine collected after overnight recumbency does not demonstrate any protein. Patients should be instructed to collect a urine sample on first arising in the morning and then after 2 hours of ambulation. If protein is detectable only in the "ambulant" specimen, no further workup is required. The prognosis is excellent; patients with postural proteinuria do not develop any subsequent renal disease with any greater frequency than that seen in the general population. It is also worth noting that urinary protein occasionally increases during febrile illness.

The laboratory investigation of pathologic proteinuria depends on the clinical setting (Table 63–2). Not all these tests are required in all patients with proteinuria. If this workup gives no indication of the cause of the proteinuria, a renal biopsy should be considered. However, not all patients with proteinuria require a renal biopsy, and the decision whether to perform this procedure depends on the likelihood that a treatable disease will be found.

TABLE 63–2.   Laboratory Investigations in Proteinuria

Test	Test Significance
24-hour urine protein, urine protein/ creatinine ratio	Indicates the extent of proteinuria
Urine culture	Excludes the presence of urinary infection
Erythrocyte sedimentation rate (ESR)	Elevated in myeloma, vasculitis, infections, etc.
Hepatitis B surface antigen, Hepatitis C antibody	Hepatitis B and C may cause proteinuria
Complement C3, C4	Levels decreased in lupus, endocarditis, membranoproliferative nephritis, poststreptococcal glomerulonephritis
Cryoglobulins	Cryoglobulinemia may cause nephrotic syndrome
Sickle cell preparation	Sickle cell disease may cause nephrotic syndrome
Rapid plasma reagin (RPR)	Positive in syphilis and sometimes lupus
Antinuclear antibody (if positive, consider anti-DNA antibody, anti-Smith antibody)	Positive in lupus
Serum and urine protein electrophoresis	Monoclonal spike present in myeloma and light chain nephropathy
Rheumatoid factor	Usually positive in rheumatoid arthritis, sometimes positive in endocarditis
Antineutrophil cytoplasmic antibody	Positive in some vasculitides
Antistreptolysin O titer	Supports the diagnosis of poststreptococcal glomerulonephritis
HIV	May indicate HIV nephropathy

MANAGEMENT

The **edema** associated with the nephrotic syndrome, the most common symptom, may be the most difficult to treat. Diuretics are frequently required at some point. It must be remembered, however, that the intravascular volume in nephrotic patients is often decreased as a result of hypoalbuminemia, and diuretics should be administered with considerable care. Nephrotic patients are frequently resistant to the effects of diuretics. Edema of the bowel wall may be one causal factor; intravenous diuretic administration may circumvent this problem.

The resolution of **minimal change disease** can be speeded with glucocorticoid administration. The outcome of patients with **membranous disease** may be improved with combinations of glucocorticoids and alkylating agents (e.g., cyclophosphamide, chlorambucil). The management of patients with active **lupus nephritis** and the **vasculitides** includes similar agents. Because all these agents have significant toxicity, the risk/benefit ratio needs to be carefully weighed before use.

Efforts to reduce protein excretion involve administration of angiotensin-converting enzyme (ACE) inhibitors, which may reduce proteinuria by reducing intraglomerular pressure. NSAIDs may have the same effect but are less often used because of their other adverse renal effects. Although dietary protein restriction may also reduce proteinuria, this method is clearly not suitable for patients who are already protein malnourished as a result of their preceding urinary protein loss.

Early and aggressive treatment of infections, management of hypercholesterolemia, and treatment of thrombotic episodes are important in the care of patients with the nephrotic syndrome.

PATIENT AND FAMILY EDUCATION

Management of the edema that may accompany proteinuria requires careful avoidance of dietary sodium. Any sudden increase in edema, which could result from cellulitis, deep leg vein thrombosis, or renal vein thrombosis, should be reported to the physician immediately.

Patients should avoid taking NSAIDs if these agents might be the cause of the proteinuria. These drugs may also cause the glomerular filtration rate (GFR) to decrease.

Patients with diabetic nephropathy should be instructed that strict diabetic control is associated with a slower progression of diabetic kidney disease.

Hypercholesterolemia, which frequently occurs as a result of the nephrotic syndrome, requires dietary restriction of cholesterol and saturated fats.

NATURAL HISTORY/PROGNOSIS

The underlying disease causing the nephrotic syndrome may result in renal failure, which may require separate management (see Chapter 64). The proteinuria itself may also result in the following problems.

Hypercoagulability may be the major cause of mortality in patients with the nephrotic syndrome. Thromboses that occur in the deep leg veins and renal veins may result in thromboemboli to the pulmonary vasculature; arterial thromboses may also occur. Increased platelet activity and possible alterations in the fibrinolytic system are possible causes of this phenomenon.

Reduced resistance to infection may result from low IgG concentrations, loss of complement in the urine, and impaired lymphocyte function. Primary peritonitis and cellulitis are common although patients with the nephrotic syndrome have an increased risk of infection in any site. *Streptococcus pneumoniae* (pneumococcus) is a particular problem in nephrotic patients.

Hypercholesterolemia is seen in nephrotic patients, who have increased total and low-density lipoprotein (LDL) cholesterol levels compared with the normal population. In the most severe cases, triglycerides may be elevated and high-density lipoprotein (HDL) cholesterol reduced. Increased lipoprotein synthesis and decreased activity of lipoprotein lipase are possible causes. Whether nephrotic patients are at increased risk of adverse cardiovascular events as a result of this lipid profile remains controversial. The majority of clinicians treat nephrotic patients with hypercholesterolemia in the same way they treat nonnephrotic patients with hypercholesterolemia.

Research Questions

1. Does protein restriction slow the progression of the nephrotic syndrome and renal failure?
2. How common is renal vein thrombosis, and how does it contribute to renal dysfunction in patients with the nephrotic syndrome?
3. What is the best way to treat a primary glomerular disease such as membranous nephropathy?

Case Resolution

The patient's BUN and creatinine were normal. The ibuprofen was discontinued, and he was brought back 4 weeks later. The proteinuria had entirely resolved and did not recur. These findings support the diagnosis of an NSAID-induced minimal change nephrotic syndrome. Had the proteinuria not resolved, the patient should have had a serologic workup and possibly a renal biopsy.

Selected Readings

Bernard, D. B. Extrarenal complications of the nephrotic syndrome. Kidney Int 33:1184–1202, 1988.

Cameron, J. S. Clinical consequences of the nephrotic syndrome. In J. S. Cameron, A. M. Davison, J. P. Grunfeld, D. Kerr, and E. Ritz (eds.). Oxford Textbook of Clinical Nephrology. Oxford, Oxford University Press, 1992, pp. 276–98.

Fine, L. G. Preventing the progression of human renal disease: Have rational therapeutic principles emerged? Kidney Int 33:116–28, 1988.

Keane, W. F., and B. L. Kasiske. Hyperlipidemia in the nephrotic syndrome. N Engl J Med 323:603–44, 1990.

Lewis, E. J. Management of the nephrotic syndrome in adults. In J. S. Cameron and R. J. Glassock (eds.). The Nephrotic Syndrome. New York, Marcel Dekker, 1988, pp. 461–521.

C H A P T E R   6 4

CHRONIC RENAL FAILURE

Mark C. Saddler, M.D.

H$_x$ A 35-year-old male soil conservationist has had diabetes for 16 years and is known to have severe retinopathy. His blood urea nitrogen (BUN) and creatinine levels have been gradually climbing, although his glucose and blood pressure have been carefully controlled for the last 7 years. Seven years ago, his creatinine was 1.1 mg/dL; 2 years ago, it had climbed to 3.2 mg/dL; and 3 months ago, it was 5.2 mg/dL. The patient now complains of having had a poor appetite for 2 weeks. He had an episode of vomiting yesterday. His laboratory values are as follows: sodium 140 mEq/L, potassium 5.2 mEq/L, chloride 106 mEq/L, bicarbonate 19 mEq/L, BUN 58 mg/dL, creatinine 5.6 mg/dL, glucose 129 mg/dL, calcium 8.9 mg/dL, phosphate 5.8 mg/dL, hematocrit 26%.

Questions

1. Why did the patient's renal function deteriorate? Could anything have been done to try to minimize the progression of the renal disease?
2. What complications of chronic renal failure are evident from his laboratory values?
3. What is the appropriate management of his condition now? What renal replacement options are available to patients with end-stage renal disease?

Chronic renal failure is the clinical syndrome characterized by a progressive and usually irreversible decline in glomerular filtration rate (GFR). When this progresses to the point at which the patient requires renal replacement therapy (chronic dialysis or transplantation), the condition is called end-stage renal disease (ESRD). African Americans are at four times greater risk of developing chronic renal failure than are whites. It is also common in Native Americans. The most common causes of chronic renal failure in the United States are shown in Figure 64–1. Some of the less frequent causes include renal artery stenosis (which may be common but is less frequently diagnosed with certainty), infective pyelonephritis, systemic lupus erythematosus, myeloma, amyloidosis, and acute tubular necrosis (ATN) due to hypovolemia or toxins. ATN is a common cause of acute renal failure, but the majority of cases do not progress to a chronic phase.

PATHOPHYSIOLOGY

Once renal function is chronically impaired, the dysfunction ultimately progresses to ESRD even if the cause of the original renal insult is removed. For example, patients with glomerulonephritis may recover from the

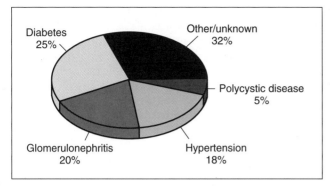

FIGURE 64–1. *Causes of chronic renal failure in the United States.*

initial disease with only a modest decrease in renal function, but renal failure is likely to progress. One possible reason is that when the number of functioning nephrons decreases, the remaining nephrons have an increased workload (i.e., filtration in each of the remaining nephrons [single-nephron GFR] is increased). The result is further damage to the remaining nephrons, possibly because of increased intraglomerular pressure.

The rise in the creatinine is exponential. Plotting the value of 1/creatinine against time can be helpful; this function is close to a straight line in the majority of patients. If patients progress faster than expected (as shown on the 1/creatinine versus time graph), this should prompt a search for a new cause of worsening renal function. For example, a patient may have developed urinary obstruction or may have started taking a new medication (e.g., an NSAID) that may adversely affect renal function. Although progression of renal failure cannot be halted, it may be possible to *slow* the deterioration. Tight blood pressure control, especially with angiotensin-converting enzyme (ACE) inhibitors, is important in this regard.

Azotemia is the condition in which the serum creatinine is above the normal range owing to a decrease in the GFR. A patient with uremia, on the other hand, has progressed to the stage where symptoms or signs are present. This distinction is important, because usually it is only when clinical signs or symptoms are evident (i.e., when the patient is uremic) that dialysis is undertaken. The clinical features of the uremic syndrome are shown in Table 64–1. All body systems may be affected by uremia.

EVALUATION

History

Patients should be asked about any symptoms of **uremia** (e.g., nausea, vomiting, anorexia, abnormal taste, itching, hiccups, fatigue, poor sleep, episodes of confusion, seizures). Symptoms of **volume overload** (e.g., shortness of breath on exertion or at night, decreased exercise tolerance) may also be important indicators that dialysis will be necessary in the near future. The duration and progression of the renal failure are important. Renal disease is often asymptomatic, but hypertension may be a clue to the presence of previous renal disease. Patients should be asked about **urinary symptoms** (e.g., dysuria, hematuria, nocturia, poor stream, incontinence, difficulty in initiating urination) because urinary obstruction is an important and treatable cause of renal failure. Polyuria and thirst are frequent in patients with chronic renal failure.

The previous presence of vascular disease in the coronary, carotid, or peripheral vascular beds may be an important clue to renal vascular disease. A family history of renal failure may be seen in polycystic kidney disease and hereditary nephritis (Alport's syndrome). A drug history is essential because of the frequency with which drugs, especially NSAIDs, cause or worsen renal failure. Illicit drug use and other risk factors for HIV infection should be asked about. The occupational history may reveal exposure to toxins (e.g., lead or other heavy metals) that may have caused the renal disease. A history of smoking should be determined, since this habit predisposes to renal vascular disease. Alcohol has an etiologic association with IgA nephropathy and is associated with hypertension.

Physical Examination

The physical examination should involve all systems. The skin should be checked for signs of scratching. A yellow-brown discoloration of the skin is characteristic of uremia; cutaneous dryness (xerosis) is also common. Pallor resulting from anemia may be present in both acute and chronic renal failure. The appearance of "uremic frost" (urea crystals on the skin) is now rare because this late sign is preventable by dialysis. "Half and half" nails, with a brownish discoloration of the distal parts of the nails, are seen in azotemic patients. The mental status of patients is important to assess; characteristically, uremic patients are drowsy, and this may progress to confusion, coma, dementia, or seizures. Peripheral neuropathy may be present in patients with long-standing renal failure. In patients with diabetes, the optic fundus should be examined, since diabetic retinopathy almost invariably accompanies diabetic nephropathy. A flapping tremor is an ominous sign in uremia and signifies an urgent need for dialysis if there is no other reason for the presence

TABLE 64–1. Clinical Features of the Uremic Syndrome

System	Clinical Signs and Symptoms
Cardiovascular	Pericarditis, myocardial dysfunction
Hematologic	Bleeding diathesis due to platelet dysfunction, susceptibility to infections (leukocyte dysfunction), anemia (erythropoietin deficiency)
Gastrointestinal	Anorexia, nausea, vomiting, gastroparesis; gastrointestinal bleeding, abnormal taste
Bones	Osteitis fibrosa, renal osteodystrophy
Neurologic	Insomnia, fatigue, asterixis, decreased mental status, seizures, peripheral neuropathy, day/night sleep inversion
Muscle	Proximal myopathy
Dermatologic	Pruritus, soft tissue calcification, uremic frost

TABLE 64–2. Significant Urinary Sediment Findings in Patients with Chronic Renal Failure

Urinary Sediment Finding	Significance
Red blood cells*	Bleeding anywhere in the urinary tract
White blood cells*	Seen in urinary tract infections (cystitis, pyelonephritis, renal tuberculosis), interstitial nephritis
Hyaline casts	May be present in normal urine
Granular casts	Present in a wide variety of renal disorders
Red blood cell casts	Indicate glomerular bleeding, strongly suggestive of glomerulonephritis
White blood cell casts	Seen in pyelonephritis, interstitial nephritis
Eosinophils	Seen in interstitial nephritis, cholesterol emboli syndrome

*May be present artifactually as a contaminant if the urine is not a "clean-catch" specimen.

of the flap (e.g., hepatic encephalopathy or carbon-dioxide retention). Pericarditis is also an urgent indication for dialysis. Signs of heart failure should be sought, and careful measurement of the blood pressure is essential in any patient with renal disease.

The abdominal examination should include a careful search for palpable kidneys; these most often indicate polycystic disease. Hydronephrosis may also result in palpable renal masses. The presence of abdominal bruits may be a clue to renal vascular disease. An enlarged bladder may signify obstructive uropathy.

Examination of the urine is one of the most important aspects of patient evaluation. Standard test strips (dipsticks) rapidly indicate whether protein, blood, glucose, ketones, or nitrite are present in the urine. Heavy proteinuria is usually indicative of glomerular disease. The examination of a "clean-catch" urinary sample (after centrifugation for 5 minutes) is also useful in distinguishing the type of renal disease present (Table 64–2).

Additional Evaluation

Laboratory Tests

The initial laboratory tests to be ordered for patients with renal failure depend to a great extent on the likely cause of the renal failure. Most patients require assessment of electrolytes, BUN, and creatinine to determine the severity and progression of disease. If the initial evaluation suggests glomerular disease, appropriate tests might include antinuclear antibodies to look for systemic lupus erythematosus; hepatitis serologies, because both hepatitis B and C are associated with glomerular disease; serum and urine protein electrophoresis to exclude multiple myeloma and other causes of amyloidosis; cryoglobulins to look for mixed essential cryoglobulinemia; antistreptolysin O titer if the history suggests poststreptococcal glomerulonephritis; and HIV serology, because HIV nephropathy usually causes heavy proteinuria. In addition, complement components C3 and C4 can help narrow the possible causes of nephrotic syndrome. Decreased complement is typically seen in lupus nephritis, poststreptococcal glomer-

ulonephritis, infective endocarditis, and membranoproliferative glomerulonephritis.

A 24-hour urine collection is usually necessary to quantify the extent of the proteinuria. In patients with pulmonary as well as renal disease, antiglomerular basement membrane antibody (for Goodpasture's syndrome) and antineutrophil cytoplasmic antibody (for Wegener's granulomatosis and polyarteritis nodosa) can also be helpful. If the urine sediment shows white blood cells, a urine culture should be performed to look for pyelonephritis. Eosinophils are typically present in the urine of patients with interstitial nephritis.

Imaging Studies

Most patients presenting with renal failure undergo renal ultrasound to assess renal size and to help rule out urinary obstruction. Other imaging tests depend on the likely cause of the renal failure. For example, if renal vascular disease is suspected, an arteriogram may be indicated, and a CT scan may be appropriate in cases of suspected polycystic disease.

MANAGEMENT

The objectives of caring for a patient with chronic renal failure include the following:

1. Attempting to determine the cause of the renal failure, so that if a treatable cause is present, it can be removed or appropriately managed.
2. Assessing whether uremia is present; if so, dialysis may be imminently indicated.
3. Paying attention to any electrolyte disturbances and treating them appropriately.
4. Assessing the patient for the endocrinologic disorders associated with chronic renal failure and treating these appropriately.
5. Attempting to slow the progression of the renal failure.
6. Assisting the patient with psychosocial issues, providing information about the likelihood of progression of the disease, and, where appropriate, making arrangements for dialysis.

The follow-up evaluation of patients with established renal failure usually includes a history of any new uremic symptoms (changes in appetite are often first) or any new urinary symptoms. Changes in medications are important; ask about over-the-counter medications (e.g., NSAIDs). The blood pressure should always be measured, and new signs of uremia need to be looked for. Laboratory tests usually performed at each visit include a chemistry panel, including potassium, bicarbonate, urea, creatinine, calcium, and phosphate. Creatinine levels should be compared with previous values to ensure that an unexpected worsening in renal function has not occurred. The hematocrit should be checked because of the frequent association of anemia with renal failure. Measurement of the parathyroid hormone level is usually done annually to assess for the presence of secondary hyperparathyroidism.

Renal Replacement Therapy

In a patient with chronic renal failure, the usual indication for starting dialysis is the onset of uremia. Other indications for starting dialysis include hyperkalemia or metabolic acidosis not treatable by medical therapy and volume overload not responsive to diuretics. Two types of dialysis are available.

Hemodialysis is usually performed in a dialysis center, although home hemodialysis is sometimes an option. Hemodialysis requires an access procedure (usually an arteriovenous fistula) to facilitate the considerable blood flow required to perform efficient dialysis. The disadvantages of hemodialysis are that patients are usually dependent on the dialysis staff, the patient has to spend about 3–4 hours three times per week on the dialysis machine, and clotting of access sites may require repeated surgical procedures.

Peritoneal dialysis uses the peritoneum as the membrane through which removal of nitrogenous substances occurs into a dialysis solution that is perfused into and out of the peritoneal cavity. This method, which is usually performed at home through a surgically implanted Tenckhoff catheter, may involve nighttime exchanges only or can be done with daytime exchanges. Although peritoneal dialysis needs to be done four times every day, patients can usually continue their usual activities, including employment, once the solution is in the peritoneum. The major disadvantage is the occurrence of peritonitis, which usually is mild and can be treated with antibiotics on an outpatient basis. More severe cases may require inpatient treatment and even removal of the catheter.

Kidney transplantation is an option preferred by many patients because it is more compatible with a normal life-style. Transplanted kidneys may come from a blood relative of the patient ("living related transplantation") or from a cadaver ("cadaveric renal transplantation"). Opportunistic infections and an increased incidence of tumors, both a result of the immunosuppression, are the main disadvantages. Rejection of the transplanted kidney remains a problem despite advances in immunosuppressive drugs.

Complications

Complications of chronic renal failure may be treated as follows.

Anemia may be treated with subcutaneous or intravenous erythropoietin. In addition, iron replacement is usually needed.

Administration of 1,25-dihydroxyvitamin D_3 may be beneficial in treating **renal osteodystrophy**. Keeping the serum phosphate level down is important; this is achieved by limiting dietary phosphate and using phosphate binders such as calcium salts and aluminum hydroxide. The latter has the disadvantage of causing aluminum bone disease with prolonged use. Parathyroidectomy is occasionally required to treat secondary hyperparathyroidism.

A low potassium diet (60–80 mEq/d) and potassium-binding resins (sodium polystyrene sulfonate) may be helpful in patients with significant **hyperkalemia**. It is important to remember that ACE inhibitors increase serum potassium.

Sodium bicarbonate may be helpful in preventing the bone disease associated with persistent acidemia.

PATIENT AND FAMILY EDUCATION

Care of the patient with chronic renal failure requires the coordinated efforts of the patient, family, medical and nursing team, and community. These patients require a considerable amount of resources and time, especially once dialysis is started. Once the chronicity and therefore the irreversibility of the renal failure is established, patients need to be told tactfully but honestly about the prognosis of the disease, in particular that the renal failure will eventually progress to ESRD, so that plans can be made for this eventuality. However, patients should also be told that the progression of the disease may be slow and that everything possible will be done to further slow its progression. Patients should be advised to report the use of new medications, since dose modifications may be needed if these agents are excreted by the kidneys. NSAIDs should be avoided, and magnesium-containing antacids should be taken only if the serum magnesium is checked frequently. Dialysis is provided free in the United States through the Medicare system, but financial concerns are still a major issue for many patients. Continuation of a career is generally encouraged, but career choices may be influenced by the time required to perform dialysis treatments and by a patient's general health.

Each clinic visit is an opportunity to reinforce the education of the patient about the possibility of dialysis and options such as transplantation.

Research Questions

1. What interventions effectively slow the progression of chronic renal failure?
2. What is the best form of renal replacement therapy?
3. What is the best way to determine whether a dialysis patient is receiving enough dialysis; i.e., how should adequacy of dialysis be measured?

Case Resolution

The patient's clinical diagnosis was uremia. Because the physician felt that there was no acute reversible component of his renal failure, the patient was started on hemodialysis, which resulted in resolution of his symptoms. After 1 year on dialysis, he received a cadaveric renal transplant.

Selected Readings

Cameron, S., A. M. Davidson, J. P. Grunfeld, et al. (eds.). *Oxford Textbook of Clinical Nephrology,* Section 9. Oxford, Oxford University Press, 1992, pp. 1147–402.

Fine, L. G. Preventing the progression of human renal disease: Have rational therapeutic principles emerged? Kidney Int 33:116–28, 1988.

Hakim, R. M., T. A. Depner, and T. F. Parker. Adequacy of hemodialysis. Am J Kidney Dis 20:107–21, 1992.

Held, P. J., N. W. Levin, R. R. Bovbjerg, et al. Mortality and duration of hemodialysis treatment. JAMA 265:871–5, 1991.

Jacobson, H. R. Chronic renal failure: Pathophysiology. Lancet 338: 419–23, 1991.

Klahr, S. Chronic renal failure: Management. Lancet 338:423–7, 1991.

Rose, B. D. *Pathophysiology of Renal Disease.* New York, McGraw-Hill Book Company, 1987, pp. 120–39.

CHAPTER 65

KIDNEY STONES

Curtis O. Kapsner, M.D.

H$_x$ A 44-year-old male sewage plant operator presented to the emergency department with a 2-hour history of excruciating left flank pain. Examination showed a very anxious man with left costovertebral angle tenderness. Urinalysis revealed many red blood cells with a few white blood cells and no bacteria. The serum creatinine was normal, and an abdominal radiograph showed a calcified density in the area of the left ureter. The patient said that he had experienced two similar episodes in the past year both of which resolved spontaneously. Metabolic evaluation done several weeks after the emergency department visit demonstrated that the patient had 1200 mg of uric acid in a 24-hour urine collection.

Questions

1. What treatment and evaluation should be performed on a patient with acute renal colic?
2. What are the common types of kidney stones, and what metabolic evaluation needs to be done to identify risk factors for these common stones?
3. What are effective therapies for preventing kidney stones?

Approximately 5% of the U. S. population has passed at least one kidney stone, with an incidence of about 16 cases per 1000 population per year. Twenty percent of these episodes result in hospitalization. Most kidney stones can be prevented with appropriate dietary and pharmacologic intervention. Kidney stones are composed of a variety of substances (Table 65–1), and since specific approaches to stone prevention depend on the type of stone, it is important that stones be sent for analysis. Because three fourths of all stones are composed of calcium oxalate, this chapter focuses primarily on calcium stones.

CLINICAL PRESENTATION

Patients with kidney stones (nephrolithiasis) frequently present with flank pain, which is initially mild but over time can become very severe. The pain is constant. As the stone moves down from the kidney through the ureter, the pain moves lower. Stones in the distal ureter may cause pain that radiates to the testicle or labia. When the stone passes into the bladder, the pain vanishes suddenly. Most patients also have hematuria.

PATHOPHYSIOLOGY

The urine of normal people who do not form kidney stones has a concentration of calcium oxalate that is four times its solubility; supersaturation without stone formation can occur because of the presence of inhibitors of stone formation in the urine (especially a urinary protein called nephrocalcin). When the urinary calcium oxalate concentration reaches 7 to 11 times its solubility, stone formation may begin.

An increase in the urinary calcium concentration will increase the risk of stone formation. Three common predisposing conditions are the following. (1) The most common cause is decreased water intake. (2) Hypercal-

TABLE 65–1. Types of Kidney Stones		
Composition	Percentage	Comments
Calcium oxalate	75%	Common, < 2 cm in diameter
Uric acid	5%	Radiolucent
Calcium phosphate	5%	Occur with renal tubular acidosis
Cystine	< 1%	Autosomal recessive, hexagonal crystals
Struvite	15%	Urine infections with urease-producing bacteria

cemia, usually due to primary hyperparathyroidism, will cause increased glomerular filtration of calcium and hypercalciuria. (3) Idiopathic hypercalciuria is a familial disorder in which patients have normal serum calcium concentrations but more than 250 mg (in women) or 300 mg (in men) of calcium in the urine per 24 hours. Because of the loss of calcium in the urine, these patients are at risk for osteoporosis.

An increase in the amount of oxalate in the urine will also increase the likelihood of forming a calcium oxalate stone. Normal excretion of oxalate is up to 45 mg/d; oxalate-containing foods such as rhubarb, cocoa, peppers, peanuts, and chocolate can increase this to 60 mg/d. In patients with small bowel malabsorption, the colonic mucosa is exposed to bile salts and fatty acids that normally are absorbed in the small bowel. This exposure increases the permeability of the colon to oxalate, resulting in urinary excretion rates of greater than 100 mg/d. Primary hyperoxaluria is a rare inherited disorder which results in massive amounts of urinary oxalate and stone formation that begins in childhood.

Citrate is an anion, normally present in urine, that binds calcium, thus decreasing urinary supersaturation with calcium oxalate. For this reason, a low urinary citrate concentration is a risk factor for calcium stone formation. However, no well-designed clinical trials have demonstrated that oral therapy with citrate salts significantly decreases the incidence of calcium stones.

The presence of preexisting surfaces in the urine will allow calcium oxalate crystals to form at a lower saturation. When uric acid is present in large amounts in the urine, small uric acid crystals form and serve as the nidus upon which calcium oxalate crystals can form, even in the absence of hypercalciuria. Hyperuricosuria is defined as greater than 800 mg/d in men and 750 mg/d in women. A well-controlled clinical trial has shown that administering allopurinol (which decreases uric acid production and thus decreases the amount of uric acid in the urine) to patients with calcium oxalate urolithiasis and hyperuricosuria significantly lowers the incidence of calcium oxalate stone formation.

DIFFERENTIAL DIAGNOSIS

Whenever patients present with acute unilateral flank pain, a variety of etiologies, including musculoskeletal problems and pyelonephritis, need to be considered. The presence of hematuria narrows this differential. Kidney stones are an obvious consideration. Other causes of hematuria and flank pain include papillary necrosis with the sloughed papilla blocking the ureter (diabetes mellitus, sickle cell anemia, and analgesic nephropathy are risk factors for papillary necrosis), renal cell carci-

noma, and polycystic kidney disease with bleeding into a cyst that breaks into the collecting system.

The pain associated with acute stone passage usually starts suddenly and increases to a severe, constant pain over 15 to 20 minutes. When the stone is located in the renal pelvis or upper ureter, the pain is localized to the flank. However, when the stone moves down into the mid or lower ureter, the pain often radiates to the testicle or labia on the same side. Stones that lodge within the intravesicular portion of the ureter can mimic cystitis, causing both frequency and dysuria. Passage of an acute stone is often associated with nausea and vomiting and can cause fever, especially in children.

EVALUATION

Evaluation of the patient with a possible kidney stone includes a urinalysis to document hematuria and rule out infection (the only crystals seen on urinalysis that are diagnostic for nephrolithiasis are cystine crystals, which are hexagonal; calcium oxalate and other crystals can occur normally in the urine). A plain radiograph of the kidneys, ureters, and bladder (KUB) may document calcifications consistent with kidney stones (the only radiolucent stones are composed of uric acid). Either a renal ultrasound or an intravenous pyelogram (IVP) can be performed to verify the presence of a stone; however, since the IVP is more sensitive for obstruction, it is usually the preferred imaging procedure.

After kidney stone disease has been diagnosed, a diagnostic evaluation should be initiated for identifying preventable causes of recurrent stone disease. Since the odds of recurrence increase substantially after two stones have been passed, the metabolic evaluation (Table 65–2) of a patient who has had a single stone should be limited to several measurements of serum calcium and phosphate to rule out primary hyperparathyroidism, which is eminently treatable and can cause

TABLE 65–2. Metabolic Evaluation of Calcium Oxalate Stones

	Test (Perform Each Twice)	Interpretation
Patients Who Have Passed a Single Stone	Serum calcium	>10 mg/dL suggests hyperparathyroidism
	Serum phosphate	<2 mg/dL suggests hyperparathyroidism
Patients With Recurrent Stones	Two 24-hour urine collections for:	
	Volume	>2000 mL implies inadequate fluid intake
	Calcium	Hypercalciuria defined as >300 mg/d in males and >250 mg/d in females
	Oxalate	Normally up to 45 mg/d
	Uric acid	Hyperuricosuria defined as >800 mg/d in men and >750 mg/d in women
	Creatinine	Measures adequacy of urine collection; males excrete about 20 mg/kg/d and females about 15 mg/kg/d

TABLE 65–3. Strategies for Prevention of Calcium Oxalate Stones

Abnormality	Intervention
Low volume	Increased fluid intake
Hypercalciuria	Thiazide diuretics
Hyperoxaluria	Dietary manipulation; evaluate for bowel disease
Hyperuricosuria	Allopurinol
No abnormality	Thiazide diuretics

serious bone disease. In primary hyperparathyroidism, the serum calcium is usually above 10 mg/dL and the phosphate less than 2 mg/dL. For patients who have had more than one kidney stone, two or three 24-hour urine collections should be obtained for volume, calcium, oxalate, and uric acid to rule out the various treatable causes of calcium stone disease. A creatinine measurement is also performed on the urine collection to help assess adequacy of the collection (males produce approximately 20 mg, and females about 15 mg, of creatinine per kilogram of body weight per 24 hours).

MANAGEMENT

Acute Management

Once the diagnosis of acute renal colic secondary to a kidney stone has been made, management usually is conservative and consists of adequate hydration and narcotic-containing pain medications while the stone is given time to pass spontaneously. Stones that are less than 5 mm in diameter generally pass spontaneously and thus rarely require surgical intervention. Stones larger than 7 mm rarely pass and may have to be removed by either extracorporeal shock wave lithotripsy, cystoscopy, or nephrolithotomy. The presence of complete obstruction or infected urine makes removal of the stone more urgent.

Prevention

Rational therapy for prevention of calcium oxalate stones depends on the underlying abnormality that put the patient at risk for developing the stones (Table 65–3). If the urinary volume is less than 2000 mL/d, the patient should be instructed to increase fluid intake appropriately. Primary hyperparathyroidism is usually treated surgically by parathyroidectomy, which results in cessation of stone formation. Idiopathic hypercalciuria is treated by administration of thiazide diuretics, which decrease the amount of calcium in the urine.

Interestingly, patients with no underlying abnormality also benefit from the administration of thiazide diuretics, presumably because the urinary calcium concentration drops below the baseline value. If hyperoxaluria is present, modest dietary restriction of oxalate-containing foods can be advised. Of note, patients with bowel disease severe enough to increase urinary oxalate levels almost always have diarrhea. Thus, if diarrhea is present, an evaluation for small bowel disease should be performed. Finally, patients who have documented hyperuricosuria should be given allopurinol, usually at a dosage of 300 mg/d.

PATIENT EDUCATION

The most important aspect of education for all patients with nephrolithiasis, regardless of frequency or type of stone, is reinforcing the need for adequate fluid intake. Urine output should be approximately 2000 mL/d, which implies that fluid intake should be approximately 2500 mL/d.

Research Question

1. In patients with hyperoxaluria secondary to bowel disease, what treatments might be effective in reducing the amount of oxalate in the urine?

Case Resolution

The patient was found to have hyperuricosuria as a risk factor for calcium oxalate stones. He was told to drink at least 2.5 L of fluid per day and was given allopurinol. Over the next 2 years, he experienced no further symptoms.

Selected Readings

Coe, F. L., J. H. Parks, and J. R. Asplin. The pathogenesis and treatment of kidney stones. N Engl J Med 327:1141–52, 1992.

Curhan, G. C., W. C. Willett, E. B. Rimm, and M. J. Stampfer. A prospective study of dietary calcium and other nutrients and the risk of symptomatic kidney stones. N Engl J Med 328:833–8, 1993.

Ettinger, B., J. T. Citron, B. Livermore, and L. I. Dolman. Chlorthalidone reduces calcium oxalate calculous recurrence but magnesium hydroxide does not. J Urol 139:679–84, 1988.

Ettinger, B., A. Tang, J. T. Citron, et al. Randomized trial of allopurinol in the prevention of calcium oxalate calculi. N Engl J Med 315:1386–9, 1986.

CHAPTER 66

PROSTATE DISORDERS

Douglas Egli, M.D.

H$_x$ A 53-year-old male welder with an unremarkable medical history presents for a general medical examination. The review of systems reveals complaints of decreased force of the urinary stream, postvoid dribbling, and nocturia that has been present without progression for 3 years. He has heard of a "PSA blood test" to check for prostate cancer. He wonders whether he needs this test. His family medical history is unremarkable. His blood pressure is 150/98 mm Hg. He has arteriovenous nicking and an S$_4$ on cardiac examination. His prostate is slightly enlarged globally without nodules, focal induration, or irregularity. The remainder of his physical examination is normal.

Questions

1. What is the differential diagnosis for this man's urinary complaints?
2. Is any further diagnostic evaluation required?
3. What are the currently available treatments for prostatism?
4. What should the patient be told about screening for prostate cancer?

The prostate gland lies inferior to the bladder and superior to the urogenital diaphragm and is bordered anteriorly by the symphysis pubis and posteriorly by the rectum. It may be affected by inflammation, hypertrophy, and cancer. Fifty percent of men complain of symptoms of prostatism in their lifetime, and 25% of men aged 55 years will have complaints of decreased force of the urinary stream. In the United States, 400,000 men per year will undergo transurethral resection of the prostate (TURP) for symptoms of prostatism.

As of 1990, prostatic carcinoma was the most common cancer in men in the United States. In 1993, 165,000 cases were diagnosed, with 35,000 deaths. The incidence of detectable prostate carcinoma ranges from 0.8:100,000 in men in China to 44:100,000 in white men in the United States to 88:100,000 in African American men in California.

PATHOPHYSIOLOGY

The prostate enlarges rapidly at puberty, reaching a size of 20 g (walnut size). The gland secretes fluid that presumably protects or enhances spermatic function. Because of its anatomic location, the prostate may provide some protection against urinary tract infections (UTIs) in men.

After the age of 30 years, the prostate grows at a rate of 0.4 g/year. Despite progressive hyperplasia, not all men will have symptoms related to prostatic enlargement.

The etiology of **benign prostatic hypertrophy** is unclear, but it is known that functioning testes are required and that the aging process also plays a role. Growth of prostate tissue is under the control of androgens. Men who are castrated do not develop benign prostatic hypertrophy. Estrogens may also play a role in the hyperplastic process.

Bladder outlet obstruction is the primary complication of benign prostatic hypertrophy. Several factors are involved: prostate mass, smooth muscle tone of the prostate, the state of the adrenergic nervous system, and the condition of the detrusor muscle of the bladder.

The static component of outlet obstruction is related to the mass of the prostate. Prostatic tissue may encroach upon the urethra, causing increased resistance. Hyperplasia can compress the prostate against its capsule, so that if the capsule does not enlarge with the growing tissue, compression of the urethra will occur. Therefore, symptoms of benign prostatic hypertrophy do not entirely correlate with the size of the prostate.

The dynamic component of benign prostatic hypertrophy is produced by the smooth muscle tone within the prostatic stroma. Smooth muscle constitutes a significant component of the prostatic capsule, stroma, and bladder neck. This smooth muscle is innervated by the adrenergic and cholinergic nervous systems, so smooth muscle tone may increase as a result of adrenergic stimulation. This dynamic aspect of obstruction accounts for a significant amount of the variability in patients' symptoms.

As outlet obstruction increases, the bladder compensates by increasing its force of contraction. Over time this leads to detrusor hypertrophy, which may be accompanied by detrusor muscle instability or loss of normal reflex detrusor response as well as a decrease in functional bladder capacity.

The etiology of **prostatic carcinoma** is not understood. No chromosomal abnormalities have been detected. Men with a positive family history of prostate cancer do have a higher risk of developing prostate cancer. There is no definite correlation between prostate cancer and benign prostatic hypertrophy. Most theories link the cancer to androgens. An interesting observation is that African American males have a 15% higher average level of serum testosterone than do white males, and they also have a higher incidence of prostate cancer. However, a direct correlation between androgen stimulation and prostate cancer has yet to be definitely proved.

Prostatitis

Prostatitis is a vague term used to describe a variety of complaints involving the lower urinary tract and pelvis, including dysuria and hematuria. Only 5% of men with this complaint will have objective evidence of a bacterial infection. It is essential to differentiate those patients who have objective evidence of bacterial infection from the majority who do not. Symptoms of dysuria, frequency, and prostatic tenderness can be due to (1) acute bacterial prostatitis, (2) chronic bacterial prostatitis, or (3) nonbacterial prostatitis or prostadynia.

EVALUATION

Acute bacterial prostatitis usually presents with rapid onset of dysuria, frequency, lower abdominal pain, and fever. The patient usually feels ill. There is pyuria, and the prostate is usually tender on rectal examination. Typically this disorder is caused by gram-negative bacteria or enterococci.

Chronic bacterial prostatitis is a more indolent process. The causative microorganisms are usually gram-negative organisms, but gram-positive organisms have been implicated as well, including *Staphylococcus saprophyticus*. The patient has a variable degree of urinary symptoms. Patients may present with recurrent UTIs or epididymitis.

Careful assessment of the lower urinary tract is required to establish the diagnosis of **chronic bacterial prostatitis**. Prostatic secretions are consistent with an inflammatory process (>10 WBC/hpf). Midstream pyuria and bacteriuria are often present. The prostate may feel normal or boggy, or there may be focal induration.

Nonbacterial prostatitis is diagnosed when symptoms of prostate inflammation are present in the absence of objective evidence of bacterial infection. The patient may have a variety of subacute symptoms including frequency, dysuria, and ejaculatory complaints. Physical examination is usually unremarkable. Prostatic secretions will show an inflammatory response. The etiology of these symptoms is unclear. Some researchers have implicated *Chlamydia* or *Ureaplasma* as the cause, but this remains controversial. Other researchers believe this is not an infection but rather an autoimmune inflammatory process.

Prostadynia occurs when a man has complaints consistent with prostatitis but all secretions and fluids are benign. Some of these patients are found to have dysfunctional voiding due to a functional obstruction of the bladder neck. In most cases, the cause is unclear.

MANAGEMENT

The treatment for prostatitis is antibiotic therapy. The antibiotic should be able to penetrate the prostatic stroma. Trimethoprim/sulfamethoxazole is the most commonly used antibiotic. For acute prostatitis, a 14-day regimen is usually adequate. Chronic prostatitis requires long-term therapy of 8 to 12 weeks. Other commonly used antibiotics include doxycycline and the fluoroquinolones.

Current therapy for nonbacterial prostatitis is limited. There is little objective evidence that antibiotics are of value.

Obstruction of the bladder neck in prostadynia can be treated medically with α-receptor blockade.

Complications

Complications of chronic bacterial prostatitis include recurrent UTIs, pyelonephritis, and infected prostatic calculi. Occasionally it is impossible to eradicate an infection; this can ultimately lead to bladder neck contracture and bladder outlet obstruction. Patients who are not cured by extended courses of full-dose antibiotics may be candidates for suppressive therapy. The goal of suppressive therapy is not to eradicate the infection but rather to keep the patient asymptomatic. Surgical measures are the last resort for patients whose symptoms cannot be controlled by antimicrobials. Radical prostatectomy is curative but undesirable. TURP can be helpful if all the infected tissue is resected.

Benign Prostatic Hypertrophy

EVALUATION

History and Physical Examination

Symptoms related to mechanical obstruction include hesitancy, trouble initiating the urinary stream, decreased force of the stream, postvoid dribbling, fullness, and double voiding. Detrusor instability leads to nocturia, urgency, frequency, and incontinence. These so-called irritative symptoms of prostatism are particularly bothersome.

The symptoms of prostatism vary widely over time, probably secondary to the dynamic component. Any medication that affects the adrenergic nervous system can affect the patient's symptoms. For instance, decongestants often worsen symptoms of prostatism, while α-receptor blockers improve symptoms. Only 50% of men with symptoms of prostatism will have an enlarged prostate on digital rectal examination, and not all men with large prostate glands on examination will have symptoms of prostatism.

Additional Evaluation

Attention should be paid to nonurologic factors that may cause urologic dysfunction, such as medication use, congestive heart failure, diabetes mellitus, and neurologic disease. Urinalysis and digital rectal examination can usually rule out infection. For men with symptoms of long duration, serum BUN and creatinine measurements may be helpful in evaluating for renal insufficiency. Measurement of prostate-specific antigen (PSA) is controversial (see below). Urodynamics and postvoid residuals can give helpful information with respect to flow rates. However, these are not usually required unless the physician is uncomfortable with the diagnosis. Imaging of the prostate or urinary tract is not routinely required.

MANAGEMENT

At this time, no treatment for benign prostatic hypertrophy has proved more effective than TURP. However, considering the complication rate of TURP (5%–30%), some patients may be interested in other therapies.

Transurethral incision of the prostate (TUIP) can be effective and has a lower complication rate. This office procedure is limited to patients with lesser degrees of prostatic enlargement.

Balloon dilatation of the prostatic urethra is an option with fewer complications than TURP. However, it is not as effective in relief of symptoms. Symptomatic improvement may be transient, with symptoms returning within 2 years. This method is also used in patients with smaller prostates.

Medical therapy can be effective in those patients without absolute indications for surgery. α-Adrenergic blockers block adrenergic input to the smooth muscle of the prostatic stroma and bladder neck, thereby decreasing muscular tone and reducing the dynamic component of prostatic obstruction. Terazosin (a long-acting α-blocker) and prazosin have been shown to improve both symptoms and urinary flow rates.

The 5α-reductase inhibitor finasteride is a newer agent that inhibits conversion of testosterone to dihydrotestosterone (DHT). It appears to be effective in improving symptoms, increasing urinary flow by decreasing prostate size. However, limited information is available about long-term follow-up.

Other medications such as GnRH analogs and antiandrogens can also decrease prostate size. However, they are not commonly used because of their expense and adverse effects.

Treatment modalities under investigation (but not currently available) include laser therapy, stents, coils, and microwave hyperthermia.

NATURAL HISTORY/PROGNOSIS

The course of symptoms is not necessarily one of progressive decline; many patients remain stable or improve. Definite indications for surgical intervention are relatively few: chronic urinary retention, hydronephrosis, overflow incontinence, severe hematuria, and recurrent infections. A single episode of urinary retention, an increased postvoid residual (PVR), or symptoms of prostatism do not necessarily indicate an immediate need for operative intervention.

Prostate Cancer

EVALUATION

History and Physical Examination

The clinical presentation of prostate cancer is usually insidious, with the majority of patients presenting with obstructive symptoms including urgency, hesitancy, and decreased force of the urinary stream. Unfortunately, these symptoms are indistinguishable from those of benign prostatic hypertrophy. Symptoms that present in a rapid fashion may be more suggestive of cancer. Other presentations can include new onset of impotence or erectile dysfunction, acute urinary retention, or back pain due to bony metastasis.

The examination of the prostate may be entirely normal or reveal a discrete nodule or focal induration, or the prostate may be hard and irregular.

Screening

Screening for prostate cancer is an area of intense debate and investigation. PSA is a protease produced by prostate epithelial cells. Its function is unknown. It is secreted into the prostatic ducts and is found in high concentrations in seminal fluid. Malignant tissue may produce higher levels of PSA per gram than benign tissue does. Serum PSA levels can also be elevated in benign prostatic hypertrophy or prostatitis, as well as following trauma to the prostate. Currently, PSA is used as a tumor marker for patients with established prostatic carcinoma, but it is not universally accepted as a screening test. The American Cancer Society currently recommends an annual digital rectal examination for men over the age of 40 years, with a PSA measurement done annually after the age of 50 years. However, the U.S. Preventive Services Task Force does not recommend PSA screening.

At present, no prospective randomized data show PSA or digital rectal examination to be useful screening tools. Research in progress should shed more light on this controversy. Transrectal ultrasound (TRUS) has no place in screening for prostate cancer at this time.

Grading and Staging

Once a tissue diagnosis has been confirmed, the cancer is graded histologically. The most widely used system at present is the Gleason system, which grades the cancer on a scale of 1 to 5 (1 denoting well-differentiated cancer, 5 denoting anaplastic cancer). The histologic pattern helps predict overall survival.

The patient is then "staged" to determine the extent of spread of the cancer. Staging can be done noninvasively by physical examination, laboratory tests, and x-ray studies, or it can be done during a surgical procedure. The clinical value of surgical staging is controversial. Staging systems in current use include the TNN and the A–D system. The A–D system is less confusing and easier to remember. 'A' denotes localized disease; 'D' denotes metastatic disease.

MANAGEMENT

Patients with localized disease (stages A–C) have two treatment options: radical prostatectomy or radiation therapy. The goal is to eliminate the tumor. However, another option for localized disease is observation. A recent study by Swedish investigators followed 223 patients with limited disease for a mean of 10 years with observation only. Nineteen of 223 patients died of prostate cancer in the 10 years of follow-up. The 10-year survival rate was 86.8%. There is currently no consensus regarding the management of localized disease. Investigation continues.

Management of node-positive disease without distant metastasis (stage D1) is controversial as well. In the past, observation only has been standard treatment. However, 80% of these patients will have diffuse disease within 5 years. Retrospective data from the Mayo Clinic indicate that patients treated more aggressively with hormonal manipulation have increased survival.

Patients with distant metastatic disease (stage D2) at diagnosis are candidates for hormonal manipulation. This can be achieved surgically by orchiectomy or medically by a variety of medications that block androgens. First-line therapy is controversial and varies from center to center.

Stage D3 is metastatic disease that is refractory to first-line hormonal manipulation. The patient should be reassessed to make sure androgens have been effectively blocked, as measured by serum testosterone. If testosterone is at appropriately low levels, additional hormonal manipulation is usually ineffective.

Several newer agents are under investigation for stage D3 disease. These include suramin, an antiparasitic having *in vitro* activity against prostate cancer, somatostatin analogs, bisphosphonates, and radionucleotides. Chemotherapeutic agents now available have not been effective against prostate cancer.

Patients with prostate cancer and new-onset back pain with neurologic symptoms should be evaluated for spinal cord compression. The test of choice is MRI of the spine. However, CT scanning or CT myelography is acceptable. This situation is one of the few true emergencies in cancer management. Treatment includes prompt institution of high-dose dexamethasone and consideration of radiation therapy. Occasionally, the patient may require decompression laminectomy.

Patients with metastatic disease to weight-bearing joints should be evaluated by an orthopedist and a radiation therapist to prevent pathologic fractures. Urinary tract obstruction can be relieved by catheterization.

Pain due to bony metastasis may require aggressive pain management measures. These include nonsteroidal antiinflammatory agents, narcotics, and palliative radiation therapy. Psychosocial support with involvement of social workers, home health care, and hospice (if available) is essential.

NATURAL HISTORY/PROGNOSIS

Eighty percent of patients with positive pelvic nodes at diagnosis will develop metastatic disease in 5 years. Patients with negative pelvic nodes at diagnosis have a 27% chance of developing metastatic disease in 5 years.

Many patients with a diagnosis of prostate cancer do not die of this disease but of other illnesses.

PATIENT AND FAMILY EDUCATION

Patients should understand that the treatment of prostate cancer is not well defined at present. Each patient must be considered individually. Overall assessment should include the extent of disease and symptomatology, the patient's age, and his performance status. Options for treatment should be thoroughly discussed prior to any intervention. The patient's wishes and overall goals should be a primary component of any treatment plan.

Research Questions

1. What is the natural history of prostatism?
2. What types of testing will be needed to definitively prove the value or lack thereof of PSA screening?

Case Resolution

The patient's urinalysis, BUN, and serum creatinine were normal. After extensive discussion, he elected to have a PSA test, which was low at a level of 2.0 (normal, 0-4). The physician determined that the patient had long-standing mild essential hypertension. After discussion they mutually agreed to initiate terazosin therapy to treat the hypertension and possibly decrease the symptoms of prostatism. Over the next several months, the patient's home blood pressure recordings were good and his symptoms of prostatism improved. At 1-year follow-up, his blood pressure remained controlled, prostatism symptoms had improved further, and the PSA remained normal at 1.8.

Selected Readings

Barry, M. J., F. J. Fowler, M. P. O'Leary, et al. (Measurement Committee of the American Urologic Association). The American Urologic Association symptom index for benign prostatic hyperplasia. J Urol 148:1549–57, 1992.

Benign Prostate Hyperplasia Guideline Panel. Benign prostatic hyperplasia: Diagnosis and treatment. Am Family Phys 49:1157–65, 1994.

Christianson, M. M., and R. C. Bruskewitz. Clinical manifestations of benign prostatic hyperplasia and indications for therapeutic intervention. Urol Clin North Am 17:509–16, 1990.

Garnick, M. B. Prostatic cancer: Screening, diagnosis and management. Ann Intern Med 118:804–18, 1993.

Johansson, J. E., H. O. Adami, S. O. Anderson, et al. High 10-year survival rate in patients with early, untreated prostate cancer. JAMA 267:2191–6, 1992.

Kramer, B. S., M. L. Brown, P. C. Prorok, et al. Prostate cancer screening: What we know and what we need to know. Ann Intern Med 119:914–23, 1993.

Voss, J. D. Prostate cancer, screening and prostate-specific antigen: Promise or peril? J Gen Intern Med 9:468–74, 1994.

COMMON SEXUALLY TRANSMITTED DISEASES

CHAPTER 67

SEXUALLY TRANSMITTED DISEASES

Josephine Williams, M.D.

H$_x$ A 22-year-old male carpenter presents with a 3-day history of a painful penile rash. His initial symptoms were itching and tingling of the penis followed several hours later by a cluster of blisters, which over the next day eroded to form painful ulcers. He denies a history of genital herpes or known exposure to herpes. His last sexual contact was 10 days ago with a new partner. A condom had not been used. On physical examination, he has slightly enlarged, tender inguinal nodes bilaterally. On the dorsal aspect of the penile shaft, there are multiple shallow painful ulcers as well as several intact vesicles and pustules.

Questions

1. What additional historical information should be gathered from this patient?
2. Which sexually transmitted diseases present with ulcers and lymphadenopathy?
3. What laboratory studies are needed?
4. What education does this patient need about reducing risk for sexually transmitted diseases?

Patients with symptoms suggestive of sexually transmitted diseases (STDs) present to a variety of clinical settings including outpatient clinics and primary care physicians' offices. An organized approach to the evaluation of such patients is necessary, since individuals at risk for one STD are at risk for multiple STDs.

PATHOPHYSIOLOGY

Sexually transmitted organisms must breach the protective barriers of mucosal or epidermal epithelium to cause disease. Those organisms (e.g., *Treponema pallidum* and herpes simplex virus) that produce ulcers on epidermal surfaces like the penile shaft most likely do so by gaining access to underlying cells via abrasions of the outermost horny layer of the epidermis. On mucosal surfaces, organisms must be able to *adhere* to mucosal cells before they can cause a local inflammatory response. Organisms which possess pili or fimbriae may cause disease more efficiently than those which do not. The normal flora of the genital mucosa most likely plays a role in defending against infection, but the exact mechanisms are unclear. In addition to microbial interaction, the presence and composition of mucus and various secretory antibodies all play a part in protecting against the acquisition of STDs.

DIFFERENTIAL DIAGNOSIS

The most commonly encountered STD syndromes in men are urethritis and epididymitis and in women, cervicitis, the acute urethral syndrome, pelvic inflammatory disease (PID), and vaginitis (Table 67–1). Genital ulcer disease, proctitis, and genital warts are seen in both men and women.

Urethritis

Urethritis is the most common STD syndrome in men and may be gonococcal or nongonococcal. Gonococcal urethritis is caused by *Neisseria gonorrhoeae*, while nongonococcal urethritis (NGU) is most commonly caused by *Chlamydia trachomatis*, with *Ureaplasma urealyticum* the next most common cause. Herpes simplex virus and *Trichomonas vaginalis* are less common causes of NGU. Other organisms such as *Bacteroides ureolyticus* and *Mycoplasma genitalium* have also been implicated as possible causes of NGU. Symptoms of urethritis are urethral discharge, dysuria, and urethral or meatal itching. On examination, a discharge may or may not be evident. On Gram's stain of urethral discharge (or the material obtained with a urethral swab), more than four polymorphonuclear leukocytes (PMNs) per oil immersion field ($\times1000$ magnification) is usually diagnostic of urethritis. The presence of gram-negative intracellular diplococci is diagnostic of gonococcal urethritis. If these organisms are absent on Gram's stain and there are more than four PMNs per oil immersion field, then the diagnosis is NGU.

TABLE 67–1. STD Syndromes and Causative Organisms

Syndrome	Organism
Infections in Men	
Urethritis	*N. gonorrhoeae*
	C. trachomatis
	U. urealyticum
	Mycoplasma species
	Herpes simplex virus
	T. vaginalis
	Undetermined
Epididymitis	*N. gonorrhoeae*
	C. trachomatis
Infections in Women	
Cervicitis	*N. gonorrhoeae*
	C. trachomatis
	Herpes simplex virus
Acute urethral syndrome	*C. trachomatis*
Pelvic inflammatory disease (PID)	*N. gonorrhoeae*
	C. trachomatis
	Mycoplasma species
	Anaerobic bacteria
	Facultative bacteria
Vaginitis	*T. vaginalis*
Infections in Men and Women	
Genital ulcer disease	
Syphilis	*T. pallidum*
Genital herpes	Herpes simplex virus
Chancroid	*H. ducreyi*
Lymphogranuloma venereum	*C. trachomatis*
Granuloma inguinale	*C. granulomatis*
Proctitis	*N. gonorrhoeae*
	C. trachomatis
	Herpes simplex virus
	T. pallidum
Genital warts	Human papillomavirus

Epididymitis

Epididymitis in young (< 35 years old) sexually active men is usually caused by either *N. gonorrhoeae* or *C. trachomatis,* with the latter organism responsible for the majority of cases. In men over 35 years of age, most cases of epididymitis are caused by coliform bacteria or *Pseudomonas aeruginosa.* The main symptom of epididymitis is pain in the epididymis. A urethral discharge may or may not be present. On examination, the epididymis is warm, swollen, and tender on the involved side. The swelling is usually localized posterior to the testis.

Cervicitis

Cervicitis is most commonly caused by infection of the endocervix with *C. trachomatis* or *N. gonorrhoeae.* Herpes simplex virus may cause endocervicitis as well as ectocervicitis. PID is a complication of cervicitis resulting from spread of infection from the endocervix to the upper genital tract. In addition to the well-established evidence for *C. trachomatis* and *N. gonorrhoeae* as etiologic agents in PID, *Mycoplasma* species and anaerobic and facultative bacteria also have been implicated. Infection may involve the endometrium, fallopian (uterine) tubes, ovaries, and pelvic peritoneum. The fallopian tubes and ovaries

are involved in tubo-ovarian abscesses. In severe cases of PID, the process may extend beyond the pelvis.

Many women with cervicitis are asymptomatic. Those with symptoms may complain of increased vaginal discharge, dysuria, or vaginal spotting. On examination, the cervix appears erythematous, is often friable, and frequently has a mucopurulent discharge from the os. Ulcerative lesions on the ectocervix suggest involvement with herpes simplex virus. If the upper genital tract is involved (PID), additional symptoms include lower abdominal pain and dyspareunia. Fever, nausea, and vomiting may be present. On physical examination, pain on cervical motion can usually be elicited. Uterine and adnexal tenderness, adnexal swelling, and direct or rebound tenderness of the lower abdomen may also be present.

Acute Urethral Syndrome

C. trachomatis has been implicated in the acute urethral syndrome in young, sexually active women. Urinary frequency, dysuria, and pyuria without bacteriuria are the typical manifestations.

Vaginitis

Sexually transmitted vaginitis is usually caused by *T. vaginalis.* Symptoms include increased vaginal discharge and often severe vaginal itching. Some women infected with *T. vaginalis* are asymptomatic. On examination, copious vaginal discharge is typically present, and the vaginal walls are erythematous. The diagnosis is usually made by examining a saline preparation of vaginal discharge under the microscope at medium (×400) magnification. The one-celled, flagellated, motile organism can be easily recognized. Strictly defined, candidal vaginitis and bacterial vaginosis are not sexually transmitted diseases.

Genital Ulcer Disease

In the United States, the three most common genital ulcer diseases (in order of prevalence) are (1) genital herpes caused by herpes simplex virus, (2) syphilis caused by *T. pallidum,* and (3) chancroid caused by *Haemophilus ducreyi.* Lymphogranuloma venereum caused by *C. trachomatis* is uncommon, and granuloma inguinale caused by *Calymmatobacterium granulomatis* is rare.

Genital Herpes

Genital herpes presents as multiple, small vesicular lesions that rapidly evolve through a pustular stage to ulcerative lesions. The lesions are typically painful, and with first episodes there is usually tender inguinal adenopathy as well. Recurrent genital herpes tends to be not so severe as the first episode. The diagnosis can usually be made on clinical grounds. Laboratory confirmation can be achieved by viral cultures, cytologic analysis, or antigen detection studies.

Primary Syphilis

Primary syphilis manifests itself as a chancre, which is a painless ulcer with a clean base and well-defined, indurated borders. Painless inguinal adenopathy is usually present. The diagnosis of syphilis can be made by darkfield microscopic examination of serous exudate from the chancre to demonstrate the presence of *T. pallidum,* which is recognized by its spiral morphology and characteristic motility.

Chancroid

Chancroid causes very tender, deep ulcers with irregular borders and a purulent base. Tender inguinal adenopathy is usually present, and nodes may eventually become fluctuant.

Lymphogranuloma Venereum

The ulcer of lymphogranuloma venereum may be fleeting, and the most prominent finding is lymphadenopathy that is usually tender. Nodes may become fluctuant and rupture through the skin.

Proctitis

Proctitis, or infection of the rectum, may be caused by *N. gonorrhoeae, C. trachomatis,* herpes simplex virus, or *T. pallidum.* Symptoms include rectal discharge or bleeding, tenesmus, and constipation. Anoscopy may reveal mucus in the rectum, erythema of the rectal mucosa, or mucosal ulceration.

Genital Warts

Genital warts are caused by the several different types of human papillomavirus. Skin or mucous membrane may be involved. Lesions may be cauliflower-like (condylomata acuminata) but may also be smooth and papular. Warts may be flesh-colored to hyperpigmented. Subclinical lesions are not visible without colposcopy or other magnification after application of 3%–5% acetic acid.

EVALUATION

Several factors must be kept in mind: (1) the patient may be asymptomatic, (2) the patient may be infected with multiple sexually transmitted organisms, and (3) the patient may be infected at more than one anatomic site.

History

Symptomatic male patients may complain of urethral discharge, dysuria, or pain in the testicles or epididy-mis. Symptoms in females include new vaginal discharge or change in the usual vaginal discharge, vulvar or vaginal irritation or itching, dysuria, lower abdominal pain, and abnormal menses. Both males and females may complain of rectal symptoms including discharge, bleeding, or tenesmus. They may also complain of genital lesions or a nongenital rash.

The history should include (1) time of last sexual contact, (2) number of sexual partners in the recent past, (3) sexual preference, (4) sites of exposure (penile, vaginal, rectal, oral), (5) previous STDs, and (6) recent antibiotic therapy. Patients should be asked about intravenous drug use, needle sharing, sex with intravenous drug users, exchange of sex for drugs or money, and condom use.

Physical Examination

In men, the physical examination includes inspection of the penis, with retraction of the foreskin in the uncircumcised, and inspection of the scrotum, with palpation of the testicles and epididymis. In women, the external genitalia and the perineum should be inspected. Speculum examination should be done for inspection of the vagina and cervix, and a bimanual pelvic examination should be performed.

In all patients, the skin, including the palms, should be carefully inspected; in addition, the pubic area should be examined for pubic lice or nits and the inguinal regions palpated for lymphadenopathy. In patients with a history of receptive anal intercourse, anal inspection should be done, and anoscopy should be performed on those complaining of rectal symptoms. The mouth and pharynx of patients with a history of orogenital contact should receive a thorough examination.

Additional Evaluation

Certain screening tests are routine. The studies that should be done for women are (1) cultures for *N. gonorrhoeae* from the endocervix, rectum, and pharynx (the last if there is a history of orogenital contact); (2) culture or antigen detection test for *C. trachomatis* from the endocervix; (3) Gram's stain of an endocervical smear; and (4) potassium hydroxide and saline wet mountings of vaginal secretions. In women who have had a hysterectomy, samples for gonorrheal and chlamydial testing should be taken from the urethra.

The studies that should be done for men are (1) urethral culture for *N. gonorrhoeae,* (2) culture or antigen detection test for *C. trachomatis* from the urethra, (3) rectal and pharyngeal cultures for *N. gonorrhoeae* if there is a history of anogenital or orogenital contact, and (4) Gram's stain of a urethral smear.

If there are genital lesions, other tests that may be warranted are viral culture for herpes simplex or darkfield examination for *T. pallidum.* All patients should have blood drawn for syphilis serology, and a human immunodeficiency virus (HIV) antibody test should be offered, especially to patients in high-risk groups. Those groups include (1) men who have sex with other men

(2) intravenous drug users, (3) commercial sex workers, (4) female partners of bisexual men, and (5) sexual contacts of intravenous drug users, commercial sex workers, and hemophiliacs.

MANAGEMENT

The reader is referred to the current STD treatment guidelines from the Centers for Disease Control and Prevention for a complete listing of management strategies, including alternative regimens. Table 67–2 lists the recommended regimens for the more common STD syndromes.

Epidemiologic Treatment of Sexual Partners

For some sexually transmitted diseases, treatment of the individual patient is not complete if sexual partners are not treated epidemiologically. Epidemiologic treatment of partners is treatment administered when a diagnosis is considered likely on clinical, laboratory, or epidemiologic grounds but before results of confirmatory tests are known. Epidemiologic treatment is an important tool in the control of STDs and should be given to sexual partners of individuals with gonococcal infection, chlamydial infection, nongonococcal urethritis, mucopurulent cervicitis, early syphilis (less than 1 year's duration), chancroid, and trichomoniasis. It is important that individuals being treated epidemiologically be examined and tested before treatment. It is

---

TABLE 67–2. Recommended Regimens for Common STDs*

Uncomplicated Chlamydial Infections
Doxycycline, 100 mg orally twice a day for 7 days
or
Azithromycin, 1 g orally in a single dose
Uncomplicated Gonococcal Infections
Ceftriaxone, 125 mg IM in a single dose
or
Cefixime, 400 mg orally in a single dose
or
Ciprofloxacin, 500 mg orally in a single dose
or
Ofloxacin, 400 mg orally in a single dose
plus
A regimen effective against *C. trachomatis*, such as doxycycline, 100 mg orally twice a day for 7 days
Genital Herpes
First episode: acyclovir, 200 mg orally 5 times a day for 7–10 days
Recurrent episode (within 2 days of onset of lesions): acyclovir, 200 mg orally 5 times a day for 5 days
Primary Syphilis
Benzathine penicillin G, 2.4 million units IM in a single dose
Chancroid
Azithromycin, 1 g orally in a single dose
or
Ceftriaxone, 250 mg IM in a single dose
or
Erythromycin base, 500 mg orally 4 times a day for 7 days
Genital Warts
Cryotherapy with liquid nitrogen
Trichomoniasis
Metronidazole, 2 g orally in a single dose

*For a complete listing of treatments, as well as alternative regimens, see the current STD treatment guidelines from the Centers for Disease Control and Prevention.

---

preferable not to prescribe medication for the partner if that person has not been seen.

Reporting Requirements

Some sexually transmitted diseases are reportable, and most states and territories have requirements for reporting. Reporting by clinician, by laboratory, or by both may be required. In the United States, gonorrhea, syphilis, chancroid, lymphogranuloma venereum, and granuloma inguinale are reportable at the federal level, and chlamydial disease is reportable in some states. Reporting is an important part of disease control efforts and is usually directed to local health departments. These organizations are staffed with disease intervention specialists who can track sexual contacts in order to get them treated.

PATIENT EDUCATION

Education is a key component of the management of a patient with an STD. In addition to basic information on the specific STD identified and on the medication prescribed, some general principles should be stressed. These include the importance of referring partners for treatment and not having sexual contact with untreated partners. The point should be made to the patient that if one is at risk for contracting one STD, one is also potentially at risk for contracting all the others, including infection with HIV. Strategies to reduce risk of infection should be discussed with the patient. Briefly, apart from abstinence, mutual monogamy between two uninfected partners is the least risky situation. Outside of mutual monogamy, one should avoid having multiple partners, avoid casual sexual contacts, and use barrier protection (condoms) for all sexual encounters.

PROGNOSIS

If patients are promptly diagnosed and appropriately managed, the prognosis for the majority of non-HIV sexually transmitted diseases is very good and infections are usually cured. Two exceptions should be noted: (1) All herpesviruses have the property of latency, and recurrent outbreaks of genital herpes are common. Recurrences tend to be less severe and less frequent over time. (2) None of the currently available therapies for genital warts has been shown to be completely effective in eradicating the human papillomavirus from underlying tissue, and recurrent disease is often seen.

Research Questions

1. *Ureaplasma urealyticum* is one cause of NGU, and *Mycoplasma genitalium* has been implicated as a possible cause. What role, if any, do these organisms play in the etiology of cervicitis?

2. What approaches other than those mentioned above could health care providers enlist to diminish the prevalence of STDs?

Case Resolution

The young man presented with classical symptoms and findings of genital herpes. The physician made the decision to initiate acyclovir therapy, resulting in rapid resolution of the active infection. The physician also made a point of educating the patient about this and other STDs.

Selected Readings

Arya, O. P., H. Mallison, B. E. Andrews, and M. Sillis. Diagnosis of urethritis: Role of polymorphonuclear leukocyte counts in Gram-stained urethral smears. Sex Transm Dis 11:10, 1984.

Bowie, W. R. Urethritis in males. *In* K. K. Holmes, et al (eds.). *Sexually Transmitted Diseases.* New York, McGraw-Hill Book Company, 1990.

Brunham, R. C., J. Paavonen, C. E. Stevens, et al. Mucopurulent cervicitis: The ignored counterpart in women of urethritis in men. N Engl J Med 311:1, 1984.

Centers for Disease Control and Prevention. *1993 Sexually Transmitted Diseases Treatment Guidelines.* MMWR 1993:42.

Corey, L., and P. G. Spear. Infections with herpes simplex virus. Parts 1 and 2. N Engl J Med 314:686, 749, 1986.

Holmes, K. K. Lower genital tract infections in women: Cystitis, urethritis, vulvovaginitis and cervicitis. *In* K. K. Holmes, et al (eds.). *Sexually Transmitted Diseases.* New York, McGraw-Hill Book Company, 1990.

Hutchinson, C. M., and E. W. Hook. Syphilis in adults. Med Clin North Am 74:1389, 1990.

Peterson, H. B., E. I. Galaid, and W. Cates. Pelvic inflammatory disease. Med Clin North Am 74:1603, 1990.

Schmid, G. P. Approach to the patient with genital ulcer disease. Med Clin North Am 74:1559, 1990.

Stamm, W. E., S. M. Kaetz, M. B. Bierne, and J. A. Ashman. *The Practitioner's Handbook for the Management of STDs.* Seattle, University of Washington Press, 1988, pp. 1.1–1.7.

CHAPTER 68

APPROACH TO THE HIV-POSITIVE PATIENT IN THE OUTPATIENT SETTING

Bruce Williams, M.D., M.P.H.

H$_x$ The patient is a 33-year-old female public school teacher who has come in a few times over the past year for a number of minor problems, including recurring candidal vaginitis, which responded promptly to topical therapy. She has been otherwise healthy and has come in today for a routine Pap test and to discuss contraceptive options, since she is starting a new relationship. Because a complete medical history, including a sexual history, has never been taken, it is done now. The patient reveals that 3 years ago she was intimately involved with a man whom she later discovered had also been having sexual relations with other women at the time. She broke off the relationship and has had no contact with him since. The physician suggests that, in addition to the Pap test, she be tested for syphilis, hepatitis B, and human immunodeficiency virus (HIV). The patient says that she had been thinking of being tested for HIV and agrees to do so. Her examination is normal except for a small amount of yeast on the vaginal smear. The laboratory results are normal except for the HIV serology, which is reactive by both ELISA and Western blot.

Questions

1. What questions is the patient likely to ask you about the test results and HIV disease?
2. What further laboratory tests should you order, and how will you use them to develop a management plan?
3. What are the social and emotional consequences of her diagnosis? What are your responsibilities in helping her and her friends and family?

For the first half of its 10- to 15-year natural history, HIV infection is a *silent* disease, raising few, if any, suspicions of its presence. Early intervention medically, socially, and emotionally with both the infected person and those in his or her social environment can significantly reduce morbidity and is often best done by a primary care clinician skilled in integrating medical, social, psychological, and emotional support services into a coherent interdisciplinary management plan.

PATHOPHYSIOLOGY

HIV is one of a group of RNA retroviruses exhibiting tropism for CD4-bearing cells known to cause disease in several mammalian species.

In humans, the cells predominantly affected belong to the helper/inducer subpopulation of T lymphocytes, although others such as monocytes/macrophages, Langerhans cells, follicular dendritic cells, and microglial cells can also be involved.

Infection by either of the two major strains of HIV (HIV-1, HIV-2) results in a slowly progressive depletion of the CD4 (helper) lymphocyte subpopulation and, for unclear reasons, the CD8 (cytotoxic) lymphocyte subpopulation.

The patient becomes susceptible to a wide variety of "opportunistic" infections whose onset apparently requires a profound deficiency of the CD4-mediated immune response. The pathogenesis of other manifestations of HIV disease, such as wasting syndrome, HIV encephalopathy (dementia), and HIV enteropathy is less clear and is the subject of current investigation. Recent research suggests that direct infection may not be the only mechanism of CD4 cell depletion. *In vitro* studies suggest that in the presence of HIV, uninfected T helper cells are also depleted, possibly through activation of a genetically encoded "programmed cell death" (apoptosis) with or without complement activation. The mechanism and clinical significance of this phenomenon are at present speculative.

Transmission of HIV appears to require the intimate exchange of cellular body fluids such as blood, semen, vaginal secretions, breast milk, cerebrospinal fluid, pleural fluid, and peritoneal fluid. Outside this environment, the virus's ability to cause infection disappears within hours. No reservoir outside of humans is known to exist, including arthropods such as mosquitoes, ticks, and mites. Urine, feces, and saliva, although cellular, do not appear to transmit the virus, probably because their chemical environment prohibits virus survival. Only through behaviors in which the exchange of "risk" fluids occurs can individuals become infected.

DIFFERENTIAL DIAGNOSIS

Diagnosis of HIV disease requires a high index of clinical suspicion based on a history of risk behavior, possible exposure, characteristic symptoms, and occasionally physical findings on routine examination (Table 68–1).

Clinical clues to the presence of HIV disease in **asymptomatic patients** may become apparent only if an adequate history is obtained. It is helpful to keep in mind that HIV transmission does not happen in "categories" but in a *network* of contacts. Exposure to the "risk" fluids of another person is, epidemiologically, the same as being exposed to all of that person's previous exposures.

Symptomatic patients may present with a number of nonspecific symptoms. On physical examination, generalized lymphadenopathy, oral thrush, shingles, or seborrheic dermatitis, especially in a young person (< 50 years), should raise the suspicion of HIV infection, even in the absence of a clear history of possible exposure.

Depending on the presenting signs and symptoms, alternatives to HIV disease include other infections (tuberculosis; deep fungal, occult abscesses; mononucleosis; cytomegalovirus [CMV]; rubella; secondary syphilis; *Rickettsia;* hepatitis), malignancy, connective tissue diseases, and drug reactions.

TABLE 68–1. Clues to Possible HIV Infection

History
Man having sex with other men (homosexual or bisexual)
Injection drug user
Transfusion/transplant recipient (before 1985)
   Blood or blood product recipient
   Hemophiliac
   Sperm recipient
   Organ transplant recipient
Occupational exposure
   Health care
   Fire/emergency
   Law enforcement/corrections
   Commercial sex worker (male/female)
Heterosexual partner of any of the above
Infant born to at-risk mother

Laboratory
Anemia (normocytic)
Lymphopenia
Thrombocytopenia
Elevated liver transaminases
Decreased total cholesterol
Increased total protein

Physical Examination
"Constitutional" symptoms
   Fevers
   Night sweats
   Unexplained weight loss
   Chronic diarrhea
   Fatigue
Generalized lymphadenopathy
Oral thrush
Shingles (especially multidermatomal)
Tuberculosis
Aseptic meningitis
Other sexually transmitted diseases
Seborrheic dermatitis
Dementia
Opportunistic disease
In women:
   Recurrent vaginal candidiasis
   Recurrent pelvic inflammatory disease
   Invasive cervical cancer

EVALUATION

History

A focused history for HIV patients (Box 68–1) is useful in providing a data base vital to the development of a comprehensive management plan. Because HIV disease is often associated with sexual, drug use, or occupational activities, other associated risks may be present and may have an impact on the patient's management.

A standard medical history including history of present illness, past medical and surgical history, immunizations, allergies, current medications (including "alternative" ones), substance use (including tobacco and alcohol), family history, and sexual history should be obtained.

A detailed social history is valuable in ascertaining the patient's living circumstances, next of kin, insurance status, and possible occupational risks.

A comprehensive review of systems may not only uncover current problems but also help in assessing the degree of immunodeficiency.

BOX 68-1. Questions to Ask to Assess Risk for HIV Disease

Sexual history

Do you have sex with men, women, or both sexes?

When you have sex do you engage in oral sex? Vaginal sex? Anal intercourse?

Do you always use condoms when you have sex?

As far as you know, have any of your sexual partners ever injected drugs? Had sex with homosexual men? Had sex with others who might have been exposed to HIV through drug use or sexual activity?

Have you ever had sex with a hemophiliac?

Drug use history

Have you used drugs in the past? If so, did you inject them? Did you share injecting equipment with anyone else? Which drugs have you used?

When did you use drugs?

History of sexually transmitted diseases

Have you ever been infected with gonorrhea? Syphilis? Herpes? *Chlamydia* (nongonococcal urethritis, cervicitis)? Hepatitis B? If so, when?

Other

Have you ever had a blood transfusion? If so, when?

Do you have hemophilia?

Have you ever had an organ or tissue transplant? If so, when?

Been artificially inseminated? If so, when?

Been exposed to someone else's blood or sexual fluids in your occupation?

A comprehensive physical examination (Table 68–2) should be conducted on all new HIV-positive patients, followed by a shorter, more focused examination at follow-up visits.

Additional Evaluation

Diagnosis of HIV infection in adults is made through serologic (anti-HIV Ab) testing. An initially positive screening test (ELISA) is followed by a confirmatory test (Western blot, radioimmunoprecipitation assay [RIPA], or indirect immunofluorescence assay [IFA]). Sensitivity and specificity of this combination exceed 99%, and it is thought to be diagnostic of HIV infection. Because these are antibody tests, false-negative results may occur if exposure to HIV is too recent for adequate antibody response to have occurred. This "window period" is approximately 6–12 weeks, with 95% of exposed individuals seroconverting by 6 months after exposure. False-positive results can occur if the patient has another type of infection at the time of testing, since antibodies elicited may "look like" HIV antibodies tested for by the ELISA. For a confirmatory test to be considered positive, two of three "diagnostic" antibodies (p24, gp41, gp160/120) must be detected. A difficult diagnostic dilemma is encountered when only one HIV-related antibody is detected on the confirmatory test following a reactive ELISA. In these "indeterminate" cases, nonantibody tests such as immune-complex dissociated (ICD) p24 Ag assay, HIV co-culture, and polymerase chain reaction (PCR) may be helpful.

Because HIV disease has important social and legal implications, many states and institutions require that patients be fully apprised of these before *and* after being tested for HIV. At a minimum, this counseling should include

1. A description of the tests and their interpretation.
2. Prognosis and options for medical care in the event of a positive test.
3. Possible social implications (discrimination in housing, occupation, insurance) of being tested, regardless of test results.
4. Mechanisms of disease transmission and measures recommended to prevent it.

For those testing positive, arrangements for medical care as well as social and emotional support should be made as soon as possible.

Laboratory tests to be ordered after diagnosis will vary somewhat depending on clinical circumstances. Baseline laboratory tests commonly obtained are listed in Table 68–3. HbcAb is obtained to ascertain the need for active HBV vaccination. A baseline chest radiograph may be useful at a later date for comparison purposes, i.e., in cases of equivocal pulmonary disease, especially *Pneumocystis carinii* pneumonia (PCP).

Although not specific for HIV, certain laboratory abnormalities are frequently present in otherwise asymptomatic HIV patients. Lymphopenia, normocytic anemia, thrombocytopenia, mildly elevated hepatic transaminases, decreased total cholesterol, or increased triglycerides may be present relatively early.

MANAGEMENT

Management of HIV patients need not be overwhelming. It is important to approach problems systematically and singly. By developing and updating a problem list that includes social, mental health, and nutritional as well as medical problems, a complete plan can be formulated. In this process, the patient is a partner, contributing not only history and symptoms but often solutions as well.

Not everything needs to be done at once. Frequent follow-up visits often are necessary at first to tackle all the problems as well as cement the therapeutic relationship. Table 68–3 summarizes the management of adults with HIV disease.

Strategies for the use of antiretroviral therapies are evolving rapidly. Consensus is emerging that aggressive combination therapy with two or perhaps three agents initiated early in the disease process may improve outcome. Although definitive studies are still in progress, combinations of reverse transcriptase inhibitors (zidovudine [ZDV], didanosine [ddI], zalcitabine [ddC], stavudine [d4T], lamivudine [3TC]) and protease inhibitors are likely to be the antiretroviral regimens of choice in coming years. Common side effects such as

TABLE 68–2. Physical Examination in HIV-infected Patients

Examine	Watch for	Think
Vital signs		
Temperature	Fever	Infection, malignancy
Respirations	Tachypnea	*Pneumocystis carinii* pneumonia (PCP), other causes of pneumonia, lymphoma, Kaposi's sarcoma (KS)
Weight	Weight loss	Wasting, malignancy, tuberculosis
Skin	Rash	KS, seborrheic dermatitis, infection, folliculitis
	Nodules	KS, fungal infection, warts, malignancy, molluscum contagiosum
	Petechiae, bruising	Idiopathic thrombocytopenic purpura
Nodes	Enlargement	Persistent generalized lymphadenopathy (PGL), lymphoma, *Mycobacterium avium* complex (MAC), tuberculosis
Eyes		
Visual acuity	Vision loss	Cytomegalovirus (CMV) retinitis
Pupils	Argyll-Robertson	Neurosyphilis
Retina	Cotton wool spots	Benign
	Periarteriolar lesions	CMV retinitis
Oropharynx	White lesions	Thrush, oral hairy leukoplakia
	Red lesions	KS, thrush
	Ulcers	Herpes simplex virus (HSV), aphthous ulcers
	Nodules	Warts, KS, lymphoma
	Gingivitis	Dental referral
Chest	May be clear	PCP, lymphoma, KS
Cardiovascular system	Murmur, S_3/S_4	Congestive heart failure, IV drug use–related valvular disease
Abdomen	Hepato(spleno)megaly	Hepatitis, KS, MAC, lymphoma
Genitourinary system	Ulcers	HSV, syphilis
Rectum	Ulcers	HSV, gonorrhea
	Heme + stool	Infection, KS, lymphoma, fissures, hemorrhoids
	Masses	Condyloma acuminatum, malignancy
Extremities	Decreased perfusion	Vasculitis
	Joint effusion	Septic arthritis, autoimmune disease
Neurologic system		
Mental status examination	Delirium, cognitive deficits	AIDS dementia, (meningo)encephalitis, metabolic disorder
Cranial nerves	Focal deficits	Lymphoma, vasculitis, meningitis, encephalitis
Motor function	Focal deficits	Same as above, progressive multifocal leukoencephalopathy (PML)
Sensory function	Focal deficits	Peripheral neuropathy, vasculitis
Cerebellar function	Focal deficits	PML, infection

headache, peripheral neuropathy, nausea, diarrhea, anemia, and neutropenia may limit compliance.

For patients with CD4 cell counts <200, prophylaxis against *P. carinii* pneumonia with trimethoprim-sulfamethoxazole, dapsone, or, for sulfa-intolerant patients, aerosolized pentamidine is considered standard care. The advisability and efficacy of prophylaxis against fungal diseases or disseminated *Mycobacterium avium* complex (DMAC) are less clear, and as yet no regimen is universally accepted.

PATIENT AND FAMILY EDUCATION

Perhaps more important than medical intervention are patient and family education and counseling. Especially at the time of diagnosis, fears of death, isolation, pain, and contagion frequently arise. Patients are often sure they are going to become invalids and die within days or weeks. Families are often afraid they might have already been exposed and are torn between the desire to be supportive and fear of becoming infected. All are frightened of what friends and colleagues will say or do. They are faced with a socially stigmatized disease that will be progressively disabling and ultimately fatal. The role of the primary care clinician in these circumstances should be to provide a safe context in which these fears can be dealt with in a realistic, mutually supportive way.

Conferences first with the patient and then the entire family can be extremely helpful in clarifying questions about medical management, prognosis, confidentiality, patient responsibility, emotional issues, and terminal care (Table 68–4).

It is important to remember that a "therapeutic" relationship requires both trust and time. It is not possible to "fix" things all at once. Patients and families need time to process both the information they receive and their feelings about it. The most helpful thing the primary care clinician can do is be available when needed.

NATURAL HISTORY/PROGNOSIS

In general, staging systems have not proved to be clinically useful in managing HIV disease. The 1993 CDC HIV Classification System and Expanded AIDS Surveillance Definition for Adolescents and Adults and the Walter Reed Staging Classification for HIV Infection are cumbersome to apply and of limited clinical value.

Accurate, objective measurement of disease progression has been elusive with regard to HIV disease. A number of "surrogate" laboratory markers, including direct measurement of viral burden (PCR, p24 Ag), immune system activation (β_2-microglobulin, neopterin), and quantitative measurements of T-lymphocyte

TABLE 68–3. Health Care Maintenance for Adults with HIV Disease

	Initial Contact	CD4 Count			
		> 500	< 500	< 200	< 100
Complete history and physical examination	X				
Follow-up		6 months	3 months	3 months	3 months
Laboratory					
CBC (differential, platelet count)	X	6 months	3 months	1 month	1 month
SMA-20	X		3 months	3 months	3 months
HBcAb	X				
Syphilis serology	X				
CD4 count	X	6 months	1–3 months	1–3 months	X
Chest x-ray (baseline)				X	X
PPD/control	X				
Immunizations					
Influenza		1 year	1 year	1 year	1 year
Pneumovax	X				
HBV*	If HbcAb negative				
Td	As indicated (every 10 years)				
Antiretroviral therapy			X	X	X
PCP prophylaxis†				X	X
MAC prophylaxis‡					X
Fungal prophylaxis§					X
AIDS case report	At diagnosis			X	X
Referrals					
Case manager	X				
Ophthalmologist‡					6 months
Dentist	Every 6 months or as indicated				
Women only					
Pap smear	Every year or as indicated				

*Dosage of HBV vaccine should be that indicated by the manufacturer for renal dialysis patients.
†PCP prophylaxis is indicated in adult patients with CD4 < 200, prior PCP, or symptomatic HIV disease.
‡Not universally accepted as standard of care.
§Not universally accepted as standard of care. Most regimens utilize fluconazole at various doses and frequencies.

TABLE 68–4. Counseling Patients and Families

Medical
Pathogenesis
Transmission
Natural history and prognosis
Therapies
Follow-up schedule
Confidentiality
Medical records
Family/friends
Workplace
Patient Responsibility
Safer sex, including informing partners of HIV status
Avoid
  Blood transmission
  Needle sharing
  Toothbrush sharing
  Razor sharing
  Invasive procedures (health care workers)
Notify all health care providers of HIV status
Emotional Support
Isolation
Fear of dying
Guilt
Shame
Therapeutic resources, including support groups
Death and Dying
Control of symptoms (e.g., pain, nausea, diarrhea)
"Code status" (living will)
Medical decisions (durable medical power of attorney)
Care of surviving dependents

subpopulations (CD4, CD8) have been investigated. It should be remembered that regardless of the relative merit of other markers, nearly all studies establishing the efficacy and timing of currently recommended therapeutic and prophylactic interventions have used absolute CD4 counts as the relevant surrogate marker. For the foreseeable future, this marker will remain the standard for use in clinical care although new viral burden assays (RT-RNA, bDNA) are attracting considerable interest.

Acute Primary Infection

Within approximately 2–4 weeks after exposure to HIV, an acute clinical syndrome lasting 1–2 weeks may develop, characterized by fever, night sweats, lethargy and malaise, myalgias, arthralgias, generalized lymphadenopathy, pharyngitis, maculopapular rash, or headache. These symptoms vary in both frequency and severity and are often similar in presentation to other viral syndromes. This phase is self-limited, usually resolving within 1–2 weeks. Transient lymphopenia followed by lymphocytosis with or without atypical lymphocyte morphology, mild thrombocytopenia, and an elevated erythrocyte sedimentation rate (ESR) may be noted during the first several weeks after exposure. Serum chemistries are generally normal.

BOX 68-2. Diagnostic Approach to Opportunistic Disease

1. Do not rely on a "unifying diagnosis" to explain all signs and symptoms. HIV patients can, and often do, have more than one opportunistic disease simultaneously.
2. Think categorically and systematically. List each problem separately, then consider *by category* the most likely possibilities.
3. Don't try to do everything at once. Start with the most likely possibility, and work toward the less likely later. When you make a diagnosis, treat it and observe. If the problem goes away, further diagnostic tests may be unnecessary.
4. If too many things are happening at once and they appear to be dangerous, hospitalize the patient.
5. Therapy can sometimes be the most effective diagnostic maneuver you can make. Treat the most likely diagnosis; if the problem resolves, you have the diagnosis. If not, keep looking.
6. Know the difference between what is curable, what is treatable, and what is neither. You can't fix everything, but you *can* help people feel better.

Asymptomatic Disease

This prolonged phase (months to years after exposure) was once thought to represent a dormant "latent" phase during which proviral DNA was sequestered in the infected CD4-cell genome with little pathogenic activity occurring, although transmission was still possible.

Recent evidence, however, strongly suggests that viral replication and transcellular infection does in fact occur during this phase but remains relatively localized to the reticuloendothelial system, although person-to-person transmission still occurs.

BOX 68-3. Terminal Care of HIV Patients

1. Start with a frank, private discussion with the patient regarding current clinical status and prognosis. Usually the patient will know before you do that death is coming soon and is often relieved when you ask, "Do you think you are dying?"
2. Reaffirm that even if further therapeutic and diagnostic efforts are suspended, "comfort" care will continue. Patients need to know that you will not abandon them just because they no longer need medical therapies and that they will not suffer pain or discomfort.
3. Make sure that a current living will and durable power of attorney have been completed and signed by the patient.
4. Mortuary arrangements should be made.
5. Arrange (with the patient's permission) a family conference to discuss prognosis, the patient's decisions regarding further care, and feelings of family members. Try to catalyze a consensus between patient and family; encourage them to talk (and cry) together about their feelings. The possibility of postmortem examination may also be discussed.
6. Meet with other involved health care providers to discuss the plan.
7. Arrange for location of care (home, hospice, skilled nursing facility, etc).
8. Visit the patient regularly, and discuss care with the health care team.

Typically, physical signs and symptoms are few or absent. Generalized lymphadenopathy and occasional bouts of fatigue, fevers, or anorexia may occur but generally are mild and self-limited. Most often, patients are unaware of their illness. Laboratory tests (often obtained for other reasons) may show nonspecific abnormalities.

Symptomatic Disease

Although symptoms referable to HIV disease (see Table 68–1) may occur at any time, they emerge more frequently with CD4 ≤ 500 cells/mm^3. Often, constitutional symptoms such as fevers, night sweats, fatigue, diarrhea, and anorexia will occur cyclically, becoming prominent for several months, then disappearing entirely for several months.

In patients with CD4 <200–300 cells/mm^3, symptoms may be due to an underlying opportunistic disease. A comprehensive review of the recognition and management of these infections and malignancies is beyond the scope of this chapter. In general, though, several observations can be made (Box 68–2).

Terminal Care

Although catastrophic, rapidly lethal events do occur, the terminal stage of HIV disease is typically a slow, progressive decline of somatic and neuropsychologic function. Rapid weight loss, numerous opportunistic diseases, and profound mental deterioration are common.

Decisions about where and how to treat dying patients can be very challenging. The patient, family, other involved health care workers, and the primary care physician may have different feelings about the best way to proceed. Each case will be different, but the patient must be empowered to make his or her own choice about quality versus quantity of life. The physician must respect that decision, provide care accordingly, and help the patient's family live with this choice, all within the ethical constraints of the medical profession (Box 68–3).

Research Questions

1. Can more effective antiretroviral strategies be developed? Current areas of investigation include molecular targets in the HIV replication cycle other than reverse transcriptase, and immunotherapy (cytokines, clonal CD8 expansion).
2. Can effective vaccines be developed to either prevent or treat HIV disease?
3. Can better prophylaxis and treatment of opportunistic diseases be developed?
4. What social interventions are necessary to prevent the spread of the epidemic and decrease its psychological impact on survivors?
5. Is the demographic character of the epidemic in the United States changing, and if so, what implications does this have for prevention efforts and future medical care?

Case Resolution

At the follow-up visit, the physician informed the patient of her diagnosis and spent an hour discussing the nature of HIV disease, its pathogenesis, transmission, and natural history. The physician listened carefully to her fears, answered her questions, and assured her of continued care. The physician offered to meet with her new boyfriend to help him adjust to the situation. She received instruction about safer sex practices and was referred to a local AIDS service organization that has a special support program for HIV-positive women.

Further laboratory work and a follow-up visit for the following week were scheduled. Her CD4 count was 337. The patient declined to take zidovudine (ZDV) because she had heard that the side effects were intolerable and that "it probably doesn't help anyway." She agreed to think about it further, though, and another follow-up visit was scheduled in 2 weeks' time.

Selected Readings

Bartlett, J. G. *The Johns Hopkins Hospital Guide to Medical Care of Patients with HIV Infection,* 5th ed. Baltimore, Williams & Wilkins, 1995.

DeVita, V. T., S. E. Hellman, and S. A. Rosenberg (eds.). *AIDS: Etiology, Diagnosis, Treatment and Prevention.* Philadelphia, J. B. Lippincott, 1992.

Edison, T. (ed.). *The AIDS Caregiver's Handbook* (rev. ed.). New York, St. Martin's Press, 1993.

Sande, M. A., and P. A. Volberding (eds.). *The Medical Management of AIDS,* 4th ed. Philadelphia, W.B. Saunders Company, 1995.

Sanford, J. P., M. A. Sande, D. N. Gilbert, and J. L. Gerberdig. *The Sanford Guide to HIV/AIDS Therapy.* Dallas, Antimicrobial Therapy, 1995.

COMMON ISSUES IN WOMEN'S HEALTH

CHAPTER 69

BREAST DISORDERS

Carolyn Voss, M.D., and John H. Saiki, M.D.

H_x   A 48-year-old female personnel manager notices a slightly tender nodular area in her left breast during her monthly breast self-examination. She has had one pregnancy and bore a child at age 30 years; she continues to have regular menstrual cycles. On physical examination, a 1.5-cm, firm nodule is felt in the upper outer quadrant of the left breast. A mammogram shows "dense fibroglandular changes, unchanged from a previous examination done 1 year ago."

Questions

1. What are the diagnostic possibilities?
2. How should further evaluation proceed?
3. What other historical information would help you assess the patient's risk for breast cancer?

Breast disease is commonly seen in primary care practice, with over 50% of women being affected in some way during their lives. Breast biopsy is the most common of all surgical procedures. Benign breast diseases consist of both fibrocystic complex (the name given to a large group of proliferative and nonproliferative disorders) and inflammations of various types (including infections). Breast cancer is the most common malignancy affecting women.

PATHOPHYSIOLOGY

Healthy, normal women experience tenderness and engorgement of the breasts prior to the menstrual period that resolve spontaneously following menses. This is due to swelling of the epithelial lobular cells of the breast as a result of hormonal changes. With fibrocystic change, these manifestations are more pronounced, and palpation can reveal nodular thickening and even masses or cysts. The etiology of fibrocystic change is not clear, but hormones may play a role. Fibrocystic change (e.g., chronic inflammation, mild epithelial hyperplasia, fibrosis, cyst formation) is present to a varying degree in most women. Cysts may be single or multiple and can present as a lump or lumps.

They result from obstructed ductules and the accumulation of entrapped secretions within lobules.

Cancer is not a sequel of fibrocystic change. However, florid hyperplasia and atypical epithelial hyperplasia are associated with an increased risk of breast cancer, 1.5–2 and 5 times the normal risk, respectively. The BRCA1 gene on chromosome 17 is a tumor suppressor gene, and a mutation of this gene carries a 90% risk of breast cancer development. The gene is more prevalent in familial breast cancer and is almost always present in families in which both breast cancer and ovarian cancer develop. In addition, it is believed to be almost always present in women with breast cancer who are younger than age 30 years. Breast cancers most commonly develop in the upper outer quadrant of the breast. The characteristic hardness is due to their propensity to induce desmoplasia (proliferation of fibrous tissue). They metastasize most commonly to the axillary lymph nodes by invasion of lymphatics and also can spread systemically through vascular invasion. Tumors less than 1 cm in diameter are associated with metastasis in less than 10% of patients. Tumors larger than 1 cm without evidence of spread to the regional lymph nodes will show recurrence in 20% of patients. When the lymph nodes are positive for metastatic tumor, the risk of systemic recurrence increases with the number of nodes involved.

DIFFERENTIAL DIAGNOSIS

Pain in the breast, as well as breast lumpiness or a breast mass, can signify many different things, ranging from normal cyclic changes to breast cancer. Although nodularity, lumps, and even nipple discharge can occur as part of normal menstrual breast changes, other diagnoses must always be considered.

Inflammatory disorders of the breast are listed in Table 69–1. Acute inflammation typically occurs in lactating women or in the setting of trauma; more chronic inflammatory disorders are most commonly seen in the perimenopausal years (ages 40–60 years).

Fibrocystic complex is the term used to describe a large group of breast abnormalities (Table 69–2). Other terms are fibrocystic breast disease, fibrocystic

TABLE 69–1. Inflammatory Disorders of the Breast

Disorder	Clinical Features
Lactating Women (Infectious)	
Acute mastitis	Postpartum, during lactation. Usually *Staphylococcus aureus*, may be *Streptococcus*.
Mammary abscess	Progression of acute mastitis. Painful, red mass.
Nonlactating Women (Noninfectious)	
Chronic periductal mastitis	Asymptomatic biopsy finding.
Duct ectasia	Nipple pain, burning, discharge. Palpable subareolar swelling.
Granulomatous mastitis	Result of chronic duct ectasia, especially with trauma.
Fat necrosis	Painful, tender mass, often post-traumatic.
Mammary duct fistula	Inflamed duct erodes through skin, usually near areola.
Periductal fibrosis	Follows long-standing inflammation. May present as mass.
Superficial thrombophlebitis	Pain, recent trauma. May cause skin retraction.

TABLE 69–2. Categories of Fibrocystic Complex, with Corresponding Risk Levels for Invasive Breast Carcinoma

Category of Histologic Change	Specific Entities	Risk Category (Relative Risk)
Nonproliferative (70% of cases of fibrocystic complex)	Adenosis (sclerosing or florid) Apocrine metaplasia Cysts (macro or micro) Duct ectasia Fibroadenoma Fibrosis Hyperplasia (mild: not more than 4 cells in depth) Mastitis Periductal mastitis Squamous metaplasia	No increased risk (1)
Proliferative without atypia (20% of cases)	Hyperplasia (moderate or florid, solid or papillary) Papilloma with fibrovascular core	Slightly increased risk (1.5–2)
Proliferative with atypia (7% of cases)	Atypical hyperplasia (borderline lesion, ductal or lobular)	Moderately increased risk (4–5)
Carcinoma in situ (3% of cases)	Ductal Lobular	Significantly increased risk (8–10)

change, and proliferative breast disease. In the majority (70%) of women with fibrocystic complex, the breast biopsy shows nonproliferative changes. In this situation, the risk for developing subsequent breast cancer is not increased compared to that of women without such changes.

Breast cancer should always be considered when a breast lump is found on physical examination. However, most lumps in premenopausal women are benign, whereas a lump in a postmenopausal woman is most likely malignant. Importantly, no historical, physical, or mammographic finding can reliably rule out malignancy. Benign cysts can be identified by ultrasonography or by

aspiration. A biopsy should be performed on all solid lumps.

Very rarely, metastatic disease, tuberculosis, and chest wall tumors can present as pain or lumps in the breast. Pain in the breast can also arise from any disease process involving the intercostal nerves.

EVALUATION

History

The physician should ask the patient how long she has noticed the pain or lump, whether the finding comes and goes, and how it is related to her menstrual cycle. The patient's menstrual status should be noted. A lump or area of lumpiness that disappears completely after a menstrual period is likely to be a manifestation of fibrocystic complex. Inflammation and fibrocystic change often result in pain in the breast; although breast cancer is usually painless, the presence of pain does not rule out a malignant process.

Every woman's breast cancer risk should be assessed (Table 69–3). A family history of breast cancer in a first-degree relative (mother or sister) is the single most important risk factor. It is especially significant if the mother was premenopausal at the time of her diagnosis or if she had bilateral breast cancer. The majority of women who develop breast cancer, however, have no known risk factors.

Physical Examination

Breast self-examination should be as routine for a woman as brushing her teeth, and her physician should reinforce this concept. Getting to know how her breasts feel normally will greatly improve a woman's ability to know when an abnormality occurs.

A thorough breast examination should be done by a physician annually. This examination should include (1) inspecting the breasts and nipples for asymmetry (which is often a normal finding), skin changes, and nipple discharge; (2) palpating the entire breast with the woman in both the sitting and the lying position; and (3) checking the axillae for lymph nodes.

Any area of the breast that feels irregular warrants further consideration, but symmetric, diffuse, bilateral nodularity (often tender) is the typical finding in

TABLE 69–3. Risk Factors for Breast Cancer

Family history of breast cancer
Previous history of breast cancer
Early menarche (before age 12 years)
Late menopause (after age 53 years)
Nulliparity
Delayed childbearing (after age 30 years)
Increased age
Biopsy-proven ductal or lobular hyperplasia, especially with atypia
High-fat diet
Excessive alcohol intake
Higher socioeconomic status
Obesity

fibrocystic complex. A solitary lump always requires further assessment, whether or not it is tender.

Additional Evaluation

Laboratory tests are generally unhelpful in the initial evaluation of breast problems, except in the case of nipple discharge. In this situation, a Sudan B fat stain can be done to confirm galactorrhea. If galactorrhea is confirmed, thyroid function and a prolactin level should be measured. Cytologic examination of nipple discharge is rarely useful.

Mammography is key in evaluating the breast. Although the use of routine screening mammography in the age group 40–49 years is controversial, it is the authors' belief that screening mammograms should be done every 2 years between the ages of 40 and 49 years, and every year thereafter. A woman with a family history of breast cancer should have a baseline study in her thirties and a mammogram every year after age 40 years. A negative mammogram in a woman with a breast lump does *not* rule out cancer.

Since neither the physical examination nor the mammogram definitively rules out cancer, fine-needle aspiration or biopsy of the suspicious area is necessary. An experienced surgeon is crucial in the evaluation of breast abnormalities. Algorithms for the workup of premenopausal and postmenopausal women with breast lumps are shown in Figures 69–1 and 69–2, respectively.

MANAGEMENT

Infections of the breast are usually caused by skin flora and may be severe enough to require intravenous antibiotic therapy.

Once a diagnosis of fibrocystic complex has been established, the goals of treatment are to slow progression and to decrease pain and tenderness. A well-fitted bra with good support can help somewhat, especially for women who are active in athletics. There is some evidence that dietary modification (including supplementation with certain vitamins) can improve symptoms in certain subpopulations of women (Table 69–4).

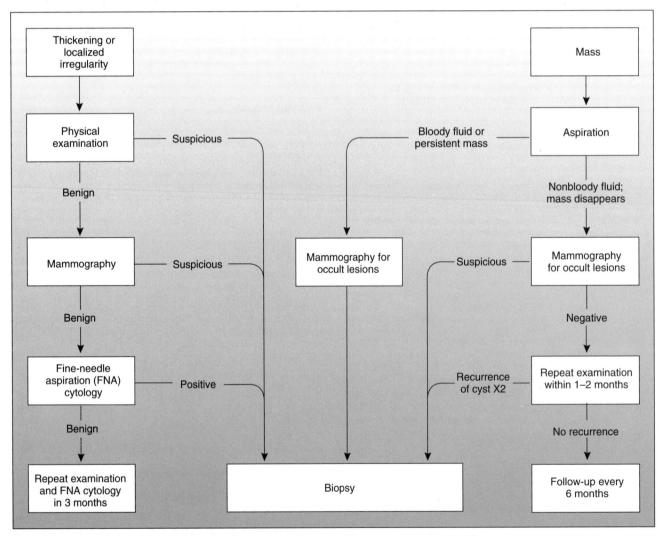

FIGURE 69–1. *Algorithm for evaluation of breast abnormalities in premenopausal women. (Reproduced, with permission, from P. J. Deckers and A. Ricci. Pain and lumps in the female breast. Hosp Pract 27[A]:87, 1992.)*

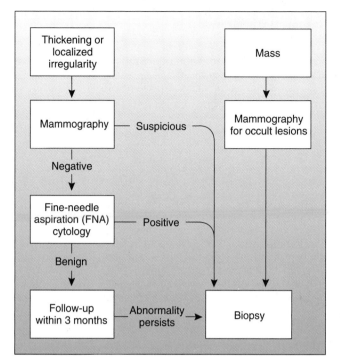

FIGURE 69–2. *Algorithm for evaluation of breast abnormalities in peri- and postmenopausal women. (Reproduced, with permission, from P. J. Deckers and A. Ricci. Pain and lumps in the female breast. Hosp Pract 27[2A]:88, 1992.)*

The most consistently effective therapy for premenopausal women is oral contraceptive medication. It will decrease tenderness, and perhaps nodularity, in 60%–70% of women by 6 months. Danazol, an androgen, is also effective but has more adverse effects (including amenorrhea, headache, acne, and edema). For postmenopausal women, lowering or discontinuing estrogen replacement therapy may be necessary. Increasing the amount of progesterone relative to the amount of estrogen given for hormonal replacement therapy can also alleviate symptoms. Tamoxifen has also been effective.

When a diagnosis of breast cancer is made, the patient should consult with both a radiation oncologist and a medical oncologist in addition to her surgeon. Lumpectomy with primary radiotherapy provides equivalent

TABLE 69–4.   Treatment of Fibrocystic Breast Disease

Effective Therapies
Oral contraceptives (lower estrogen, higher progesterone)
Danazol
Luteal-phase progesterone
Tamoxifen
Lowering dosage of or discontinuing estrogen replacement therapy
Possibly Effective Therapies
Vitamin E supplementation
Abstinence from methylxanthines (e.g., tea, coffee, chocolate)
Bromocriptine
Unproved Therapies (Probably Ineffective)
Diuretics
Thyroid hormone
Vitamins A, B

results to a modified radical mastectomy in the local control of breast cancer. However, when the cancer is multicentric or the lesion is so large that lumpectomy would significantly deform the breast, a modified radical mastectomy is the treatment of choice. Additionally, if there is significant axillary lymph node metastasis, a modified radical mastectomy is the preferred approach. When the lymph nodes are not involved by tumor and the breast primary lesion is less than 1 cm in diameter, systemic treatment is not necessary. If the primary is greater than 1 cm, with or without positive lymph nodes, adjuvant chemotherapy (CMF: cyclophosphamide, methotrexate, fluorouracil) should be administered. All patients with positive lymph nodes should receive adjuvant chemotherapy (CMF). More aggressive chemotherapy (FAC: fluorouracil, doxorubicin [Adriamycin], cyclophosphamide) should be considered in women with more than three lymph nodes involved. When there is a diagnosis of inflammatory carcinoma or there is extensive lymph node metastasis (> 8 nodes), high-dose chemotherapy with or without stem cell harvesting or marrow transplantation is required. All of these treatment approaches apply to the premenopausal and young postmenopausal woman, regardless of hormone receptor status. In the elderly woman with positive estrogen or progesterone receptors, regardless of the extent of disease, treatment with tamoxifen (an estrogen blocker) alone should be considered. Tamoxifen should also be considered for all women with tumors positive for estrogen or progesterone receptors; i.e., at the completion of systemic chemotherapy. The risk of metastatic disease and the risk of a second primary breast cancer are both reduced with the addition of tamoxifen.

PATIENT AND FAMILY EDUCATION

All women should receive instruction and reinforcement regarding the techniques and importance of breast self-examination. Women should be instructed to obtain a second opinion when they feel a lump they believe is significantly abnormal and their physician believes (without a biopsy) it is benign. If the second opinion is that the lump is benign and the patient still feels uneasy, she should request a biopsy.

When a breast biopsy shows a malignancy, communication with the patient and family is as important as the medical treatment of the cancer. The nature of the disease, its risk in other female members of the family, its evaluation, its treatment, and its prognosis must be discussed in detail. The potential complications of treatment should also be discussed.

Finally, an intimate discussion of the social and emotional problems associated with having breast cancer is crucial to the well-being of the patient and her family. This discussion might first take place with the patient and her spouse, but a second discussion should include all family members. Open and frank communication between patient and spouse is the most important factor in living with cancer. This means not only sharing each other's concerns, but also each other's emotions or feelings. Patients and families have a need to cry together, and they should not feel compelled to constantly protect each other.

NATURAL HISTORY/PROGNOSIS

For the large majority of women who have fibrocystic complex without proliferative changes, the natural history is usually characterized by waxing and waning pain and tenderness. For most women, menopause results in relief of symptoms (unless estrogen replacement is prescribed), although nodularity of the breasts may remain. If proliferative changes are found on breast biopsy, the woman's increased risk for subsequent breast cancer must be taken into account when planning frequency of screening mammography and clinical follow-up.

The most important clinical parameter influencing prognosis in breast cancer is the number of axillary lymph nodes involved by metastasis. The next most important factor is the size of the primary lesion. Finally, the pathologist's evaluation plays a key role in predicting the behavior of the tumor (see below).

When the lymph nodes are negative and the primary lesion is less than 1 cm in diameter, the long-term survival is > 90%. If the primary lesion is greater than 1 cm and the lymph nodes are negative, the long-term survival is > 80%. The presence of estrogen or progesterone receptors (or both) is a favorable prognostic sign. A high S-phase fraction and high DNA content portend a poorer prognosis. The risk of recurrence is markedly reduced after 5 years, but the possibility of recurrence always exists.

Research Questions

1. Can noninvasive tests be devised for women with fibrocystic complex to differentiate those with proliferative changes from those without?
2. Can dietary modification prevent breast cancer?

Case Resolution

The patient was referred to a surgeon with expertise in breast disease. A biopsy of the breast nodule was positive for cancer. The patient underwent a lumpectomy with lymph node dissection, and a 1.1-cm tumor was removed. All lymph nodes were negative, and both estrogen and progesterone receptors were positive. Radiation therapy followed. The patient was then referred to a medical oncologist for possible systemic chemotherapy.

Selected Readings

Deckers, P. J., and A. Ricci. Pain and lumps in the female breast. Hosp Pract 27(2A):67–94, 1992.

Eddy, D. M. Screening for breast cancer. Ann Intern Med 111:389–99, 1989.

Harris, J. R., M. E. Lippman, U. Veronesi, and W. Willett. Breast cancer. N Engl J Med 327:390–8, 1992.

CHAPTER 70

VAGINITIS

Lesley W. Janis, M.D.

H$_x$ A 23-year-old female student teacher presents with a 3-day history of a foul-smelling vaginal discharge, vaginal irritation, and itching. She is sexually active with one partner and is quite concerned about her current symptoms. She has never been pregnant, uses oral contraceptives, and has regular menses. Her last period ended 1 week ago. She has never had an abnormal Pap test or a sexually transmitted disease. She takes no medications and denies significant medical problems or past surgeries. On pelvic examination, the cervix is erythematous and a thin discharge is pooled in the vaginal vault.

Questions

1. What additional questions do you want to ask this patient?
2. What diagnostic tests should be performed?
3. What patient education issues are important to address with this patient?

Vaginitis has been estimated to account for over half of all outpatient visits made to primary care physicians by their female patients. Although there are numerous potential causes of vaginitis and abnormal vaginal discharge, approximately 90% of cases are caused by a few conditions. With a thorough history, a focused physical examination, and a few basic diagnostic procedures, the diagnosis can often be made in the office.

PATHOPHYSIOLOGY

The normal vaginal environment includes vaginal secretions, cellular elements, and microorganisms existing in balance. Normal vaginal mucosa consists of glycogen-rich epithelial cells that are supported by estrogen. Normal vaginal flora consists of numerous bacteria, with lactobacilli being the most common. Through a complex process involving enzymatic breakdown of glycogen by local bacteria and other factors, lactic acid is produced. This results in the normally acidic pH of the vaginal environment, which inhibits the growth of potentially pathogenic microorganisms.

Many factors can disrupt this balance, among them, trauma to the epithelium, changes in hormonal levels, the use of certain douches or soaps, and the introduction of sexually transmitted microorganisms. These events often result in a change in the normally acidic pH or an overgrowth of potentially pathogenic organisms that normally are held in check. Local irritation and a change in vaginal secretions prompt the patient to seek treatment.

DIFFERENTIAL DIAGNOSIS

Vaginitis is defined as inflammation of the vulvovaginal mucosa; this inflammation can have a number of causes and result in a variety of symptoms. The symptoms commonly encountered in vaginitis (abnormal vaginal discharge, irritation, itching, malodor, dysuria, dyspareunia) are also seen in a variety of other settings (Table 70–1).

True vaginitis is most commonly due to bacterial vaginosis, candidiasis, or trichomoniasis. Atrophic vaginitis is common in postmenopausal women. Viral infections such as herpes simplex and human papillomavirus can also present as vaginal/vulvar irritation with discharge. While cervicitis related to sexually transmitted organisms can result in similar symptoms, particularly vaginal discharge, it is important to remember that it is a separate entity. It is also important to realize that multiple infectious agents are commonly present at the same time.

TABLE 70–1. Differential Diagnosis of Vaginitis

Common Causes	Less Common Causes
Candidiasis	Foreign body (retained tampon or sponge)
Bacterial vaginosis	Lice, pinworms
Trichomoniasis	Vaginal fistulas
Atrophic vaginitis	Allergic reaction (e.g., detergent, perfume)
Cervicitis (*Chlamydia*, gonorrhea)	Cystitis
Normal vaginal secretions	Oral contraceptive use

EVALUATION

History

Initially, the history should focus on the onset and nature of the patient's symptoms: what are the characteristics of the vaginal discharge (color, odor, amount), and are there any associated symptoms such as itching, burning, dysuria, spotting, or dyspareunia? It should be kept in mind that the volume and consistency of normal vaginal secretions change throughout a woman's cycle as hormone levels vary.

Items in the past medical history that are of particular importance include (1) the gynecologic and sexual history, (2) the presence of any chronic medical illnesses, (3) allergies and current medications, and (4) diet and personal habits.

It is important to know whether the patient has been treated for vaginitis or sexually transmitted diseases in the past. Recurrent episodes should alert the physician to the possibility of more serious underlying illnesses, to problems with medication compliance, or to gaps in the patient's understanding of sexually transmitted diseases. This is an excellent time for the health care provider to counsel the patient about the importance of safe sexual habits.

Diabetes, HIV infection, antibiotics, and chronic corticosteroid use are associated with candidiasis. Inflammatory bowel disease and prior gynecologic surgery are associated with the development of enterovaginal fistulas. Excessive use of douches or deodorants, local tissue trauma, and the atrophy that often accompanies postmenopausal changes can disrupt the normal vaginal environment and may lead to the overgrowth of organisms that normally exist in a balanced state.

Physical Examination

The first step is close visual inspection of the external genitalia and perineum. The mons, vulva, and perianal area should be examined for signs of irritation, inflammation, or the presence of organisms such as scabies, lice, or pinworms. Inspect closely for lesions commonly associated with sexually transmitted diseases, such as genital warts, herpetic vesicles, or ulcerated areas of mucosa.

The vaginal mucosa should be examined for the same signs during the speculum examination. Thin, friable tissue that bleeds easily and is accompanied by diminished secretions is indicative of atrophic changes. The presence, location, and nature of any vaginal discharge should be noted. The discharge associated with candidiasis is typically thick, is white to yellow in color, and adheres to the vaginal wall, whereas the discharge associated with bacterial vaginosis and trichomoniasis is thin, is gray to green in color, and either pools in the vault or is easily swabbed off the vaginal wall.

The appearance of the cervix should be noted, particularly the presence or absence of discharge coming from the os. Mucopurulent discharge is associated with sexually transmitted disease-related cervicitis. Finally, samples should be collected for wet mount

TABLE 70–2. Diagnosis of Vaginitis

Features	*Candida*	*Trichomonas*	Bacterial Vaginosis
Discharge	Thick, white	Thin, green	Thin, gray
pH	< 4.5	> 4.5	> 4.5
Amine odor	Absent	Often present	Always present
WBCs	+/–	+	–
Lactobacilli	+	+/–	–
Trichomonads	–	+	–
Clue cells	–	–	+
Hyphae	+	–	–

evaluation in the office and, if necessary, appropriate cultures should be sent to the laboratory.

After the speculum examination, a bimanual examination should be performed. Tenderness on cervical motion as well as adnexal fullness and tenderness are associated with pelvic inflammatory disease. Inguinal lymph nodes should be assessed for increased size and tenderness.

Additional Evaluation

The simple tests performed as part of the routine office-based evaluation of vaginitis are both cost effective and invaluable in diagnosing the etiology of vaginitis; they should never be omitted. It is best to collect a sample of the vaginal discharge with a cotton swab and place it in a small test tube with a drop or two of normal saline. This solution should then be evaluated in the following manner: (1) Check pH with a test strip. (2) Perform the "whiff test" by adding a drop of 10% KOH and checking for the release of a fishy, amine odor. (3) Prepare a microscope slide to look for the presence of WBCs, clue cells, bacilli, yeast forms, and specific organisms (e.g., trichomonads). While it is important to remember that there may be more than one cause of a patient's symptoms (e.g., cervicitis and bacterial vaginosis), certain characteristics of vaginal discharge are extremely helpful in arriving at a diagnosis (Table 70–2).

MANAGEMENT

Medications are available to treat the four most common causes of vaginitis: bacterial vaginosis, candidiasis, trichomoniasis, and atrophic vaginitis (Table 70–3). Trichomoniasis is treated with metronidazole. Sexual partners must also be treated, and the patient must abstain from drinking alcohol while taking the medication. Bacterial vaginosis also is treated with metronidazole, but treatment of partners has not been shown to reduce the rate of recurrence. Various topical imidazoles are available for the treatment of candidiasis. Atrophic vaginitis is treated with topical estrogen cream, if the patient's symptoms warrant it.

Recurrent candidal infections are sometimes a problem. If recurrence is not related to chronic disease or medication use, the patient may need to be counseled to avoid the use of douches, vaginal deodorant sprays, or nylon underwear. Including yogurt in the diet on a regular basis (two to three times a week) has been shown to decrease the incidence of recurrent candidal infections.

Treatment choices are fairly straightforward for cervicitis (i.e., treatment of the underlying organism) as well as for the less common etiologies of vaginitis. Foreign bodies, such as retained tampons or contraceptive sponges, must be removed and the patient counseled. Medications are available to treat urinary tract infections, lice, and pinworms. Vaginal fistulas should be referred to a gynecologist for further evaluation. Women who feel that their normal vaginal secretions are excessive or abnormal need to be educated and reassured.

PATIENT EDUCATION

All women should be counseled periodically about sexually transmitted diseases, HIV infection, safe sexual practices, and contraceptive choices.

NATURAL HISTORY/PROGNOSIS

With a thorough history, physical examination, and selected testing done in the office, most cases of vaginitis can be diagnosed and successfully treated. If treatment failures occur, the examiner should consider the following: multiple infections, poor compliance or reinfection, and a more serious underlying condition (such as diabetes or AIDS).

TABLE 70–3. Treatment of Vaginitis

Diagnosis	Organism	Medication	Comment
Candidiasis	*Candida* sp.	Miconazole, clotrimazole, butoconazole, terconazole	Topical creams or intravaginal tablets; treatment regimens vary according to agent chosen
		Fluconazole	150 mg orally, single dose
Trichomoniasis	*Trichomonas*	Metronidazole (contraindicated during pregnancy)	2 g orally as a single dose *or* 500 mg orally twice a day for 7 days; treat partner
Bacterial vaginosis	*Gardnerella, Mobiluncus,* anaerobes	Metronidazole (contraindicated during pregnancy)	500 mg orally twice a day for 7 days *or* 2 g orally as a single dose
Atrophic vaginitis		Estrogen cream	Topical

Research Questions

1. What preventive measures can be taken to maintain an acidic vaginal pH (to prevent recurrent candidiasis)?
2. Compliance is a common cause of treatment failure. What can be done to improve compliance?

Selected Readings

Deutchman, M. E., D. Leaman, and J. L. Thomason. Vaginitis: Diagnosis is the key. Patient Care 28:39–61, 1994.

Grossman, J. H., and J. W. Larsen. Pelvic infections. *In* N. G. Kase, A. B. Weingold, and D. M. Gershenson. *Principles and Practice of Clinical Gynecology.* New York, Churchill Livingstone, 1990.

Hatcher, R. A., et al. Sexually transmitted diseases. *In* R. A. Hatcher et al. *Contraceptive Technology.* New York, Irvington Publishers, 1994.

Hilton, E., H. D. Isenberg, P. Alperstein, et al. Ingestion of yogurt containing *Lactobacillus acidophilus* as prophylaxis for candidal vaginitis. Ann Intern Med 116:353–7, 1992.

Reed, B. D., and A. Eyler. Vaginal infections: Diagnosis and management. Am Fam Physician 47(8):1805–18, 1993.

Shaw, G. N., and N. D. Sullivan. Vulvovaginitis. *In* C. S. Hafvens, N. D. Sullivan, and P. Tilton. *Manual of Outpatient Gynecology.* Boston, Little, Brown & Co., 1991.

CHAPTER 71

VAGINAL BLEEDING

Maxine H. Dorin, M.D.

H$_x$ A 35-year-old female cosmetologist presents with a history of irregular, prolonged vaginal bleeding. She notes that her menses had been regular up until 3 months ago, but now she has almost daily spotting. She denies hot flashes, vaginal dryness, or other symptoms. The patient had a tubal ligation following her third delivery. She used barrier methods of contraception before her sterilization because of a history of a possible pulmonary embolism while taking oral contraceptives at the age of 19 years. There were no complications with any of her pregnancies. She does not smoke and takes no medications. The general physical examination is normal. On the pelvic examination, the uterus seems slightly enlarged and mildly tender and there is a small quantity of old blood at the cervical os. The ovaries are of normal size and nontender.

Questions

1. What would be your differential diagnosis at this time?
2. What other questions might you ask to narrow the differential?
3. What other physical findings might be pertinent?
4. What tests are you considering? Why?

PATHOPHYSIOLOGY

Dysfunctional vaginal bleeding is abnormal bleeding from the uterine endometrium unrelated to anatomic lesions of the genital tract. It is caused by a hormonal imbalance due to derangements in the hypothalamic-pituitary-ovarian axis. It is usually associated with anovulatory cycling but occasionally occurs in ovulatory cycles.

Anovulatory dysfunctional vaginal bleeding most often occurs at the beginning or end of a woman's reproductive life. In adolescence, the cause is probably an immature hypothalamic-pituitary system that fails to respond to the positive feedback effect of estrogen. In perimenopausal patients with abnormal bleeding, diminished ovarian response to gonadotropin stimulation results in variable cycle length and bleeding, possibly due to imminent ovarian failure.

In obese patients, fat metabolizes ovarian and adrenal androstenedione into estrone. Estrone is a weak estrogen that probably depresses the function of the hypothalamic-pituitary axis through a negative-feedback mechanism, a situation that interferes with the proper fluctuations of estrogen essential for the development of normal ovulatory cycles. Hirsute patients secrete an abnormally high amount of testosterone, androstenedione, dehydroepiandrosterone, or a combination of these androgens. A rise in the blood level of any of these androgens, particularly testosterone, may prevent adequate function of the hypothalamic-pituitary axis as a result of the negative-feedback mechanism.

Although any endocrine disease can disturb the normal hypothalamic-pituitary-ovarian axis, the two most common are hyperprolactinemia and hypothyroidism. Hyperprolactinemia (whether idiopathic or secondary to medication, hypothyroidism, or a pituitary adenoma) will inhibit the synthesis and secretion of gonadotropin-releasing hormone (GnRH).

DIFFERENTIAL DIAGNOSIS

After completion of the history, physical examination, and a few selected tests, the differential diagnosis of abnormal uterine bleeding can be narrowed significantly by answering two questions: (1) Is the patient pregnant? (2) Could the problem be a cancer? Other causes of vaginal bleeding are listed in Table 71–1.

Pregnancy

If the pregnancy test is positive, either an intrauterine pregnancy exists that is threatening or about to abort (which is the most common cause of first trimester bleeding) or the pregnancy is ectopic. If the blood is coming from the uterus, the use of ultrasound and serial β-hCG (human chorionic gonadotropin) measurements will help determine the diagnosis.

Pregnancy does not exclude the possibility of cancer.

Cancer

After the age of 35 years, any woman who presents with abnormal uterine bleeding should be evaluated for uterine and cervical cancer. Uterine or endometrial cancer is diagnosed by endometrial sampling in the office or minor surgery suite.

Before the age of 35 years, only a selected group of patients would need to undergo an endometrial biopsy.

TABLE 71–1. Common Organic Causes of Abnormal Vaginal Bleeding

Anovulation
  Hypothalamic dysfunction
  Polycystic ovary disease
  Hyperprolactinemia
Pregnancy complications
  Abortion
  Ectopic pregnancy
  Gestational trophoblastic disease
Benign neoplasm
  Submucosal fibroid
  Endometrial polyp
  Cervical polyp
  Endometriosis
Malignant neoplasm
  Endometrial carcinoma
  Cervical carcinoma
Genital tract infection
  Endometritis
  Cervicitis
  Vaginitis
Intrauterine contraceptive device (IUD)
Foreign body
Adenosis
Theca or granulosa cell tumor producing estrogen
Coagulopathy
Cirrhosis
Thyroid dysfunction
Trauma

BOX 71–1. Questions for the Patient with Vaginal Bleeding

1. How old is the patient, and when was the last normal menses?
2. How long has the problem of vaginal bleeding been present?
3. For how many days has she been bleeding, and how much, e.g., number of pads or tampons used during last episode?
4. Does she have cramping or abdominal pain?
5. Does she have any symptoms of pregnancy, e.g., nausea or breast tenderness? Is she sexually active? Does she use birth control?
6. Does she have bleeding during or after intercourse?
7. When was her last Pap test and pelvic examination? Were both normal?
8. Does she have any history of IUD use, infertility, sexually transmitted disease, or pelvic inflammatory disease?
9. How many times has she been pregnant? How many live births, stillbirths, miscarriages, pregnancy interruptions, or ectopic pregnancies have there been?
10. Does the patient take any medications?
11. Does she have any other medical problems?
12. Has she had any surgery, especially abdominal or vaginal procedures such as a D&C, cesarean section, or tubal ligation?

Patients who have unopposed estrogen, either exogenous or endogenous, would be candidates. Rarely, an ovarian estrogen-producing tumor will be the offender. The unopposed estrogen would cause unchecked proliferation of the endometrium, possibly precipitating adenomatous hyperplasia and eventually leading to endometrial adenocarcinoma.

Cervical cancer is diagnosed by a cervical biopsy, but clues to the possibility are a lesion on the cervix—ulcerated, fungating, or friable—or an abnormal Pap test.

EVALUATION

History

The history should focus on the questions listed in Box 71–1. The patient's age, date of last normal menstrual period, and method of birth control should be documented. The amount and duration of bleeding episodes should be quantitated as accurately as possible along with relationship to coitus and abdominal cramping. A question such as "How many pads or tampons were used daily during this episode?" helps in approximating the amount. Blood flow lasting longer than 8 days, menstrual intervals shorter than 21 days, or blood loss exceeding 80 mL per menstrual period (quantitated by pad count) is considered abnormal.

With the possibility of pregnancy, inquiry into any tissue passed, nausea, appetite changes, and breast tenderness should be made. Concern about ectopic pregnancy should lead to questions regarding any type of abdominal pain and its description. A complaint of dizziness or fainting spells is extremely worrisome in the context of a possible ruptured ectopic pregnancy or hemorrhage from a miscarriage in that it may signify major blood loss.

Past gynecologic and obstetric history may help raise or lower the suspicion for a particular diagnosis. A history of weight loss, abdominal mass, postcoital bleeding, and no pelvic examination in the past 9 years raises the suspicion for a gynecologic malignancy.

Anovulatory dysfunctional uterine bleeding lacks most of the features usually associated with ovulatory cycles, such as midcycle pain, midcycle vaginal mucus, premenstrual breast tenderness, and dysmenorrhea.

Physical Examination

The physical examination should focus on the height, weight, blood pressure, pulse rate, general appearance, abdomen, pelvis, and lymph nodes.

Patients who have a significant amount of hemorrhage may have changes in their vital signs. Tachycardia should trigger a check of orthostatic vital signs and a concern for a ruptured ectopic pregnancy.

On abdominal examination, it is important to palpate for masses and areas of pain or tenderness. It is not uncommon for a patient in the third trimester to claim she is not pregnant. Listening for fetal heart tones will clarify the diagnosis. An abdominal mass may be an estrogen-producing ovarian tumor, inducing uterine endometrial proliferation and vaginal bleeding. If the mass is uterine, a leiomyoma should be considered.

Abdominal tenderness should be assessed for location and intensity. If obvious peritoneal signs are present, rupture of a viscus should be considered.

On speculum examination, signs of infection, trauma, or lesions should be sought in the vagina and cervix. A biopsy should be made of any obvious abnormalities such as cervical polyps, ulcers, or discolorations. With diffuse erythema, vaginitis or cervicitis is suspected. Atrophy in menopausal patients can be so severe that the examination can cause pain and significant bleeding. If possible, it should be documented whether the blood is coming from the cervical os or elsewhere.

On bimanual examination, the consistency, mobility, size, tenderness, position, and shape of the uterus should be noted. The size, position, and tenderness of the adnexa (ovaries) bilaterally should be documented. A rectovaginal examination should be performed to confirm previous findings and to discern the existence of a mass or tenderness behind the uterus. A stool test for occult blood is performed to rule out a gastrointestinal source of bleeding.

TABLE 71–2. Evaluating Vaginal Bleeding

Most Helpful Selected Tests
Hemoglobin/hematocrit
β-hCG (pregnancy test), either urine or blood
Often Helpful Tests
Endometrial biopsy
Prolactin level
Thyroid function tests
Occasionally Helpful Tests, Used Only When Indicated
Colposcopy and cervical biopsy
Cervical cultures (e.g., *Chlamydia, N. gonorrhoeae*)
Helpful Tests in Selected Situations
Partial thromboplastin time, prothrombin time, and bleeding time
Hysteroscopy
Dilatation and curettage (D&C)

Additional Evaluation

Laboratory work should include hematocrit/hemoglobin, platelet count, and pregnancy test (Table 71–2). For severe recurrent bleeding, a partial thromboplastin time, prothrombin time, and bleeding time should be requested.

Endometrial biopsy or dilatation and curettage (D&C) to assess for endometrial cancer is done for high-risk patients. Colposcopy and cervical biopsy are performed when cervical malignancy is suspected.

Occasionally, hysteroscopy is performed in conjunction with D&C to optimize the diagnosis of a submucosal fibroid or a polyp.

Hormonal evaluation should be ordered only when the history and physical examination warrant. Tests should be selective, based on the differential diagnosis. A prolactin level and thyroid function tests typically are the most helpful.

MANAGEMENT

Pregnancy Complications

In threatened abortion, the cervical os is closed on examination and the patient is sent home for bed rest with a 50% chance that the pregnancy will progress normally into the third trimester. Ultrasound and serial β-hCG tests will document whether it is a viable intrauterine pregnancy. D&C can be performed to remove the products of conception in nonviable cases. In inevitable abortion, the cervical os is open and the bleeding will continue until the products of conception are completely evacuated. Between 6 and 14 weeks, there is a higher chance of retained products of conception, with continued bleeding and increased likelihood of infection. Therefore, in cases in which the os is open, D&C is recommended.

In ectopic pregnancy, the treatment is either surgical or medical management. With medical management, a chemotherapeutic agent, methotrexate, is administered orally or as an injection. If a laparoscopy or laparotomy is performed, the ectopic pregnancy is removed, or methotrexate can be injected directly into the ectopic pregnancy. Removal of the ectopic pregnancy entails removing a portion or all of the fallopian (uterine) tube (salpingectomy) or making an incision into the wall of the fallopian tube and expressing the trophoblastic tissue without removing any portion of the wall (salpingostomy).

In the rare instance of gestational trophoblastic neoplasm, a careful D&C must be performed as soon as possible; blood loss at the time of the procedure can be excessive. The abnormal proliferation of placental tissue (trophoblast) can be cured 80% of the time with D&C alone. Serial β-hCG measurements must be done following the D&C to detect the 20% of cases of persistent disease. Methotrexate is routinely given to eradicate remaining trophoblasts.

Cancer

Treatment of cervical cancer depends on the stage of the disease at diagnosis. Usually, either radiation or surgery is the primary mode, sometimes with adjuvant chemotherapy or radiotherapy.

Endometrial cancer typically is treated with either surgery or radiation or both, depending on the stage and the patient's medical status. Hormonal chemotherapy is a useful adjuvant to the primary treatment.

Ovarian malignancies are first debulked and staged at exploratory laparotomy, and chemotherapy is used after the procedure. Radiation is not routinely used for most of the common radiation-resistant ovarian cancers.

Dysfunctional Uterine Bleeding

The diagnosis of anovulatory dysfunctional uterine bleeding (DUB) is one of exclusion. In most cases, the history, general physical examination, pelvic examination, and a few selected laboratory tests will yield the correct diagnosis. In acute, profuse bleeding, the exclusion of a pregnancy complication or malignancy must be made immediately, before instituting therapy for DUB.

The objectives of therapy are to control bleeding, prevent recurrence, and preserve fertility if desired. If the bleeding is not acute, the treatment is individualized to the patient's age, desire for fertility, and medical status (Table 71–3).

In teenagers, observation alone is warranted for mild cases without evidence of anemia, since the hypothalamic-pituitary-ovarian axis matures within 1 year of menarche. If the patient is not sexually active, medroxyprogesterone acetate is recommended to control bleeding. In sexually active patients, oral contraceptives should be offered.

In the reproductive age group, if dysfunctional uterine bleeding persists, the treatment is individualized according to the patient's desire for contraception or fertility. Oral contraceptives are a good choice to regulate irregular bleeding for patients desiring contraception. If fertility is desired, induction of ovulation with clomiphene citrate can be tried initially.

In perimenopausal patients or in patients who have contraindications to the use of oral contraceptives, medroxyprogesterone acetate is effective. It can be used until menopause, at which time cyclic estrogen and progesterone may be employed.

In acute moderate bleeding, a combination oral contraceptive that contains ethinyl estradiol may be given. Depending on the patient's circumstances, after the withdrawal bleeding, any of the other therapies, such as cyclic progesterone or oral contraceptives, can be utilized to establish regular menstrual cycles.

In acute severe bleeding in a stable patient, high-dose conjugated estrogen is given to stimulate rapid endometrial proliferation to "heal" the bleeding sites. When the bleeding has stopped, an oral contraceptive is given for 3 weeks, or conjugated estrogen plus medroxyprogesterone for the last 10 days of therapy is given.

Finally, surgical intervention can be used in dysfunctional uterine bleeding. D&C can be therapeutic as well as diagnostic in some cases. However, this cure is temporary and should be followed with hormonal

---

TABLE 71–3. Medical Therapy for Dysfunctional Vaginal Bleeding

In the Teenage Years
Observation in mild cases without anemia
Medroxyprogesterone if patient not sexually active
Oral contraceptive if patient sexually active
In the Reproductive Age Group
Oral contraceptive if fertility undesired
Clomiphene citrate if ovulation induction desired
In Perimenopausal Patients
Medroxyprogesterone
In Acute Moderate Bleeding
Oral contraceptive containing ethinyl estradiol
In Acute Severe Bleeding in a Stable Patient
Conjugated estrogen until bleeding stops, then estrogen with progesterone for 3 weeks

---

therapies. Endometrial ablation has been advocated in patients who are poor surgical risks or who do not desire a hysterectomy. Dysfunctional uterine bleeding by itself is rarely an indication for hysterectomy, but a hysterectomy is definitive treatment for dysfunctional uterine bleeding unresponsive to hormonal therapy.

PATIENT AND FAMILY EDUCATION

Teaching the patient about the normal menstrual cycle can be a valuable management tool for the physician. By understanding the normal physiology and then the underlying pathophysiology, the patient can comprehend the reasoning behind the therapies and cooperate more fully with management strategies.

PROGNOSIS

Medical management is successful in most cases, whether it be to supplement a hypothyroid patient or to use hormonal manipulation. Some cases may be effectively treated by D&C, and in the few refractory cases, surgery by either endometrial ablation or hysterectomy usually suffices. Vaginal bleeding secondary to dysfunctional uterine bleeding is inconvenient but not life threatening in the majority of cases.

Research Question

1. How does hypothyroidism cause menorrhagia?

Case Resolution

Endometrial biopsy revealed endometrium consistent with anovulation. Prolactin, thyroid function tests, and hemoglobin were normal. Although an oral contraceptive (or some type of hormone replacement) would have been ideal treatment, her history of possible pulmonary embolism precluded its use. The patient decided to "wait and watch" after being counseled about her options.

Selected Readings

Altchek, A. Dysfunctional uterine bleeding in adolescence. Clin Obstet Gynecol 20:633, 1977.

Baggish, M. S., and P. Baltoyannis. New techniques for laser ablation of the endometrium in high-risk patients. Am J Obstet Gynecol 159:287, 1988.

Douglas, L. W., and B. Greisman. Early hypothyroidism in patients with menorrhagia. Am J Obstet Gynecol 160:673, 1989.

Fraser, I. S., G. McCarron, R. Markham, et al. Measured menstrual blood loss in women with menorrhagia associated with pelvic disease or coagulation disorder. Obstet Gynecol 68:630, 1986.

Fraser, I. S., E. A. Michie, L. Wide, and D. T. Baird. Pituitary gonado-tropins and ovarian function in adolescent dysfunctional uterine bleeding. J Clin Endocrinol Metab 37:407, 1973.

Hall, P., N. Maclachlan, N. Thorn, et al. Control of menorrhagia by the cyclo-oxygenase inhibitors naproxen sodium and mefenamic acid. Br J Obstet Gynaecol 94:554, 1987.

Healy, D. L., and G. D. Hodgen. The endocrinology of human endometrium. Obstet Gynecol Surv 38(8):509, 1983.

Hsueh, A. J. W., E. J. Peck, and J. H. Clark. Progesterone antagonism of the estrogen receptor and estrogen-induced uterine growth. Nature 254:337, 1975.

Speroff, L., R. H. Glass, and N. G. Kase. Regulation of the menstrual cycle. *In* Speroff, L., R. H. Glass, and N. G. Kase. *Clinical Gynecologic Endocrinology and Infertility,* 5th ed. Baltimore, Williams & Wilkins, 1994.

CHAPTER 72

CONTRACEPTION

Lydia Lawson, M.D.

H$_x$ A 19-year-old female community college student comes in with her 3-month-old daughter to discuss birth control. She is not currently using any method of birth control. Her cousin recently had levonorgestrel implants, and she wonders whether she might have the same procedure. She and her boyfriend are in a monogamous relationship, and they want to postpone having more children until they complete school and get jobs.

Questions

1. What methods of birth control are available to the patient and her partner?
2. Are her choices affected by the fact that she is breast-feeding?
3. What information in her medical and social history will affect your recommendations?

Every year in the United States, 6.3 million pregnancies occur. Among never-married women, 88% of pregnancies are unintended; among married women, 40% are unintended. Of unintended pregnancies, 44% end in abortion.

It is safer to use contraception than to be pregnant. The mortality rate associated with pregnancy is 1 death per 10,000 pregnancies, as compared to 0.2 deaths for 10,000 women using contraception. In addition, one woman in five suffers a pregnancy complication serious enough to require hospitalization. Yet most women believe that taking oral contraceptives is more dangerous than giving birth.

The form of birth control most commonly used in the United States is oral contraceptives (28% of contraceptive users), followed by female sterilization (25%), condoms (13%), and male sterilization (10%). Most patients have some idea about the type of contraceptive they wish to use based on information from friends, family, mass media, and lay literature.

PHYSIOLOGY

Figure 72–1 is a schematic representation of the menstrual cycle. The highest potential for conception occurs over a 4-day period. The oocyte is maximally fertile for 12–24 hours, while sperm retain fertility for 2–7 days. Thus, maximal fertility occurs during the 3 days prior to ovulation. The next most fertile time is on the day of ovulation.

EVALUATION

History

Past medical illnesses, surgeries, medications, and allergies should be explored. Specific risk factors associated with contraceptive choice include older age, hypertension, cardiovascular disease, migraines, seizure disorders, liver disease, lipid disorders, cancer, clotting disorders, sexually transmitted diseases (STDs), pelvic inflammatory disease (PID), previous abnormal Pap tests, and abnormal vaginal bleeding. A family history of breast, ovarian, or endometrial cancer may affect a patient's choice. For women, the menstrual history (age at menarche, cycle pattern, dysmenorrhea,

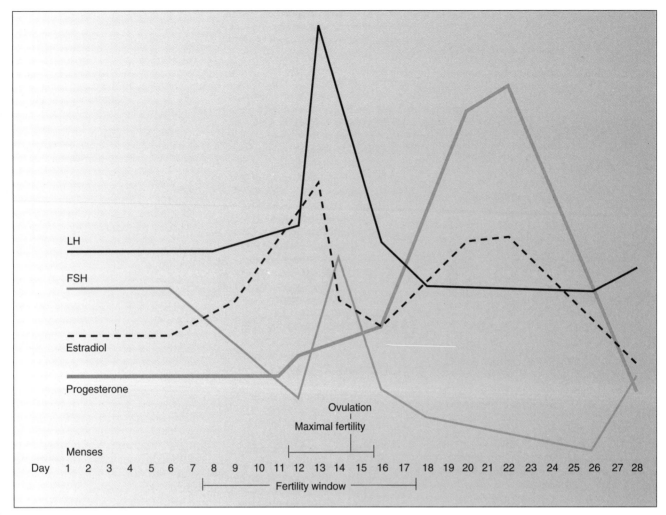

FIGURE 72-1. *The menstrual cycle.*

premenstrual syndrome) and obstetric history are important. The sexual history should include the age at first intercourse and number and sex of partners. Finally, it is important to review previous contraceptive methods utilized and how the patient felt about those methods.

Physical Examination

For women, the physical examination should include a check of blood pressure and weight, a breast examination, and a pelvic examination including inspection of the external and internal genitalia, cultures for STDs as appropriate, and a Pap test. Bimanual examination of the uterus, ovaries, and adnexa also must be done. For men, a genital examination is performed, with cultures taken for STDs as appropriate.

MANAGEMENT

Considerations affecting the contraceptive method chosen include medical history, prevention of STDs, efficacy, convenience, side effects, future fertility, partner compliance, sexual expression, and cost.

Abstinence

Abstinence is one of many options available to a patient making a well-informed choice. Abstinence is the choice of 12.4% of unmarried men and 13.2% of unmarried women aged 25–34 years in the United States. Some married couples also choose abstinence. Besides being the most effective form of birth control, abstinence prevents STDs, including infection with the human immunodeficiency virus (HIV). For those who choose abstinence from sexual intercourse, there are other ways to experience sexual touch and intimacy. These can be discussed with patients who want more information.

Coitus Interruptus

Mechanism. The male withdraws his penis from the vagina prior to ejaculation.

Effectiveness. The effectiveness is decreased by sperm released prior to ejaculation and the timing of the man's withdrawal. The failure rate among typical users in the first year is approximately 19%.

Advantages. The method has no cost, is always available, and requires no chemicals or devices.

Disadvantages. Disadvantages include interruption of pleasure, emotional consequences, difficulty with compliance, lack of protection against STDs (including HIV infection), and a relatively high rate of conception.

Rhythm Method

Mechanism. Abstention from intercourse during the maximally fertile days or use of additional forms of birth control during this vulnerable period prevents contact between sperm and oocyte. Ovulation time can be determined by calendar charting, since ovulation usually occurs on day 14 plus or minus 2 days. Basal body temperature (BBT) charting can also be used to predict ovulation because a woman's temperature drops 12–24 hours before ovulation, then rises owing to progesterone release after ovulation. BBT can be disrupted by illness, stress, travel, or lack of sleep. Other indicators of ovulation include cervical mucus changes (cervical mucus can be obtained with fingers or toilet tissue from the vaginal opening). Ovulation occurs within 1 day before, during, or after the last day of abundant, slippery, stretchy discharge. Ferning—cervical mucus allowed to dry on a microscope slide—demonstrates a fern-like pattern during fertile days; or symptothermal charting—a combination of BBT and cervical mucus changes—may be used to track fertility. Fertility is considered highest from 7 days before ovulation to 3 days after (fertility window). In addition, home urine testing for hormones related to ovulation demonstrates rises in estrone and pregnanediol and may help predict ovulation.

Effectiveness. Failure rates for typical users are 20% in the first year of use. Failure is usually due to a misunderstanding about the timing or to the mistaken belief that conception will not occur early in the fertile period.

Advantages. An increase in self-awareness and active involvement in planning pregnancy can happen for those using this method. Improved communication between partners can occur.

Disadvantages. This method does not prevent STDs, including HIV infection. Emotional strain can result from the lack of spontaneity. The method is complicated, necessitating detailed charting.

Spermicides

Mechanism. Nonoxynol-9 and octoxynol-9 are surfactants that destroy the sperm cell membrane. They come in various forms, including foam, jellies, creams, suppositories, and tablets.

Effectiveness. Failure rates are estimated to be around 21% for a typical user in the first year.

Advantages. Spermicides are available without prescription and are good adjuncts to other methods. Spermicides may enhance lubrication and protect against gonorrhea, *Chlamydia,* and other STDs.

Disadvantages. Spermicides provide little if any protection against HIV infection and can produce allergic reactions, promote vaginal candidiasis, and decrease

spontaneity. Spermicidal films, tablets, and suppositories are effective 10–15 minutes after insertion, whereas foam, cream, and jellies are immediately effective. All spermicides are effective for only 1 hour after application.

Condoms (Male and Female)

The standard male condom is a sheath that covers the penis. The oldest form of birth control, condom use can be traced as far back as 1350 BC.

Mechanism. Condoms provide a mechanical barrier. They are made of latex or other materials (5% of male condoms are made of collagenous tissue and are called "skin" or "natural membrane"). Newer synthetic materials are being developed for people who have sensitivity reactions to latex. The female condom is made of polyurethane and consists of an internal ring inserted over the cervix and connected to a sheath that is attached to an external ring placed over the labia. It contains a silicone-based lubricant but no spermicide.

Effectiveness. The failure rate for typical use of male condoms is 12%; for female condoms, 21%. For a "perfect" user of male condoms combined with a vaginal spermicide, the failure rate falls to 0.1%.

Advantages. Condoms do not require a prescription, are available in a variety of locations, are inexpensive or free, may help maintain the erection longer (rim tourniquet effect), and help prevent HIV and other STD transmission.

Disadvantages. Condoms may reduce penile sensitivity, interrupt foreplay, decrease pleasure for the woman, and cause allergic reactions. They can break, limiting their effectiveness. The male condoms made of collagenous tissue do not provide protection against STDs and HIV.

Diaphragm, Cervical Cap, Contraceptive Sponge

Mechanism. Barrier methods are used with a spermicide to provide a mechanical barrier as well as enhanced spermicidal activity.

Effectiveness. The typical failure rate for the diaphragm is 18%. For the sponge and cap, the typical failure rate for parous women is 36%; for nulliparous women, 18%.

Advantages. The sponge is available over-the-counter and provides continuous protection for 24 hours. The cervical cap provides continuous protection for 48 hours. These methods offer added protection against some STDs (but not HIV). They do not have systemic side effects.

Disadvantages. Wearing the sponge or diaphragm for longer than 30 hours or the cervical cap for longer than 48 hours increases the risk of toxic shock syndrome. The diaphragm and cap require a "fitting" and a prescription. The diaphragm requires repeated applications of spermicide at 6-hour intervals if intercourse is repeated. There is an increased risk of urinary tract infections, bacterial vaginosis, and vaginal candidiasis. Other disadvantages include allergic reactions to spermicide or latex, cramps, bladder pain, rectal pain, problems with sponge removal, and increased vaginal colonization with *Escherichia coli.*

Oral Contraceptive Pills (OCPs)

Mechanism. Combined (estrogen and progesterone) pills and progesterone-only pills are available. Estrogen suppresses FSH and LH, which in turn inhibits ovulation, alters secretions within the uterus, changes the cellular structure of the endometrium, and promotes the degeneration of the corpus luteum. Progesterone suppresses LH, creates a thick cervical mucus that hampers sperm penetration, inhibits penetration of the ovum by sperm through deactivation of enzymes, alters uterine tube secretions, and inhibits implantation by production of a decidualized endometrial bed.

Effectiveness. The failure rate for the typical user in the first year is 3%.

Advantages. When taken "perfectly," the failure rate is 0.1%. Fertility is easily restored through discontinuation of the pill. OCPs may decrease dysmenorrhea, hirsutism, menstrual blood loss, premenstrual symptoms, pelvic inflammatory disease, and ovarian and endometrial cancers.

Disadvantages. OCPs are often discontinued for nonmedical reasons. OCPs do not protect against HIV infection or other STDs. The failure rate of OCPs is influenced by poor compliance, expense, abnormal menstrual bleeding, headache, depression, decreased libido, nausea, increased breast size and tenderness, fluid retention, and weight gain. Whether or not combination oral contraceptives increase the risk of breast cancer remains controversial. Estrogen decreases while progesterone promotes breast milk production. Problems associated with estrogen use include hypertension, hypercoagulability (particularly in women with such risk factors as tobacco use, abnormal blood lipids, severe diabetes, hypertension, morbid obesity, polycythemia vera, or previous history of deep venous thrombosis), cerebrovascular accident, myocardial infarction, hepatocellular adenoma, and hepatocellular carcinoma.

Levonorgestrel Implants (Norplant System)

Mechanism. Levonorgestrel is a progestin that when diffused slowly through implanted capsules prevents pregnancy over a period of years.

Effectiveness. The typical user failure rate for the first year is 0.09%. In the second year, the rate is 0.5%; the third year, 1.2%; the fourth year, 1.6%; and the fifth year, 0.4%. Women weighing more than 69 kg (152 lb) have cumulative 5-year failure rates of 2.4%.

Advantages. The main advantage is 5 years of continuous birth control without having to remember to take a medication or use a device. Long-term fertility is not impaired. Benefits may include amenorrhea and decreased rates of dysmenorrhea, endometrial cancer, ovarian cancer, and pelvic inflammatory disease. The capsules can be removed at any time, long-term fertility is preserved, and there are no estrogen-related problems such as cardiovascular risks or thrombophlebitis.

Disadvantages. An office procedure is required to insert or remove the capsules. The most common problem associated with the Norplant system is irregular bleeding. Other disadvantages include amenorrhea, weight gain, breast tenderness, higher failure rates for women taking anticonvulsants, possible decreased bone density, possible infection at the site of insertion, allergic reaction to the capsules, and visibility of the capsules just under the skin. No protection is provided against STDs, including HIV infection.

Depot Medroxyprogesterone Acetate (DMPA)

Mechanism. DMPA is given by intramuscular injection, 150 mg every 3 months. The mechanism of pregnancy prevention is similar to that of other progesterone agents.

Effectiveness. The failure rate for typical use is 0.3%. The effectiveness can last for 2 weeks (perhaps up to 4 weeks) after the 3-month prescribed interval.

Advantages. The advantages are similar to those of the Norplant system. DMPA allows privacy, since it is undetectable by sexual partners and others. There are no major drug interactions, and it does not interfere significantly with breast-feeding.

Disadvantages. Fertility is not immediately reversible because the effect lasts for 3–4 months. Amenorrhea is a common result of DMPA use, increasing anxiety when periods are "missed." The average time to return of fertility after discontinuation is 6 months to 1 year. Other drawbacks include office visits every 3 months for injections, headache, decreased libido, breast pain, depression, weight gain, and a fall in high-density lipoprotein levels. No protection is provided against STDs, including HIV infection.

Intrauterine Devices (IUDs)

Mechanism. The IUD immobilizes sperm and interferes with sperm migration from the vagina to the uterine tubes. The IUD may speed ovum transport through the uterine tubes and inhibit implantation because of local effects on the endometrium. The Paragard T380A is a T-shaped device made of plastic surrounded by copper wire. The Progestasert system also is T-shaped but is made of an ethylene vinyl acetate copolymer containing a progesterone reservoir. These two are the only models of IUD currently approved for use in the United States.

Effectiveness. For the Paragard, the first-year typical use failure rate is 0.8%. For the Progestasert, the first-year typical use failure rate is 2%.

Advantages. Paragard is effective for 8 years and does not require daily management. Progestasert is effective for 1 year and is preferred for patients with a sensitivity to copper.

Disadvantages. IUDs increase the risk of pelvic inflammatory disease and subsequent infertility. They do not protect against HIV infection or other STDs, and they may increase dysmenorrhea and vaginal bleeding. Expulsion of the IUD may not be immediately apparent, and thus pregnancy may occur. If a woman becomes pregnant with an IUD in place, she has a 50% chance of spontaneous abortion and a 5% chance of ectopic pregnancy. Severe pelvic infections resulting in death are more likely to occur if the IUD is left in place in a pregnant woman. The IUD should be removed early in pregnancy.

Sterilization

Mechanism. In women, the uterine tubes are interrupted (tubal ligation) to prevent union of sperm and oocyte. In men, the vas deferens is ligated bilaterally (vasectomy) to prevent the passage of sperm into the ejaculate.

Effectiveness. The female sterilization failure rate averages 0.4% in the first year. The failure rate for vasectomy (reported as failure to eliminate sperm from the ejaculate) is approximately 0.1%.

Advantages. Tubal interruption is permanent and cost effective, requiring nothing to remember, purchase, or insert. Sexual activity is not interrupted, and the contraceptive choice is private. Vasectomy is a simple, inexpensive, permanent procedure.

Disadvantages. For women, the tubal ligation is not easily reversible. Sterilization requires surgery, a high initial expense, and some increase in the probability of ectopic pregnancy. It offers no protection against STDs. For men, complications include bleeding or infection from the procedure. Vasectomies have an initial moderate cost, are not easily reversed, and do not protect against STDs.

Morning-After Pill

Mechanism. The use of Ovral (2 tablets), Lo/Ovral, Nordette, Levlen, Triphasil, or Tri-Levlen (4 tablets) in two doses 12 hours apart and initiated within the first 72 hours after unprotected intercourse temporarily disrupts ovarian hormone production, causing an out-of-phase endometrial development that is unsuitable for implantation.

Effectiveness. The risk of pregnancy is reduced by 70%–80%.

Advantages. The morning-after pill offers a low-risk method to prevent unwanted pregnancy in cases of rape or mechanical failure of contraceptive devices or when a woman decides she does not want a pregnancy after the risk has been taken.

Disadvantages. Nausea, vomiting, breast tenderness, abdominal pain, headache or dizziness, and abnormal timing of the next menstrual period are the main disadvantages. Adverse effects are usually of short duration. Other disadvantages are similar to those of oral combination pills.

Lactational Amenorrhea Method (LAM)

Mechanism. Breast-feeding suppresses LH levels while a woman is amenorrheic and thus suppresses ovulation.

Effectiveness. If a woman is breast-feeding without supplementation and she remains amenorrheic, breast-feeding provides more than 98% protection from pregnancy in the first 6 postpartum months.

Advantages. LAM is considered to be a "natural" form of birth control.

Disadvantages. This method is unpredictable, and no protection is provided against STDs.

Research Questions

1. Can an effective, inexpensive oral contraceptive be developed for men?
2. What is the level of satisfaction among women using levonorgestrel implants?
3. What is the cause of "post-tubal ligation syndrome," which results in heavy menses and, ultimately, hysterectomy?

Case Resolution

The patient's history revealed no previous medical problems. The physical examination was normal, and Pap test and cervical cultures were normal. She did not want to interrupt foreplay to insert a diaphragm and worried about complications of an IUD. Because she was breast-feeding, her remaining contraceptive choices were limited; she decided to try depot medroxyprogesterone and felt she could return every 3 months for the injections.

Selected Readings

Bialy, G., et al. Introduction. Am J Obstet Gynecol 170:1483–4, 1994.

Forrest, J. D. Epidemiology of unintended pregnancy and contraceptive use. Am J Obstet Gynecol 170:1485–9, 1994.

Grimes, D. A. Breast feeding and contraception. The Contraception Report 4(5), November 1993.

Grimes, D. A. Compliance with oral contraceptives. The Contraception Report 5 (special edition), 1994.

Hatcher, R. A., et al. *Contraceptive Technology.* New York, Irvington Publishers, 1994.

PRENATAL CARE

Martha Cole McGrew, M.D.

H$_x$ A 36-year-old unemployed female, new to the clinic, presents with complaints of a missed period, nausea, and breast tenderness. She is certain that her last menstrual period (LMP) began 7 weeks before this visit. She has some concerns about pregnancy at this age and wants information about her baby's risks for birth defects. She is in a stable marriage, has no health insurance, but qualifies for Medicaid during pregnancy. Until she became pregnant, she smoked one-half pack of cigarettes per day and drank 2 to 3 beers per week. She has no known risk factors for HIV or hepatitis B. She exercises "occasionally." She was 10 kg (20 lb) overweight prior to this pregnancy. Her diet is generally good although she admits to occasionally skipping meals. Her first pregnancy 8 years ago was uncomplicated (except for the development of mild anemia) and ended in a normal vaginal delivery at 41 weeks estimated gestational age (EGA). Her daughter weighed 4 kg (8 lb, 15 oz). On physical examination, her blood pressure is 110/70 mm Hg, pulse 80/min, and weight 77 kg (170 lb). The pelvic examination is significant for a bluish appearing cervix. The uterus is 6- to 8-week size. Urine protein and glucose are negative.

Questions

1. What are the key elements of prenatal care?
2. Does early and sustained prenatal care make a difference in fetal and maternal outcome? If so, why?
3. Why and when should prenatal genetic screening be offered? What is the sensitivity, specificity, risks, benefits, and costs of these tests?

TABLE 73–1. Components of Preconception Care as Part of Primary Care Services

Risk Assessment

Individual and social conditions (age, diet, education, housing, economic status)

Adverse health behaviors (tobacco and alcohol use, substance abuse)

Medical conditions (immune status, medications, genetic illness, illnesses including infection, prior obstetric history)

Psychological conditions (personal and family readiness for pregnancy; stress; anxiety; depression)

Environmental conditions (workplace hazards, toxic chemicals, radiation contamination)

Barriers to family planning, prenatal care, and primary health care

Health Promotion

Promotion of healthy behaviors (proper nutrition; avoidance of smoking, alcohol, and teratogens; practice of "safe sex")

Counseling about the availability of social, financial, and vocational assistance programs

Advice on family planning, pregnancy spacing, and contraception

Counseling about the importance of early registration for and compliance with prenatal care, including high-risk programs if warranted

Identification of barriers to care and assistance in overcoming them

Arrangements for ongoing care

Interventions

Treatment of medical conditions, including changes in medications, if appropriate, and referral to high-risk pregnancy programs

Referral for treatment of adverse health behaviors (tobacco and alcohol use, substance abuse)

Rubella and hepatitis immunization

Reduction of psychosocial risks, which may involve counseling or referral to home health agencies, community mental health centers, safe shelters, enrollment in medical assistance, or assistance with housing

Nutrition counseling, supplementation, or referral to improve adequacy of diet

Home visits to further assess and intervene in the home environment

Provision for family planning services

Reproduced with permission, from B. W. Jack and L. Culpepper. Preconception care: Risk reduction and health promotion in preparation for pregnancy. JAMA 264:1148–9, 1990. © 1990, American Medical Association.

PRECONCEPTION CARE

Achieving the best possible health for the woman prior to pregnancy is the primary goal of preconception care. Physicians who provide care to women of childbearing age should understand the components of preconception care, including risk assessment, intervention, follow-up, and health promotion (Table 73–1).

Preconception care emphasizes the identification and reduction of risk factors that may lead to adverse pregnancy outcome. Risk factors may be social (substandard housing, lack of insurance), behavioral (alcohol and tobacco use), medical (medication use, genetic history, chronic illness or infection, past obstetric history), psychological (anxiety, depression), or environmental (workplace hazards). Another risk factor is real or perceived lack of access to prenatal care, since late or inadequate prenatal care leads to increased morbidity. The specific components of preconception risk assessment are included in Table 73–2. As risk factors are

identified, multidisciplinary interventions may reduce psychosocial or medical risk *before* pregnancy.

Preconception care promotes healthy behaviors. Educating patients about eating a nutritious diet, exercising regularly, and avoiding alcohol, tobacco, unnecessary medications, and possible teratogens is best begun prior to pregnancy. Regular pelvic examinations and Pap tests, along with advice on appropriate contraceptive use and safe sex, should be provided. Social barriers to prenatal care should be identified and addressed and the importance of early prenatal care emphasized. Finally, the woman is informed about screening and diagnostic tests that may be indicated during pregnancy.

PRENATAL CARE

Prenatal care begun in the first trimester reduces perinatal morbidity and mortality for the mother and the infant. Additionally, prenatal care offers the opportunity to (1) screen for health and social risk factors, (2) intervene when problems arise, (3) maintain optimal maternal health, and (4) give the infant a healthy start in life. Early and adequate prenatal care decreases the incidence of low-birth-weight infants, especially in high-risk women. However, the most socially at-risk women are often the least able to obtain prenatal care.

FIRST PRENATAL VISIT

Risk assessment, intervention, close follow-up, and health promotion are the components of prenatal care. The first two prenatal visits are perhaps the most important in this regard. If a preconception visit has not occurred, the issues discussed in the previous section should be addressed during the first prenatal visit.

Risk assessment activities for the first visit include a history, physical examination, and laboratory studies

**TABLE 73–2.   Risk Assessment at
Preconception/First Prenatal Visit**

HISTORY	*Physical Examination*
Medical	General physical examination
Sociodemographic data	Blood pressure*
Menstrual history	Pulse*
Past obstetric history	Height
Contraceptive history	Weight*
Sexual history	Height/weight profile
Medical/surgical history*	Pelvic examination with clinical pelvimetry
Infection history	
Family and genetic history	Pelvic examination for uterine size, dating, pathology*
Nutrition*	
Current pregnancy to date*	Breast examination*
Psychosocial	*LABORATORY TESTS*
Smoking*	*Routine*
Alcohol*	Hemoglobin or hematocrit*
Illicit drugs*	Rh factor
Social support*	Rubella titer
Stress level*	Urine dipstick
Physical/sexual abuse	Protein
Mental illness/mental status	Glucose
Pregnancy readiness	Pap smear
Exposure to teratogens	Gonococcal culture*
Housing, finances, etc.	Syphilis serology*
Extremes of physical work, exercise, and other activity*	Hepatitis B serology
	Urine culture*
	Screening, As Indicated
	Tuberculosis screen
	Chlamydia screen or culture
	Toxoplasmosis
	CMV
	Herpes simplex
	Varicella
	HIV (offer)
	Hemoglobinopathies
	Tay-Sachs disease
	Parental karyotype
	Illicit drug use
	O'Sullivan glucose determination

*If a preconception visit occurred within 6 months before the pregnancy, only the (*) items need be repeated at the first prenatal visit. If no preconception visit occurred, all items should be included during the first or second prenatal visit.

Adapted from U. S. Public Health Service Expert Panel on the Content of Prenatal Care. *Caring for Our Future: The Content of Prenatal Care.* Washington, D. C., U. S. Department of Health and Human Services, 1989.

(see Table 73–2). Risk factor assessment guides the clinician in planning the level of intervention needed during the pregnancy.

EVALUATION

History

An accurate estimate of the gestational age is important for all pregnancies. Pregnancy dating is ideally performed early in pregnancy. The first day of the last menstrual period (LMP) accurately recalled is the method for assigning an estimated date of delivery (EDD) and estimated gestational age (EGA). The EGA is confirmed by initial physical examination of uterine size. Use of ultrasound as a tool for assessing fetal age in every pregnancy is controversial. Routine ultrasound decreases induction of labor for postdate gestations (> 42 weeks). However, routine ultrasound for dating or as a screening tool does not improve perinatal outcome when compared with selective ultrasound based on clinical judgment of need.

Problems experienced during previous pregnancies may predict problems in the current pregnancy. A history of cesarean section, preterm labor, pregnancy-induced hypertension, or gestational diabetes increases their risk in subsequent pregnancies.

The medical history screens for previous or chronic illness that may impact the pregnancy. A medication history, surgical history (particularly gynecologic surgery), and anesthesia history are essential.

A history of drug and substance use (over-the-counter, prescription, or recreational) should be obtained. Alcohol and illicit drug use during pregnancy may lead to low–birth-weight infants, infants with fetal alcohol syndrome (FAS), and infants with neurologic and learning disabilities. Cocaine use has been identified as a cause of abruptio placentae. Tobacco use is associated with small-for-gestational-age infants.

The use of certain medications (e.g., isotretinoin, lithium, valproic acid, warfarin) or exposure to x-rays, chemicals (herbicides, pesticides, cleaning products), and other substances may put the fetus at risk for birth defects.

Levels of social support and stress should be explored. Family dysfunction is a significant predictor of low–birth-weight infants. A certain level of anxiety about pregnancy and birth is considered normal. In women with unusually high levels of stress or anxiety, the practitioner should look beyond the pregnancy to other life concerns, e.g., family, job, or physical or sexual abuse. The greater the stress, the more likely that obstetric complications will occur. Current mental status and a history of mental illness should be obtained.

Physical Examination

The physical examination (see Table 73–2) consists of blood pressure measurement and examination of the cardiovascular system, breasts, and pelvis (uterine size, uterine pathology, clinical pelvimetry).

Additional Evaluation

First Prenatal Visit

Laboratory tests are obtained at the first prenatal visit to screen for conditions amenable to treatment or interventions to improve pregnancy or neonatal outcome (see Table 73–2).

Genetic counseling and screening may be indicated for women 35 years of age and older or those with a family history of genetic disorders. Chorionic villus sampling and amniocentesis are genetic screening tests offered to women at higher risk of having an infant with a genetic disorder. Each test should be accurately and clearly described, including an explanation of the sensitivity, specificity, risks, and benefits. Patients opting for chorionic villus sampling must have the procedure performed at 8–11 weeks EGA. Thus, early referral is mandatory. Amniocentesis is ideally performed at 14–17 weeks.

Second Prenatal Visit

The second pregnancy visit usually follows the first by 4 weeks. In women who entered prenatal care early, this visit often occurs within the first trimester of pregnancy. In women who entered prenatal care later than the first trimester, or if abnormal test results are received, the second visit should occur sooner than 4 weeks to allow for timely response. At the second visit, the normal physiologic and emotional changes and general health habits (exercise, rest, sexual activity) during pregnancy are discussed.

The overall plan for prenatal care—scheduled visits and screening and diagnostic tests—should be discussed with the patient. Visits every 4 weeks until 30 weeks, then every 2 weeks until 36 weeks, and then weekly until delivery is a routine prenatal care schedule. Some clinicians encourage more frequent early visits to emphasize health promotion and education with fewer visits between 30 and 38 weeks. Higher risk pregnancies require more frequent visits.

Health Promotion

Throughout pregnancy, an ongoing discussion of activities that promote and maintain maternal and fetal health should occur.

A 24-hour dietary recall from a typical day is an excellent method of assessing a patient's general nutritional habits. Advising pregnant women about a nutritious food plan is an important part of early pregnancy counseling. Pregnancy is a "teachable moment" for improving eating habits. The eating plan should include foods from all four food groups—bread, fruits/vegetables (especially those rich in vitamins C and A), protein, and fats. Vegetarians may continue their vegetarian diet during pregnancy if they are careful to meet protein requirements through nonmeat sources such as soy protein and legumes. Approximately 300 extra calories per day are needed during pregnancy. Women should get their extra calories from nutritionally dense foods. For example, a peanut butter sandwich on wheat bread with a glass of milk is 300 calories and far more nutritious than pastry for the same number of calories.

Weight prior to pregnancy and weight gain during pregnancy are important factors affecting infant birth weight. Women who are underweight prior to pregnancy or have suboptimal weight gain during pregnancy are at risk for delivering low-birth-weight infants. A minimal weight gain of 22 to 24 pounds is recommended for women at 90%–120% of ideal weight. Significantly underweight women are encouraged to gain at least 30 pounds. Significantly overweight women might be encouraged to gain only 15–20 pounds. The focus for obese women should be on good nutrition and not "dieting." A consultation with a registered dietitian may be helpful.

Hemoglobin levels normally decrease throughout pregnancy owing to the increased plasma volume. This does not represent true anemia. All women should receive supplemental iron throughout pregnancy. Those with poor nutritional status should receive prenatal multivitamins with iron. The Centers for Disease Control and Prevention (CDC) currently recommends that all women of childbearing age in the United States who are capable of becoming pregnant consume 0.4 mg of folic acid per day. Folic acid supplementation has been shown to reduce the occurrence of fetal neural tube defects of women who had a previous child with a neural tube defect. Calcium intake should be monitored closely. If a woman has lactose intolerance or does not like dairy products, supplemental calcium should be given.

Physical changes of pregnancy must be taken into account when discussing exercise regimens. The enlarged uterus may obstruct venous return in the supine position. The uterus and breasts exaggerate lumbar lordosis and affect balance. Hormonal influences may soften connective tissue and increase joint laxity. Women at low risk for adverse maternal or fetal outcomes may continue mild to moderate physical activity throughout pregnancy. Regular exercise at least three times a week is preferable to intermittent exercise. Appropriate clothing and maintenance of hydration are essential. Contraindications to exercise include pregnancy-induced hypertension, premature rupture of membranes, preterm labor in the current or a previous pregnancy, incompetent cervix, persistent second or third trimester bleeding, or intrauterine growth retardation.

Some couples have anxiety about sexual activity during pregnancy. The pregnant woman may fear that she is no longer attractive. Partners may fear that the baby will be harmed during sexual activity. In a low-risk pregnancy without vaginal bleeding, ruptured membranes, or preterm labor, sexual activity may continue as a healthy part of a couple's relationship. Couples should be sensitive to each other's feelings and openly discuss concerns. Sexual activity may encompass a range of behaviors from affection and cuddling to intercourse.

The planned method of infant feeding should be discussed during the first or second prenatal visit. Breast-feeding is the ideal form of infant nutrition—it protects the infant from disease and is economical and convenient. Women should be asked how they plan to feed their baby and whether they have considered breast-feeding. Providers should be skilled in examining the breast prenatally and postnatally, teaching breast-feeding skills, and referring for breast-feeding assistance if necessary.

SECOND TRIMESTER CARE

The standard schedule of visits throughout the second trimester (14–26 weeks EGA) is every 4 weeks. Women with low-risk pregnancies may need fewer visits. A limited history is obtained, including questions about contractions, vaginal bleeding, headache, dysuria, edema, abdominal pain, and blurry vision. Undiagnosed and untreated urinary tract infections are a preventable cause of preterm labor. Abdominal pain, headache, blurry vision, and edema may be signs of preeclampsia. Vaginal bleeding may indicate placenta previa or vaginal infection. Psychosocial problems such as anxiety, abuse, and inadequate level of support should be explored.

A focused physical examination is done at each visit, including assessment of weight, blood pressure, and urine glucose and protein levels. Fundal height is measured to document appropriate fetal growth. Fetal heart tones are first heard with a Doppler stethoscope at approximately 12 weeks EGA and with a fetoscope by 20 weeks EGA. Auscultating fetal heart tones at these dates confirms the dating. Fetal heart tones not heard at these times may indicate a less advanced pregnancy or fetal demise. Fetal heart tones are auscultated with a Doppler stethoscope until 18 to 20 weeks EGA. In a correctly dated pregnancy, fetal heart tones may be auscultated with a fetoscope after 20 weeks.

Determination of maternal serum α-fetoprotein (MSAFP) to screen for neural tube defects is offered at 15–17 weeks EGA. This test and its implications should be carefully explained to the patient. If the test result is abnormal, ultrasound is performed first to look for neural tube defects (spina bifida or anencephaly). If the cause of the elevated MSAFP is not identified on ultrasound, amniocentesis is recommended. Genetic counseling should be offered prior to amniocentesis. Particularly troublesome are abnormal screening values with normal follow-up ultrasound and amniocentesis. When appropriate, amniocentesis for determination of chromosomal abnormalities is optimally performed at 14–18 weeks.

Ultrasound screening should be performed as indicated for problems such as size/date discrepancy, vaginal bleeding, or decreased fetal movement. However, some physicians routinely obtain ultrasound to confirm dating.

Health Promotion

Women often feel better during the second trimester of pregnancy. Gone are the fatigue and nausea of the first trimester, and the aches and discomforts of late pregnancy have not yet begun. Good nutrition, adequate rest and sleep, and physical activity such as walking are encouraged. Near the end of the second trimester, couples should be encouraged to enroll in prenatal classes—especially during the first pregnancy.

THIRD TRIMESTER CARE

Traditionally the pregnant patient is seen every 2 weeks from 30 to 36 weeks, and then weekly until delivery. In the low-risk pregnancy, however, patients may be seen every 4 weeks from 14 to 38 weeks, and then weekly until delivery. Greater attention is given to screening for preterm labor and preeclampsia.

A hemoglobin or hematocrit determination is recommended at 28 weeks' gestation. The hematocrit decreases normally during the second and third trimesters owing to the expanded plasma volume rather than to a deficiency of red blood cells. A hematocrit at or below 35% should not be ignored. The dietary history is reviewed, and the patient is given iron supplementation. An anemia workup may be indicated.

Infants of diabetic mothers are at greater risk for macrosomia, intrauterine death, and neonatal morbidity and mortality. All pregnant women should be screened between 26 and 28 weeks with a 50-g glucose load. Women with blood glucose values ≥ 140 mg/dL at 1 hour after a 50-g glucose load require further evaluation. Unless the primary care provider is skilled in management of gestational diabetes, a perinatologist should be consulted for assistance with management or the patient referred to an obstetrician/gynecologist, particularly for insulin-dependent diabetes mellitus.

Those at greatest risk for morbidity due to gestational diabetes are the obese patient and the patient older than 25 years. When cost and inconvenience make universal screening difficult, the CDC recommends screening women with the following risk factors: > 25 years of age, obesity, first-degree relative with diabetes, history of a stillbirth pregnancy, prior infant birth weight > 4 kg (9 lb), and a prior history of congenital malformation in a child.

Rh immunization occurs in 16% of Rh-negative mothers who deliver an Rh-positive ABO-compatible infant. ABO compatibility confers partial protection against Rh immunization. Infants of mothers with Rh immunization may develop hemolytic disease, the most severe form being hydrops fetalis. By the time of delivery, 1.5%–2% of Rh-negative mothers will be overtly sensitized. The current recommendation is that every Rh-negative, nonimmunized woman receive one prophylactic dose of Rh_o (D) immune globulin at 28 weeks unless the father is known to be Rh-negative. After birth, the same dose of immune globulin is given within 72 hours. If the patient received a second dose prenatally at 40–40.5 weeks, the postdelivery dose need not be given unless delivery occurs more than 3 weeks after the second injection. If the baby is Rh-negative, no postdelivery immune globulin is given.

At 28 weeks, the patient is instructed to monitor fetal kick counts daily after a main meal. Sitting quietly or lying on her left side, the patient should record each definite movement she feels. Eight movements should be felt in 2 hours. The patient may stop counting after eight definite movements are felt whether or not the 2 hours have passed. Further fetal surveillance is indicated if fewer than eight movements are detected, and the patient is instructed to call her physician.

As the patient nears term, an abdominal examination (Leopold's maneuvers) to determine fetal position is performed. A digital cervical examination may be done to check cervical dilatation. A digital examination is contraindicated in women with ruptured membranes or active vaginal bleeding. A sterile speculum examination is mandated with rupture of membranes. Women with active vaginal bleeding require ultrasound scanning prior to examination to rule out placenta previa.

Health Promotion

Pregnant women experience more physical discomfort during the third trimester. Musculoskeletal aches, mild edema, difficulty sleeping, and indigestion are common. Providers can offer ideas for help for these conditions (e.g., massage, lying with the feet elevated above the heart, eating smaller and more frequent meals).

For first-time parents, the thought of parenthood may be daunting. Parents should be able to discuss anxieties with their provider. Couples who are identified as at-risk for parenting must be referred appropriately.

Plans for infant feeding are reviewed. Information regarding circumcision for a male infant is given. The provider affirms the need (and the law) for infant car seat use.

The signs and symptoms of labor are reviewed, including ruptured membranes and contractions that increase in frequency and intensity over time. A "bloody show" is described for the patient but is not necessarily indicative of immediate labor. Bright red vaginal bleeding should be immediately reported to the physician.

Postterm Pregnancy

A postterm pregnancy is one that extends beyond 42 weeks (or 294 days) from the LMP. It occurs in approximately 10% of pregnancies. The risk of perinatal mortality increases markedly after 42 weeks. Pregnancies extending beyond 42 weeks require increased fetal surveillance.

Beginning at 40 weeks, the cervix should be examined for "ripening." If the cervix is inducible (Bishop score of >6), induction of labor may be undertaken by 42 weeks if fetal surveillance (kick counts, nonstress test, or biophysical profile) indicates no problems. The patient should be admitted to the hospital for closer observation and probable delivery at any time that fetal surveillance is nonreassuring. At 42 weeks, either labor is induced or twice weekly fetal surveillance is begun. A nonstress test (NST) alone at this point may not be adequate to assess fetal well-being. A biophysical profile (which includes an NST as well as fetal heart rate, amniotic fluid determination, assessment of fetal respiratory effort, limb flexion, and gross body movements) has better sensitivity and specificity than an NST alone. An alternative method of fetal assessment is a contraction stress test in combination with a determination of amniotic fluid volume. Primary care physicians not skilled in the use of ultrasound for biophysical profile or amniotic fluid determination should consult an obstetrician for these procedures. Abnormal fetal testing or oligohydramnios necessitates delivery.

Research Questions

1. Does routine ultrasound examination improve pregnancy outcome?
2. Should screening for HIV, HbSAg, neural tube defects, or gestational diabetes be performed in all pregnant women? Is such screening cost effective? Does it improve outcome?
3. How can prenatal care be made more widely accessible?

Case Resolution

Amniocentesis at 16 weeks' EGA revealed a 46,XY male, and α-fetoprotein evaluation was within normal limits. The patient had an uncomplicated prenatal course and at 40 weeks EGA delivered a 3.5-kg (8 lb, 8 oz) boy by normal, spontaneous vaginal delivery. She chose to breastfeed. She and her son were doing well at her 6-week postpartum checkup.

Selected Readings

American College of Obstetricians and Gynecologists Technical Bulletin. *Exercise During Pregnancy and the Postpartum Period.* No. 189. Washington, D.C., ACOG, 1994.

Belfrage, P., I. Fernstrom, and G. Hallenberg. Routine or selective ultrasound examinations in early pregnancy. Obstet Gynecol 69: 747–50, 1987.

Centers for Disease Control and Prevention. Public health guidelines for enhancing diabetes control through maternal and child health programs. MMWR 35(13):201–13, 1986.

Centers for Disease Control and Prevention. Recommendations for the use of folic acid to reduce the number of cases of spina bifida and other neural tube defects. MMWR 41:1–7, 1992.

Creasy, R. K., and R. Resnik (eds.). *Maternal-Fetal Medicine: Principles and Practice.* Philadelphia, W.B. Saunders Company, 1989.

Everett, W. D. Screening for gestational diabetes: An analysis of the health benefits and costs. Am J Prev Med 5:38–43, 1989.

Ewigman, B. G., J. P. Crane, F. D. Frigoletto, et al. (RADIUS Study Group). Effect of prenatal ultrasound screening on perinatal outcome. N Engl J Med 329:821–7, 1993.

Jack, B. W., and L. Culpepper. Preconception care. J Fam Pract 32:306–15, 1991.

Jack, B. W., and L. Culpepper. Preconception care: Risk reduction and health promotion in preparation for pregnancy. JAMA 264:1147–9, 1990.

U.S. Public Health Service Expert Panel on the Content of Prenatal Care. *Caring for Our Future: The Content of Prenatal Care.* Washington, D.C., U.S. Department of Health and Human Services, 1989.

AMENORRHEA AND OTHER MENSTRUAL ABNORMALITIES

Maxine H. Dorin, M.D.

H$_x$ A 20-year-old female camp counselor presents with a 10-month history of amenorrhea. Age at menarche was 16 years, but she has had only six or seven menses since then. She has gained approximately 35 kg (75 lb) in the last 5 years, denies any unusual hair growth, and has no other medical problems. She weighs 108 kg (240 lb) and is 165 cm (5 ft, 5 in) tall. She is sexually active with men, uses no birth control, and has never been pregnant. She does not smoke, takes no medications, and has never had surgery. On physical examination, she has female secondary sex characteristics with well-developed breasts. There is a small amount of hair growth on her upper lip but none on her chin, chest, or back. On pelvic examination, she has a normal female escutcheon and external genitalia. Her vagina is pink, moist, and well rugated. Her cervix is smooth, nulliparous, and without lesions. Her uterus is difficult to palpate but is nontender and mobile. There are no large masses in the adnexa, which are nontender. The rectovaginal examination is unremarkable and confirms the vaginal examination.

Questions

1. What would be the differential diagnosis at this time?
2. What other questions might you ask to narrow the differential?
3. What other physical findings might be pertinent?

Amenorrhea is defined as no menses by age 16 years (primary amenorrhea) or cessation of menses for three average cycles in a previously menstruating female (secondary amenorrhea). Amenorrhea at any time can be a source of apprehension in the reproductive age group. The diagnosis and management of amenorrhea or oligomenorrhea (infrequent menses) depend on an understanding of the physiologic mechanisms regulating normal menstrual cycles and the embryologic, genetic, and endocrinologic aberrations that can disrupt it. Three broad categories of causes can be considered: anatomic defects, ovarian failure, and hypothalamic/pituitary defects.

PATHOPHYSIOLOGY

Anatomic Defects

Abnormalities of the genital outflow tract accompanied by normal secondary sexual characteristics and normal external female genitalia signal müllerian duct anomalies (imperforate hymen, uterine or vaginal aplasia, vaginal septa) with normal ovarian function. Abnormal pubertal development and absence of a normal vagina necessitate chromosomal studies for testicular feminization.

Pregnancy or intrauterine adhesions, caused by endometrial damage usually due to postpartum dilatation and curettage (D&C), can lead to secondary amenorrhea. Pregnancy is diagnosed by β-hCG (human chorionic gonadotropin) measurement and adhesions by hysterosalpingography or hysteroscopy.

Ovarian Failure

Hypergonadotropic amenorrhea is seen when there is end-organ failure in the hypothalamic-pituitary-ovarian axis. Since the ovaries are not responsive to gonadotropins (FSH, LH), their levels increase. This is a normal event at menopause, but before the age of 35 years, it is considered premature. It can be caused by removal of or damage to the ovaries by surgery, radiation, chemotherapy, autoimmune disease, or idiopathic causes. In patients with chromosomal dysgenesis (XO, XX, mosaics), normal ovarian tissue does not develop.

Hypothalamic/Pituitary Defects

Approximately 3% of North American adolescents experience delayed puberty (up to age 16 years) and then develop normally. This constitutional defect results in normal pubertal progression and normal height, but before age 16 it is difficult to distinguish from isolated congenital gonadotropin-releasing hormone (GnRH) deficiency, which in its severe forms prevents pubertal development. Diagnosis is confirmed by low FSH and LH levels when other causes such as extreme physical, psychological, or nutritional stress, systemic illness, hyperprolactinemia, and hypothalamic or pituitary tumor all have been ruled out.

Hyperestrogenic hyperandrogenic chronic anovulation or polycystic ovary syndrome (Stein-Leventhal syndrome) can cause amenorrhea or oligomenorrhea. These patients are obese and show an increased amount of estrone being produced from conversion of androstenedione and testosterone in fat cells, resulting in a continuous positive feedback for LH production and a continuous negative feedback for FSH production. This in turn enhances LH-stimulated production of androgens from theca-lutein and stromal cells, while inhibiting the FSH-stimulated production of estrogen by aromatization of androgens in granulosa cells, which then affects intraovarian hormone regulation. The imbalance results in abnormal follicular development and anovulation.

DIFFERENTIAL DIAGNOSIS

The differential diagnosis of amenorrhea or oligomenorrhea can be narrowed significantly by conducting the history and physical examination and a few selected tests. Common causes of amenorrhea are listed in Table 74-1.

EVALUATION

History

The history should focus on the questions listed in Box 74-1. Questions regarding coital exposure, contraceptive use, and symptoms of pregnancy should be asked when relevant. If the patient has primary amenorrhea, inquiry should be made about pubertal milestones and family history of genetic anomalies.

When pregnancy is a possibility, inquiries concerning nausea, appetite changes, and breast tenderness should be made. Even with the young patient with primary amenorrhea, there is a possibility of pregnancy if she is sexually active, because she is less likely to be using contraception.

General health questions are important when considering the possibility of extreme physical, psychological, or nutritional stress. Questions regarding dietary habits, especially in the thin patient, may uncover an eating disorder. Abnormal sleep patterns may lead to the conclusion that the patient is depressed or anxious, and this can be further explored. An extreme exercise schedule can be an underlying cause of hypothalamic amenorrhea. A history of a sudden change in weight should lead to inquiries about stress level. Both obesity and anorexia nervosa can lead to amenorrhea.

A history of head trauma, galactorrhea, headache, or visual changes may indicate a pituitary source of the problem. A history of change in hair texture, tempera-

BOX 74-1. Questions for the Patient with Amenorrhea

1. How old is the patient? If this is primary amenorrhea, then pubertal milestones are important. Age at menarche? Age of pubic and axillary hair growth? Age of breast development?
2. How is the patient's general health? What are her dietary habits? What is her sleep pattern? Exercise schedule? Stress level (both environmental and psychological)? Has she experienced weight loss or gain? What is her employment? Does she use any medications?
3. Is there any history of head trauma? Galactorrhea? Change in hair texture? Headache? Visual changes? Temperature intolerance to heat or cold? Acne? Hirsutism? Temporal balding? Change in voice? Increased muscle mass? Decreased breast size?
4. If this is secondary amenorrhea, have there been hot flashes, vaginal dryness, or dyspareunia?
5. Are there any symptoms of pregnancy? Is she sexually active? Is birth control being used?
6. Are any recreational drugs being used? If so, for how long?
7. When was her last Pap test and pelvic examination? Were both normal?
8. Has she had any surgeries, especially uterine or vaginal, including D&C, cesarean section, etc.?
9. How many times has she been pregnant? How many live births, stillbirths, miscarriages, pregnancy interruptions, ectopic pregnancies have there been?
10. Are there any other medical problems?
11. Is there any family history of amenorrhea or genetic anomalies?

ture intolerance, and other hypothyroid symptoms would suggest either anterior pituitary dysfunction or primary hypothyroidism.

Although rare in puberty, symptoms of androgen excess should be sought. Temporal balding, hirsutism, increased muscle mass, and acne in a pubertal patient may point to androgen insensitivity or congenital adrenal hyperplasia. In patients who have a later onset of hirsutism or virilization, the diagnosis could be polycystic ovary syndrome, an androgen-producing tumor, or exogenous anabolic steroid use.

Patients who have secondary amenorrhea and complain of hot flashes, night sweats, and vaginal dryness or dyspareunia (pain with intercourse) may be experiencing loss of ovarian function. Premature ovarian failure is defined as the loss of ovarian function by age 35 years.

The use of certain medications can lead to amenorrhea. Suppression of the endometrium can be accomplished by oral contraceptive pills, gonadotropin agonists, danazol, and depot medroxyprogesterone. These drugs are usually given for contraception or to treat endometriosis or dysfunctional uterine bleeding. Other medications, such as phenothiazines, opiate analgesics, and cimetidine, can cause an increase in prolactin secretion by a stimulation of the lactotrophs, leading to menstrual irregularities.

A complete obstetric history (if applicable) and gynecologic history should be obtained. A patient who has cyclic abdominal pain that worsens each month and

TABLE 74-1. Common Causes of Amenorrhea

Anatomic Defects
Agenesis (Mayer-Rokitansky-Kuster-Hauser syndrome, androgen insensitivity)
Obstruction (imperforate hymen, vaginal agenesis)
Endometrial suppression (medication, intrauterine adhesions)
Ovarian Failure
Hypergonadotropic amenorrhea
Gonadal dysgenesis
Premature ovarian failure
Surgical or radiation damage
Hypothalamic/Pituitary Defects
Deficient GnRH secretion due to
  Constitutional defect
  Extreme physical, psychological, or nutritional stress
  Systemic illness
  Isolated gonadotropin deficiency
Hyperestrogenic hyperandrogenic chronic anovulation
  Polycystic ovary syndrome
Hyperprolactinemia

a history of decreased or no menstrual flow may have an outflow obstruction. A history of postpartum or post-abortal D&C suggests destruction of the endometrium (Asherman's syndrome).

Physical Examination

The physical examination should focus on the height, weight, body habitus, distribution and extent of terminal androgen-stimulated body hair, breast development, and external and internal genitalia.

Abnormalities such as a webbed neck, high-arched palate, wide carrying angle, increased arm span, short fourth metacarpal, or sexual infantilism indicate a chromosomal abnormality.

Abnormal reflexes, thyroid tenderness or mass, or an abnormal neurologic or eye examination should raise the possibility of an endocrine or hypothalamic-pituitary problem.

The approach to the pelvic examination is individualized for each patient. In the adolescent, an educational approach may be best. On examination of the external genitalia, the decision to use a speculum can be aborted in the patient with vaginal agenesis or imperforate hymen. In these cases, a rectal examination may be more informative and less traumatic.

Additional Evaluation

Typically, other diagnostic investigations are only confirmatory, since the diagnosis will have been established with a high degree of certainty based on the history and physical examination.

Initial laboratory tests should include a pregnancy test, LH, FSH, prolactin, and thyroid function tests (Table 74–2).

CT scanning or MRI can be used when hypothalamic-pituitary defects are suspected. Chromosomal analysis is needed to diagnose testicular feminization or Turner's syndrome.

Occasionally, hysterosalpingography is performed to confirm the suspicion of intrauterine adhesions. An ultrasound test can help diagnose the presence or absence of a uterus in a patient for whom the pelvic

---

TABLE 74–2.   Evaluating Amenorrhea

Most Helpful Tests
β-hCG (pregnancy test), either urine or blood
Thyroid function tests
Prolactin level

Often Helpful Tests
LH and FSH measurement
Progestin challenge test

Occasionally Helpful Tests, Used Only When Indicated
CT scan of the head
MRI of the head

Helpful Tests In Selected Situations
Chromosomal analysis (karyotype)
Pelvic ultrasound
Hysterosalpingography, hysteroscopy
Diagnostic laparoscopy
Endometrial biopsy

---

examination is difficult either because of body habitus or lack of cooperation.

Additional hormonal evaluation should be ordered only when the history and physical examination suggest problems in the neuroendocrine axis. Testing should be selective, based on the differential diagnosis.

MANAGEMENT

In most cases of vaginal aplasia with a uterus, a surgical procedure to establish a vagina is necessary to provide an outflow tract for menstrual blood and to prevent tubal damage and endometriosis with reflux into the abdominal cavity. In adolescents without a vagina and uterus, either a surgical procedure or dilators can be used to establish a vagina when regular sexual intercourse is anticipated. In the case of intrauterine adhesions, the adhesions are lysed surgically during hysteroscopy.

In ovarian failure with normal ovaries, only education and hormonal support can be given. Occasionally, hormone replacement therapy causes periodic ovulation, and this needs to be discussed. In gonadal dysgenesis, the removal of all gonadal tissue is mandatory to prevent the up to 25% chance of malignancy.

In hypothalamic chronic anovulation, as seen in anorexia nervosa or extreme psychological stress, psychological counseling, weight gain, and a change in life-style may be effective in producing ovulation. Induction of ovulation can also be accomplished by the use of clomiphene citrate. In hypoestrogenic women, estrogen can be given as hormone replacement therapy.

Although the treatment for hyperprolactinemia is controversial, a dopamine agonist for microadenomas is usually recommended, because nearly 5% progress to a macroadenoma. Macroadenomas can be treated with surgery, a dopamine agonist, irradiation, or a combination of the three. Frequent endocrine and visual field testing is generally recommended for patients who are treated with a dopamine agonist. Because the tumor will usually quickly return to pretreatment size if the medication is stopped, the dopamine agonist must be used indefinitely.

In polycystic ovary syndrome, management depends on the fertility desires of the patient. The need for endometrial biopsy prior to initiating therapy needs to be assessed because of the increased risk of endometrial hyperplasia and cancer. If the patient does not desire fertility and is at low risk for the side effects of oral contraceptives, these can be used. In patients who desire fertility, clomiphene citrate is the drug of choice for ovulation induction. Laparoscopic follicular puncture (and cortical drilling) is an unproven treatment modality for ovulation induction but may be an alternative to ovarian wedge resection to reduce the amount of ovarian stroma.

PATIENT EDUCATION

Patient education is probably the most important factor in the outcome of treatment for amenorrhea. Whether an anatomic defect has resulted in permanent infertility or the patient has anorexia nervosa, she must understand what the underlying defect is so that the appropriate therapy can be carried out. Many visits may be needed before the patient will accept treatment.

PROGNOSIS

The prognosis for restoring menstrual flow or establishing fertility depends on the cause of amenorrhea. In some cases, such as uterine aplasia, both outcomes are impossible. For polycystic ovary syndrome, use of clomiphene citrate can result in a 75% ovulation rate and 40% pregnancy rate.

Research Question

1. In the polycystic ovary syndrome, the technique of decreasing the number of cysts by cortical drilling seems to increase the fertility rate for some patients, but the mechanism is unclear. What substances in the cyst fluid or wall should be analyzed, and why?

Case Resolution

The patient had a normal prolactin level and normal thyroid function tests. LH was three times greater than FSH, suggesting polycystic ovary syndrome. After further discussion with her health care provider, she was placed on progestin for 10 days every 3 months.

Selected Readings

Aiman, J., and C. Smentek. Premature ovarian failure. Obstet Gynecol 66(1):9–14, 1985.

Batzer, F. R., S. L. Corson, B. Gocial, et al. Genetic offspring in patients with vaginal agenesis: Specific medical and legal issues. Am J Obstet Gynecol 167:1288, 1992.

Daneshdoost, L., T. A. Gennarelli, H. M. Bashey, et al. Recognition of gonadotroph adenomas in women. N Engl J Med 324:589, 1991.

Jonnavithula, S., M. P. Warren, R. P. Fox, and M. I. Lazaro. Bone density is compromised in amenorrheic women despite return of menses: A 2-year study. Obstet Gynecol 81:669, 1993.

Katznelson, L., J. M. Alexander, H. A. Bikkai, et al. Imbalanced follicle-stimulating hormone β-subunit hormone biosynthesis in human pituitary adenomas. J Clin Endocrinol Metab 74:1342, 1992.

Nestler, J. E., J. N. Clore, and W. G. Blackard. The central role of obesity (hyperinsulinemia) in the pathogenesis of polycystic ovary syndrome. Am J Obstet Gynecol 161:1095, 1989.

Reindollar, R. H., M. Novak, S.P.T. Tho, and P. G. McDonough. Adult-onset amenorrhea: A study of 262 patients. Am J Obstet Gynecol 155:531, 1986.

Speroff, L., R. H. Glass, and N. G. Kase. Amenorrhea. *In* Speroff, L., R. H. Glass, and N. G. Kase. *Clinical Gynecologic Endocrinology and Infertility,* 5th ed. Baltimore, Williams & Wilkins, 1994.

CHAPTER 75

THE ABNORMAL PAP TEST

Caryn McHarney-Brown, M.D.

Hx A 22-year-old female college student comes in for follow-up of a Pap test that reported a "high-grade squamous intraepithelial lesion." She uses an oral contraceptive, has a 5 pack-year history of cigarette smoking, and has no prior history of an abnormal Pap test. She has never been pregnant. She and her current partner have been together for 2 years, but she has had eight lifetime partners since becoming sexually active at age 15. She reports normal monthly menses without any recent abnormal vaginal bleeding or discharge. The patient is concerned about the Pap test result and has many questions.

Questions

1. What other questions would you ask the patient?
2. What does "high-grade squamous intraepithelial lesion" mean?
3. What do you tell the patient when she asks, "How did I get this?" "Can I be treated?" "Do you need to see my boyfriend?" "Do I have cancer?" "Will I have trouble having children?"

Since its introduction in the late 1940s, the Papanicolaou (Pap) test has been an important tool used in the detection of cervical abnormalities. Worldwide, cervical cancer is the most common cancer in women. In the United States, it is the eighth most common cancer in women, with an incidence of 8 to 10 cases per 100,000 population, considerably less than the 28 to 30 cases per 100,000 population seen prior to the widespread use of Pap testing.

Cervical neoplasia is one of the best studied cancers,

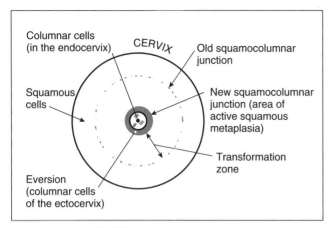

FIGURE 75–1. *Cervical anatomy.*

severe dysplasia) to cervical cancer. The challenge of caring for a patient with an abnormal Pap test is to appropriately manage the precursor stages and to prevent cervical cancer.

PATHOPHYSIOLOGY

The cervix is composed mostly of collagenous connective tissue, blood vessels, and primarily squamous epithelial and columnar glandular epithelial cells (Fig. 75–1). The columnar epithelium is primarily found in the endocervix (the cervical canal), and the tougher squamous epithelium covers the ectocervix. The columnar epithelium is everted onto the ectocervix at birth, at puberty, and during pregnancy. Environmental factors, such as pregnancy and aging, cause the transformation (metaplasia) of columnar cells into squamous epithelial cells. As metaplasia occurs, the columnar cells retreat into the endocervix. This restless region of cellular change, the squamocolumnar junction, is vulnerable to infection and environmental insult. It is the area where dysplasia usually begins.

Normal squamous epithelium consists of several cell types with the deeper cells dividing and providing cells for the more superficial layers (Fig. 75–2). Small round cells with large nuclei (basal cells) give rise to flatter

partially owing to the accessibility of the cervix for observation and sampling and the frequency of disease. From studies of cervical abnormalities, it has become clear that cervical cancer arises from precursor lesions that can be identified and treated at an early stage. Cervical lesions progress through a continuum of worsening abnormalities from low-grade lesions (atypia, mild dysplasia) to higher grade lesions (moderate and

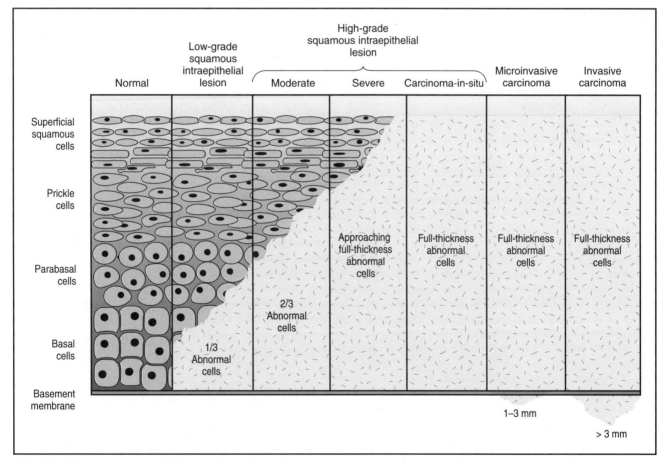

FIGURE 75–2. *Cervical squamous epithelium and the progression of squamous intraepithelial lesions. Moving from left to right, the basal cells become less differentiated, with more mitotic figures and a higher nuclear-to-cytoplasmic ratio. As these abnormal basal cells occupy more of the stroma, the severity of the squamous intraepithelial lesion (SIL) increases. Invasion occurs when the abnormal basal cells break through the basement membrane and may be present even with lower grades of SIL.*

superficial cells with small or absent nuclei as squamous maturation progresses. **Dysplasia** is disordered growth or development of the squamous epithelium. It is characterized by small cells with large nuclei, increased mitotic figures, loss of polarity, and pleomorphism. As dysplasia progresses, more and more layers of the epithelium become involved, from deeper to more superficial, until the entire stratified squamous epithelium is filled with abnormal cells.

While information about the natural histologic progression of cervical dysplasia is incomplete, recent DNA probe techniques provide clues about the etiology of these abnormalities. Human papillomavirus (HPV) has been implicated as a sexually transmitted cofactor in the development of cervical dysplasia. HPV DNA has been found in cervical smears; in cervical, vaginal, and perineal biopsies from women with genital warts (condylomata acuminata); in women with abnormal Pap tests; and in patients with genital cancer (vulvar, cervical, penile, and anal).

Certain types (e.g., types 6 and 11) of HPV are associated with external genital lesions and condyloma. Types 16, 18, 31, 33, and others are associated with dysplastic and cancerous cervical lesions. HPV, human immunodeficiency virus (HIV), and other sexually transmitted diseases (STDs) may be cofactors causing dysplasia as well as a more rapid progression of dysplasia to higher grade lesions and cancer.

The Bethesda system (Table 75–1) currently is used to categorize and describe Pap test results. The cytopathologist must comment on the adequacy of the specimen and describe pertinent pathologic findings. For example, if the endocervical cells appear atypical, the pathologist might describe the appearance as "reactive" or "inflammatory" atypia and comment on the presence of clue cells, *Trichomonas,* or other sexually transmitted disease. The presence of "dysplastic atypia" requires diagnostic workup. Results reported in this way help the clinician formulate a treatment plan.

DIFFERENTIAL DIAGNOSIS

Sometimes it is difficult to determine the cause of an abnormal Pap test, since many hormonal and environmental factors play important roles in cervical pathology.

Areas of squamous metaplasia, which is the normal transformation of columnar cells into stratified squamous epithelium on the cervix, can appear abnormal and friable.

Concurrent infection with *Chlamydia trachomatis, Neisseria gonorrhoeae, Trichomonas,* or severe yeast infection can cause the cervix to look abnormal and confuse the results of the Pap test.

Inflammation due to an identifiable STD, childbirth, or an unknown cause can make cells on the Pap test appear abnormal.

Hyperkeratosis (hyperplasia of the stratum corneum) is a microscopic description of squamous cell proliferation. Hyperkeratosis is found in cervical dysplasia and cancer but may also occur in smokers or patients who use barrier methods of contraception (e.g., diaphragm).

After menopause, estrogen stimulation of receptor cells declines. This causes loss of vaginal rugae and thinning and fragility of the mucosal skin. Cytologically, this loss of estrogen influence can resemble atypia or dysplasia. These gross and cellular alterations are called atypical changes or atrophic cervicovaginitis.

In addition to detecting precancerous and cancerous lesions of the cervix, the Pap test can sometimes detect abnormal cells from other genital tract and vulvar or vaginal cancers. The cytopathologist should comment on the possible origin of abnormal cells in the Pap test report. If any notation of abnormal or atypical cells appears on the Pap test report, follow-up is mandatory.

EVALUATION

The physician should determine the existence of conditions or medications that may influence cervical cytology, such as a decrease in immune system function (e.g., due to HIV infection), the age of the patient, and her hormone status (e.g., postmenopausal but not on hormone replacement therapy).

Inquiry should be made about the specific risk factors for cervical dysplasia:

1. Age at onset of sexual activity (including sexual abuse): early onset of sexual activity correlates with increased risk of dysplasia.

2. Number of sexual partners: incidence of cervical dysplasia increases with three or more lifetime partners.

3. Previous history of STDs, e.g., HPV, HIV, and possibly others.

4. Smoking history.

5. History of previous abnormal Pap tests: this information may provide clues about prior untreated or recurrent disease.

TABLE 75–1. Bethesda System for Reporting Cervical/Vaginal Cytologic Diagnoses

I. Statement of adequacy
II. General categorizations
  A. Within normal limits
  B. Descriptive diagnosis
    1. Infection
    2. Reactive/reparative changes
    3. Epithelial cell abnormalities
      a. Squamous cell
        i. ASCUS (atypical squamous cells of uncertain significance)
        ii. Squamous intraepithelial lesion (SIL)
          (a) Low-grade SIL (encompassing HPV, slight dysplasia/CIN1)
          (b) High-grade SIL (encompassing moderate dysplasia/CIN2, severe dysplasia/CIN3, carcinoma-in-situ/CIN3)
          (c) Squamous cell carcinoma
      b. Glandular cell
        i. Presence of endometrial cells
        ii. Atypical glandular cells of undetermined significance
        iii. Adenocarcinoma
        iv. Other epithelial malignant neoplasm: Specify
    4. Nonepithelial malignant neoplasm: Specify
    5. Hormonal evaluation (vaginal smears only)
    6. Other

CIN, cervical intraepithelial neoplasia.

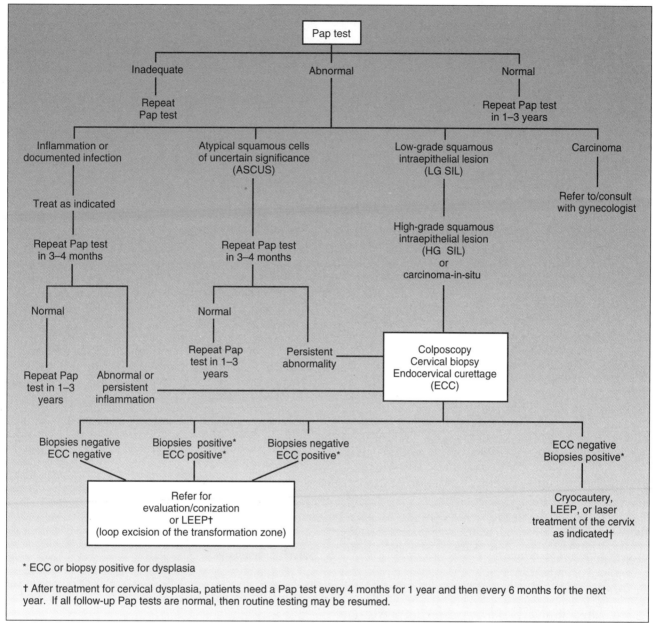

FIGURE 75-3. *Algorithm for follow-up of the Pap test.*

6. History of exposure to diethylstilbestrol (DES): this estrogen was sometimes given to pregnant women in the 1950s in an effort to prevent miscarriage. The practice was discontinued when the offspring, both female and male, were found to have an increased risk of developing clear cell adenocarcinoma of the genital tract. Women with DES exposure may have a deformed ("cockscomb") cervix and marked eversion (see Fig. 75-1), which may increase their risk for cervical dysplasia.

7. Barrier contraception: barrier methods of contraception, such as cervical caps and diaphragms, may cause inflammation and hyperkeratosis, whereas oral contraceptives may decrease the risk of cervical disease, and condoms (especially when used with spermicidal gel) may decrease the risk of dysplasia and cervical cancer.

MANAGEMENT

The majority of abnormal Pap tests can be managed in the outpatient setting by a primary care provider skilled in colposcopy and cryocautery of the cervix (Fig. 75-3).

The colposcope provides binocular magnification of the cervix. The cervix is visualized after the application of a weak acid solution to highlight potential abnormal areas. Biopsy specimens are taken of abnormal areas, and endocervical curettage (ECC) is obtained. The importance of the ECC is due to the fact that treatment is different when lesions are present in the endocervical canal than when the canal is normal. If the lesions are only on the ectocervix, local ablative treatment of the transformation zone is done. Cryocautery, laser, or LEEP (loop excision of the transformation zone) are all effective treatment modalities. If the ECC is positive, indicating abnormalities in the endocervix, then cervical conization can be carried out in the office (LEEP) or as a day surgery procedure (cold knife conization of the cervix).

Treatable causes for abnormal Pap tests should be pursued prior to colposcopy (see Figure 75–3). If the cervix appears abnormal on routine examination, a biopsy can be made of the suspicious lesion and the patient referred for colposcopy. A Pap test alone is not a sufficient diagnostic tool when an abnormal lesion is noted. Since the Pap test can have a false-negative rate of 15%–25% or more, its use is reserved for screening rather than diagnosis in a patient with a cervical lesion.

PATIENT AND FAMILY EDUCATION

Identification and treatment of cervical dysplasia are critical in the prevention of cervical cancer. Cervical dysplasia has the epidemiologic profile of HPV. HPV is an important cofactor in the development of cervical dysplasia and cancer and is extremely prevalent (about 30%) in the sexually active population.

Regular screening Pap tests can detect cervical dysplasia and guide follow-up. The U. S. Preventive Service Task Force recommends the following schedule for Pap tests:

1. Pap tests are recommended for all women who are or have been sexually active.
2. Pap tests should begin with the onset of sexual activity or at age 18 years (whichever occurs earlier) and be performed every 1–3 years, depending on the patient's history.
3. Pap testing may be discontinued at age 65 years if the previous tests have been normal.

Patient education can play a key role in the prevention of cervical cancer. By delaying the onset of sexual activity, decreasing the number of sexual partners, eliminating tobacco use, and consistently using condoms, the risk of cervical dysplasia and cancer can be reduced.

NATURAL HISTORY/PROGNOSIS

The prognosis for cervical dysplasia is excellent when treated early. Early treatment can cure cervical dyspla-

sia and prevent cervical cancer. New information is becoming available to aid the clinician in determining which cervical lesions may progress and which may resolve. Viral DNA probes are available to type HPV. HPV types 6 and 11 are generally thought to be slow growing and rarely associated with progression to more dangerous lesions. HPV types 16, 18, 31, 32, 33, and some 50s are frequently associated with high-grade lesions and cancer. At present, if the Pap test and subsequent biopsies are abnormal, treatment is the same regardless of viral type, so routine viral typing is not performed.

Research Questions

1. Should HPV viral typing be performed on every patient with an abnormal Pap test to help guide treatment?
2. How do HPV, HIV, and other cofactors interact to lead to the development of cervical cancer?

Case Resolution

The patient underwent colposcopy. ECC and biopsies of abnormal-appearing areas were performed. The ECC was normal. The cervical biopsies revealed a high-grade squamous intraepithelial lesion (HGSIL) consistent with moderate dysplasia. The patient elected to have a loop excision of the transformation zone as local ablative treatment. She also was encouraged to stop smoking and was counseled about ways to prevent recurrence of cervical dysplasia. She was advised to return for repeat Pap tests every 4 months for a year and every 6 months for the next year.

Selected Readings

Cotran, R. S., V. Kumar, and S. L. Robbins. *Robbins Pathologic Basis of Disease,* 5th ed. Philadelphia, W.B. Saunders Company, 1994.

Fowler, J. Screening for cervical cancer. Postgrad Med 57–70, February 1993.

Ham, A., and D. Cormack. *Histology,* 9th ed., Philadelphia, J.B. Lippincott Company, 1987.

Larsen, W. G., et al. The problematic Papanicolaou smear. The Female Patient 31–40, July 1992.

Koss, L. G. The Papanicolaou test for cervical cancer. JAMA 261:737–43, 1989.

National Cancer Institute Workshop. The 1988 Bethesda system of reporting cervical/vaginal cytologic diagnosis. JAMA 262:931–4, 1989.

U.S. Preventive Services Task Force. *Guide to Clinical Preventive Services: An Assessment of the Effectiveness of 169 Interventions.* Baltimore, Williams & Wilkins, 1989.

CHAPTER 76

MENOPAUSE AND POSTMENOPAUSAL SYMPTOMS

Lesley W. Janis, M.D.

H$_x$ The patient is a 51-year-old female biochemist whose chief complaint is a 2-week history of intermittent episodes of sweating and flushing. She feels warm from her neck up, her skin becomes red, and she sweats profusely. The episodes last a few minutes and now occur daily, sometimes at work or in the middle of the night. The patient denies any other recent medical problems and her past medical history is unremarkable; however, her menstrual cycles have become irregular and infrequent over the past 6 months. She takes a daily vitamin supplement but no prescription medications. She considers herself healthy and works full-time. Her last visit to the doctor was over a year ago.

Questions

1. What other questions are important to ask this patient?
2. Which elements of the physical examination do you want to include on this visit?
3. What health promotion/disease prevention issues are important to address with this patient?

The menopause is not a disease state. It is a period of physiologic transition caused by decreased levels of circulating estrogen. When women approach the menopause, they should be evaluated and counseled about several unique health care issues.

PATHOPHYSIOLOGY

The normal ovarian cycle repeats itself monthly from menarche to menopause. Under the influence of the hypothalamus, the anterior pituitary produces follicle-stimulating hormone (FSH) and luteinizing hormone (LH), which stimulate the ovary to produce a primary follicle. During this process, estrogen and progesterone are produced by the ovary and ovulation takes place. While estrogen and progesterone participate in feedback loops that keep the cycle going, they also have extensive end-organ effects. Since all women are born with a finite number of follicles, the ovary ultimately stops responding to signals from the pituitary. When this happens, the cycle is disrupted: ovulation and menstrual cycling end, circulating levels of estrogen and progesterone fall, and serum FSH and LH levels rise (Fig. 76–1).

Menopause is defined as the cessation of menses for at least 6 consecutive months. The average age at which this occurs is 50 years (average range, 45–55 years). Owing to the widespread anatomic and physiologic effects of estrogen and progesterone, the menopausal state encompasses a broad spectrum of symptoms and health implications. While the incidence and severity of symptoms vary widely, it is important to thoroughly evaluate all peri- and postmenopausal women and discuss with them the possible benefits of hormone replacement therapy.

DIFFERENTIAL DIAGNOSIS

Once a careful history has been performed, there are very few clinical entities that can be confused with the symptoms associated with the menopause. However, there are a few caveats.

If a perimenopausal woman is having irregular bleeding, other causes must be ruled out. Estrogen causes the endometrial cells to proliferate, while progesterone causes them to differentiate. Most irregular bleeding represents a disruption of the usual estrogen/progesterone balance, caused by anovulatory cycles. However, endometrial neoplasia, intrauterine tumors, and bleeding from nonuterine sites must also be considered. Unexpected pregnancy is a possibility.

Vasomotor instability, or hot flashes or flushes, is related to the sudden decrease in estrogen levels. Hot flashes occur in 75% of menopausal women and consist of a sudden feeling of warmth followed by visible erythema of the face, neck, and upper chest. Occurring at night, they can result in insomnia, fatigue, and irritability. The symptoms associated with hot flashes are unique, but night sweats associated with infectious etiologies (e.g., tuberculosis, HIV infection) and malignancy (e.g., Hodgkin's disease, non-Hodgkin's lymphoma) should be considered. Hot flashes are easily distinguished from pheochromocytoma, which is notable for cold sweats and skin pallor.

The tissue lining the vagina and distal urethra is estrogen dependent. After the menopause, urogenital atrophy often develops, with thinning of the mucosa and a decrease in secretions. While some women are asymptomatic, others develop vaginal itching, stress incontinence, dysuria, and dyspareunia. Other causes of vaginitis should be ruled out in women presenting with vaginal itching, burning, or discharge. Stress incontinence may be caused by an anatomic cystocele. Dysuria

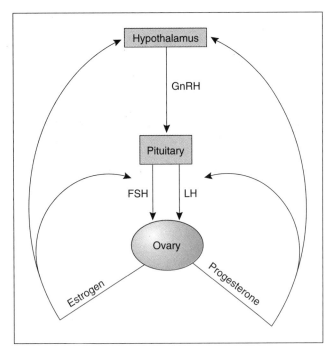

FIGURE 76–1. *The hypothalamic-pituitary-ovarian axis. FSH, follicle-stimulating hormone; LH, luteinizing hormone; GnRH, gonadotropin-releasing hormone.*

associated with urogenital atrophy should not be confused with a bacterial cystitis or urethritis. Dyspareunia that does not respond to topical estrogens or lubricants deserves further evaluation.

Depression and anxiety are frequently seen in women at the time of the menopause. The existence of a "psychological" component of menopause is a controversial issue. It was believed for many years that decreased estrogen levels lead to depression, irritability, fatigue, nervousness, and anxiety. Numerous studies seem to conclude that many of these symptoms were related to hot flashes; when hot flashes were relieved, so were many of the symptoms. Anyone presenting with symptoms of depression should be thoroughly evaluated.

The risk of developing osteoporosis increases dramatically after the menopause, with some women being at higher risk than others. Osteoporotic fractures of the spine are painful and disfiguring, while hip fractures are a leading cause of morbidity and mortality in elderly women. Other causes of bone disease, such as malignancy, should be ruled out (see Chapter 17).

Cardiovascular disease is the leading cause of death in women, and its incidence increases dramatically after the menopause. The risk factors for cardiac disease in men and women are essentially the same, except that surgical removal of the ovaries before menopause in the absence of estrogen replacement puts the female patient at especially high risk. Risk factor assessment and modification is especially important in this setting, since there are a variety other factors (e.g., hypertension, diabetes, elevated cholesterol levels, obesity, tobacco use) that have an impact on the development of cardiovascular disease.

EVALUATION

History

The most common presenting complaints of perimenopausal women who seek medical care are menstrual irregularities and hot flash symptoms. The nature, duration, and associated symptoms of hot flashes should be established, as well as any effect on sleep pattern or daily activities. A thorough menstrual history should be included. Symptoms that may be related to estrogen deficiency, e.g., dysuria, stress incontinence, vaginal dryness or irritation, vaginal discharge, and dyspareunia, should be noted. A thorough evaluation of the patient's risk factors for osteoporosis and cardiovascular disease should be performed.

The past medical history should be reviewed for any major medical or surgical problems. Gynecologic surgery, such as hysterectomy, and the reason for the procedure, should be documented. It is important to know whether the patient has a history of breast or gynecologic cancer, cardiovascular disease, osteoporosis, gallstone, liver disease, migraine headache, or lipid abnormalities.

The family history should be reviewed for breast cancer, gynecologic cancers, osteoporosis, and cardiovascular disease. The patient should be asked about smoking history, alcohol intake, dietary habits, calcium intake, and level of exercise. This information will influence advice to the patient on the relative benefits and risks of hormone replacement therapy. What medications does the patient take? Is the patient sexually active? Postmenopausal women are at increased risk for contracting sexually transmitted HIV owing to atrophy of the vaginal mucosa.

Physical Examination

If the patient has not had a complete screening physical examination during the past few years, this is a good opportunity. The focus of the examination is on the heart; assessment of height (to follow for the development of osteoporotic vertebral body fractures); breasts, and pelvis. The pelvic examination is performed to evaluate for uterine or ovarian enlargement, the presence of a cystocele or rectocele, and the status of the vaginal mucosa.

Additional Evaluation

Not all women need laboratory confirmation of their menopausal status; in most cases, the history is sufficient. When the presentation is less than classic, an elevated FSH level will confirm the diagnosis. If the patient has had heavy or irregular bleeding, an endometrial biopsy should be performed to rule out neoplasia, along with a complete blood count to rule out anemia. Prior to starting hormone replacement therapy, the patient should be checked for lipid status and should have a mammogram and Pap test.

The current recommendation is for an annual mammogram for women over the age of 50 years. Screening mammograms between the ages of 40 and 50 years are controversial; many physicians advise mammograms every 2 years for women in this age group (annually for women at increased risk for breast cancer); mammograms should be done every other year unless the woman is at high risk.

Controversy exists about performing Pap tests in older women. Women who have had a hysterectomy for benign disease probably do not need the test, nor do women over the age of 65 years who are no longer sexually active and have had three consecutive normal tests. Sexually active women with a history of normal Pap smears can be followed every 2–3 years. A woman who is sexually active and considered at high risk for cervical cancer (e.g., has multiple partners, smokes, has a history of dysplasia or STDs) should have an annual examination regardless of her age. Unfortunately, older women may not be counseled about safe sex practices because it is assumed that they are not engaging in high-risk behaviors. However, postmenopausal women with vaginal atrophy are at especially high risk for HIV infection because the vaginal mucosa is thin and bleeds easily.

MANAGEMENT

The mainstay of treatment for postmenopausal symptoms and for the prevention of osteoporosis and cardiovascular disease in postmenopausal women is estrogen replacement. The duration of treatment depends on the goal. Hot flash symptoms may need to be treated for only a few years, while disease prevention requires the use of estrogen indefinitely.

There are few absolute contraindications to estrogen replacement. These include undiagnosed vaginal bleeding, pregnancy, breast cancer, an estrogen-dependent neoplasm, active thromboembolic disorders, and a history of thrombosis related to estrogen use. Some relative contraindications are gallbladder disease, liver disease, and a history of menstrual migraines. Unopposed estrogen is known to increase the incidence of endometrial hyperplasia and cancer. Therefore, in women with an intact uterus, progesterone must be added to the regimen.

Estrogen is available in both oral and transdermal forms. Conjugated estrogen is the most commonly used oral form in the United States, but estradiol also is available. Transdermal estrogen is often used in women who have elevated triglyceride levels or liver disease or who cannot tolerate the oral dose. Progesterone also is available orally. Common dosing regimens are summarized in Table 76–1.

Side effects are few, but they should be reviewed with the patient. Bloating and breast tenderness may be experienced with both estrogen and progesterone. Nausea and abdominal discomfort sometimes occur. Localized skin irritation is fairly common with the transdermal patch. If the patient can tolerate them, most side effects resolve within a few months.

Some women are reluctant to start hormone replacement therapy (HRT) because of the fear of cancer, particularly of the breast. Although large population studies have not shown an overall increased risk of breast cancer with the use of postmenopausal estrogen replacement, they have shown a slightly increased risk in those patients who (1) take estrogens for more than 10 years, (2) have a family history of breast cancer, and (3) also take progesterone. No other cancers have been linked to the use of estrogen or progesterone (excluding the already mentioned risk of endometrial cancer with unopposed estrogen).

Another reason women may be reluctant to begin hormone replacement therapy is the possibility of resuming menses. While regular periods generally disappear after a few years, HRT does tend to prolong them for a while or cause them to reappear. Use of the continuous low-dose regimen of estrogen and progesterone may suppress withdrawal bleeding. If a woman cannot or chooses not to take estrogen, she should not be left with the feeling that there is no other help. Topical lubricants can be used to alleviate discomfort during intercourse related to vaginal atrophy. Clonidine is sometimes effective in controlling hot flashes. All women should be shown how to improve their overall health by addressing risk factors for osteoporosis and heart disease.

PATIENT EDUCATION

The perimenopause is an excellent time for a thorough assessment of a patient's health status. Information on the physical and psychological effects of the menopause should be reviewed. Topics for discussion include the symptoms of hot flashes and vaginal atrophy, the risks and benefits of hormone replacement therapy, sexuality and safe sex practices, and prevention strategies for heart disease, osteoporosis, and breast cancer.

TABLE 76–1. Dosing Regimens for Hormone Replacement Therapy

Patient Without Uterus

Continuous estrogen: 0.625 mg of conjugated estrogens or 2 mg of estradiol daily orally, or 0.05-mg transdermal patch twice a week

Patient With Uterus

Cyclic therapy: continuous estrogen (as above) plus 5–10 mg of medroxyprogesterone on days 1–10 of each month

Continuous low-dose therapy: continuous estrogen (as above) plus 2.5 mg of medroxyprogesterone daily

---

Research Questions

1. What are the long-term health effects of estrogen replacement in women who have used oral contraceptives for a number of years prior to menopause?

2. Do women who smoke receive any protective effects (antiosteoporotic, cardiovascular) from estrogen replacement therapy?

Case Resolution

This patient had a classic presentation of vasomotor instability (hot flashes). Further diagnostic evaluation was not necessary, but she should have a thorough history and risk factor assessment performed. The impact of the menopause and the risks and benefits of hormone replacement therapy should be discussed with her. Her physical evaluation should include breast and pelvic examinations, mammogram, and Pap test.

Selected Readings

Bachman, G. A. Sexual issues at menopause. Ann NY Acad Sci 592:87–94, 1990.

Belchetz, P. E. Hormonal treatment of postmenopausal women. N Engl J Med 330:1062–71, 1994.

Collins, J. B. Menopause. Prim Care 15: 593–605, 1988.

Dupont, W. D., and D. L. Page. Menopausal estrogen replacement therapy and breast cancer. Arch Intern Med 151:67–72, 1991.

Ettinger, B., H. K. Genant, and C. E. Cann. Long-term estrogen replacement therapy prevents bone loss and fractures. Ann Intern Med 102:319–24, 1985.

Grady, D., et al. Hormone therapy to prevent disease and prolong life in postmenopausal women. Ann Intern Med 117:1016–37, 1992.

Stampfer, M. J., F. Grodstein, and S. Bechtel. Postmenopausal estrogen and cardiovascular disease. Contemp Intern Med 6:47–56, 1994.

COMMON ENDOCRINE PROBLEMS

C H A P T E R   7 7

DIABETES MELLITUS

Janette S. Carter, M.D.

H$_x$ The patient is a 50-year-old, obese man with diabetes mellitus. He works afternoons in a convenience store and is a bartender at night. The patient was put on insulin 10 years ago after an unsuccessful trial of oral medication. At present, he takes 14 units of NPH and 6 units of regular insulin in the morning and 12 units of NPH and 8 units of regular insulin in the evening. Even though he reports glucose levels between 120 and 180 mg/dL, his HbA$_{1c}$ measurement is 14%. He complains of polydipsia, polyphagia, polyuria, and nocturia. He is on antihypertensive medication with poor control. He does not exercise but states that he follows a diabetic diet to assist with glucose control.

Questions

1. What type of diabetes does the patient have?
2. Is his risk of complications higher since he has poor control as demonstrated by a high HbA$_{1c}$?
3. What can be done to prevent complications in people with diabetes?
4. Is diabetes more common in certain population groups?

Diabetes mellitus is a common problem in clinical practice. It is more common in the elderly and in certain populations, such as Native Americans, Hispanics, and African Americans. There is now strong evidence that controlling glucose levels prevents or postpones complications. Additional patient and provider practices can improve outcomes. Type I diabetes is also called insulin-dependent diabetes mellitus (IDDM) or juvenile-onset diabetes mellitus. Type II diabetes is also called non–insulin-dependent diabetes mellitus (NIDDM) or adult-onset diabetes mellitus (AODM).

CLINICAL PRESENTATION

The patient with hyperglycemia presents with polydipsia, polyuria, and weight loss. The type I patient may be acutely ill with diabetic ketoacidosis (DKA) owing to complete lack of insulin. A patient with DKA may present with marked dehydration, nausea or vomiting, abdomi-

nal pain, and central nervous system depression. The type II patient may present with symptoms of hyperglycemia or may have the hyperglycemia discovered during routine evaluation while asymptomatic.

PATHOPHYSIOLOGY AND TREATMENT IMPLICATIONS

Type I diabetes (Table 77–1) occurs in people usually of normal weight at an early age (usually under the age of 40 years). The hyperglycemia is caused by destruction of islet cells, which are the insulin-producing cells of the pancreas. Although the mechanism is not entirely clear, early in the disease process insulin antibodies are present, suggesting an autoimmune phenomenon. While in the first year after diagnosis (the so-called honeymoon period) some insulin may be present, there is progressive destruction of islet cells and eventually no insulin production. These patients require insulin injections to prevent ketosis and death.

Patients with type II diabetes (Table 77–1) typically are older (over 40 years of age), are overweight (about 90% are obese), have insulin resistance rather than islet cell destruction, and usually have some insulin secretion. Type II patients are treated with exercise

TABLE 77–1. Distinguishing Characteristics of Type I and Type II Diabetes

Characteristic	Type I (IDDM)	Type II (NIDDM)
Age	Usually < 40 years	Usually > 40 years
Body habitus	Usually thin/normal weight	90% of patients overweight, especially upper body obesity
Etiology	Possibly autoimmune	Insulin resistance with relative insulin deficiency
Insulin production	None	Some
Ketosis-prone	Yes	No
Initial treatment	Insulin (required to sustain life)	Weight reduction, exercise, possibly oral agent or insulin

Dx **Diabetes Mellitus**

- Random glucose level ≥ 200 mg/dL with symptoms, or
- Fasting glucose level ≥ 140 mg/dL on at least two occasions, or
- Positive glucose tolerance test with oral administration of 75 g of glucose.

and weight loss through meal planning to improve insulin resistance and decrease hyperglycemia. Although difficult to achieve, weight reduction can significantly improve glucose control, especially in the early stages of the disease. Insulin secretion may be especially low when hyperglycemia has been severe and prolonged. Insulin secretion can often be increased through improved glucose control. When type II patients need insulin for glucose control, specialists use the term "insulin-requiring" along with "type II" or "NIDDM" to distinguish the pathophysiology from that of type I patients.

Occasionally, it is difficult to know whether a patient has type I or II diabetes. This can be determined by measuring endogenous insulin production; i.e., by obtaining a C-peptide level, which is the cleaved end of endogenous insulin and which can be measured even when the patient is receiving insulin injections.

Complications occur in both types I and II diabetes. The microvascular complications of diabetes are retinopathy, nephropathy, neuropathy, and foot pathology. A large multicenter study has shown that the level of glucose control is directly related to the progression of these chronic complications, which usually occur years after the diagnosis of diabetes has been made. Diabetes is also associated with macrovascular disease (such as cardiovascular and peripheral vascular disease) as well as periodontal disease. The acute complications of diabetic ketoacidosis (type I) and nonketotic hyperosmolar coma (type II), which are not discussed in this chapter, can be prevented by careful glucose control. Thus, both acute and chronic complications can be prevented by optimal glucose control.

DIFFERENTIAL DIAGNOSIS

Hyperglycemia is the hallmark of diabetes. While hyperglycemia is usually due to the pathogenic mechanisms noted above, it may have other causes. In some cases, removal of the offending substance or treatment of the primary disorder will return glucose control to normal. Usually, however, there has been an "unmasking" of underlying abnormal glucose tolerance. Table 77–2 lists some conditions or medications that can either cause or worsen hyperglycemia.

EVALUATION

History

Family history may reveal either type I or type II diabetes in close relatives. For patients who have family members with type I diabetes, evaluation of insulin

autoantibodies may detect early disease. Although at present this testing is primarily done in a research setting, there is hope that in the future the autoimmune phenomenon may be able to be controlled and the deterioration to frank diabetes thus prevented.

Symptoms of hyperglycemia include urinary frequency with large urinary volume, thirst, weight loss, and occasionally hunger. While these symptoms demand glucose testing, patients can have significant hyperglycemia with no symptoms. Therefore, patients with a strong family history should undergo periodic screening for diabetes, especially if they are overweight or come from a population with a high prevalence of diabetes.

Physical Examination

Physical examination is usually normal in the early stages of diabetes. However, it is not uncommon to encounter patients who have complications of diabetes at the time of diagnosis, indicating that they have had undiagnosed diabetes for more than 10 years. Therefore, funduscopic, neurologic, and foot examinations should be performed routinely in all "new" diabetic patients as well as during follow-up visits.

Additional Evaluation

Laboratory testing is needed to confirm the diagnosis of diabetes. A "positive" glucose tolerance test (measuring blood glucose fasting and then 0.5, 1, 1.5, and 2 hours after a standardized 75-g glucose dose) requires the 2-hour value and at least one other value to be ≥ 200 mg/dL. Diabetes can also be diagnosed when (1) a random glucose is ≥ 200 mg/dL in a patient with symptoms (polyuria, polydypsia) or (2) a fasting glucose is ≥ 140 mg/dL on at least two occasions. Once the diagnosis of diabetes is made, an HbA_{1c} provides an assessment of the overall glucose control over the last 1–3 months and should be done quarterly or semiannually. A baseline serum creatinine, serum lipids, urine protein or microalbumin, and ECG are all appropriate to obtain.

MANAGEMENT

Glucose control is paramount. In type I diabetes, this is accomplished with insulin therapy. These patients

---

TABLE 77–2. Medications or Conditions Causing or Worsening Hyperglycemia

Medications	Conditions
Thiazide diuretics	Pancreatic diseases
β-Blockers	Chronic pancreatitis
Calcium channel blockers	Hemochromatosis
Glucocorticoids	Cystic fibrosis
Estrogen	Endocrine diseases
Psychoactive agents	Cushing's syndrome
Catecholamines	Primary aldosteronism
Niacin	Pheochromocytoma
Phenytoin	Acromegaly
	Glucagonoma

generally require lower insulin doses than insulin-resistant type II patients. A regular schedule matching insulin to meals and exercise is absolutely essential to obtain optimal control. Glucose monitoring four times a day, with insulin adjustment based on those levels, allows the patient to achieve tighter control. Insulin administration at least twice a day, and frequently three to four times a day, taken 30–45 minutes before eating, allows optimal control. Frequent surveillance of glucose levels by the patient is necessary along with adjustments in food intake, exercise, and insulin dose to achieve tight glucose control but avoid hypoglycemia. Recent advances in insulin regimens and insulin pumps allow patients to maintain their usual life-style to a large extent.

In type II diabetes, weight reduction and exercise are the basis for control. However, socioeconomic factors may assist or impair meal planning. In addition, because exercise is not without risk in the older population, specific exercise prescriptions may be advisable. Since patients vary greatly with regard to age, ability to control glucose with healthful eating and exercise, and even ability to participate successfully in nonpharmacologic management, treatment goals need to be individualized. When these efforts fail, oral agents or subsequently insulin may be needed. Risks and benefits of medication must be weighed carefully; e.g., the risk of hypoglycemia in a 75-year-old man versus the risk of complication development in a 40-year-old man mandate different treatment goals. Overtreatment with ensuing hunger and overeating needs to be avoided in these patients, since subsequent weight gain increases insulin resistance, leading to worsening glucose control, which is treated with still higher medication doses. For this reason, the lowest possible insulin dose to reach the treatment goal is best. Since treatment is primarily healthful life-style changes, encouragement and goal setting in a supportive environment are especially important.

Patient and provider self-care practices can greatly enhance outcomes. Table 77–3 lists activities performed by the patient or the provider that are required for optimal diabetes care. Since a large proportion of patients in general practice have diabetes, clinicians must have a method of ensuring that these practices are followed. Patient information handouts and diabetes care flow sheets for office use are found in various textbooks, as well as in the Centers for Disease Control and Prevention publication listed at the end of this chapter. American Diabetes Association publications are available from regional ADA offices.

Blood pressure control and smoking cessation are essential, since they help prevent complications associated with diabetes. Hyperlipidemia will greatly improve once euglycemia is achieved; therefore, lipid-lowering medication should be based on lipid levels obtained once glucose is controlled. Influenza and pneumococcal vaccinations should be up to date in this population regardless of age.

PATIENT AND FAMILY EDUCATION

For patients with a family history of type II diabetes, it is important to provide counseling about maintaining ideal body weight and exercising regularly; both can decrease insulin resistance and perhaps prevent diabetes from developing.

Diabetes education and self-care classes for patients and family members provide necessary information and skills otherwise not available in a busy clinician's office. Individualized nutrition counseling can greatly enhance the likelihood of dietary changes. Standards for diabetes education have been established by the diabetes community. To meet these standards, a team approach is especially useful (see Chapter 124). While handouts and literature may be helpful to patients, a key factor in successful programs is usually an empathetic provider who establishes clear goals and guidelines in partnership with the patient. Goals as well as the skills and means to reach them must be within reach of the patient.

NATURAL HISTORY/PROGNOSIS

At the present time, decreased vision, end-stage renal disease, amputation, and cardiac disease are still frequent complications for people who have had diabetes for many years. Given the knowledge that optimal glucose control and complication surveillance can prevent many of these devastating and costly outcomes, their prevalence should decrease over the next decade.

TABLE 77–3.   Patient Self-Care and Provider Practices to Improve Outcomes

---

Patient Self-Care Practices

Regular medical appointments to assess control and for complication surveillance/prevention
Healthful meal planning
Regular exercise
Regular medication use as prescribed
Glucose self-monitoring (take results to appointments)
Adjustment of medication based on glucose results
Daily foot checks
Annual eye checks
Annual dental checks

Provider Office Practices

Patient education (team approach)
  Nutrition education for patient
  Exercise prescription
  Glucose self-monitoring
  Medication adjustment
  Foot care
Ask about
  Hyper/hypoglycemic symptoms
  Impotence and autonomic dysfunction symptoms
  Cardiac and vascular disease symptoms
Each visit
  Check weight, blood pressure, glucose, condition of feet
  Check glucose self-monitoring results/make recommendations
Yearly
  Vascular, neurologic, eye examinations; dental referral
Referrals
  Ophthalmologic referral as needed
  Podiatry referral as needed
Laboratory
  Hemoglobin A_{1c} measurements every 3–6 months
  Creatinine, lipids, urinalysis yearly or as needed
Baseline ECG
Influenza and pneumococcal vaccines

SUMMARY

It is important to understand the differences between the two types of diabetes and the therapeutic implications of those differences. Glucose control is of paramount importance for prevention of the acute complications of diabetic ketoacidosis and nonketotic hyperosmolar coma, as well as for prevention of chronic complications such as end-stage renal disease, blindness, and amputation. Providers must offer individualized patient education with clear and achievable goals, taking into account factors such as age, socioeconomic status, and educational level. When possible, this is best achieved through a team approach. A nonjudgmental and supportive professional environment provides patients with the education, skills, and psychological support for taking personal charge of the many demands of diabetes.

Research Questions

1. Will the availability of noninvasive glucose sensors (currently being developed) increase patients' ability to achieve tighter control of their diabetes?
2. Will early treatment of autoimmune islet cell destruction prevent type I diabetes?
3. Will early treatment of patients with impaired glucose intolerance prevent deterioration to type II diabetes?

Case Resolution

The patient had been monitoring his glucose only on his days off and taking his insulin just before he ate. He had been eating high-sugar, high-fat snacks and had a significant alcohol intake. He had also been taking a thiazide diuretic for blood pressure control. Through (1) changing his insulin injection to 30–45 minutes before meals, (2) monitoring glucose level three times a day, (3) beginning a walking program, (4) stopping alcohol consumption, and (5) substituting healthier snacks, the patient's glucose came under better control. His antihypertensive medication was switched to an ACE inhibitor for its renal protective effects and lack of adverse effects on glucose. Several months later, the patient had lost weight, the HbA_{1c} had improved significantly, and he felt better overall.

Selected Readings

American Diabetes Association. Position statement: Implications of the Diabetes Control and Complications Trial. Diabetes 42:1555–8, 1993.

Diabetes Control and Complications Trial Research Group. The effect of intensive treatment of diabetes on the development and progression of long-term complications in insulin-dependent diabetes mellitus. N Engl J Med 329:977–86, 1993.

Lebovitz, H. E. (ed.). *Therapy for Diabetes Mellitus and Related Disorders.* Alexandria, Virginia, American Diabetes Association, Inc., 1991.

Physician's Guide to Insulin-Dependent (Type I) Diabetes: Diagnosis and Treatment. Alexandria, Virginia, American Diabetes Association, Inc., 1988.

Physician's Guide to Non-Insulin-Dependent (Type II) Diabetes: Diagnosis and Treatment, 2nd ed. Alexandria, Virginia, American Diabetes Association, Inc., 1988.

The Prevention and Treatment of Complications of Diabetes: A Guide for Primary Care Practitioners. Atlanta, Georgia, Department of Health and Human Services, Public Health Service, Centers for Disease Control, Center for Chronic Disease Prevention and Health Promotion, 1991.

Santiago, J. V. Perspectives in diabetes: Lessons from the Diabetes Control and Complications Trial. Diabetes 42:1549–54, 1993.

CHAPTER 78

THYROID DISORDERS

Patricia Kapsner, M.D.

Hx The patient is a 54-year-old female graphic artist who was found to have multiple thyroid nodules on a routine examination 5 years ago. The majority of the nodules were small except for a prominent one on the right side. She had no symptoms, and thyroid function tests were normal. Fine-needle aspiration of the dominant nodule was performed and was negative for malignancy. The nodules remained unchanged on yearly examinations. Five years later she is complaining of shortness of breath. On further questioning, she admits to an intermittent racing heart and the ability to eat whatever she wants without gaining weight. Her lifelong constipation has resolved. She denies chest pain, orthopnea, paroxysmal nocturnal dyspnea, and edema. Her heart rate is 104 bpm. Her thyroid gland examination is unchanged from 5 years ago. Her palms are warm and moist. The remainder of the physical examination is normal.

Questions

1. What additional information should you obtain from the history and physical examination?
2. What are the diagnostic possibilities?
3. Do you think laboratory tests are necessary? If so, which ones?

PATHOPHYSIOLOGY

The thyroid gland is a bilobar structure located in the neck. The two lobes are connected by an isthmus at the level of the cricoid cartilage. When examining the thyroid gland it is important to locate the cricoid cartilage, for it serves as a landmark for the isthmus. It is important to appreciate that the thyroid gland moves up with the larynx on swallowing.

The function of the thyroid gland is to produce and store thyroid hormone. To produce a sufficient quantity of thyroid hormone, adequate ingestion of iodide is necessary. The thyroid gland is able to regulate its iodide uptake. Once within the thyroid cell, inorganic iodide is rapidly oxidized by peroxidase in the presence of hydrogen peroxide. This intermediate is then incorporated into the tyrosine residue of several proteins, mainly thy-

roglobulin. Thyroglobulin is a large glycoprotein molecule and the precursor of all thyroid hormones. It is secreted by thyroid cells and stored in viscous gel called colloid. Colloid is located in thyroid follicles; these hollow spheres of cells are the basic functioning units of the thyroid gland. Coupling of the iodinated tyrosine residues occurs to form triiodothyronine (T_3) and thyroxine (T_4). Following these coupling reactions, the thyroglobulin molecule, which is stored extracellularly, reenters the thyroid cell and undergoes proteolysis; thyroid hormone is then secreted into the circulation.

Synthesis and secretion of thyroid hormone are regulated mainly by thyrotropin (TSH, thyroid-stimulating hormone), secreted by the anterior pituitary gland. TSH in turn is positively regulated by thyrotropin-releasing hormone (TRH) produced by the hypothalamus. Its secretion is inhibited by circulating T_4 and T_3 (Fig. 78–1). The major thyroid hormone secreted into the circulation is T_4. T_4 is then converted in the periphery to T_3 or reverse T_3 (rT_3) depending on whether the outer ring (T_3) or the inner ring (rT_3) is deiodinated. Reverse T_3 is essentially metabolically inactive, and its formation is increased in severe illness, starvation, and by certain medications. Free thyroid hormone must enter the cell and bind to nuclear receptors to exert its metabolic activity. T_3 is the most metabolically active hormone and occupies approximately 80% of bound receptor sites.

FIGURE 78–1. *Hypothalamic-pituitary-thyroid feedback mechanisms. Thyroid hormone production by the thyroid gland is under the control of TSH produced by the pituitary gland. Thyroid hormone (primarily T_3) negatively feeds back, suppressing pituitary TSH. TRH is responsible for adjusting the set point for pituitary responsiveness to T_3 levels and is under the control of higher brain centers and T_3.*

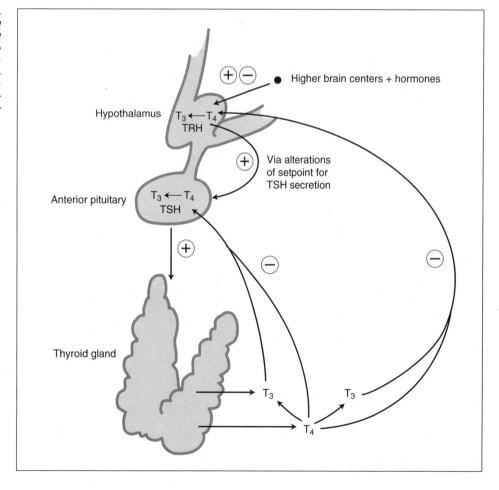

Thyroid hormones in plasma are largely bound to proteins (thyroid hormone–binding globulin, prealbumin, and albumin). Thyroid hormone–binding globulin (TBG) has the highest affinity for thyroid hormone (T_4, T_3), and even though present in the smallest concentration, it carries 70% of circulating thyroid hormone. Bound hormone serves as a readily accessible reservoir for free hormone.

THYROID FUNCTION AND THYROID IMAGING

TSH measures the pituitary's response to peripheral levels of thyroid hormone. The sensitive immunoradiometric assays are able to detect levels as low as 0.05 µU/mL. If the hypothalamic-pituitary axis is intact, the TSH will be suppressed in hyperthyroidism and elevated in hypothyroidism.

Serum T_4 can be determined by obtaining a **free T_4 level**, which determines the free T_4 present, usually by immunometric techniques. If a T_4 is ordered, a measurement of total T_4 bound and free is provided by radioimmunoassay techniques. Binding globulin abnormalities need to be considered when interpreting T_4 results. Alternatively, the **free T_4 index** (FTI) can be used as an estimate of free T_4. This is calculated by taking the measured total T_4 (bound + free) and multiplying it by the **T_3 resin uptake** (T_3 RU), which is an indirect measurement inversely related to the amount of TBG present. The FTI usually correlates well with the free T_4. T_3 RU has nothing to do with the amount of T_3 present (radiolabeled T_3 is used to perform the assay, hence the origin of the assay name). **Total T_3** (free + bound) and **free T_3** may also be measured by radioimmunoassay techniques.

Ultrasound can measure size and evaluate the architecture of the thyroid gland. It can assess whether the gland is homogenous, whether nodules are present, and whether the nodules are solid or cystic. It is of benefit when the clinical examination is difficult or questionable.

Thyroid scans provide a picture of the gland based on the uptake by the thyroid of the isotope used. Size and function of the thyroid tissue can be assessed by scans. If a nodule is present and hyperfunctioning, it will appear as a hot area; a nodule that is hypofunctioning will appear as a cold area. Even though the risk of malignancy is increased in the presence of a cold nodule, thyroid scans are not particularly helpful in euthyroid patients, since most nodules are cold. A thyroid scan is indicated if a patient is hyperthyroid and a hyperfunctioning nodule is suspected.

The **radioactive iodine uptake** is an important test in the diagnosis of certain causes of hyperthyroidism. The radioactive iodine uptake is a measure of the percentage of the administered dose of radioactive iodine taken up by the thyroid gland. It is elevated when there is an increased stimulus to take up iodine by the thyroid gland (e.g., Graves' disease, toxic multinodular goiter, and TSH-secreting adenoma) and low when there is a decreased stimulus (e.g., factitious hyperthyroidism from exogenous thyroxine ingestion and subacute thyroiditis, a painful postviral inflammatory condition

TABLE 78–1. Etiologies of Hypothyroidism

Autoimmune thyroiditis (Hashimoto's disease)
Idiopathic (end-stage autoimmune disease, silent thyroiditis, congenital, inborn errors in thyroid hormone synthesis)
Radioactive iodine therapy
Surgical thyroidectomy
Medications (thioamides, amiodarone, lithium, and others)
Diet (iodine deficiency, iodine excess, goitrogens)
Subacute thyroiditis
Peripheral resistance to thyroid hormone
Pituitary/hypothalamic disease

associated with leakage of preformed hormone into the circulation).

HYPOTHYROIDISM

DIFFERENTIAL DIAGNOSIS

Causes of hypothyroidism are given in Table 78–1.

EVALUATION

Hypothyroidism is the clinical result of low levels of circulating thyroid hormones. The clinical manifestations are listed in Table 78–2. Hashimoto's disease, an autoimmune process resulting in lymphocytic infiltration of the thyroid gland, is the most common cause of hypothyroidism. It is more common in women and is usually associated with a goiter. In primary (thyroidal) hypothyroidism, the TSH level is elevated. If the TSH is normal or low, a secondary (pituitary) or tertiary (hypothalamic) cause should be suspected. Some patients have slightly elevated TSH and normal thyroid hormone levels—a situation that is sometimes referred to as subclinical hypothyroidism.

Myxedema coma is a rare condition with a high mortality rate in which an untreated or inadequately treated hypothyroid patient becomes obtunded or comatose. Usually hypothermia and hypoventilation

TABLE 78–2. Clinical Features of Hypothyroidism

Symptoms	Signs
Arthralgias	Anemia
Breathlessness	Bradycardia
Constipation	Brittle hair
Cold intolerance	Cool skin
Depression	Delayed relaxation of reflexes
Dry skin	Dementia
Fatigue	Dry skin
Memory impairment	Effusions (pericardial, peritoneal, and pleural)
Menstrual irregularities	Gravelly voice
Mental impairment	Hyponatremia
Muscle cramps	Hypoventilation
Paresthesias	Lateral eyebrow thinning
Psychosis	Neuropathies
Somnolence	Puffy face and hands
Weight gain	Slow speech

exist along with the symptoms and signs of hypothyroidism. Frequently, a coexisting condition such as infection, narcotic use, anesthesia use, or systemic illness precipitates myxedema coma. Myxedema coma is a medical emergency.

MANAGEMENT

Treatment of hypothyroidism consists of replacement with L-thyroxine. Average daily doses are 0.075 mg to 0.15 mg. Occasionally, lower or higher doses are required. Those with underlying heart disease should be started at lower doses (0.025 mg/d) and gradually advanced to a full replacement dose. After 6–8 weeks of therapy, TSH should be measured to assess adequacy of replacement. Occasionally, a longer period of time is required for the TSH to normalize. The dose of thyroxine prescribed should not suppress the TSH to below normal levels, even if T_4 levels are normal, since this may put patients at risk for osteoporosis.

HYPERTHYROIDISM

DIFFERENTIAL DIAGNOSIS

Causes of hyperthyroidism are given in Table 78–3.

EVALUATION

Hyperthyroidism is the clinical result of excess circulating thyroid hormones. As a result of feedback suppression by thyroxine on the hypothalamic pituitary axis, the TSH level is below the lower normal limit. (The only exception is the rare TSH-secreting tumor.) The clinical manifestations of hyperthyroidism are listed in Table 78–4. Graves' disease is the most common cause of hyperthyroidism in North America. It is the result of a stimulatory antibody directed against the TSH receptor on the thyroid follicular cells. It is associated with a diffuse goiter and exophthalmos secondary to infiltration of the orbital muscles by various antibody-antigen complexes. Dermopathy of the distal lower extremities (which may range from slight discoloration to elephantiasis) may also occur. Usually both T_4 and T_3 are elevated. Rarely, a patient may have T_3 thyrotoxicoses and a normal T_4 level.

Thyroid storm is the extreme of the hyperthyroid state. Clinically, patients have severe thyrotoxicosis,

---

TABLE 78–3. Etiologies of Hyperthyroidism

Graves' disease (most common)
Factitious or iatrogenic disease
Toxic multinodular goiter
Single toxic nodule
Excess iodide (jodbasedow phenomenon)
Functioning thyroid carcinoma
Hashitoxicosis
Hydatidiform mole
Struma ovarii
TSH-secreting tumor

TABLE 78–4. Clinical Features of Hyperthyroidism

Symptoms	Signs
Appetite increased	Anxious
Double vision, bulging eyes (specific to Graves' disease)	Bruit over thyroid
	Dermopathy (specific to Graves' disease)
Fine, thin hair	Exophthalmos (specific to Graves' disease)
Heat intolerance	Finger clubbing (thyroid acropathy)
Hyperdefecation, diarrhea	Goiter
Insomnia	Gynecomastia
Itching	Lymphadenopathy (specific to Graves' disease)
Loss of libido	
Menstrual irregularities	Onycholysis
Muscle weakness	Palmar erythema
Nausea, vomiting	Proximal myopathy
Nervousness, anxiety, irritability	Pulmonic scratching sound
Rapid heart rate, palpitations	Pulse pressure increased
Shakiness	Warm, smooth, moist skin
Shortness of breath	Splenomegaly
Sweating	Fine tremor

---

tachycardia, fever, and central nervous system abnormalities (confusion, delirium, coma). It is commonly precipitated by surgery, infection, or medical problems. Like myxedema coma, it is a medical emergency.

MANAGEMENT

Medical management with thioamides (propylthiouracil and methimazole) is commonly initially employed followed by radioactive iodine ablation of the overactive gland. β-Blockers, if not contraindicated, are used to treat systemic symptoms. Surgical thyroidectomy is occasionally employed in extenuating circumstances or because of patient preference. Thioamides inhibit the formation, release, and conversion of T_4 to T_3 (propylthiouracil); when treatment is stopped, most patients (70% to 80%) have recurrence of symptoms. However, some physicians recommend medication for long-term therapy. Others think that the risks (e.g., agranulocytosis, hepatitis) outweigh the benefits.

NODULES

DIFFERENTIAL DIAGNOSIS

Thyroid nodules are relatively common, occurring clinically in 4% to 7% of adults. The majority are benign. The causes are listed in Table 78–5.

EVALUATION

Most endocrinologists obtain thyroid function tests and perform a fine-needle aspiration as the initial evaluation of a solitary thyroid nodule or a dominant nodule in a multinodular goiter. This is the most cost effective approach and has an overall accuracy of about 90%. The procedure is well tolerated, and complications are uncommon. The results fall into four categories: malignant, benign, suspicious, and inadequate. In the case of a follicular neoplasm, vascular or lymphatic

TABLE 78–5. Etiologies of Thyroid Nodules

Benign	Malignant
Acute thyroiditis	Primary
Colloid nodule	Papillary
Cysts	Follicular
Follicular adenoma	Papillary-follicular
Hashimoto's thyroiditis	Medullary
Nodular Graves' disease (Marie-Lenhart syndrome)	Anaplastic
Subacute granulomatous thyroiditis	Hurthle cell
	Metastatic
	Lymphoma

invasion must be demonstrated to confirm malignancy; since this cannot be done with fine-needle aspiration specimens, nodules containing follicular neoplasms may be read out as indeterminate.

MANAGEMENT

Malignant (and frequently suspicious and indeterminate) lesions require surgery. If the lesion is malignant on frozen section, total thyroidectomy is usually performed. Exceptions are small (< 1.5 cm), localized, papillary carcinomas, for which there is no difference in survival between lobectomy and total thyroidectomy. If treated correctly, these thyroid cancers usually have little impact on life span. Medullary carcinoma originates in the parafollicular cells, or C cells, of the thyroid. It may be familial or associated with the multiple endocrine neoplasia (MEN) syndromes and has a worse prognosis. Screening for premalignant lesions in family members is important. Anaplastic carcinoma, most commonly presenting as a very rapidly growing nodule in an older patient, has a poor prognosis.

Once surgical thyroidectomy is performed for thyroid cancer, the patient is rendered hypothyroid and a ^{131}I body scan is performed to evaluate for residual thyroid tissue (normal or carcinoma) and for metastatic disease. If any uptake is demonstrated, the patient is treated with higher doses of [131]I. The ^{131}I body scan is repeated in 6 to 12 months to verify successful ablation of all thyroid tissue. If uptake persists or new uptake develops, the patient is again treated. This process is repeated periodically. Additionally, serum thyroglobulin levels are monitored as a means of diagnosing cancer recurrences. Elevations correlate well but not perfectly with ^{131}I body scans.

Thyroid hormone replacement is also given to patients with thyroid cancer to treat the hypothyroid state as well as to suppress TSH, since differentiated cancers are TSH dependent. Patients should be followed with sensitive TSH assays to ensure that TSH is suppressed to the lower limit of normal. If tumors continue to persist in spite of ^{131}I and thyroid hormone suppressive therapy, or if they fail to trap iodine, alternative treatments such as external beam radiation or systemic chemotherapy can be considered.

Research Question

1. Using modern bioengineering technology, how might you circumvent the necessity to render a patient hypothyroid prior to performing a ^{131}I body scan to evaluate for persistent or recurrent thyroid cancer?

Case Resolution

The patient was biochemically hyperthyroid. [131]I uptake was increased, and a scan revealed a single nodule. The patient was treated with radioactive iodine and is now euthyroid. The nodule has resolved.

Selected Readings

Burrow, G. N., J. H. Oppenheimer, and R. Volpe. *Thyroid Function and Disease.* Philadelphia, W.B. Saunders Company, 1989.

Greenspan, F. S., and B. Rapoport. Thyroid gland. *In* F. S. Greenspan (ed.). *Basic and Clinical Endocrinology,* 3rd ed. Norwalk, Connecticut, Appleton & Lange, 1991.

Helfand, M., and L. M. Crapo. Screening for thyroid disease. Ann Intern Med 112:840–9, 1990.

Martinez, M., D. Derksen, and P. Kapsner. Making sense of hypothyroidism: An approach to testing and treatment. Postgrad Med 93(6):135–45, 1993.

McDougall, I. R. *Thyroid Disease in Clinical Practice.* New York, Oxford University Press, 1992.

Rojesk, M. T., and R. Gharib. Nodular thyroid disease. N Engl J Med 313:428–36, 1985.

Surks, M. I., I. J. Chopra, C. N. Mariash, et al. American Thyroid Association guidelines for use of laboratory tests in thyroid disorders. JAMA 263:1529–32, 1990.

Wartofsky, L. The thyroid gland. *In* K. L. Becker, J. P. Bilezikian, W. J. Bremner, et al. (eds.). *Principles and Practice of Endocrinology and Metabolism.* Philadelphia, J.B. Lippincott Company, 1990.

HYPERLIPIDEMIA

B. Sylvia Vela, M.D.

H$_x$ A 36-year-old male engineer presents for a routine annual physical examination. His history includes a myocardial infarction 5 years ago, mild hypertension, and an episode of gouty arthritis last summer. He is a nonsmoker and nondrinker. He does not have diabetes. He was told at the time of his myocardial infarction that he had "high cholesterol" and has been "watching" his diet ever since. The physical examination is remarkable only for an elevated blood pressure of 152/92. The laboratory lipid profile is remarkable for a total cholesterol of 279, triglycerides of 220, HDL of 26, and calculated LDL of 209.

Questions

1. How do you interpret this lipid profile? What effect does the patient's myocardial infarction have on your interpretation?
2. Is further testing needed? If so, what?
3. Why is his history of hypertension and gout important?
4. What are your treatment options?

Hyperlipidemia is a major health problem frequently encountered by primary care physicians in the United States. Hyperlipidemia is present when serum cholesterol or triglycerides reach levels that are associated with coronary heart disease (CHD) or pancreatitis. While most Americans are aware of the need to lower their cholesterol level, many health care providers are ill equipped to diagnose and aggressively manage hyperlipidemia.

PATHOPHYSIOLOGY

The principal plasma lipids, **triglycerides** and **cholesterol,** represent a basic metabolic resource for living cells. Triglycerides function as an energy source, and cholesterol is a component of cell membranes and a precursor of steroid hormones and bile acids. Because cholesterol and triglycerides are not water soluble, they are transported in the plasma attached to proteins in the form of lipoproteins.

Lipoprotein particles consist of a central core composed of triglycerides and cholesteryl esters, surrounded by a surface coat of phospholipids and apolipoproteins (apoproteins; abbreviated Apo). Four main types are recognized according to their density (Table 79–1): (1) **chylomicrons,** a triglyceride-rich particle that transports exogenous fatty acids; (2) **very low density lipoproteins** (VLDLs), which consist largely of triglycerides and transport endogenous triglycerides; (3)

low-density lipoproteins (LDLs), which are cholesterol rich and are associated with CHD risk; and (4) **high-density lipoproteins** (HDLs), which contain mostly cholesterol but are inversely proportionate to CHD risk and are felt to be protective against CHD.

Apoproteins have three main functions: (1) they act as structural elements in the shell of the lipoprotein, (2) they serve as ligands for specific lipoprotein receptors, and (3) they activate enzymes that play a role in lipoprotein metabolism. Apoproteins are divided into five classes (A–E), some of which have subdivisions. Many defects of lipid metabolism involve abnormal apoproteins.

Exogenous, or **dietary, fat** is absorbed in the small intestine and converted to chylomicrons that enter the blood via the lymphatics. Once in the bloodstream, chylomicrons exchange apoproteins with HDL, which allows the chylomicron particle to activate the lipoprotein lipase (LPL) enzyme located in the wall of the capillary bed. LPL hydrolyzes the triglyceride in the chylomicrons, and the free fatty acid released is taken up for oxidation or storage by adipocytes and muscle cells. The chylomicron remnant is taken up by the liver through the Apo-E receptor and cleared from the circulation.

Endogenously synthesized triglycerides and **cholesterol** from the liver are transported to the periphery by VLDL. Like chylomicrons, VLDL is hydrolyzed by LPL, and the VLDL remnant (also called intermediate-density lipoprotein or IDL) is either taken up by the liver through the Apo-B–100/E receptor or converted to LDL by hepatic lipase.

HDL is generated in both liver and intestine. HDL takes up excess free cholesterol from peripheral tissues, such as the coronary arteries, and transports it to the

TABLE 79–1.   Hyperlipoproteinemias

Type	Lipoprotein	Major Elevated Lipid	Incidence (%)
I	Chylomicrons	Exogenous triglycerides	< 1
IIa	LDL	Cholesteryl esters	10
IIb	LDL, VLDL	Cholesteryl esters, endogenous triglycerides	40
III	IDL, VLDL remnants	Cholesteryl esters and triglycerides	< 1
IV	VLDL	Endogenous triglycerides, cholesteryl esters	45
V	VLDL, chylomicrons	Endogenous and exogenous triglycerides, cholesteryl esters	5
	HDL2	Cholesteryl esters, phospholipids	
	HDL3	Cholesteryl esters, phospholipids	
	Lp(a)	Cholesteryl esters	

TABLE 79–2. Secondary Lipoprotein Disorders

Laboratory Test	Disease or Agent	Lipid Pattern*
Glucose	Diabetes	↑ TG, ↓ HDL, and/or ↑ cholesterol
BUN, creatinine, urinalysis	Uremia	↑ TG
	Nephrotic syndrome	↑ TG and cholesterol
Transaminases, alkaline phosphatase, bilirubin	Biliary obstruction	↑ Cholesterol
	Acute hepatitis	↑ TG
TSH, T₄, T₃RU	Hypothyroidism	↑ Cholesterol and/or TG
Protein electrophoresis	Myeloma, systemic lupus erythematosus	↑ Cholesterol and/or TG
γ-Glutamyl transferase, transaminases	Alcoholism	↑ TG
Cortisol, ACTH	Cushing's syndrome	↑ Cholesterol and/or TG
	Anorexia nervosa	↑ Cholesterol
	Ethanol	↑ TG and HDL
	Oral contraceptives	↑ TG and HDL
	Corticosteroids	↑ TG
	β-Blockers	↑ TG, ↓ HDL
	Thiazide and loop diuretics	↑ TG, ↓ HDL, ↑ cholesterol
	Phenothiazines	↑ Cholesterol
	Cyclosporine	↑ Cholesterol
	Isotretinoin	↑ TG, ↓ HDL, ↑ cholesterol

*TG—triglycerides, HDL—high-density lipoprotein.

liver for disposal. This movement of cholesterol from the periphery to the liver is known as **reverse cholesterol transport** and illustrates why HDL has the unique status of being antiatherogenic.

Genetic or environmental conditions may influence lipoprotein metabolism. Genetic conditions that affect the function of enzymes, apoproteins, and receptors have been identified. Likewise, environmental factors such as obesity or alcohol may increase input and retard disposal of lipoproteins, leading to hyperlipidemia. Regardless of the underlying cause, the **hyperlipoproteinemias** can be classified into phenotypic patterns. Fredrickson recognized six classes based on the type of lipoprotein accumulated (see Table 79–1). While useful as a guide to therapy, this classification does not identify the hyperlipoproteinemias according to causative genetic defects, nor does it distinguish primary from secondary causes.

Hyperlipidemias can be classified as either primary or secondary causes. Common **secondary etiologies** include diabetes, excess alcohol intake, hypothyroidism, nephrosis, liver disease (Table 79–2), and concomitant drug use such as corticosteroids, diuretics, and β-blockers. **Primary etiologies** are due to genetic conditions (Table 79–3) that result in altered lipoprotein metabolism. Examples include the following: (1) **familial hypercholesterolemia,** which results from an inherited defect in the LDL receptor gene in which there are either absent (homozygous form) or decreased numbers of (heterozygous form) LDL receptors, leading to decreased clearance of LDL; (2) **familial combined hyperlipidemia,** an autosomal dominant condition in which family members may have increased VLDL, LDL, or both, but all are at risk of premature CHD; (3) **familial dysbetalipoproteinemia,** a condition in which Apo-E on chylomicron remnants and IDL are defective and cannot bind to the Apo-E hepatic receptor for clearance; and (4) **familial mixed hypertriglyceridemia,** an autosomal dominant condition in which chylomicrons and VLDL are overproduced.

EVALUATION

History

A history of pancreatitis, coronary heart disease, peripheral vascular disease or carotid disease is important, since this is the population that can most benefit from lipid lowering. A family history of both hyperlip-

TABLE 79–3. Primary Lipoprotein Disorders

Genetic Lipid Disorder	Lipoprotein Profile	Clinical Manifestations
Hypercholesterolemia		
Familial heterozygous	↑↑ LDL-cholesterol	Tendinous xanthomas, premature atherosclerosis
Familial homozygous	↑↑↑ LDL-cholesterol	Planar xanthomas, aortic stenosis, premature catastrophic atherosclerosis
Familial defective apo B-100		
Polygenic	↑ LDL cholesterol	Xanthomas absent ; often associated with obesity, diet
Hypertriglyceridemia		
Familial hypertriglyceridemia	↑ Triglycerides ↓ HDL cholesterol	Usually asymptomatic
Familial combined hyperlipidemia		Xanthomas absent; family history of ↑ VLDL, LDL or both; premature atherosclerosis
Fasting hyperchylomicronemia	↑↑↑ Triglycerides	Eruptive xanthomas, lipemia retinalis, recurrent pancreatitis
Familial dysbetalipoproteinemia	Mild fasting chylomicronemia, ↑ IDL, VLDL, β-VLDL	Palmar/planar xanthomas are pathognomonic. Tuberoeruptive xanthomas are common. Premature coronary and peripheral vascular disease
Familial mixed hypertriglyceridemia	Mild fasting chylomicronemia, ↑↑↑ triglycerides, ↓ HDL	Eruptive xanthomas, recurrent pancreatitis
Hypoalphalipoproteinemia	↓ HDL	Asymptomatic
Hyperalphalipoproteinemia	↑↑ HDL	Extremely rare
Hypobetalipoproteinemia	↓ LDL, VLDL; ↑ HDL	Associated with longevity, reduced coronary heart disease
Abetalipoproteinemia	Absence of VLDL, LDL	Malabsorption of fat and fat-soluble vitamins; neurologic lesions; erythrocyte abnormalities
Diabetic dyslipidemia	↑↑↑ Triglycerides, ↓ HDL with or without ↑ LDL	Premature atherosclerosis

idemia and premature CHD is especially important in order to determine genotype and risk factor status (Table 79–4). Risk factor modification should be a primary goal of any treatment program.

Physical Examination

The physical examination should focus on the eyes, skin, musculoskeletal system, cardiovascular system, and extremities. A corneal arcus, if detected in an individual less than 55 years of age, is specific for hyperlipidemia and reflects lipid deposition in the cornea. Lipemia retinalis, or salmon-colored vessels in the retina, is seen in severe hypertriglyceridemia. The skin examination can be remarkable for lipid deposition in the skin or tendons. Specific patterns of deposition are seen with certain conditions. Tendinous xanthomas (lipid deposition in the Achilles and extensor tendons of the hand) and planar xanthomas (deposition in a plaque-like fashion) are seen only in familial hypercholesterolemia (LDL receptor deficiency) and familial defective Apo-B–100. Eruptive xanthomas (small papules on arms, buttocks, and thighs) are seen in severe hypertriglyceridemias. Palmar xanthomas (yellow-orange discoloration of hand creases) and tuberous xanthomas (raised, nodular, 0.5-cm lesions) are seen in type III hyperlipoproteinemia. Carotid bruits and peripheral pulses help establish whether atherosclerosis is present. Peripheral edema may be present in the hyperlipidemia of nephrotic syndrome.

Additional Evaluation

Secondary causes (see Table 79–2) of hyperlipidemia should be ruled out. Thyroid function tests; liver function tests; glucose; BUN and creatinine levels; and a urinalysis should be performed to detect hypothyroidism, liver disease, diabetes mellitus renal failure, and the nephrotic syndrome, respectively.

Screening Evaluation

Everyone over the age of 20 years should be screened for hyperlipidemia every 5 years. Screening consists of nonfasting total cholesterol and HDL levels. If the total cholesterol is > 240 mg/dL, or the HDL is < 35 mg/dL, a fasting lipid profile should be performed. The lipid profile includes a triglyceride level and a calculated LDL level in addition to total cholesterol and HDL. Patients

---

TABLE 79–4. Major Coronary Heart Disease Risk Factors

LDL cholesterol > 160
HDL cholesterol < 35
Hypertension
Cigarette smoking
Diabetes
Familial history of myocardial infarction or sudden death before age 55 years in males or 65 years in females
Male > 45
Female > 55
Subtract one risk factor if HDL cholesterol > 60

---

with established coronary heart disease or diabetes should have yearly fasting lipid profiles. Interpretation of the lipid profile depends on the coronary risk status of the patient (see Table 79–4). In general, desirable levels are total cholesterol < 200 mg/dL, triglycerides < 200 mg/dL, HDL cholesterol > 35 mg/dL, and LDL < 160 mg/dL. If two or more risk factors are present, the LDL should be < 130 mg/dL. If CHD is present, the LDL should be < 100 mg/dL.

MANAGEMENT

The immediate goal of treatment of hyperlipidemia is to reduce lipid levels, with the long-term goal of reducing the risk of coronary heart disease and pancreatitis. Initial management should always begin by modifying any exacerbating factors, followed by diet and risk factor modification. For example, discontinuation of amiodarone, anabolic steroids, and diuretics may help alleviate hypercholesterolemia, while discontinuation of estrogen, β-blockers, alcohol, and glucocorticoids may improve hypertriglyceridemia. For patients who have concomitant hypertension, a lipid-neutral agent should be chosen, such as an ACE inhibitor, a calcium channel blocker, or an α-blocker. Patients with diabetes should first improve glucose control before the need for lipid-lowering drug treatment is considered. Smokers should stop smoking.

Dietary factors that elevate LDL include saturated fats, excess calories, and dietary cholesterol. All patients should receive instruction about a low-fat, low-cholesterol diet from a dietitian. After 3–6 months of dietary therapy, the lipid profile should be repeated, and if still elevated, drug therapy should be considered.

At present there are five classes of lipid-lowering drugs: niacin, bile acid resins, fibrates, probucol, and hydroxymethylglutaryl–coenzyme A (HMG–CoA) reductase inhibitors.

Niacin (vitamin B_3) is first-line therapy for all types of hyperlipidemia except hyperchylomicronemia. It effectively lowers cholesterol, triglycerides, LDL, and is the only agent shown to lower Lp(a), a lipoprotein believed by some investigators to predispose to CHD. In addition, niacin is the most potent agent for raising HDL levels. Its mechanism of action is largely unknown, but niacin appears to decrease VLDL synthesis and release from the liver. Both regular and slow-release forms of niacin are available. The most common adverse effect is flushing, which is mediated by prostaglandins and can be attenuated with aspirin ingestion 20–30 minutes before the niacin dose. Other side effects include hepatitis (especially with the slow-release preparation) and hyperuricemia; consequently, liver function tests and uric acid levels should be monitored. Niacin can precipitate gouty attacks and bleeding ulcers and can worsen insulin resistance and glucose control in patients with gout, active peptic ulcer disease, and diabetes, respectively. Niacin can be effectively combined with other agents such as fibrates and bile acid resins. Combining niacin with HMG–CoA reductase inhibitors has been associated with a 2% risk of myositis, potentially leading to rhabdomyolysis, and should be used with caution.

Bile acid resins (e.g., cholestyramine, colestipol) are first-line therapy for hypercholesterolemia only. They typically reduce LDL cholesterol concentrations by approximately 25%. The resins bind bile acids in the gut, causing a compensatory increase in bile acid synthesis and an increase in the number of hepatic LDL receptors, resulting in increased LDL clearance. Adverse effects are predominantly gastrointestinal and include constipation and indigestion. Bile acid resins can exacerbate hypertriglyceridemia. Effective combinations include bile acid resins with niacin, HMG-CoA reductase inhibitors, or gemfibrozil.

HMG–CoA reductase inhibitors (e.g., lovastatin, pravastatin, simvastatin, fluvastatin) are effective for patients with the type IIa or IIb phenotype. They are not indicated for isolated hypertriglyceridemia. These agents decrease cholesterol by inhibiting HMG–CoA reductase and therefore cholesterol synthesis, which leads to up-regulation of the number of LDL receptors in the liver and increased clearance of LDL. Side effects are few but include hepatitis and myositis. Myopathy and rhabdomyolysis have occurred in 5% of patients when one of these drugs is taken in combination with gemfibrozil, compared with a 2% risk when taken with niacin and a 0.1% risk when used alone. For the first 12–18 months of therapy, transaminase and creatine kinase levels should be monitored frequently. These agents can be combined with bile acid resins.

Fibrates (e.g., gemfibrozil, clofibrate, fenofibrate) are most effective at lowering VLDL and are therefore first-line therapy for hypertriglyceridemia. Possible mechanisms of action include lipoprotein lipase activation and inhibition of lipolysis. Side effects include cholelithiasis, nausea, diarrhea, hepatitis, and myositis. Fibrates may increase LDL levels. Combining a fibrate with niacin is useful for severe hypertriglyceridemia. Bile acid resins can be added for LDL lowering if needed.

Probucol is used for type IIa and IIb phenotypes. In animal studies, it has been shown to have antioxidant properties. Its mechanism of action is unknown. One side effect of unknown consequence is lowering of HDL cholesterol.

PATIENT AND FAMILY EDUCATION

All patients with hyperlipidemia should receive instruction about a low-fat, low-cholesterol diet, along with other risk factor modification techniques, such as exercise and smoking cessation. Family members of patients who have hereditary conditions should be screened for underlying hyperlipidemia. Early institution of proper diet and exercise may prevent the long-term sequelae of hyperlipidemia.

NATURAL HISTORY/PROGNOSIS

Several studies have demonstrated that treating hypercholesterolemia reduces cardiovascular morbidity and mortality, especially in patients with established heart disease. Now, multiple studies have shown that atherosclerotic lesions can regress with aggressive lipid lowering. This regression appears to be associated with significant declines in recurrent cardiac events, occurring perhaps as a result of stabilization and deactivation of atherosclerotic plaques.

Research Question

1. How should hyperlipidemia be managed in the elderly?

Case Resolution

Because the patient has known premature coronary disease with a type IIb phenotype, as well as hypertension, he would benefit from lipid-lowering therapy (LDL cholesterol < 100 mg/dL) and blood pressure control. He was sent to the dietitian for a low-cholesterol, low-saturated-fat, low-salt diet. After 3 months of dietary therapy, his LDL improved to 185 mg/dL but he remained hypertensive. Thyroid disease, nephrosis, liver disease, and diabetes were ruled out, and he was given an HMG–CoA reductase inhibitor with excellent results. Antihypertensive therapy was started with a calcium channel blocker.

Selected Readings

Gotto, A. M. (ed.). Hypercholesterolemia: New findings and clinical applications. (Proceedings of a Symposium.) Am J Med 91:1B–36S, 1991.

Grundy, S. M., and G. L. Vega. Causes of high blood cholesterol. Circulation 81:412–27, 1990.

Hunninghake, D. B. Drug treatment of dyslipoproteinemia. Endocrinol Metab Clin North Am 90:345–60, 1990.

Jones, P. H. A clinical overview of dyslipidemias: Treatment strategies. Am J Med 93:187–98, 1992.

Margolis, S. Diagnosis and management of abnormal plasma lipids. J Clin Endocrinol Metab 70:821–25, 1990.

Schonfeld, G. Inherited disorders of lipid transport. Endocrinol Metab Clin North Am 19:229–57, 1990.

Summary of the Second Report of the National Cholesterol Education Program (NCEP) Expert Panel on Detection, Evaluation, and Treatment of High Blood Cholesterol in Adults (Adult Treatment Panel II). JAMA 269:23, 1993.

CHAPTER 80

HYPERCALCEMIA

Mark R. Burge, M.D.

Hx A 55-year-old female retired school teacher has an elevated serum calcium level of 11.0 mg/dL (normal, 8.5–10.5 mg/dL) on a routine chemistry panel. She has no complaints about her health and denies weakness or mental status changes. The serum phosphate level is 2.4 mg/dL (normal, 2.7–4.5 mg/dL), and renal function is normal. Past medical history is significant for an episode of painless hematuria 5 years ago. She suffered a Colles fracture last year while playing tennis, and she has been treated with fluoxetine over the past 3 years for mild depressive symptoms. Other medications are limited to estrogen replacement therapy, and she does not take calcium supplements. Physical examination reveals a mildly elevated blood pressure of 144/89 mm Hg and a slight haziness of the corneas bilaterally.

Questions

1. Is a mildly elevated calcium level significant?
2. Does the serum phosphate level help in the evaluation of hypercalcemia?
3. What is the significance of the history of Colles' fracture?
4. What are your next steps in the evaluation of this patient?

Calcium is one of the most tightly regulated substances in the human body, and multiple processes are in place to maintain normocalcemia. Any apparent perturbation in calcium homeostasis is an indicator of potentially severe underlying disease and deserves a thorough evaluation. Moreover, hypercalcemia is common, occurring in roughly 0.5% of hospitalized patients and more than 0.1% of asymptomatic outpatients. The role of the primary care physician is to identify hormonal and malignant causes of hypercalcemia so that proper therapy can be initiated, as well as to prevent secondary complications and unnecessary surgery. Hypercalcemia should be confirmed by repeat testing, since serum protein levels and the freshness of the blood sample may artificially affect calcium levels.

PATHOPHYSIOLOGY

Calcium levels are regulated by three principal hormones: parathyroid hormone, 1,25-dihydroxyvitamin D_3, and calcitonin. These hormones act on the three organ systems responsible for maintaining calcium homeostasis: the gut, kidney, and skeletal system. All these hormones are regulated in turn, either directly or indirectly, by serum calcium levels. Calcium is highly protein bound in the circulation, and only the free (or ionized) fraction is biologically active. Of the bound fraction, 80% is bound to albumin and 20% to globulin.

Parathyroid hormone (PTH) is an 84-amino-acid polypeptide hormone produced by four pea-sized parathyroid glands located immediately posterior to the thyroid gland. PTH secretion is stimulated by low calcium levels in the blood, and PTH acts by binding to specific membrane-bound receptors located on the surface of PTH-sensitive cells. Upon binding of the hormone to its receptor, cyclic AMP is generated by adenylate cyclase; cyclic AMP subsequently acts at the subcellular level to result in the biologic effects of PTH.

PTH has specific actions on kidney and bone as well as indirect actions on the gut. At the kidney, PTH increases tubular reabsorption of calcium and decreases reabsorption of phosphate and bicarbonate. These latter actions explain the hypophosphatemia and mild metabolic acidosis commonly observed in PTH-mediated hypercalcemia. Additionally, PTH acts at the kidney to increase production of 1,25-dihydroxyvitamin D_3. In bone, PTH acts to increase osteoclastic bone resorption, resulting in a net release of calcium and phosphate. At the gut, PTH acts through 1,25-dihydroxyvitamin D_3 to stimulate calcium and phosphate absorption. All these factors work in complementary fashion to increase serum calcium levels. When calcium homeostasis is reestablished, PTH secretion is inhibited.

Vitamin D is absorbed from the diet or formed by the action of ultraviolet irradiation on vitamin D precursors in the skin. Vitamin D is subsequently converted to 25-hydroxyvitamin D_3 (25-OHD$_3$) in the liver through the action of microsomal enzymes. This prohormone is finally converted to the active hormone 1,25-dihydroxyvitamin D_3 [1,25(OH)$_2$D$_3$] in the kidney by the enzyme 1α-hydroxylase. This last step is rate limiting. A schematic representation of vitamin D metabolism is shown in Figure 80–1.

1,25(OH)$_2$D$_3$ is a steroid hormone that exerts its biologic effects by first binding to an intracellular receptor. The hormone-receptor complex then binds DNA directly and thus affects gene transcription. 1,25(OH)$_2$D$_3$ probably has some direct effects on proper bone mineralization, and 1,25(OH)$_2$D$_3$ receptors have been demonstrated in many tissues, including parathyroid cells. The main effect of this hormone, however, is to increase calcium and phosphate absorption from the gut in order to provide adequate substrate for new bone formation. Thus, phosphate levels tend to be normal or elevated in purely 1,25(OH)$_2$D$_3$-mediated hypercalcemia.

The effect of **calcitonin** on calcium homeostasis is weak compared to that of PTH or 1,25(OH)$_2$D$_3$. Calcito-

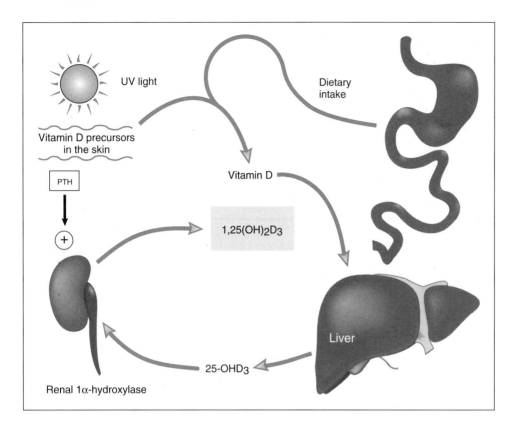

FIGURE 80–1. *Schematic summary of vitamin D metabolism. Vitamin D is derived from the diet or is converted from precursors in the skin by ultraviolet light. 25-Hydroxylation of vitamin D occurs in the liver, resulting in formation of 25-hydroxyvitamin D_3. This prohormone is subsequently converted to the active hormone, 1,25-dihydroxyvitamin D_3, in a rate-limiting step by the renal enzyme 1α-hydroxylase. 1α-hydroxylase activity is, in turn, regulated by PTH levels.*

nin is a 32-amino-acid polypeptide hormone produced by the parafollicular cells of the thyroid gland that also employs cyclic AMP as a second messenger to produce biologic effects. Calcitonin weakly antagonizes the effects of PTH by decreasing bony resorption and by facilitating renal calcium excretion. Clinical syndromes of calcitonin excess or deficiency do not exist in humans.

TABLE 80–1. Causes of Hypercalcemia According to Pathophysiologic Mechanism

PTH Mediated
Primary hyperparathyroidism*
Chronic renal failure (tertiary hyperparathyroidism)
Vitamin D Mediated
Vitamin D intoxication
Granulomatous diseases
Hodgkin's lymphoma
Medication Mediated
Thiazide diuretics*
Lithium
Milk-alkali syndrome
Malignancy Mediated
PTH-RP (squamous cell of lung, renal cell)
Local osteolysis (breast, multiple myeloma)*
Genetically Mediated
Familial hypocalciuric hypercalcemia*
MEN I, MEN II
Miscellaneous
Immobilization
Hyperthyroidism

*A common condition.

Some **cancers** produce a humoral factor that causes hypercalcemia in humans. Recently this substance has been characterized and has been termed "PT-related peptide," or PTH-RP. PTH-RP is a 141-amino-acid peptide produced by certain solid tumors that has a high degree of homology with PTH and is thus able to exert the biologic effects of PTH in bone and kidney. Since PTH-RP production by a tumor is not under the influence of negative feedback from calcium, hypercalcemia is a frequent finding with malignancies that produce this substance.

DIFFERENTIAL DIAGNOSIS

Primary Hyperparathyroidism

Hyperparathyroidism is the most common cause of hypercalcemia among otherwise healthy people (Table 80–1). Moreover, the proliferation of screening chemistry panels and improvements in the PTH assay have led to a marked increase in the diagnosis of hyperparathyroidism as well as in earlier diagnosis when symptoms tend to be mild or nonexistent. Inappropriate secretion of PTH usually (80% of cases) results from a benign tumor (adenoma) in one of the four parathyroid glands. These lesions secrete PTH in an unregulated fashion. Four-gland hyperplasia accounts for about 20% of cases of primary hyperparathyroidism. Correct identification of the cause of hyperparathyroidism is critical, since surgical removal of a single parathyroid gland will not be curative in four-gland hyperplasia, whereas surgical removal of a solitary parathyroid adenoma usually results in resolution of the hypercalcemia.

Hypercalcemia of Malignancy

Cancer is the second most common cause of hypercalcemia, and at least three different mechanisms of hypercalcemia have been identified in this heterogeneous group of disorders. PTH-RP–mediated hypercalcemia is most common and is associated with solid tumors, such as squamous cell carcinoma of the lung and renal cell carcinoma. Other tumors, such as multiple myeloma and breast carcinoma, produce hypercalcemia through the action of local osteolytic substances such as interleukin-1 and tumor necrosis factor. Finally, some hematopoietic tumors, such as Hodgkin's lymphoma, produce hypercalcemia through inappropriate production of $1,25(OH)_2D_3$. In any event, hypercalcemia may be the first presenting manifestation of an underlying malignancy, and this fact should be remembered when evaluating any otherwise unexplained hypercalcemia.

Nutritional Causes

Most cases of vitamin D intoxication occur when a form of vitamin D is ingested in pharmacologic doses. Vitamin D intoxication resulting purely from dietary intake is unusual. One nutritional cause of hypercalcemia known as the milk-alkali syndrome (MAS) occurs when calcium supplements are ingested along with large quantities of absorbable alkali. Although MAS was more common in the era when milk and bicarbonate were used to treat peptic ulcers, the recent popularity of self-medication with calcium supplements and over-the-counter antacids assures that this condition will continue to occur. Thus, it is important to carefully question hypercalcemic patients about all the medications they are taking.

Drugs

Certain medications are well known for their ability to cause hypercalcemia. Patients taking therapeutic doses of a vitamin D preparation must be followed carefully for the development of hypercalcemia and the permanent kidney damage that can result. Thiazide diuretics cause reduced renal calcium excretion in all patients who take them, but probably only those with subtle underlying defects in parathyroid or renal function develop hypercalcemia. Lithium therapy causes hypercalcemia by increasing the "set point" around which PTH regulates serum calcium levels. The hypercalcemia observed with thiazides and lithium is typically mild, rarely exceeding 11 mg/dL.

Granulomatous Diseases

Diseases such as sarcoidosis and tuberculosis have long been associated with hypercalcemia, but only within the past decade has it become clear that this hypercalcemia is mediated by $1,25(OH)_2D_3$. Macrophages in these granulomatous lesions have active 1α-hydroxylase activity, leading to the unregulated production of the active form of vitamin D. Additionally, Hodgkin's and other lymphomas occasionally cause hypercalcemia through this mechanism.

Familial Hypocalciuric Hypercalcemia

Familial hypocalciuric hypercalcemia (FHH) is a common and benign cause of hypercalcemia that is transmitted as an autosomal dominant trait. Affected individuals usually have asymptomatic hypercalcemia that is discovered during the course of a workup for another problem or as the result of routine screening tests. Such patients have an inherited defect in renal calcium clearance as well as an apparent increase in the "set point" for PTH regulation. Thus, PTH levels may be normal or mildly elevated despite the presence of hypercalcemia. Hyperparathyroidism may thus be erroneously diagnosed, which is unfortunate because isolated parathyroidectomy will not cure the hypercalcemia. It is important to clearly identify the indication and expected benefit of parathyroid surgery preoperatively so that needless surgery is not performed.

Miscellaneous Causes

Immobilization may cause hypercalcemia in young patients, who have a high rate of bone turnover. Similarly, diseases that increase the rate of bone turnover, such as hyperthyroidism, may cause mild hypercalcemia. Chronic renal failure may cause severe hypercalcemia owing to inappropriate secretion of PTH stimulated by high phosphate levels and decreased $1,25(OH)_2D_3$ levels, often despite the presence of hypercalcemia. This disorder is termed tertiary hyperparathyroidism.

EVALUATION

History

Patients with hypercalcemia should be questioned about its physical manifestations. Many patients with hyperparathyroidism will relate a prior history of nephrolithiasis or hematuria with renal colic. Hyperparathyroidism occurs most commonly after the age of 50 years, is more common in women than in men, and is associated with both hypertension and peptic ulcer. Because hypercalcemia may induce a nephrogenic diabetes insipidus, polyuria and polydipsia may be seen. Severe hypercalcemia may cause muscle weakness, fatigability, and mental status changes (e.g., confusion, depression, memory loss, or subtle alterations in personality). Even patients with no neuropsychiatric complaints may have an improved sense of well-being and improved thinking after hypercalcemia resolves. A family history of calcium problems should be elicited, and risk factors for an underlying malignancy should be assessed.

Physical Examination

Blood pressure, mental status, and muscle strength should be assessed, although these parameters will frequently be normal in mildly hypercalcemic patients. Calcification of the cornea may occur with any cause of hypercalcemia, leading to a clouding termed "band keratopathy."

Additional Evaluation

The total serum calcium level should always be interpreted in relation to the serum albumin level, since a disturbance in the level of this protein may artificially elevate or depress the calcium level. An easy way to correct for hypoalbuminemia is to multiply the difference between the observed albumin level and a normal albumin level (approximately 4 g/dL) by 0.8, then add the result to the measured serum calcium level. If doubt exists, an ionized calcium level should be obtained. Serum phosphate levels and measurement of renal function (e.g., BUN and creatinine) should always be obtained when evaluating potential causes of hypercalcemia. A 24-hour urine collection for creatinine clearance and total calcium excretion is helpful in distinguishing hyperparathyroidism from FHH, since 24-hour urine calcium levels rarely exceed 300 mg/day in the latter. Calculating a calcium:creatinine clearance ratio will further help delineate these two entities. In cases of suspected vitamin D intoxication, 25-OHD$_3$ rather than 1,25(OH)$_2$D$_3$ levels should be obtained, since the latter is tightly regulated and may be normal even during toxicosis.

Most patients with hypercalcemia of unknown cause should have the PTH level measured. Currently, a reliable and accurate immunoradiometric assay (IRMA) for the intact PTH molecule exists, and this is the test of choice when evaluating for hyperparathyroidism. PTH levels should always be interpreted in relation to a simultaneously obtained calcium level, and the application of a nomogram helps in this interpretation (Fig. 80–2). If PTH levels are low in the setting of hypercalcemia, a PTH-RP level should be obtained.

Radiographs of the hands in hyperparathyroidism frequently reveal pathognomonic subperiosteal resorption. In more severe hyperparathyroidism, a typical bony lesion termed osteitis fibrosa cystica is observed. In conditions in which calcium and phosphate concentrations are both elevated, such as renal failure or vitamin D intoxication, radiographs of the extremities may reveal ectopic calcification of the soft tissues and joints. Bone densitometry of areas high in cortical bone (such as the wrist) may reveal a marked decrease in bony integrity in hyperparathyroidism. Finally, nuclear imaging studies of the parathyroid glands may reveal a single large parathyroid adenoma and help exclude the possibility of four-gland hyperplasia, but this test may not be necessary in centers with experienced parathyroid surgeons.

MANAGEMENT

Mild Hypercalcemia

Medications that can contribute to hypercalcemia should be discontinued, and immobility should be

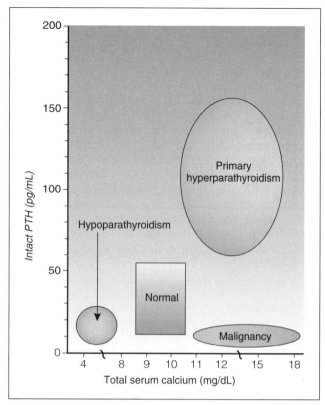

FIGURE 80–2. *Representative nomogram used in the interpretation of serum intact PTH levels.*

discouraged. Estrogen replacement therapy may prove helpful in postmenopausal women with mild hypercalcemia, since estrogen helps ameliorate active bony resorption. Oral phosphate therapy may decrease serum calcium levels but must be weighed against the theoretical danger of ectopic calcification of tissues. Adequate hydration to facilitate renal calcium excretion is the mainstay of therapy. Hydration also prevents supersaturation of the urine with calcium salts and subsequent nephrolithiasis. For refractory cases, a loop diuretic, such as furosemide, may be added to the regimen.

Severe Hypercalcemia

Aggressive intravenous hydration with normal saline and subsequent furosemide diuresis are the initial steps in the treatment of severe hypercalcemia (calcium levels > 14 mg/dL, or the presence of severe symptoms). Therapy should be directed at the underlying cause, but that is often unclear initially. Regardless of the cause, saline hydration and diuresis should be attempted first. In advanced malignancy, these maneuvers are merely temporizing, however, and therapy should be aimed at slowing osteoclastic bony resorption. Many therapeutic agents are available that interfere with osteoclast function, including calcitonin, bisphosphonates (e.g., etidronate, pamidronate), and gallium nitrate. Unfortunately, patients become tolerant to the therapeutic effects of calcitonin relatively quickly, so the other agents may be preferable. Vitamin D–mediated cases of hypercalcemia, such as sarcoidosis, frequently respond rapidly to treatment with glucocorticoids. Older chemotherapeutic agents such as mithramycin (plicamycin) reduce serum calcium levels rapidly, but thrombocytopenia, hepatotoxicity, and nephrotoxicity may result. Nephrotoxicity is a risk with all bisphosphonates and gallium nitrate, and adequate hydration during therapy is essential.

PATIENT AND FAMILY EDUCATION

Hyperparathyroidism is a component of both types of multiple endocrine neoplasia (MEN). MEN I is typified by hyperparathyroidism, pituitary tumors, and pancreatic islet cell tumors (gastrinomas, insulinomas), while MEN II is a syndrome of hyperparathyroidism, medullary thyroid carcinoma, and pheochromocytoma. Hyperparathyroidism occurs in approximately 80% of MEN I and 50% of MEN II cases. Hyperparathyroidism typically results from four-gland hyperplasia in these settings, although isolated adenomata may occur in MEN I. Since the MEN syndromes are propagated in autosomal dominant fashion, a family history focusing on endocrine disease should be obtained in all patients with hyperparathyroidism. If suspicion arises, appropriate screening tests should be obtained in both the patient and the family members.

NATURAL HISTORY/PROGNOSIS

FHH and asymptomatic hyperparathyroidism tend to follow a benign course, although patients with hyperparathyroidism should be followed over time for the possible development of an indication for surgery. Symptomatic hyperparathyroidism, if left untreated, causes significant morbidity in the form of nephrolithiasis, renal failure, crippling bone disease, or psychological sequelae. The outcome of most cases of hypercalcemia of malignancy is grim, and hypercalcemia may be the ultimate cause of death when patients opt for no specific anticancer therapy.

Research Questions

1. Can PTH antagonists be developed for use in the treatment of severe malignancy-associated hypercalcemia?
2. Can a simple and affordable genetic marker for FHH be developed that will allow confirmation of this diagnosis?
3. Can reliable genetic markers for the MEN syndromes be developed that will allow diagnosis of these conditions before tumors develop?

Case Resolution

Given the findings of hypertension and corneal calcifications, as well as the prior history of hematuria (which was suspicious for nephrolithiasis), a diagnosis of primary hyperparathyroidism was suspected. Bone densitometry of the left wrist confirmed a marked decrease in bone mineral density at this location, and 24-hour urine calcium excretion was elevated at 856 mg. The intact serum PTH level was elevated at 134 pg/mL (normal, 10–55 pg/mL) with a concomitant serum calcium level of 11.3 mg/dL. At exploratory parathyroid surgery, a 1.3-gram right superior parathyroid adenoma was identified and resected. After the surgery, the hypercalcemia resolved and the patient felt much improved.

Selected Readings

Bilezikian, J. P. Management of acute hypercalcemia. N Engl J Med 326:1196–1203, 1992.

Broadus, A. E., M. Mangin, K. Ikeda, et al. Humoral hypercalcemia of malignancy: Identification of a novel parathyroid hormone–like peptide. N Engl J Med 319:556–63, 1988.

Heath, H. III. Primary hyperparathyroidism: Recent advances in pathogenesis, diagnosis and management. Adv Intern Med 37:275–93, 1992.

Law, W. M. Jr., and H. Heath III. Familial benign hypercalcemia (hypocalciuric hypercalcemia): Clinical and pathogenetic studies in 21 families. Ann Intern Med 102:511–19, 1985.

Mallette, L. E. Management of hyperparathyroidism in the multiple endocrine neoplasia syndromes and other familial endocrinopathies. Endocrinol Metab Clin North Am 23:19–36, 1994.

Orwoll, E. S. The milk-alkali syndrome: Current concepts. Ann Intern Med 92:242–8, 1982.

CHAPTER 81

MALE SEXUAL DYSFUNCTION

B. Sylvia Vela, M.D.

Hx   A 66-year-old male dentist complains of the inability to maintain an erection. Over the past year, he has noticed progressive loss of erectile function, with intact libido. At present, he can obtain an erection with masturbation, but loses his erection when he attempts intercourse. He denies difficulties in his marital relationship. Over the last several months, he has not had any spontaneous erections during the night or upon early wakening. He has a history of hypertension and adult-onset diabetes mellitus and underwent coronary artery bypass surgery 14 months ago. He has never had pelvic trauma or surgery. He neither smokes nor uses recreational drugs. His diabetes is "diet-controlled," and he takes a β-blocker for hypertension. Since his bypass surgery, he has not had any angina. The physical examination is remarkable for a blood pressure of 159/88 mm Hg and pulse of 59/min. The rest of his examination is normal except for retinal hemorrhages on funduscopy, diminished peripheral pulses, and decreased vibratory sensation in both feet.

Questions

1. Is the patient's erectile dysfunction organic, psychogenic, or both?
2. What aspects of the medical history are pertinent to the chief complaint?
3. What further information is needed?
4. What tests would you order?

Sexual dysfunction is a common problem for men of all ages. Ejaculation disturbances (e.g., premature ejaculation, retrograde ejaculation, inability to ejaculate) and erectile dysfunction are the two general categories of sexual dysfunction in males. These problems are often initially discussed, diagnosed, and treated by the primary care provider. Ejaculation disturbances are most frequently due to sexual ignorance, anxiety, guilt, depression, and interpersonal maladaptation. Treatment involves both behavioral therapy and psychotherapy. Organic causes of ejaculatory disturbances include sympathetic nerve dysfunction due to surgery or trauma or to drugs that interfere with sympathetic tone. Of all the sexual dysfunctions, erectile dysfunction is the condition most likely to have an organic basis.

Erectile dysfunction, or "impotence," is the inability to achieve or maintain an erection suitable for sexual intercourse on more than 50% of attempts for at least 3 months. The prevalence of impotence in the United States is at least 10 million men, or more than 10% of the adult male population. Above the age of 60 years, approximately 30% of men are affected. Moreover, certain disease states, such as diabetes mellitus, predispose the patient to developing impotence in as many as 50% of cases.

In the last decade, large gains have been made in the diagnosis and treatment of impotence. Most cases are now considered to have an organic cause, and many problems previously felt to be beyond help respond to current therapies. Unfortunately, most clinicians are insufficiently trained in the evaluation and treatment of impotence.

PHYSIOLOGY

Erection is a complex physiologic function under psychologic, neurologic, endocrine, and vascular control. Erections are elicited by both sensory stimulation (reflexogenic erections) and by central psychogenic stimuli (psychogenic erections). Reflexogenic erections are mediated by a spinal reflex pathway with peripheral innervation through T11–L2, sympathetic nerves, and S2–4 parasympathetic nerves. Psychogenic erections are less well understood. Erections occur following relaxation of penile smooth muscle from cholinergic stimulation and release of nitric oxide from endothelial cells. This relaxation causes dilatation of the penile cavernosal arteries, which increases blood flow within the cavernosal tissue and results in engorgement of the penis. Once the blood pressure is elevated significantly, penile veins are compressed and venous outflow ceases. Detumescence occurs when sympathetic constrictor nerves cause contraction of penile smooth muscle, which leads to reduction of arterial inflow and collapse of the lacunar spaces.

DIFFERENTIAL DIAGNOSIS

The functional classification of impotence can be grouped according to psychogenic, neurogenic, endocrinologic, vascular, and pharmacologic causes (Tables 81–1 and 81–2). A combination of causes may play a role in an individual patient. Once a patient develops organic impotence, a psychogenic overlay often adds to the difficulty. Psychogenic impotence has many causes including performance anxiety, depression, marital conflict, childhood sexual abuse, and religious beliefs.

EVALUATION

Given the many nonsurgical options for the management of impotence, it can be argued that an expensive diagnostic workup is not necessary for most patients. In most cases, a thorough history, physical examination, and minimal laboratory work can determine the cause of the impotence. In more than 25% of cases, a reversible cause will be found or a previously undiagnosed medical condition detected.

TABLE 81–1. Causes of Erectile Dysfunction

Neurogenic	*Psychogenic*
Spinal cord disorders	Performance anxiety
Multiple sclerosis	Depression
Traumatic nerve injury	Religious inhibition
Peripheral neuropathies	Sexual phobia
Alcoholism	Marital discord
Diabetes	
Amyloidosis	*Vasculogenic*
B vitamin deficiencies	Arterial insufficiency
	Congenital
Endocrinologic	Traumatic
Diabetes mellitus	Atherosclerosis
Hypogonadism	Endothelial dysfunction
Hyperprolactinemia	Hypertension
Hyper- or hypothyroidism	Hypercholesterolemia
Pharmacologic	
See Table 81–2.	

TABLE 81–2.   Agents That Produce Impotence

Diuretics

Hydrochlorothiazide
Chlorthalidone
Spironolactone

Antihypertensives *

β-Blockers
Methyldopa
Reserpine
Clonidine

Anxiolytics, Antipsychotics

Phenothiazines
Butyrophenones

Antiandrogens

Cyproterone acetate
Flutamide
Cimetidine
Digoxin
Ketoconazole

Habituating Substances

Alcohol
Amphetamines
Barbiturates
Cocaine
Nicotine
Marijuana
Opiates

Tricyclic Antidepressants
Anticholinergics
Estrogens

---

*Note that any antihypertensive can have adverse sexual effects.

History

Evaluation begins with a detailed medical, sexual, and psychosocial history in order to evaluate underlying factors that may be affecting erectile function. First, the sexual problem should be defined; many patients confuse impotence with premature ejaculation or disorders of orgasm such as retrograde ejaculation. If the patient does have erectile dysfunction, he should be questioned regarding the progression of the dysfunction. Acute onset, as well as a history of early-morning erections or erections with masturbation, suggest a psychogenic cause. On the other hand, a slow insidious onset, with progressive inability to sustain an erection with masturbation, is suggestive of an organic cause. Decreased libido is suggestive of either hypogonadism or depression. Psychosocial stressors should be explored, such as the patient's relationship with his partner, outside stressors, or a history of sexual abuse.

The medical history should focus on vascular disorders and risk factors such as hypertension, hyperlipidemia, diabetes mellitus, coronary artery disease, claudication, pelvic or vascular surgery, pelvic radiation, or pelvic/perineal trauma. Neurologic dysfunction should be explored, such as changes in sensation or bowel or bladder function. A detailed history of medications as well as recreational drug use should be obtained.

Physical Examination

The endocrinologic, neurologic, and cardiovascular systems are emphasized. Examination of secondary sexual characteristics including hair distribution, voice, muscle mass, and skeletal proportions can give clues regarding the presence of hypogonadism. Gross visual field examination should be performed to screen for a pituitary tumor. The thyroid gland should be palpated, and the breasts checked for gynecomastia. The abdomen and genitalia should be carefully examined for sensory testing of the penis and perineum, inguinal hernias, adenopathy, and adequate peripheral and femoral pulses. The penis should be palpated for evidence of corporal plaques (Peyronie's disease, or fibrous thickening of the penile shaft), and the scrotum and testes should be examined for testicular volume as well as the presence of hydrocele, varicocele, and epididymitis. A rectal examination is performed to detect abnormalities of anal sphincter tone and of the prostate.

Additional Evaluation

Laboratory evaluation includes urinalysis, liver and renal function tests, and CBC to detect underlying systemic disease; glucose level for diabetes detection; thyroid function tests, and prolactin, testosterone, luteinizing hormone (LH), and follicle-stimulating hormone (FSH) levels to assess for abnormalities of thyroid or hypothalamic–pituitary–gonadal function.

If the etiology is unclear, nocturnal penile tumescence (NPT) testing can be performed. NPT was the first test to differentiate between psychogenic and organic causes of impotence. In formal NPT laboratories, mercury strain gauges are placed at the tip and base of the penis while the patient is sleeping, to monitor circumference changes and tumescence. In normal men, three to five erections per night occur in association with REM sleep. Patients with organic impotence have impaired or absent erectile activity, whereas patients with psychogenic causes usually have a normal pattern. Portable devices for home testing are also available. However, interpretation is often difficult, and test results may not be reliable in patients with depression, sleep disorders, or neurologic disease.

If neurologic factors are suspected, biothesiometry (measurement of the threshold of perception of vibration) or dorsal nerve conduction studies can be performed. To diagnose arteriogenic impotence, the penile brachial index (PBI), combined injection stimulation (CIS) tests, or duplex ultrasound scanning can be performed. PBI measures blood pressure in the penis compared to that in the arm. A ratio of penile to brachial blood pressure below 0.6 indicates arteriogenic impotence. CIS tests the erectile response to intracavernous injection of vasodilators. A prompt and sustained response eliminates the need for further testing. Patients with venous leaks can be evaluated by radiographic cavernosography and cavernosometry prior to surgical repair. At present, these studies are best performed in referral centers with this specific expertise.

MANAGEMENT

If a dysfunctional relationship is suspected as the cause of erectile dysfunction, couples counseling might

TABLE 81–3. Options for Management of Impotence

Treatment	Comments
Counseling	Helpful in psychogenic causes.
Vacuum pump device	Safe, effective, and inexpensive over the long-term.
Yohimbine hydrochloride	Response usually within 4 weeks. Adverse effects include water retention and blood pressure alterations.
Penile injection treatment	Preparations include phentolamine, phenoxybenzamine, prostaglandin E_1, papaverine, and mixtures. Complications include priapism, fibrosis, pain. Can be expensive.
Testosterone therapy	For use in hypogonadal men only. Intramuscular or patch administration recommended. Oral administration causes hepatotoxicity. Adverse effects include prostate hypertrophy.
Bromocriptine	For use in hyperprolactinemia only.
Venous ligation	Poor long-term success rate.
Arterial revascularization	Varying success rate.
Penile implant	Mechanical breakdown, infection, extrusion may necessitate reoperation. Should be reserved for patients who failed another therapy.

be indicated. If psychodynamic factors are thought to be contributory, psychotherapy may be the treatment of choice. Sexual therapy with both partners present is often helpful if the problem is performance anxiety or distractions. A prerequisite for successful therapy is accurate identification of the cause of the sexual dysfunction. Treating organic impairment with psychological methods alone is of little benefit.

Medical or noninvasive pharmacologic management of impotence can be successful (Table 81–3). In hypogonadism, androgen replacement (e.g., testosterone enanthate) can restore libido and erectile function. Testosterone delivered in the form of scrotal patches may better approximate physiologic secretion of testosterone. Hyperprolactinemia can be treated with bromocriptine. Hypothyroidism and hyperthyroidism can be treated with thyroid hormone or antithyroid drugs, respectively. In patients with psychogenic impotence, yohimbine decreases outflow of blood from the corporeal tissue and is more effective than placebo.

Penile injection therapy with vasoactive drugs is probably the most important advance made in the treatment of impotence during the past decade. Vasoactive substances used include papaverine hydrochloride, phentolamine, prostaglandin E_1, and combinations of the three. These drugs either relax the smooth muscle directly or block adrenergically induced tone. Patients are instructed in self-injection to be administered whenever they desire intercourse. Patients with neurogenic or psychogenic causes achieve the best results; patients with severe arterial insufficiency are the least likely to respond. Patients with mild to moderate vasculogenic causes can respond because of the long-acting nature of the smooth muscle relaxation provided by the vasoactive agents. Adverse effects include local discomfort, fibrosis, and priapism.

External vacuum pump therapy is perhaps the safest and most economical therapy. Vacuum pumps consist of a vacuum source connected to a plastic cylinder, which is placed over the flaccid penis. The negative pressure generated by the vacuum in the cylinder causes blood to accumulate in the penis, resulting in erection. Constriction bands are then placed around the base of the penis to impede drainage of the blood and maintain tumescence.

The three basic types of penile prosthesis are rigid, semirigid, and inflatable models. Selection of a type is influenced by cost, the surgeon's familiarity with the device, the patient's manual dexterity, and the extent of sensory function. Penile prostheses will not restore libido, the ability to ejaculate, or penile sensation. Pain, infection, erosion, mechanical breakdown, or wear of the product may necessitate removal or reoperation.

Penile revascularization may be indicated in young patients who have suffered pelvic or perineal trauma. Success rates vary. This procedure is not generally successful in patients with arteriosclerosis.

PATIENT AND FAMILY EDUCATION

Most of the public remains uninformed or misinformed about erectile dysfunction. This lack of information and a reluctance on the part of physicians to deal candidly with sexual matters have resulted in patients being denied the benefits of diagnosis and treatment of their sexual problems. Accurate information on sexual function and the management of dysfunction must be provided to affected men and their partners. Most importantly, patients and their partners should be reassured that treatments are available that can restore a healthy sex life.

PROGNOSIS

The prognosis is excellent with the appropriate therapy when the correct etiology is determined.

Research Questions

1. How do androgens affect male erectile function?
2. What is the most cost-effective approach to the diagnosis and treatment of erectile dysfunction?

Case Resolution

Diabetes, hypertension, an antihypertensive agent, and coronary heart disease all contributed to this patient's erectile difficulties. Laboratory analysis was remarkable for proteinuria, a glucose level of 289, and normal hormone studies. The physician's recommendations included better control of diabetes with an oral hypoglycemic agent and treatment of his hypertension with an ACE inhibitor, an agent that is less likely to contribute to impotence. After several months, his erections had improved but were not sufficient for intercourse. After discussing the various treatment options with the physician, the couple chose to use a vacuum pump device.

Selected Readings

Carrier, S., G. Brock, N. W. Kour, and T. Lue. Pathophysiology of erectile dysfunction. Urology 42:468–81, 1993.

Cookson, M. S., and P. W. Nadig. Long-term results with a vacuum constriction device. J Urol 149:290–4, 1993.

Krane, R. J., I. Goldstein, and I. Saenz de Tejada. Impotence. N Engl J Med 321:1648–58, 1989.

Lerner, S. E., A. Melman, and G. J. Christ. Review of erectile dysfunction: New insights and more questions. J Urol 149:1246–55, 1993.

Montague, D. K. Impotence therapy. J Urol 149:1313, 1993.

Virag, R., K. Shoudry, J. Floresco, et al. Intracavernous self-injection of vasoactive drugs in the treatment of impotence: 8-year experience with 615 cases. J Urol 145:287–93, 1991.

CHAPTER 82

GLUCOCORTICOID THERAPY

Richard I. Dorin, M.D., and Laura M. Ferries, M.D.

"Never take prednisone unless you absolutely have to."

—A patient on chronic glucocorticoid therapy

H$_x$ A 61-year-old male electrical engineer with a history of asthma complains of aching joints, loss of appetite, nausea, and dizziness upon standing of 1 week's duration. For 20 years his asthma has been treated with bronchodilators as well as inhaled and systemic glucocorticoids. He takes a 10-mg maintenance dose of prednisone daily but requires intermittent steroid bursts during asthma exacerbations. Recently, he was hospitalized with bronchitis and asthma exacerbation that responded to antibiotic and intravenous steroid therapy. Upon hospital discharge, he was maintained on prednisone 40 mg/d for 3 weeks before reverting to his maintenance dose for the past week. The patient is afebrile with a respiratory rate of 20/min; blood pressure of 100/60 mm Hg, which drops to 85/50 upon standing; and pulse of 80/min, which goes to 94 upon standing. He has a cushingoid appearance with a round face and central obesity. The pulmonary examination is normal, and there is no evidence of arthritis.

Questions

1. What should be the goal for this patient—maintenance or discontinuation of systemic glucocorticoid therapy?
2. How does the chronic use of prednisone affect this patient?
3. What are three conditions that limit the taper or discontinuation of chronic glucocorticoid therapy?
4. What is the most likely explanation for his complaints of arthralgia, anorexia, and dizziness?

Following the discovery of cortisone and recognition of its antiinflammatory properties in 1948, glucocorticoids have become a standard therapeutic modality used in a diverse array of clinical conditions. In general, the use of pharmacologic doses of corticosteroids is directed toward three related effects: (1) antiinflammatory, (2) immunosuppressive, and (3) lymphocytotoxic properties. Common disorders for which corticosteroids are used include asthma and rheumatologic conditions.

Clinical experience has emphasized that these potent compounds are a two-edged sword, with the beneficial therapeutic effects on immune and inflammatory cells inextricably linked to undesirable and serious side effects on other tissues. In spite of efforts to develop alternative immunosuppressive or antiinflammatory modalities, glucocorticoids remain an essential and irreplaceable agent in the therapeutic armamentarium. The challenge to the clinician is to balance treatment efficacy with efforts to minimize side effects of pharmacologic glucocorticoids.

PATHOPHYSIOLOGY

The cortex of the adrenal gland produces three classes of naturally occurring steroid compounds: (1) glucocorticoids (e.g., hydrocortisone), (2) mineralocorticoids (e.g., aldosterone), and (3) androgens (e.g., dehydroepiandrosterone). Of these, glucocorticoids are quantitatively and physiologically the most important. Glucocorticoids are required for normal physiologic function and adaptation to physiologic stress. The only site of glucocorticoid synthesis is the adrenal cortex, thus ex-

TABLE 82–1. Half-life and Daily Replacement Dose of Some Commonly Used Glucocorticoids

Drug	Circulating Half-Life (Hours)	Biologic Half-Life (Hours)	Equivalent Daily Replacement Dose (mg)
Hydrocortisone (IV or PO)	1.5	3	20
Prednisone (PO)	3.5	4	5
Methylprednisolone (IV) (Solu-medrol)	3	4	4
Dexamethasone (IV or PO) (Decadron)	4	8	0.75

IV, intravenous; PO, oral.

plaining the term "corticosteroids." In humans, the principal glucocorticoid produced by the adrenal is hydrocortisone, also known as cortisol.

Glucocorticoids circulate in two forms: either bound to serum proteins, such as cortisol binding globulin (CBG), or in a free, unbound state. Free hormone diffuses across cell membranes and binds with high affinity to a specific cytosolic receptor (the glucocorticoid receptor). After binding glucocorticoid, the hormone-receptor complex enters the cell nucleus, where it binds to the regulatory regions of specific target genes. Thus, glucocorticoids alter cell phenotype by regulating the rate of transcription of specific genes and synthesis of their cognate protein products.

What are the clinical implications of receptor-mediated glucocorticoid action? First, the biologic activity of glucocorticoids depends on receptor binding. Accordingly, the potency and biologic half-life of glucocorticoids is influenced by their affinity and duration of binding to the glucocorticoid receptor. For example, hydrocortisone has a relatively low affinity and rapidly dissociates from the receptor, conferring relatively weak glucocorticoid activity and short-lived biologic effects. Dexamethasone has a much greater affinity for the glucocorticoid receptor and so is more potent; in addition, dexamethasone dissociates more slowly and has a longer duration of action (Table 82–1). Second, because glucocorticoid effects are mediated through regulation of gene expression, the biologic activity of glucocorticoids does not correlate with circulating half-life (see Table 82–1). Third, the number of glucocorticoid receptors limits the maximum biologic effect of glucocorticoids. Once glucocorticoid concentrations are sufficient to saturate all receptors, little additional benefit is likely to be achieved by increasing the dose of glucocorticoid.

Glucocorticoid receptors are expressed in almost all tissues, and therefore the biologic effects of glucocorticoids are generalized. Because therapeutic as well as deleterious side effects of glucocorticoids are mediated by the same receptor molecule, it is difficult to target glucocorticoid effects to specific tissues, such as the immune system, or to dissociate beneficial effects of glucocorticoids from unwanted effects in other tissues.

EVALUATION

Clinical evaluation should be directed initially at the status of the underlying condition for which glucocor-

ticoids were prescribed, such as asthma or arthritis, and secondarily at glucocorticoid status.

Useful objective data include temperature and orthostatic blood pressure and pulse measurements. Blood pressure can be elevated in the steroid excess state and low (with orthostatic changes) during steroid withdrawal and adrenal insufficiency. Evidence of hypercortisolism should be sought. The finding of specific complications of glucocorticoid therapy (e.g., hyperglycemia or hypertension) may require directed therapy until such time that glucocorticoids can be decreased or discontinued. Evaluation for signs of infection should also be performed, since patients receiving supraphysiologic steroid doses are at higher risk for both common and opportunistic infections. Usual signs and symptoms of an infectious process may not be evident owing to suppression of the inflammatory and immune responses.

The ACTH stimulation test is useful in establishing the presence or absence of secondary adrenal insufficiency. Serum cortisol levels are determined at baseline and 60 minutes after intravenous or intramuscular administration of one ampule (0.25 mg) of cortrosyn ($ACTH_{1-24}$). A stimulated cortisol of > 20 μg/dL usually indicates normal adrenal function. Since prednisone cross-reacts in the cortisol assay, it is useful to discontinue prednisone therapy for 24 hours prior to performing the short ACTH stimulation test in patients on replacement therapy.

MANAGEMENT

Principles of Glucocorticoid Therapy

One of the most important maneuvers for avoiding the complications of glucocorticoid therapy is appropriate **patient selection**. Glucocorticoid therapy should be reserved for conditions in which therapeutic efficacy has been established. It also is useful to document objective clinical benefit of corticosteroid therapy in individual patients. This is important because many patients treated with glucocorticoids experience an initial euphoria or subjective sense of well-being that is independent of objective improvement.

A second principle is to use the **lowest possible glucocorticoid dose** required to achieve clinical efficacy. Whenever possible, less toxic alternative therapies should be instituted before chronic glucocorticoids. Alternative routes of administration, such as topical glucocorticoids for dermatologic conditions or inhaled aerosolized glucocorticoids for respiratory conditions, may provide therapeutic efficacy with fewer side effects than systemic therapy. In some circumstances, use of "steroid-sparing" cytotoxic agents or alternate-day therapy may produce clinical efficacy while reducing side effects of glucocorticoids.

A third principle involves **continuity of care**. Glucocorticoid therapy is a long-term undertaking that benefits from mutual familiarity and understanding between patient and clinician. Serial evaluation also facilitates assessment of the underlying condition, including objective measures of disease activity, in a stable clinical setting. In addition, continuity of care facilitates patient education, institution of measures to prevent complications of glucocorticoid therapy, and integration of quality-of-life issues into clinical management and decision making.

A fourth principle is that glucocorticoid therapy should be **individualized** to be both disease- and patient-specific. Various immunologic and inflammatory conditions differ in their response to specific doses or tapering schedules, as well as their response to alternate-day therapy. Individual patients with the same disorder also tend to differ in their response to glucocorticoids. Other principles include **patient and family education** and institution of **preventive measures** to avoid complications of glucocorticoid therapy.

Complications of Glucocorticoid Therapy

Patients on chronic supraphysiologic glucocorticoid therapy are at risk for development of clinical manifestations of hypercortisolism similar to those seen in endogenous adrenal overactivity (Cushing's syndrome). These include characteristic body habitus with moon facies, buffalo hump, supraclavicular fat pads, and central obesity. Other manifestations of glucocorticoid excess are expressed in organ systems such as skin (easy bruising, acne, striae, poor wound healing), musculoskeletal (osteoporosis, myopathy), cardiovascular (hypertension, coronary artery disease), neuropsychiatric (mood changes, psychosis), immune (immunosuppression), and endocrine-metabolic (hyperlipidemia, glucose intolerance).

Another complication of glucocorticoid therapy is suppression of the hypothalamic-pituitary-adrenal (HPA) axis and development of adaptation and dependence on supraphysiologic glucocorticoids. Following an extended course of glucocorticoid therapy, the HPA axis remains suppressed after removal of glucocorticoids, with gradual recovery over 12 to 18 months. During this period, patients may have decreased adrenal reserve and develop relative adrenal insufficiency during times of physiologic stress, such as surgery or illness.

The steroid withdrawal syndrome is a multisystem disorder with clinical manifestations similar to those of adrenal insufficiency (Table 82–2). In contrast to frank adrenal insufficiency, however, glucocorticoid withdrawal syndrome occurs during glucocorticoid replacement. The syndrome can be viewed as an acquired "habituation" or "tolerance" to glucocorticoids. In addi-

TABLE 82–2.   Clinical Manifestations of Glucocorticoid Withdrawal Syndrome

Fatigue
Weakness
Anorexia
Nausea/vomiting
Diarrhea
Arthralgia
Myalgia
Weight loss
Postural hypotension
Skin desquamation

tion, some patients may develop a psychological dependence on glucocorticoids.

Dosage and Administration

The acute phase of glucocorticoid treatment is typically initiated using oral prednisone (or equivalent doses of IV methylprednisolone) at doses of 1–4 mg/kg/d administered in 2–4 divided doses. The supraphysiologic nature of this therapy is illustrated by comparison with physiologic glucocorticoid replacement therapy in patients with adrenal insufficiency (see Table 82–1). Once the acute phase of the disease has been controlled, maintenance therapy can be initiated with lower doses of prednisone, typically 25–60 mg, administered as a single daily dose. When the patient is clinically stable, gradual steroid taper is initiated in order to empirically determine the lowest, therapeutically effective dose of glucocorticoid.

The ability to decrease the dose of daily steroid is typically prevented by development of one of three conditions: (1) recurrence or activation of the underlying disease, (2) steroid withdrawal syndrome, or (3) adrenal insufficiency. In general, a relatively rapid reduction in the daily prednisone dose, e.g., 5–10 mg of prednisone per week, is well tolerated in patients receiving high doses of prednisone. However, the rate of steroid taper usually becomes more gradual as the total daily dose is decreased below 20 mg/d, and slower yet at doses of 5–10 mg/d. Glucocorticoid taper is achieved more easily after a short course of intensive therapy as compared to chronic glucocorticoid therapy. Generally, a taper is not necessary if the duration of therapy has been less than 2 weeks and if there is no prior history of steroid use.

Glucocorticoid withdrawal syndrome is managed by an increase in the dose of prednisone or by addition of a short-acting glucocorticoid, such as hydrocortisone. The latter has the advantage of producing less marked suppression of the HPA axis. Patients may require small amounts of supplemental glucocorticoid for extended periods of time to prevent symptoms of steroid withdrawal prior to termination of steroid therapy. Many patients have decreased adrenal reserve following steroid taper and require glucocorticoid supplement at times of physiologic stress, such as surgery or medical illness, to prevent manifestations of adrenal insufficiency.

Because of the long duration of glucocorticoid action, it is possible in some cases to achieve adequate anti-inflammatory or immunosuppressive effects using an alternate-day schedule of prednisone administration. This regimen is associated with fewer side effects of glucocorticoids. Alternate-day therapy can be initiated by gradually decreasing the dose of prednisone on the "off" day; at times this requires a commensurate increase in prednisone dose for the "on" day.

Prevention

Many of the undesirable effects of glucocorticoids occur in a predictable fashion. These complications should be anticipated and, if appropriate, preventive strategies initiated. For example, skin testing for tuberculosis should be performed in patients prior to instituting an anticipated course of chronic, high-dose glucocorticoid therapy. Similarly, glucocorticoid therapy predictably increases the rate of bone loss, leading to osteoporosis in susceptible individuals. This decrease in bone mass can be slowed, but not prevented, by simple measures such as adequate intake of vitamin D (400 IU/d in multivitamins) and calcium (1500 mg/d of elemental calcium). Other therapies that decrease the rate of bone resorption, such as bisphosphonates or calcitonin, are currently under investigation and may also prove to be effective in prevention or treatment of steroid-induced osteoporosis.

PATIENT AND FAMILY EDUCATION

It is useful for patients to have a clear understanding of the potential benefits and risks of glucocorticoid therapy from the outset. Patients frequently respond enthusiastically to the often dramatic clinical benefits and improved sense of well-being associated with glucocorticoid therapy. It is important that they also appreciate the complications of chronic steroid use and the rationale for minimizing the dose and duration of glucocorticoid exposure. This will help enlist their interest and cooperation in the process of steroid taper and withdrawal. This is particularly important because patients frequently feel worse when their steroid dose is lowered.

Patient education is also useful in maximizing alternative therapies that may facilitate reduction in glucocorticoid dose.

Patients and their families need to be advised of the potential for adrenal insufficiency during times of physiologic stress, which may necessitate supplemental steroid administration. A medical emergency bracelet, identifying the patient as one on chronic glucocorticoid therapy with adrenal suppression, may be indicated.

Research Questions

1. What is the role of new treatment modalities, such as bisphosphonates and calcitonin, in prevention and treatment of steroid-induced osteoporosis?
2. Which advances in gene therapy and molecular medicine would permit targeting of glucocorticoid effects to selected tissues?

Case Resolution

The patient's prednisone dose was increased to 25 mg/d, with prompt resolution of signs and symptoms during close outpatient follow-up. The clinical course was consistent with glucocorticoid withdrawal syndrome, which did not recur when a more gradual taper schedule was instituted subsequently.

Selected Readings

Axelrod, L. Corticosteroid therapy. *In* K. Becker (ed.). *Principles and Practice of Endocrinology and Metabolism.* Philadelphia, J.B. Lippincott Company, 1990.

Baxter, J. D. The effects of glucocorticoid therapy. Hosp Pract 27:111–18, 1992.

Boumpas, D. T., G. P. Chrousos, R. L. Wilder, et al. Glucocorticoid therapy for immune-mediated diseases: Basic and clinical correlates. Ann Intern Med 119:1198–1208, 1993.

Kendall, E. C. *Cortisone.* New York, Charles Scribner's Sons, 1971.

Sambrook, P., J. Birmingham, P. Kelly, et al. Prevention of corticosteroid osteoporosis: A comparison of calcium, calcitriol, and calcitonin. N Engl J Med 328:1747–52, 1993.

COMMON HEMATOLOGIC-ONCOLOGIC PROBLEMS

CHAPTER 83

ANEMIA

William R. Hardy, M.D.

Hx A 56-year-old female economist presents with intermittent joint pain and swelling, primarily in the proximal interphalangeal (PIP) joints of both hands, both wrists, left shoulder, and right knee, that have bothered her for 3 months. She complains of morning stiffness. Local heat and over-the-counter analgesics provide some relief. Except for joint pain, the woman says she feels well, and she denies rash, fever, anorexia, and weight loss. She had a total hysterectomy at age 40 years for fibroids, and she has been taking thyroxine for 8 years for "low thyroid." Physical examination reveals a healthy woman with normal vital signs. The only findings of note include slight fusiform swelling and capsular thickening of the PIP joints of both hands. Initial laboratory studies show hemoglobin, 10.5 g/dL; mean corpuscular volume (MCV), 81 fL; red cell distribution width (RDW), 17.8%; WBC, 7400/μL (76% neutrophils); platelets, 454,000 μL; erythrocyte sedimentation rate (ESR), 47 mm/h; and rheumatoid factor, 1:320. Urinalysis is normal.

Questions

1. What other information concerning the patient's history might be helpful?
2. What is the most likely cause of the anemia?
3. What additional information is necessary for confirmation of this hypothesis?

Anemia, which is detected and defined on the basis of a blood count, is a sign of an underlying disease. The diagnosis of anemia is based on obtaining a value—hematocrit, hemoglobin, or red blood cell (RBC) count—below the defined normal range for the patient's age, sex, and altitude of residence. The recognition of anemia is important on two levels. First, anemia that is severe, is abrupt in onset, or occurs in individuals with preexisting compromised oxygen delivery may result in significant morbidity and mortality. Second, identification

and treatment of the etiologic process causing the anemia is key to overall management of the patient. This discussion focuses on establishing the cause of the most common types of anemia; anemia due to acute hemorrhage is not considered.

PATHOPHYSIOLOGY

Normally, erythrocytes (RBCs) survive about 120 days, which means that about 0.8% of the circulating red cell mass must be replaced and catabolized every 24 hours. The normal marrow readily effects replacement, although erythroblast maturation is not 100% efficient (about 15% of RBC precursors die within the marrow). Marrow reserve is sufficient to allow RBC production to increase 2 to 3 times the basal level following acute blood loss and up to 6 to 8 times the basal level in chronic hemolysis. Both normal and enhanced erythropoiesis require (1) an intact marrow microenvironment; (2) a fully functional erythropoietin mechanism; (3) uncompromised DNA synthesis, which is necessary for nuclear maturation; and (4) hemoglobin (Hb) production unimpaired by either lack of iron or inhibition of the rate of globin synthesis. Compromise of the microenvironment or of the erythropoietin mechanism principally impedes erythroblast proliferation (i.e., marrow shows decreased numbers), and compromise of DNA synthesis or of Hb production primarily interferes with maturation (i.e., marrow erythroblasts are increased in number but do not develop properly). In healthy individuals, RBCs that are newly released from the marrow contain residual RNA for about 24 hours, which means that they can be counted with special ("vital") stains as reticulocytes; this count is a useful index of the rate of delivery of new RBCs from the marrow. A normal count is approximately 1%.

At the conclusion of their 4-month life span, approximately 85% of senescent RBCs are engulfed by cells of the macrophage-monocyte system. Hb is processed to

TABLE 83–1.   Kinetic Classification of Anemia

Kinetic Category	Reticulocyte Count	Indirect Bilirubin	Marrow and Blood Count	Common Clinical Settings	Confirming/Associated Findings
Impaired erythroblast proliferation	< 2 times basal	Normal	Marrow normal, anemia only	Chronic renal failure; hypothyroidism	Azotemia, acidosis; increased TSH
			Marrow hypocellular, pancytopenia	Stem cell injury	Aplastic anemia, radiation, myelosuppressive drugs
			Marrow infiltrated, leukoerythroblastosis	Leukemia, other cancers, fibrosis (e.g., tuberculosis)	Diagnostic features of infiltrating process
Impaired erythroblast maturation	< 2 times basal	Normal	Marrow normal (except absent iron); anisocytosis early, microcytosis late	Iron deficiency (chronic blood loss)	↓Serum iron/↑TIBC; ↓Serum ferritin
		Normal to ↑	Erythroid hyperplasia; microcytosis constant, anisocytosis if severe	Thalassemia syndromes	Family studies; ↑hemoglobin A$_2$ and/or F
			Megaloblastic hyperplasia; macrocytosis/anisocytosis, hypersegmented neutrophils	B$_{12}$ or folate deficiency, myelodysplasia (idiopathic, drug-induced)	Serum B$_{12}$ or erythrocyte folate↓, clinical setting
Hemolytic Anemia Chronic	> 3 times basal	↑	Erythroid hyperplasia; prehemolytic forms (e.g., spherocytes, fragments, sickle cells)	Hereditary spherocytosis, sickle cell disorders, immune hemolytic anemias, fragmentation syndromes	Clinical setting, appropriate tests (e.g., hemoglobin electrophoresis, Coombs' test)
Acute	< 2–> 3 times basal	Normal to ↑	Marrow normal initially; ± spherocytosis, agglutination	G6PD* deficiency, cold agglutinin syndromes	Clinical setting, appropriate tests (e.g., G6PD assay)
Anemia of chronic disease	< 2 times basal	Normal	Normal erythroid marrow; little anisocytosis, occasional microcytosis	Chronic inflammatory or infectious disease, advanced malignancy	Clinical setting

*G6PD, glucose-6-phosphate dehydrogenase.

conserve the amino acids of the globin chains and the iron for reuse, but the protoporphyrin ring of the heme prosthetic group is catabolized to become unconjugated bilirubin, which is transported to the liver, where it is conjugated and excreted into the bile. The remaining 15% of RBCs undergo lysis in the circulation; the released Hb is bound to carrier proteins (haptoglobin, hemopexin), transported to the liver, and processed as above. In certain types of anemia, an increased level of serum unconjugated bilirubin suggests an increase in the amount of Hb undergoing degradation.

From the above considerations it is apparent that, kinetically, anemia may result from decreased RBC production, premature destruction (hemolysis), or blood loss. Decreased production can be considered a failure of either erythroblast proliferation or maturation. In most chronic anemias, a single pathophysiologic mechanism is operative. This kinetic view can be used, in conjunction with cytologic information (described below) from the blood count, to pinpoint the cause of most anemias (Table 83–1).

DIFFERENTIAL DIAGNOSIS

During the past decade, the widespread use of accurate, precise electronic counters has led to a cytologic classification of anemia based on red cell size (MCV) and degree of variation in RBC size (anisocytosis, which is expressed as RDW). This cytologic classification shown in Table 83–2 complements the kinetic classification in Table 83–1. Although electronic counters provide other red cell indices—mean corpuscular hemoglobin

TABLE 83–2.   Cytologic Classification of Anemia

Laboratory Finding	Microcytic (< 80 fL)	Normocytic (80–100 fL)	Macrocytic (> 100 fL)
RDW < 15 (normal)	Thalassemia minor, anemia of chronic disease (some)	Hypothyroidism, malnutrition, chronic renal failure, marrow injury (most), marrow infiltration (most), anemia of chronic disease (most)	Aplastic anemia, chronic liver disease, chronic alcohol excess, zidovudine therapy
RDW > 15 (increased)	Iron deficiency (late), thalassemia major, fragmentation hemolysis (some)	Iron deficiency (early), vitamin B$_{12}$/folate deficiency (early), chronic hemolytic disorders (most)	Vitamin B$_{12}$/folate deficiency (late), chronic hemolytic disorders (some), myelodysplastic disorders, antimetabolite therapy

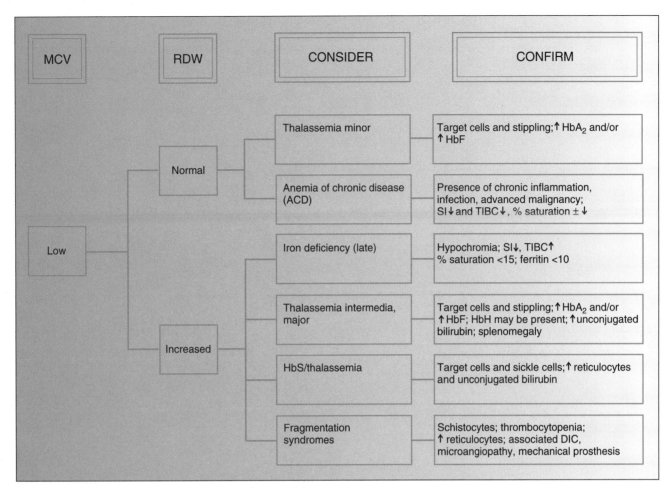

FIGURE 83–1. *Algorithm for diagnosis of microcytic anemia. DIC, disseminated intravascular coagulation; SI, serum iron; TIBC, total iron-binding capacity.*

(MCH) and mean corpuscular hemoglobin concentration (MCHC)—they infrequently provide additional useful information.

The goal of all diagnostic techniques is identification of a specific etiology. The list of potential causes for anemia is long and continually growing. This necessitates a diagnostic approach using easily available and inexpensive information to narrow the possibilities efficiently. The presence of one or more potential etiologic factors in a given patient does not necessarily indicate a cause-and-effect relationship.

EVALUATION

The algorithms in Figures 83–1, 83–2, and 83–3 for microcytic, normocytic, and macrocytic anemias, respectively, combine cytologic and kinetic classifications and allow a specific etiology to be identified expeditiously for most situations.

This approach appears to minimize the importance of the history and physical examination. Certainly, some patients present with symptoms (fatigue, exertional dyspnea) or signs (pallor) suggestive of anemia, but confirmation requires a blood count. Nonetheless, both history and physical examination may provide important clues to etiology (e.g., a history of hematochezia,

concurrent illness, or drug exposure or physical findings such as atrophic glossitis, splenomegaly, or an abdominal mass may be suggestive). Often the results of the CBC lead to a more critical historical or physical evaluation.

MANAGEMENT AND PROGNOSIS

Management depends on an accurate diagnosis. Since anemia is *always* a sign of an underlying disorder, failure to identify that process is likely to result in inappropriate management, prognosis, and advice to patients. Indeed, the anemia is often managed easily, whereas treatment of the underlying process is usually much more difficult. The outlook and management for some of the common anemias are shown in Table 83–3.

> **Research Questions**
>
> 1. Can better (accurate, inexpensive, available) techniques be developed to define the rates of RBC production and destruction?
> 2. Is the anemia of chronic disease always an appropriate biological response?

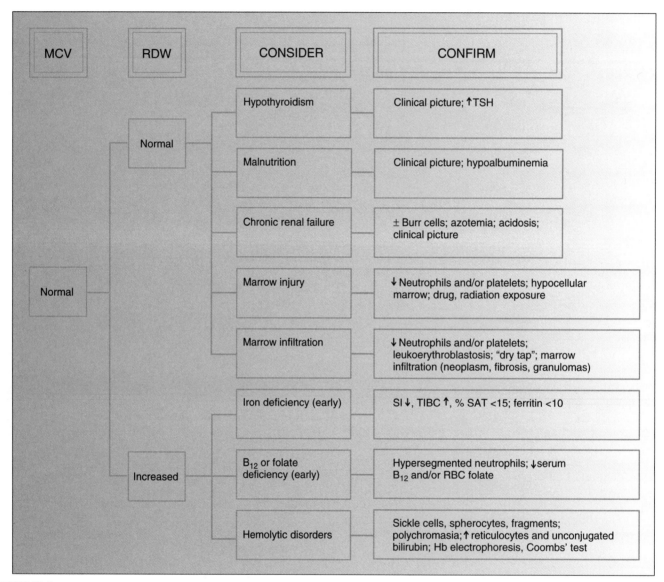

FIGURE 83–2. *Algorithm for diagnosis of normocytic anemia. SAT, saturation; SI, serum iron; TIBC, total iron-binding capacity; TSH, thyroid-stimulating hormone.*

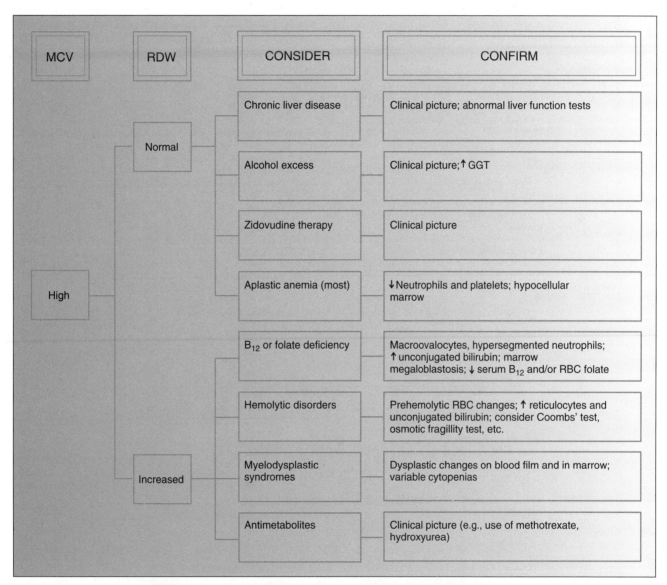

FIGURE 83–3. *Algorithm for diagnosis of macrocytic anemia. GGT, γ-glutamyltransferase.*

TABLE 83–3. Etiology, Management, and Prognosis of Common Anemias

Etiology	Management*	Prognosis for the Anemia
Chronic renal failure	Erythropoietin, transfusion, renal transplant	Good
Hypothyroidism	Thyroxine	Excellent
Aplastic anemia	Discontinuation of potential exposures; marrow transplant (young people), antilymphocyte globulin (older people)	About 50% mortality with therapy for aplastic anemia
Iron deficiency	Iron salts	Good; overall outcome depends on cause
Thalassemia minor	None necessary	Excellent
Thalassemia major	Transfusion, marrow transplant	Poor
Megaloblastic anemia	Vitamin B_{12} or folic acid	Excellent
Hereditary spherocytosis	Splenectomy	Excellent
Sickle cell disorders	Supportive; transfusions	Significant morbidity, some early mortality for sickle cell disease
Immune hemolysis	Discontinuation of drug; corticosteroids; splenectomy	Good; overall outcome depends on underlying disease
Fragmentation hemolysis	Treatment of underlying disease/mechanism; transfusion	Guarded to poor

*Transfusion may be appropriate in some additional situations.

Case Resolution

Additional questioning revealed that the patient had taken 6 to 10 aspirins daily for pain and had occasionally experienced mild epigastric distress. Her MCV was at the lower limit of normal and her RDW was elevated, suggesting iron deficiency rather than anemia of chronic disease as the cause. Iron deficiency was confirmed by the following studies: serum iron (SI) decreased; total iron-binding capacity (TIBC) increased; percent saturation decreased; serum ferritin decreased. Repeat stool guaiac tests were positive, and an upper GI x-ray study revealed the presence of a gastric ulcer. Treatment included stopping NSAID use and administering an H_2 blocker and oral iron. The anemia was corrected, and the ulcer healed.

Selected Readings

Bessman, J. D. *Automated Blood Counts and Differentials.* Baltimore and London, Johns Hopkins University Press, 1986.

Hillman, R. S., and K. A. Ault. *Hematology in Clinical Practice: A Guide to Diagnosis and Management.* New York, McGraw-Hill, Inc., 1995.

Hillman, R. S., and C. A. Finch. *Red Cell Manual,* 6th ed. Philadelphia, F.A. Davis Company, 1992.

CHAPTER 84

BLEEDING DISORDERS

William R. Hardy, M.D.

H$_x$ A 24-year-old female flight attendant is seen in the emergency room with a 1-week history of recurrent epistaxis. She had also noted "decreased energy" for 4 to 6 weeks and "very heavy" menstrual flow for 8 to 12 months. She was taking an oral contraceptive preparation and took occasional aspirin for headaches. Vital signs were normal. Physical examination was normal except for conjunctival pallor and clotted blood in both nostrils. Laboratory studies revealed the following: hematocrit 29%, hemoglobin 8.9 g/dL, mean corpuscular volume (MCV) 87 fL, red cell distribution width (RDW) 19.1%, WBC 10,400/µL (with a normal differential), and platelets 7800/µL. Urinalysis revealed 2+ protein and 30–40 RBC/hpf.

Questions

1. Do the history and physical examination suggest a bleeding disorder? If so, do they suggest the most likely type?
2. What additional laboratory information would be helpful?

Hemostasis is the term for body processes that prevent or arrest bleeding. Bleeding usually results from injury or diseases that disrupt blood vessels but also may result from faulty hemostasis alone or in combination with disease or injury. When bleeding appears to be

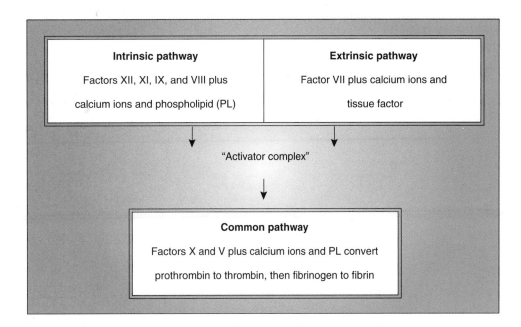

FIGURE 84–1. *Coagulation pathways.*

spontaneous or excessive (in amount or duration) or when it occurs from multiple sites, the integrity of the hemostatic mechanism should be questioned. Identification (or exclusion) of a hemostatic defect is essential for appropriate management and to minimize the risk of excess morbidity or mortality.

PATHOPHYSIOLOGY

Disruption of a vessel wall results in endothelial cell (EC) injury or loss. Local vasoconstriction and activation of platelets result. The latter respond by adhering to the wound and by sticking to one another (aggregation) to form a temporary "platelet plug" to arrest the bleeding. The injured vessel wall and activated platelets join forces to initiate coagulation (clotting). The coagulation system consists of some 12 plasma proteins that interact (proenzyme-to-enzyme cascade) to convert fibrinogen (a sol) to fibrin (a gel). Fibrin deposition in the platelet plug converts it to a longer lasting hemostatic plug. Vessel patency may be restored subsequently by dissolution of the fibrin by the plasminogen or fibrinolytic system.

Vascular disorders associated with abnormal bleeding (e.g., anaphylactoid purpura, various vasculitides) are distinctive clinically (palpable purpura) and are not discussed further.

Platelets are derived from bone marrow megakaryocytes and survive about 10 days in the absence of increased hemostatic needs (e.g., surgery, trauma). The normal platelet count ($150–350 \times 10^3/\mu L$) underestimates the total circulating number, since about one third are slowly perking through the spleen and are not counted. Platelet functions include adhesion to injured endothelial cell or subendothelium and aggregation. Both processes require specific membrane receptors plus bridging plasma proteins (von Willebrand factor [vWf] and fibrinogen). Activated platelets also produce and release proaggregatory substances (thromboxane

A_2, adenosine diphosphate) and provide membrane phospholipid (PL) for coagulation. Platelet evaluation is based on (1) counts, (2) bleeding time (BT; time required for cessation of bleeding from a standardized superficial skin incision), and (3) in vitro studies of aggregation. Platelet-related bleeding disorders may be quantitative (thrombocytopenia), qualitative (thrombocytopathia), or both.

The coagulation cascade is more easily understood if viewed as consisting of three separate, but linked, pathways: intrinsic, extrinsic, and common (Fig. 84–1).

Fibrin formation is the end point of the two main clotting tests used clinically—prothrombin time (PT) and partial thromboplastin time (PTT)—to evaluate coagulation. The PT is the interval to fibrin formation after tissue factor (TF) and calcium are added to citrated plasma (normal, 11–13 seconds), thus reflecting activity/concentration of VII, X, V, prothrombin, and fibrinogen (extrinsic and common pathways). The PTT is the interval to fibrin formation after phospholipid (PL) and calcium are added to citrated plasma (normal, 25–35 seconds); it indicates activity/concentration of XII, XI, IX, VIII, X, V, prothrombin, and fibrinogen (intrinsic and common pathways). Because the interval to clotting is shorter, the PT is more sensitive than the PTT to common pathway abnormalities. All clotting factors, except for a portion of the factor VIII molecule (the von Willebrand factor, which is of endothelial cell origin), are made in the liver. Four clotting factors (prothrombin, VII, IX, and X) are dependent on vitamin K for their activity.

Abnormal bleeding may be due to lesions involving the platelets, the coagulation mechanism, or a combination of the two (Tables 84–1, 84–2, and 84–3).

DIFFERENTIAL DIAGNOSIS

The differential diagnosis of the more common bleeding disorders is listed in Table 84–4.

TABLE 84–1.   Platelet Disorders

Mechanism	Associated Hematologic Features	Common Clinical Settings
Thrombocytopenias		
Decreased production	↓Megakaryocytes; ±↓RBC/WBC precursors; ±marrow infiltration or hypoplasia.	Aplastic anemia, chemotherapy leukemia, alcoholism
Splenic pooling	Normal megakaryocytes; evidence of myeloproliferative disorder.	Marked splenomegaly (e.g., portal hypertension, chronic granulocytic leukemia)
Increased consumption	RBC fragmentation and platelet consumption from endothelial abnormalities. Normal or ↑ megakaryocytes.	Microangiopathic hemolytic disorders
Accelerated immune destruction	Antiplatelet antibodies (or antigen-antibody complexes) lead to rapid destruction. Normal or ↑megakaryocytes.	Autoimmune thrombocytopenic purpura (ATP) (idiopathic, drug-related), human immunodeficiency virus infection (HIV), systemic lupus erythematosus (SLE).
Thrombocytopathias		
Decreased adhesion, aggregation, or release on activation	Platelets not reduced; BT* usually increased; in vitro aggregation studies may be abnormal.	Uremia, severe liver disease, myeloproliferative disorders, drugs (especially aspirin)

*BT, bleeding time.

EVALUATION

Clinical bleeding due to disordered hemostasis correlates reasonably well with the severity of the abnormality as seen in laboratory tests. For example, petechiae are not seen in isolated thrombocytopenia until the platelet count is < 20,000 μL and the severity of bleeding is clearly related to the VIII level in classic hemophilia. While history and physical findings may provide helpful clues to the etiology, laboratory studies

TABLE 84–2.   Coagulation Disorders

Mechanism	Associated Hematologic Features	Common Clinical Settings
Hereditary		
Decreased or abnormal gene product	(1) Decreased or defective VIII or IX (2) Decreased or defective vWf	(1) Hemophilia A or B (X-linked) (2) von Willebrand's disease (vWd) (autosomal)
Acquired		
Impaired hepatic synthesis	Mild—decreased prothrombin, VII, IX X Severe—also decreased fibrinogen, V	Any significant liver disease
Vitamin K deficiency	Decreased prothrombin, VII, IX, X	Decreased K availability, malabsorption

TABLE 84–3.   Mixed Platelet and Coagulation Disorders

Mechanism	Associated Hematologic Features	Common Clinical Settings
Increased hemostatic requirements and/or loss	Thrombocytopenia, variable decrease in clotting factors	Major trauma, surgery, hemorrhage with multiple transfusions
Systemic thrombin generation	Decreased platelets and clotting factors, increased fibrin degradation products (FDP)	Disseminated intravascular coagulation (DIC)
Decreased clotting factor synthesis and splenic pooling	Thrombocytopenia; variable decrease in clotting factors	Liver disease with portal hypertension

are always necessary for confirmation, beginning with platelet count, PT, and PTT (Table 84–4).

Clinical information is often helpful to predict or interpret laboratory data as well as to counsel and manage the patient. Most hereditary disorders result in decreased production of a single coagulation protein and are X-linked (i.e., expressed in males) (hemophilia A and B) or autosomal (i.e., expressed in both males and females) (von Willebrand's disease). The more severe the deficiency is, the earlier the age of clinical expression. Less severe inherited deficiencies may not be identified until a traumatic hemostatic challenge occurs after childhood. The platelet disorders are almost always acquired, as are the mixed platelet and coagulation disorders.

The nature of the clinical bleeding may be helpful in diagnosis. For example, in hemophilia the bleeding is usually deep (retroperitoneal, joint or muscle), spreading (hematoma, ecchymosis), and often delayed (hours after injury). Thrombocytopenic bleeding typically is into skin (petechiae, purpura) or mucosal surfaces (epistaxis, menorrhagia, hematuria), and begins immediately after injury.

MANAGEMENT AND PROGNOSIS

Individuals with a hemostatic disorder may not require therapy if their bleeding is not life threatening and the outlook for spontaneous recovery is good. The patient should avoid exposure to agents (e.g., aspirin) that may add to the bleeding diathesis. In most patients with a hemostatic disorder, the abnormal bleeding is secondary to an underlying disease (e.g., liver disease, systemic lupus erythematosus); in these patients, management and prognosis of the underlying problem are usually the critical determinants (Table 84–5). Platelet transfusions provide transient benefit when decreased production is the mechanism but little benefit in situations of ongoing increased destruction or increased splenic pooling. The same concept holds true for coagulation factor transfusion therapy. Nonetheless, in acute life-threatening situations (e.g., fulminant disseminated intravascular coagulation), transfusions of platelets, coagulation factors, or both may be appropriate.

TABLE 84–4. Diagnostic Approach to Bleeding

Platelets	PT	PTT	Consider	Confirmatory Data
N	N	N	Thrombocytopathy	↑BT*, abnormal aggregation
			Vascular purpura	?Skin biopsy
N	↑	N	Mild liver disease	Liver function tests
			Vitamin K deficiency	Response to treatment
N	N	↑	Hemophilia	Factor VIII, IX assays
			von Willebrand's disease	Factor VIII assay, ↑BT*, vWf assay
N	↑	↑	Severe liver disease	Liver function tests; ↓Fibrinogen
↓	N	N	↓Production	Marrow: ↓megakaryocytes, marrow infiltration/hypoplasia
			Splenic pooling	Marked splenomegaly
			↑Consumption	Fragmented RBCs on blood film
			Immune destruction	Normal/↑megakaryocytes; associated condition (e.g., SLE, HIV); response to therapy
↓	↑	↑	↑Hemostatic demand, loss, dilution	Clinical setting (major trauma, hemorrhage, multiple transfusions)
			Systemic thrombin generation (DIC)	↓Fibrinogen, ↑FDP†; clinical setting (e.g., sepsis, malignancy)
			Severe liver disease with portal hypertension	Liver function tests, splenomegaly

*BT, bleeding time.
†FDP, fibrin degradation products.

PATIENT AND FAMILY EDUCATION

Patients with bleeding disorders should be informed that substances which may compromise platelet function (e.g., aspirin) or number (e.g., alcohol in alcohol-induced thrombocytopenia) or which may inhibit hepatic synthesis of coagulation factors (e.g., alcohol) will increase the risk of bleeding.

TABLE 84–5. Management of Bleeding Disorders

Diagnosis	Management
Thrombocytopathy	(1) Uremia: dialysis, erythropoietin, DDAVP.* (2) Drug-induced: stop putative drug.
Vascular purpura	Give corticosteroids, immunosuppressants.
Liver disease	Treat underlying disease, ?FFP.†
Hemophilia	Give FFP,† VIII/IX concentrates, recombinant VIII.
von Willebrand's disease	Give FFP,† VIII concentrate, DDAVP (some).
↓Platelet production	Treat underlying disease, platelet transfusions.
↑Platelet pooling	Treat underlying disease, ?splenectomy.
↑Platelet consumption (fragmentation)	Treat underlying disease (e.g., treat TTP‡ with plasmapheresis, replace defective prosthetic valve).
↑Platelet destruction (e.g., autoimmune thrombocytopenic purpura [ATP])	Seek underlying disease (e.g., SLE) or drug (e.g., quinine). Treat with corticosteroids, splenectomy, immunosuppressants, intravenous immunoglobulin.
Hemostatic demand; dilution	Manage trauma, hemorrhage; give fresh whole blood, FFP,† platelets to correct deficits.
Systemic thrombin generation (DIC)	Identify and treat primary process; give FFP†/platelet transfusions to correct hemostatic deficits.

*Desmopressin (induces release of vWf from endothelial cells).
†Fresh-frozen plasma (contains all coagulation factors).
‡Thrombotic thrombocytopenic purpura.

Research Questions

1. Can clinically useful tests be developed to allow rapid identification of specific clotting factor deficiencies and to determine whether the deficiency is due to decreased production, increased consumption, or both?
2. Will thrombopoietin be of value in treating thrombocytopenia due to decreased platelet production?

Case Resolution

The history suggested excessive bleeding from two mucosal sites (nasal and endometrial), raising the question of a systemic disorder, probably involving platelets. The initial blood count identified a severe thrombocytopenia plus anemia (with RBC indices suggestive of iron deficiency). Additional studies revealed a normal PT and PTT, no fragmented RBCs on the blood smear, and increased marrow megakaryocytes. The physician made a presumptive diagnosis of autoimmune thrombocytopenic purpura (ATP). The patient was treated with corticosteroids, and improvement occurred within 2 weeks.

Selected Readings

Hathaway, W. E., and S. H. Goodnight, Jr. *Disorders of Hemostasis and Thrombosis.* New York, McGraw-Hill, Inc., 1993.
Hillman, R. S., and K. A. Ault. *Hematology in Clinical Practice: A Guide to Diagnosis and Management.* New York, McGraw-Hill, Inc., 1995.
Rapaport, S. I. *Introduction to Hematology,* 2nd ed. Philadelphia, J.B. Lippincott Company, 1987.

CHAPTER 85

LYMPHADENOPATHY AND SPLENOMEGALY

John H. Saiki, M.D.

H$_x$ A 22-year-old female presented to the student health service with left supraclavicular lymphadenopathy. The lymphadenopathy was first noted 2 months previously. She became concerned because of continued enlargement. No other symptoms were noticed. Physical examination revealed a healthy young woman with an obvious fullness in the left supraclavicular fossa. A 4-cm nodal mass was palpable. Other lymphadenopathy was not noted. Her spleen tip was palpable just below the left costal margin.

Questions

1. What are the diagnostic possibilities?
2. Which physical finding serves as the best handle on the diagnosis—lymphadenopathy or splenomegaly?
3. What are the causes of lymphadenopathy, and what simple laboratory tests would you order for this patient?
4. Would you biopsy the node? When? What are the indications for a lymph node biopsy?
5. If a diagnosis of lymphoma is made, what additional information would be important to obtain?

Lymphadenopathy is an abnormal increase in size, change in consistency, or increase in number of palpable lymph nodes. It is the principal manifestation of malignant lymphoma but can be a secondary manifestation of other disease.

Splenomegaly is the presence of an enlarged spleen, identified by feeling the spleen on physical examination or seeing the enlargement on radiologic imaging studies. Its clinical significance is that it serves as a diagnostic clue, and its involvement influences the clinical staging of the malignant lymphomas. Splenomegaly can cause thrombocytopenia (50,000–150,000 platelets/mm^3) owing to increased splenic pooling of peripheral blood platelets. It can cause neutropenia, as in Felty's syndrome (rheumatoid arthritis), or pancytopenia (hypersplenism). Enlargement of the spleen leaves it unprotected by the rib cage and more vulnerable to trauma. Isolated splenomegaly is an uncommon finding. Most frequently it is identified in association with other primary disease, e.g., chronic hemolytic anemia, chronic liver disease, or an advanced lymphoma. Its presence always requires explanation.

PATHOPHYSIOLOGY

Lymphadenopathy

Normal lymph nodes are bean shaped, measuring 1–1.5 cm in diameter, nontender, and soft. Normally just a few nodes are palpable in the cervical regions. There are a few more in the axillae. There is a normal prominence of lymph nodes in the groin.

Lymph nodes may enlarge from reactive hyperplasia secondary to inflammation or from infiltration by granulomatous or neoplastic tissue. Hyperplasia occurs with infection and other inflammatory disorders such as rheumatoid arthritis. Infiltrative disorders can be benign (e.g., sarcoidosis) or malignant (e.g., primary lymphoma or metastatic carcinoma).

Splenomegaly

The spleen can enlarge from vascular congestion, hyperplasia, and infiltrative diseases. Obstruction of the portal vein can result in congestion and enlargement of the spleen. The obstruction to flow is frequently secondary to primary liver disease or to chronic passive congestion due to heart failure. Hyperplasia, or "work hypertrophy," of the spleen occurs with the chronic hemolytic anemias. Reactive hyperplasia also occurs with collagen-vascular disease and infectious diseases. Finally, infiltration of the spleen by benign or malignant tissue is an important cause of splenomegaly.

DIFFERENTIAL DIAGNOSIS

Lymphadenopathy

An elderly person with lymphadenopathy is likely to have a malignant lymphoma. A young adult is likely to have infectious mononucleosis. An asymptomatic patient is more likely to have malignant lymphoma, whereas a symptomatic patient is more likely to have reactive disease (Table 85–1).

The rate of growth or of change in a lymph node is helpful in differentiating benign from malignant disease. Infectious processes generally result in rapid change of size (days to a few weeks). Lymphomas, on the other hand, usually take several weeks or months. Lymph nodes associated with infection are frequently tender, whereas in malignant lymphoma, the nodes are not tender.

The consistency of a normal lymph node is soft. In low-grade lymphomas and chronic lymphocytic leukemia, they also are soft. In large cell lymphomas and Hodgkin's disease, lymph nodes are significantly firmer and rubbery in consistency. In metastatic carcinoma, they frequently are very firm and sometimes stone-hard.

The pattern of lymphadenopathy (whether localized or generalized) may be helpful. Acute bacterial infections often are associated with localized lymphadenop-

---

TABLE 85-1. Causes of Lymphadenopathy

Reactive Hyperplasia

Infectious
  Bacterial
    Pyogenic infections, tuberculosis
  Viral
    Infectious mononucleosis, cytomegalovirus
  Fungal
    Coccidioidomycosis
  Parasitic
    Toxoplasmosis
Noninfectious
    Connective tissue disease, dermatopathic, drug-induced (e.g., phenytoin)

Infiltration

Benign
    Sarcoidosis
Malignant
    Primary lymphoma (i.e., Hodgkin's and non-Hodgkin's lymphomas), chronic
      lymphocytic leukemia

---

athy in the area of infection. Viral infections and toxoplasmosis frequently have a generalized pattern. Posterior cervical triangle lymphadenopathy is said to be characteristic of infectious mononucleosis. Large-cell lymphomas and Hodgkin's disease frequently have a regional pattern, but the low-grade lymphomas and chronic lymphocytic leukemia are associated with a generalized pattern. Hodgkin's disease is commonly associated with a mediastinal mass. Non-Hodgkin's lymphomas generally are not associated with a mediastinal mass with the exception of the young adult patient with primary B-cell lymphoma with sclerosis.

Systemic symptoms characteristic of lymphoma occur in advanced disease. They include fever, drenching sweats, excoriating pruritus, and significant weight loss (10% of body weight). Characteristically patients presenting with lymphoma are asymptomatic. The presence of fever and tender lymphadenopathy favors infection.

Certain normal and abnormal anatomic structures can be mistaken for enlarged lymph nodes; e.g., the lateral spinous processes of the cervical vertebrae, the lateral ends of the hyoid bone, and tortuous carotid arteries. A fullness in the absence of a discrete mass in the supraclavicular region must not be mistaken for an enlarged lymph node, since a blind biopsy could injure the brachial plexus. A prominence in the supraclavicular region is most commonly related to either a fat pad or distortion of the rib cage due to scoliosis.

Splenomegaly

A palpable spleen is abnormal, though a small percentage (3%) of young adults may have a palpable spleen tip in the absence of underlying disease. The following aphorism is important: "If you think you feel the spleen, it means that you didn't feel it . . . for when you feel the spleen, you don't 'think,' you 'know.'" The finding of a palpable spleen must be confirmed by imaging studies, since other masses, such as an enlarged polycystic kidney, can masquerade as a palpable

spleen. Identification of the cause of splenomegaly is made on the basis of "the company it keeps," since biopsies of the spleen are rarely done and splenectomy should be avoided. Splenomegaly is often a secondary finding, identified during the course of the underlying disease, such as cirrhosis of the liver, rheumatoid arthritis, or a chronic hemolytic anemia. However, when isolated splenomegaly is the only clinical manifestation, a systematic evaluation of the various causes is necessary (Table 85-2).

In the young adult, both infectious mononucleosis and Hodgkin's disease must be considered. A middle-aged person is more likely to have primary liver disease, a lymphoproliferative disorder (malignant lymphoma or Hodgkin's disease), or a myeloproliferative disorder (chronic granulocytic leukemia). The elderly person is most likely to have a lymphoproliferative disorder (lymphoma or chronic lymphocytic leukemia) or a myeloproliferative disorder (myelofibrosis with myeloid metaplasia).

Massive splenomegaly is associated with hairy cell leukemia, myelofibrosis with myeloid metaplasia, late-stage polycythemia vera, and late-stage chronic granulocytic leukemia.

Chronic splenomegaly (since childhood) suggests a congenital disorder; e.g., a hereditary hemolytic disorder such as sickle cell anemia, hereditary spherocytosis, thalassemia, or a storage disease such as Gaucher's disease.

The peripheral blood smear will help identify a primary hematologic disorder (e.g., chronic hemolytic anemias).

Hepatomegaly, portal hypertension, abnormal liver function tests, a history of alcoholism, or positive serologic tests for hepatitis suggest primary liver disease as the cause of splenomegaly.

TABLE 85-2. Causes of Splenomegaly

Congestion

Congestive heart failure, portal hypertension

Reactive Hyperplasia

Chronic hemolytic anemias
    Hereditary (e.g., hereditary spherocytosis and sickle cell anemia), acquired
      (e.g., autoimmune hemolytic anemia)
Infections
  Bacterial
    Subacute bacterial endocarditis, tuberculosis, brucellosis
  Viral
    Infectious mononucleosis, cytomegalovirus
  Fungal
  Parasitic
    Toxoplasmosis, malaria
Connective tissue diseases
    Rheumatoid arthritis, systemic lupus erythematosus
Serum sickness

Infiltrative Diseases

Nonneoplastic
    Lipidosis (Gaucher's disease), sarcoidosis, amyloidosis
Neoplastic
    Leukemia (acute and chronic), Hodgkin's disease, non-Hodgkin's lymphomas,
      polycythemia vera, myelofibrosis with myeloid metaplasia, metastatic tumor
      (rare)

EVALUATION

History

Where is the lymphadenopathy located? Is it localized or generalized? Has it developed over days, weeks, or months? Is it stable, or has there been steady progression? How old is the patient? How is the patient's general health? Has the patient had an upper respiratory tract infection? Has there been fever, drenching sweats, itching, or weight loss? Has the patient had lymphadenopathy before? Is the patient taking any medications, particularly drugs such as phenytoin? Does the patient have pets?

The above questions apply to splenomegaly as well. However, in addition it is important to elicit information related to hepatitis or alcoholic liver disease. Does the patient have a history of rheumatoid arthritis or a familial anemia?

Physical Examination

What is the size of the adenopathy? What is the consistency of the nodes? How many nodes are there? What is their location? Is the pattern localized or generalized? Is there evidence of infection; e.g., fever, inflammation of the oropharynx, or cutaneous inflammatory lesions? Is there splenomegaly? Is there evidence of petechiae or bruising? Is there gingival hypertrophy? Are there physical manifestations of other disease such as chronic liver disease or rheumatoid arthritis?

Additional Evaluation

CBC, platelets, and peripheral blood smear evaluation are helpful in identifying evidence of a reactive problem, i.e., activated lymphocytes, as seen in infectious mononucleosis, toxoplasmosis, and phenytoin-induced lymphadenopathy or splenomegaly. The morphology of the red cells and the presence of increased polychromasia can identify a hemolytic anemia.

A chemistry profile will identify liver function abnormalities. A mononucleosis test (e.g., Monospot) and *Toxoplasma* titer are simple screening tests for not uncommon causes of lymphadenopathy and splenomegaly. If the patient has splenomegaly without lymphadenopathy, a reticulocyte count, Coombs' test, and hepatitis profile should be obtained.

A chest x-ray is helpful in identifying evidence of parenchymal infiltrates or a mediastinal mass.

Biopsy of the largest node should be done if the lymphadenopathy is grossly abnormal and the above studies are negative. Histopathology, special stains, immunologic marker studies, and tissue cultures are important. If lymphadenopathy is not accessible for biopsy, a bone marrow aspirate and core biopsy should be done. If these studies do not yield a diagnosis, a CT scan of the chest, abdomen, and pelvis should be done. If significant lymphadenopathy is identified, an exploratory laparotomy with multiple biopsies should be performed.

Primary lymphoma of the spleen is exceedingly rare. Biopsy of the spleen is virtually never done. Splenectomy for diagnosis should be avoided, unless all clinical studies are negative and the spleen continues to enlarge.

MANAGEMENT

Treatment of secondary lymphadenopathy or splenomegaly is directed at the primary disease.

When a diagnosis of **Hodgkin's disease** is made, the next step is to determine the extent of the lymphoma, since treatment specifically relates to the clinical and pathologic stage (Table 85–3). Specific laboratory studies include CBC and platelet count, complete chemistry profile, bone marrow aspirate and core biopsy, and CT scans of the chest, abdomen, and pelvis. Some centers do routine lymphangiograms. Exploratory laparotomies, which have been routine in the past, are now being questioned. Clearly, if a laparotomy would not influence the type of treatment, it should not be performed. The treatment of clinical stage I and II Hodgkin's disease is extended-field radiotherapy. If the patient has a large mediastinal mass (greater than one-third the transverse diameter of the thorax), combined chemotherapy and radiotherapy must be given. Stage III-A disease could be managed with radiotherapy alone. Stage III-B disease should be managed with combined chemotherapy and radiotherapy to areas of bulky disease. Stage IV disease is managed with chemotherapy. Standard chemotherapy is MOPP (mechlorethamine, vincristine [Oncovin], procarbazine, and prednisone). Because of the associated risk of sterility and leukemia, alternative approaches are being used: ABVD (doxorubicin [Adriamycin], bleomycin, vinblastine, dacarbazine), MOPP/ABV hybrid, and MOPP alternating with ABVD. The MOPP/ABV hybrid may be the most effective regimen. Studies of these regimens are ongoing.

Low-grade non-Hodgkin's lymphomas are benign in behavior, almost always advanced, and incurable. More than 80% of patients have bone marrow involvement at

---

TABLE 85–3.   Staging of Hodgkin's Disease

Stage	Criteria
I	Single lymph node region (I) or a single parenchymal lesion (I-E)
II	Two or more lymph node regions (II) or localized parenchymal disease with one or more node regions on the same side of the diaphragm (II-E)
III	Lymph node involvement above and below the diaphragm (III)
	Above plus splenic involvement (III-S)
	Above plus localized parenchymal involvement (III-E) and when spleen is involved (III-SE)
IV	Disseminated foci of one or more parenchymal organs with or without lymph node disease. A single lesion in liver or bone marrow is defined as IV.
Subclassification	
A	Asymptomatic
B	Symptomatic*

*Symptoms are fever, sweats, weight loss > 10% of body weight.

the time of initial diagnosis. In most patients, a watchful-waiting attitude is the best approach, since chemotherapy has not been shown to influence the prognosis. Chlorambucil is used, but only when the patient is symptomatic with bulky adenopathy.

The large-cell lymphomas are more localized and more aggressive but are potentially curable with intensive chemotherapy using the CHOP (cyclophosphamide, doxorubicin [Hydroxydaunorubicin], vincristine [Oncovin], prednisone) regimen. The addition of radiotherapy to bulky disease may also be important and is under study.

Chronic lymphocytic leukemia is a benign disease and in some cases never requires treatment and never progresses. Indications for treatment are systemic manifestations of weakness or weight loss, hematologic suppression of hemoglobin or platelets, or the presence of bulky, uncomfortable lymphadenopathy. Standard treatment is chlorambucil; newer agents with significant activity are fludarabine and chlorodeoxyadenosine.

PATIENT AND FAMILY EDUCATION

A patient who presents with a lump in the neck is concerned that "something very serious is going on." It is important to be frank at all times regarding the potential seriousness but also to assure the patient that there are many possible causes, including various infections. Not infrequently, preliminary tests for an infectious agent are negative, but over a couple of weeks they become positive. During this waiting period, the patient must be informed to return immediately if a clear progression of the adenopathy is noticed. The patient should be told that if the enlarged node cannot be explained by blood tests and if it significantly progresses in size, a biopsy will have to be performed. When all studies, including biopsy, are negative, the patient should be informed that if recurrent or increasing adenopathy develops, biopsy will have to be repeated. In some patients, nonspecific granulomatous change may be a precursor of malignant lymphoma, especially Hodgkin's disease. Therefore, in any patient who has recurrent adenopathy, another biopsy must be done.

When a diagnosis of malignancy is made, the nature of the disease, its investigation, its treatment, and its prognosis must be discussed in detail. The potential complications of treatment must be addressed. If the disease is a low-grade lymphoma or chronic lymphocytic leukemia and observation is the management of choice, time needs to be spent helping the patient understand that he or she has cancer and that the wisest approach is avoidance of chemotherapy, which might be difficult for the patient to comprehend. When the disease has a potential for cure (e.g., Hodgkin's disease and the diffuse large-cell lymphomas), the patient should be informed that certainty of cure will be known only with time. As each day, month, and year passes, the chance for relapse becomes less and less, but the possibility of relapse probably always exists.

An intimate discussion of the social and emotional problems associated with having cancer is crucial to the well-being of the patient and family. This discussion might first take place with the patient and spouse or another close family member, but a second discussion should include all family members. Open, frank communication between patient and spouse is the most important remedy in living with cancer. This means sharing not only each other's concerns, but also each other's emotions or feelings. Living one day at a time was a philosophy of life for Sir William Osler, and it is essential in the setting of malignant disease, perhaps even in good health as well.

PROGNOSIS

The prognosis depends on the underlying disease. Cure rates in Hodgkin's disease are fairly high and should be expected in clinical stage I (90%) and II (80%–90%) disease. Stage III disease also has the potential for cure, but on the order of 60% to 70%—lower in patients with "B" symptoms (see Table 85–3) and higher in patients without symptoms. Cure rates for stage IV disease are low (40%–65%). The histologic type influences the prognosis, being best with lymphocyte-predominant and nodular sclerosing Hodgkin's disease, less good with mixed cellularity, and worst with lymphocyte-depleted Hodgkin's disease. Low-grade non-Hodgkin's lymphomas and chronic lymphocytic leukemia are incurable but may have an excellent prognosis even without treatment. The aggressive large-cell lymphomas have a high potential (> 90%) for cure in early-stage disease with a less favorable cure rate (approximately 60%) in advanced stages.

Research Questions

1. What is the etiology of Hodgkin's disease?
2. How can chemotherapy-induced sterility and cardiotoxicity be prevented?
3. A current theory of the molecular mechanism of the low-grade lymphomas is inhibition of apoptosis (natural cell death). What genetic approaches to therapy might be considered?

Case Resolution

The patient was found to have clinical stage II-A Hodgkin's disease with a small mediastinal mass. She was treated with extended-field radiation therapy and is in complete remission.

Selected Reading

Saiki, J. H. White blood cell abnormalities: Erythrocytosis (polycythemia); splenomegaly; lymphadenopathy. *In* H. H. Friedman (ed.). *Problem-Oriented Medical Diagnosis,* 5th ed. Boston, Little, Brown & Co., 1991.

CHAPTER 86

APPROACH TO THE CANCER PATIENT IN THE PRIMARY CARE SETTING

Walter B. Forman, M.D.

Hx A 75-year-old male retired geologist visited his primary care physician 3 years ago because of rectal bleeding. His physical examination was unremarkable except for the presence of guaiac-positive stool. Colonoscopy demonstrated a 3-cm mass in the splenic flexure, and a biopsy of the mass revealed a poorly differentiated adenocarcinoma. After discussing the various options, the patient elected to have a laparotomy, and an oncologic surgeon performed a partial colectomy. The pathologist reported that 10 of the 16 lymph nodes biopsied were positive for adenocarcinoma. After discussing this issue with both his primary care physician and a consulting medical oncologist, the patient began a 1-year course of adjuvant chemotherapy. During this period, he was hospitalized twice for complications related to his chemotherapy, once for severe diarrhea and once for painful oral ulcerations. He felt well during the next 3 years, fully enjoying his retirement. One week prior to the current visit, however, he noticed that his urine had become dark and his stools light in color. Further evaluation reveals that he has recurrent colorectal carcinoma with hepatic metastases. Resection is not feasible, and the patient refuses other antineoplastic treatment. He asks to be kept comfortable, and a living will and durable power of attorney for health care are executed.

Questions

1. What is the role of the primary care physician in the diagnosis of cancer in symptomatic patients?
2. What is the role of the primary care physician in recognizing and managing complications, i.e., either of the disease or its treatment?
3. What is the role of the primary care physician in the long-term follow-up care of cancer patients?
4. What is the role of the primary care physician in treating the terminally ill?

the patient and family; (6) providing follow-up care; (7) recognizing—and sometimes managing—complications, either during or following treatment; and (8) providing palliative and terminal care to those who require it. Prevention of cancer is discussed in Chapter 15 and detecting occult cancer in asymptomatic patients in Chapter 11. This chapter focuses on the remaining six issues.

DETECTING CANCER IN PATIENTS WITH SUSPICIOUS SYMPTOMS

The primary care physician must be aware of how common malignancies present, especially in the early stages (Table 86–1). Without such knowledge, a delay in diagnosis might occur, thus denying the patient the opportunity for cure. When the diagnosis of cancer is suspected, the practitioner needs to order the appropriate test or procedure to establish (or rule out) the diagnosis with certainty. Physicians thus need to understand the sensitivity and specificity of the test in question (see Chapter 3); in addition, they must be cognizant of any adverse effects of the test or procedure. Lastly, the aggressiveness of the evaluation will depend, at least in part, on the physician's sense of the patient's overall health status. For example, an elderly nursing home patient with advanced Alzheimer's disease might not be a suitable candidate for colonoscopy if he or she exhibits relatively mild rectal bleeding. Ideally, however, such medical decisions should be made jointly, after a full and open discussion with the patient (if possible) or the patient's family or health care surrogate.

Although most patients with cancer are treated by specialists (e.g., medical oncologists, radiation oncologists, or surgical oncologists), primary care physicians offer a variety of cancer-related services to their patients, including (1) providing information and advice on how the risk of developing specific types of cancer can be decreased; (2) detecting occult cancer in asymptomatic patients; (3) detecting cancer in patients with suspicious symptoms; (4) discussing the diagnosis and arranging for appropriate specialty care; (5) providing emotional and (if needed) social service support to

TABLE 86–1. Some Common Presenting Symptoms in Cancer Patients

Symptom	Cancer
Enlarging or changing "mole"	Melanoma
Persistent hoarseness	Laryngeal cancer
Persistent cough or change in chronic cough	Lung cancer
Early satiety, weight loss	Any cancer, particularly pancreatic or gastric
Rectal bleeding or change in bowel habits	Colorectal cancer
Irregular vaginal bleeding	Endometrial cancer

DISCUSSING THE DIAGNOSIS AND ARRANGING FOR APPROPRIATE SPECIALTY CARE

Informing a patient of the diagnosis of cancer can be a daunting challenge for even the most experienced physician. For many people, the mere mention of the word "cancer" is so frightening that much information from the first discussion will not be understood or remembered. One approach is to make a special appointment to convey the news. A family member or other advocate should accompany the patient to assist in remembering important details of the conversation.

To communicate effectively with the cancer patient, what does the primary care physician need to know? At the very least, the physician needs to know something about the cancer itself, including its type, grade, invasiveness, metastatic potential, and prognosis. Ideally, the primary care physician will also have an understanding of the therapeutic options available, including the pros and cons of each treatment approach. It is important that the physician maintain an up-to-date knowledge base related to this ever-changing area. Computer programs (e.g., GRATEFUL MED or PDQ) are invaluable for accessing the latest information regarding treatment.

Why is it important for the primary care physician to keep well informed? First, a clear discussion with the patient and family may spare them from engaging in a fruitless, expensive search for the "latest cure." Second, a full discussion with the patient and family will assist them in making a wise decision regarding the initial treatment of the cancer. This is especially important because the initial "therapeutic window" might be the only opportunity for cure. Third, keeping well informed will enable the primary care physician to knowledgeably explain the risks and benefits of each treatment option.

Maintaining excellent communication with the oncologic specialist is also critical. Initially, this can be accomplished by an introductory phone call or letter in which the details of the patient's situation are presented. It is essential that all key information be forwarded to the oncologist, including x-rays, CT scans, biopsy reports, and the actual biopsy slides. In return, the oncologist should be expected to provide information back to the primary care physician; this should include a phone call and letter after the first consultation visit and periodic updates thereafter. By maintaining close communication with the oncologic specialist, the primary care physician can remain an active member of the therapeutic team and can knowledgeably respond to the patient's (and family's) concerns and questions.

PROVIDING EMOTIONAL AND OTHER SUPPORT TO THE PATIENT AND FAMILY

Another important reason for maintaining an active role in the cancer patient's care is to provide ongoing emotional support to the patient and family. Although the oncologic specialist will nearly always participate in this task, the primary care physician, almost by definition, is the health care provider who knows the patient

TABLE 86–2. Recommended Follow-up for Successfully Treated Common Cancers*

Cancer Site	Recommended Follow-up
Prostate (early stage)	Prostatic specific antigen (PSA) (interval not certain)
Breast	Annual mammogram
Colon	Colonoscopy every 6 months for one year then annually
Lung	Unknown

*In addition to periodic follow-up visits including a focused physical examination.

and family the best. In the early phase of decision making and management, when the relationship with the oncologic specialist is just being established, the patient and family may need the primary care physician's emotional support as much as—or even more than—his or her knowledge and technical expertise. One aspect of providing psychosocial support is to discuss with the patient and family the benefits of drawing up a living will and a durable power of attorney (if these documents have not been drawn up previously). The existence of a living will and durable power of attorney assures patients that their wishes regarding care—especially terminal care—will be listened to and honored.

PROVIDING FOLLOW-UP CARE

Depending on a variety of factors (including the personal preference of the patient, the oncologic specialist, and the referring physician), some cancer patients may receive their ongoing follow-up care from their primary care physician. This is especially likely to occur after the initial course of treatment (either radiation, surgery, or chemotherapy) has been completed. A key element in providing follow-up care to cancer patients is knowing exactly what to look for and when. For example, breast cancer patients are at increased risk of developing a second cancer in the other breast and should therefore be advised to (1) perform a monthly breast self-examination, (2) have a yearly breast examination by a health care professional, and (3) undergo a yearly mammogram. Similarly, colon cancer patients need to have a periodic colonoscopy performed for surveillance purposes. Additional information about follow-up care for common cancers is provided in Table 86–2. Since this, too, is an ever-changing area, the primary care physician needs to keep abreast of the relevant literature. The American Cancer Society represents one excellent source of current information and can greatly assist primary care physicians in their efforts to keep up to date.

RECOGNIZING COMPLICATIONS

Although some cancer patients will be cured by the initial therapeutic intervention, others will develop complications related to the metastatic spread of the original cancer. Still other patients will develop complications related to their treatment. The primary care physician must therefore be able to diagnose a variety

TABLE 86–3. Common Complications Encountered in Cancer Patients

Fever
Infection
    Granulocytopenia-related
    Related to indwelling venous (or other) catheters
    Secondary to unrelated concurrent infection
Inflammation
    Related to treatment; e.g., drug-induced phlebitis
    Secondary to unrelated concurrent inflammatory process
Secondary to neoplasm itself
Metabolic Disorders
Hypercalcemia
Electrolyte abnormalities (e.g., hypokalemia, hyponatremia)
Hyperglycemia (e.g., pancreatic cancer)
Acute tumor necrosis syndrome
Vascular Complications
Superior vena cava syndrome
Superficial/deep thrombophlebitis
Compromise of Specific Organ Systems
Neurologic
    Brain metastases
    Spinal cord compression
    Neuropathy/myopathy
Pulmonary
    Pleural inflammation and/or effusion
    Pulmonary fibrosis
Cardiac
    Cardiomyopathy
    Pericardial effusion
    Endocarditis
Renal
    Renal failure
    Nephrotic syndrome
    Bladder dysfunction
Hepatobiliary
    Hepatic failure
    Biliary obstruction
    Pain secondary to hepatic metastases
Gastrointestinal
    Oral ulcerations
    Diarrhea and/or constipation
    Bowel obstruction
Orthopedic
    Bone pain
    Pathologic fracture

TABLE 86–4. Common Symptoms Seen in Terminally Ill Cancer Patients

Pain
Weight loss
Dyspnea
Weakness/fatigue
Dysphagia
Depression
Constipation
Anorexia

cancer cannot be cured using currently available treatment modalities. In these situations, symptom relief and the provision of terminal care become paramount. Because of rapidly expanding knowledge concerning care of the dying, a new field of palliative medicine has developed. The goals of palliative medicine are to (1) control pain and other end-of-life symptoms; (2) integrate medical, psychosocial, and spiritual care; and (3) attend to the bereavement experienced by the patient and the patient's family. The philosophy of palliative medicine is to neither hasten death nor prolong dying; the overriding goal is to provide the patient and the family the best quality of life possible for whatever time remains.

The relief of pain and other end-of-life symptoms can help shift the focus from suffering and despair to enjoyment of life. Principles of palliative care include (1) careful evaluation of the patient's symptoms, (2) a clear understanding of the pathophysiologic mechanisms involved, (3) a judicious approach to diagnostic testing (with the aim of avoiding "overtesting" and testing that will not affect management), and (4) establishment of a treatment plan that is simple and also subject to continual reevaluation.

Table 86–4 lists some common symptoms encountered when providing palliative and terminal care. Some symptoms (e.g., cough) can be controlled relatively easily, whereas others (e.g., weight loss) can be more problematic. It is useful to begin the evaluation of a symptom by asking whether it is secondary to the disease or related to the therapy. If it is related to the therapy, can the treatment be adjusted in some way or should it be discontinued?

The management of end-of-life symptoms often represents a significant challenge to the physician, but it is a challenge that can usually be met by skillfully combining the science of medicine with the art of medicine. A frequent problem is how best to deliver medication, especially in the home or hospice setting when the patient's oral intake is negligible or nonexistent. Table 86–5 lists the variety of routes by which medications can be administered in such situations.

of cancer-related complications as well as understand the principles of management.

Table 86–3 lists a number of common problems that can develop in cancer patients. A frequently encountered challenge in primary care is deciding whether a cancer patient's symptom (e.g., low back pain) is due to metastatic disease or to a benign process (e.g., a simple muscle strain). Similarly, a symptom such as fever might represent a complication of chemotherapy (e.g., sepsis related to granulocytopenia) or a straightforward viral syndrome. How can the primary care physician be certain of not "missing" an important cancer-related symptom? A prudent approach is to maintain a high index of suspicion; the physician should assume that the problem at hand might be cancer-related and then obtain sufficient information from the history, physical examination, and (if need be) ancillary testing to either rule in or rule out this possibility.

PROVIDING PALLIATIVE AND TERMINAL CARE

Approximately 55% of all patients presenting with

TABLE 86–5. Possible Routes of Drug Administration in the Terminally Ill Patient

Oral
Sublingual
Intravascular
Transcutaneous
Subcutaneous
Local deposition (e.g., intrathecal, intrapleural)

When caring for terminally ill patients, the physician usually needs to work in concert with a number of other professionals, including social workers, pharmacists, home care nurses, and the clergy. Although traditional medical education has not emphasized the notion of physician as "team player," such a team approach is mandatory if effective palliative and terminal care is to be delivered.

Research Questions

1. Can symptoms in the terminally ill be controlled and the patient still "suffer"?
2. What are the pharmacokinetics of subcutaneous versus intravenous opioids?

Case Resolution

Over the next several weeks, the patient began to experience increasing pain in the right upper abdomen secondary to hepatic metastases. He was started on oral morphine sulfate, which adequately controlled his discomfort. Over the subsequent few weeks, his condition progressively deteriorated, and he and his family informed the primary care physician of his strong preference not to be hospitalized and to die at home. Working with a hospice team, the physician arranged for a hospital bed for home use. As the patient's oral intake decreased, he was switched from oral morphine to a continuous subcutaneous infusion. The patient died a week later, with his family at his bedside. His son called to inform the physician of his father's death and to thank the physician for the care provided during the latter stages of his father's life.

Selected Readings

Cleland, C. Barriers to cancer pain management. Oncology 1:19–26, 1987.

Doyle, D., W. C. Hanks, and N. MacDonald (eds.). *Oxford Textbook of Palliative Medicine.* New York, Oxford University Press, 1993.

Harris, I. B., E. C. Rich, and T. W. Crowson. Attitudes of internal medicine residents and staff physicians toward various patient characteristics. J Med Educ 102:60–5, 1985.

Holleb, A. I., D. J. Fink, and G. P. Murphy (eds.). *American Cancer Society Textbook of Clinical Oncology.* Atlanta, American Cancer Society Publications, 1991.

Twycross, R. G., and S. A. Lack (eds.). *Therapeutics in Terminal Cancer.* New York, Churchill Livingstone, 1990.

COMMON MUSCULOSKELETAL PROBLEMS

C H A P T E R   8 7

APPROACH TO THE PATIENT WITH ARTHRITIS

Wilmer L. Sibbitt, Jr., M.D.

Hx A 22-year-old female college student complains of aches and pains that have persisted for 2 weeks. She states that 2 days previously her right knee became swollen and stiff. She complains of 1 hour of morning stiffness affecting her hands, feet, knees, ankles, and shoulders. The tenderness in her joints awakens her at night. Three days previously she had some shaking chills and fever. The patient is sexually active, and her sexual partner uses condoms. The physical examination demonstrates tenderness in multiple joints; in addition, tenderness is present in several extra-articular locations that is consistent with bursitis or tenosynovitis. The right knee is warm and swollen with a large effusion. Full range of motion is present in all other joints with no evidence of effusion, synovial thickening, or deformity.

Questions

1. Does the patient have myalgias, arthralgias, arthritis, bursitis, or tenosynovitis?
2. What other questions should you ask her?
3. Is further testing required? If so, which tests would you recommend?
4. What would be the proper empiric therapy?

PATHOPHYSIOLOGY

The inflammation of arthritis is mediated by the same cellular and humoral factors that cause and maintain inflammation in other tissues of the body. Examples of inflammatory mediators are prostaglandins, leukotrienes, interferon alpha, interleukin-1, and tumor necrosis factor. Implicated cellular elements include neutrophils, monocytes, macrophages, lymphocytes, plasma cells, and dendritic cells. The symptoms of arthritis are also related to mechanical changes in the joints and the presence of effusion. Mechanical changes include (1) erosion of cartilage and bone, (2) loss of joint stability, (3) contracture of muscle and tendon, and (4) joint deformity. Effusion within the joint, caused by increased synovial membrane permeability, may induce mechanical discomfort and restrict the range of motion.

DIFFERENTIAL DIAGNOSIS

The broadest etiologic classification of the diseases of joints comprises (1) noninflammatory, (2) inflammatory, and (3) miscellaneous diseases (Table 87–1). The most common forms of arthritis are osteoarthritis, rheumatoid arthritis, septic arthritis, and gout.

Arthritis is characterized by signs of inflammation—pain, swelling, decreased function, and redness or signs of locally increased blood flow—in one or more joints. Acute arthritis is arbitrarily defined as having been present for 6 weeks or less, while chronic arthritis has persisted for greater than 6 weeks. Monarticular arthritis refers to involvement of only one joint, pauciarticular (or oligoarticular) arthritis to involvement of two to four joints, and polyarticular arthritis to involvement of more than four joints. Patterns of joint involvement include symmetrical (both sides of the body), asymmetrical (one side of the body), small joint (joints of the hands and feet), large joint (ankle, knee, hip, shoulder, elbow, wrist), and axial skeleton (spine, including neck).

TABLE 87–1. Diseases of Joints

Noninflammatory	Inflammatory	Miscellaneous
Osteoarthritis	Tenosynovitis	Primary fibrositis
Osteonecrosis syndrome	Autoimmune disease	Restless leg syndrome
Amyloidosis	Reactive arthritis	Hysteria
Metabolic arthropathy	Crystal synovitis	
Neuroarthropathy	Polymyalgia rheumatica	
Tumors	Palindromic rheumatism	
Mechanical abnormalities	Viral arthritis	
Sympathetic dystrophies	Septic joint	
Periarthritis	Immune complex arthritis	
Tendinitis		
Blood dyscrasias		

TABLE 87–2.   Analysis of Synovial Fluid

Criteria	Normal	Noninflammatory (Group I)	Inflammatory (Group II)	Purulent (Group III)	Hemorrhagic (Group IV)
Volume (mL)	< 4	Often > 4	Often > 4	Often > 4	Often > 4
Color	Clear yellow	Xanthochromic	Xanthochromic or white	White	Hemorrhagic
Clarity	Clear	Transparent	Translucent or opaque	Opaque	Opaque
Mucin clot	Good	Fair to poor	Poor	Poor	Good
Spontaneous clot	None	Often	Often	Often	Often
Leukocytes (mm^3)	< 150	< 3000	3000–50,000	50,000–300,000	Variable
Red cells	Low	Low	Low	Low	Extremely high
Glucose	Normal	Normal	Normal or low	Low	Normal

Infectious Arthritis

The category of infectious arthritis includes septic arthritis and arthritis associated with systemic infections. **Septic arthritis** is a purulent, exudative process that rapidly destroys cartilage, bone, and ligaments. Septic arthritis tends to be monarticular or oligoarticular and requires arthrocentesis (joint aspiration) for diagnosis. Blood cultures should always be performed because hematogenous spread is the most common route for bacteria to enter and infect the joint. The most common etiologic organisms in adults are (1) *Neisseria* species (50%), (2) *Staphylococcus aureus* (35%), (3) streptococcal species (10%), and (4) gram-negative bacilli (5%). Infections with fungi and mycobacteria are unusual but should be suspected in immunosuppressed patients.

Systemic infections associated with polyarthritis include bacterial endocarditis, other systemic bacterial infections, Lyme disease, and syphilis. **Viruses** that are associated with acute polyarthritis include parvovirus B19, hepatitis B, rubella (including the vaccine), alpha virus, cytomegalovirus, human immunodeficiency virus (HIV), Epstein-Barr virus, and varicella-zoster virus.

Osteoarthritis

Osteoarthritis (degenerative joint disease, osteoarthrosis) is the most common form of arthritis and is associated with (1) old age, (2) a family history of osteoarthritis, (3) obesity, (4) joint trauma, (5) inflammatory joint disease, (6) metabolic diseases, (7) joint instability, and (8) diabetes mellitus. On physical examination, the presence of bony enlargement of the distal interphalangeal joints (Heberden's nodes), proximal interphalangeal joints (Bouchard's nodes), or base of the thumb (first carpometacarpal joint) strongly suggests osteoarthritis. The joint fluid is typically noninflammatory (Tables 87–2 and 87–3).

Rheumatoid Arthritis

Rheumatoid arthritis is a symmetrical polyarthritis that affects the small joints of the hand and wrist, the corresponding joints of the foot, and large joints such as the knee, hip, shoulder, and elbow. Rheumatoid arthritis is more common in women than in men and is often associated with a family history of rheumatoid arthritis and the HLA antigen DR4. Morning stiffness lasting greater than 45 minutes, night pain, the presence of subcutaneous nodules, and multiple swollen joints with synovial thickening strongly suggest its presence. The diagnosis is confirmed by the presence of rheumatoid factor in the blood and by radiographs demonstrating osteopenia, marginal bony erosions, and loss of cartilage.

Rheumatoid-like diseases (rheumatoid variants) superficially resemble rheumatoid arthritis. They include ankylosing spondylitis, Reiter's syndrome, reactive ar-

TABLE 87–3.   Joint Disease and Synovial Fluid Analysis

Noninflammatory (Group I)	Inflammatory (Group II)	Purulent (Group III)	Hemorrhagic (Group IV)
Osteoarthritis	Rheumatoid arthritis	Bacteria	Trauma
Trauma	Reactive arthritis	Fungi	Neuroarthropathy
Osteochondritis dissecans	Viral arthritis	Tuberculosis	Blood dyscrasias
Osteonecrosis	Rheumatic fever		Tumor
Osteochondromatosis	Behçet's syndrome		Anticoagulants
Crystal synovitis	Fat droplet synovitis		Joint prosthesis
Systemic lupus erythematosus	Crystal synovitis		Thrombocytosis
Polyarteritis nodosa			Sickle cell
Scleroderma			Myeloproliferative diseases
Amyloidosis			
Polymyalgia rheumatica			
Corticosteroid therapy			

thritis (arthritis related to systemic infection or other stimuli), psoriatic arthritis, Whipple's disease, and arthritis associated with inflammatory bowel disease. These joint diseases tend to be large-joint oligoarthritides but may also affect the axial skeleton (spine), particularly the sacroiliac joints (sacroiliitis), resulting in fusion. When spine inflammation occurs in these diseases, the human histocompatibility antigen HLA-B27 can frequently be demonstrated by HLA testing.

Crystal-induced Diseases

The most common crystal-induced diseases are gout and calcium pyrophosphate deposition disease (CPPD). Acute gouty arthritis, intercritical (subacute) gout, and chronic tophaceous gout are recognized as various stages of the gout syndrome. Confirmatory tests include an elevated serum uric acid level and an arthrocentesis that demonstrates strongly negative birefringent needle-shaped sodium urate crystals. A 24-hour urine collection for uric acid should be obtained to differentiate overproducers of uric acid from underexcretors.

CPPD is caused by crystals of calcium pyrophosphate dihydrate. CPPD can appear as pseudogout, an acute gout-like arthritis, or can resemble rheumatoid arthritis or osteoarthritis. Diagnosis requires the demonstration of weakly positive birefringent crystals in synovial fluid. Hypercalcemia and other metabolic diseases must be excluded.

Systemic Lupus Erythematosus and Related Diseases

Systemic lupus erythematosus (SLE) is a systemic inflammatory condition seen predominantly in women that often is complicated by (1) arthritis, (2) rashes (malar, photosensitive, discoid, or nonspecific), (3) serositis (pleuritis, pericarditis, or peritonitis), (4) oral or nasopharyngeal ulcers, (5) glomerulonephritis, (6) hematologic disorders, (7) seizures, (8) psychosis, (9) a positive antinuclear antibody, or (10) other positive serologies. Related diseases include systemic sclerosis (scleroderma), polymyositis, dermatomyositis, Sjögren's syndrome, overlap syndromes, mixed connective tissue disease, and Raynaud's disease.

EVALUATION

History

The duration and pattern of joint complaints should be documented. Morning stiffness is especially important to quantitate, since it usually lasts less than 45 minutes in noninflammatory arthritis and greater than 45 minutes in inflammatory arthritis. Complaints of rash, other mucocutaneous lesions, back pain, fever, weight loss, myalgias, arthralgias, and fatigue should also be sought. A careful medication history should be taken, since a variety of drugs can induce toxic reactions characterized by arthritis, urticaria, rash, vasculitis, or lupus-like manifestations. Raynaud's phenomenon is a reversible three-phase reaction (sequential blanching, cyanosis, and rubor) caused by digital vasospasm and often associated with lupus or other systemic or toxic inflammatory diseases.

Symptoms related to the genitourinary, neurologic, gastrointestinal, or ocular systems should be recorded. The patient should be asked about a history of preceding illness or trauma. The age and sex of the patient and a family history of arthritis also provide diagnostic clues.

Physical Examination

The general medical examination should consist of screening examinations of each organ system. The musculoskeletal examination should include (1) inspection of both involved and uninvolved joints, (2) joint palpation, (3) active and passive range of motion, (4) examination for ligamentous instability, (5) observation of the patient during activities, and (6) a neurologic examination (including an assessment of muscular strength).

The following should also be determined: (1) the pattern of joint involvement (symmetrical, asymmetrical, small joint, large joint, spine); (2) the presence of joint or bony deformity (ulnar deviation, Heberden's and Bouchard's nodes, etc.); (3) crepitus; (4) decreased range of motion (active and passive); (5) synovial thickening; (6) synovial effusion; (7) cutaneous or subcutaneous nodules; (8) muscle weakness or tenderness; (9) rashes; (10) alopecia; (11) mucocutaneous lesions; (12) splenomegaly or hepatomegaly; (13) cardiac or pulmonary abnormalities; and (14) neurologic abnormalities.

Additional Evaluation

Radiologic Examination

X-ray examination should focus on those affected joints with the greatest diagnostic specificity for a particular condition. Erosive changes may suggest a chronic inflammatory arthritis (especially rheumatoid arthritis), septic arthritis, erosive osteoarthritis, or gout. Degenerative changes (irregular joint space narrowing, subchondral sclerosis, pseudocyst formation, and osteophyte formation) imply osteoarthritis, posttraumatic arthritis, metabolic disease, or chronic crystal-induced disease. Periarticular osteopenia implies inflammatory arthritis. Fragmentation occurs with neuropathic joints, avascular necrosis, septic joints, or trauma. Chondrocalcinosis suggests crystal-induced arthritis, particularly CPPD. Ankylosis (fusion) of a joint occurs with ankylosing spondylitis, reactive arthritis, or rheumatoid arthritis. Normal radiographs do not exclude arthritis, since all early forms of arthritis show normal radiographs.

Synovial Fluid Analysis

All joint effusions of unknown etiology should be aspirated and the synovial fluid analyzed. Immediately after arthrocentesis, the fluid should be transferred to a

TABLE 87–4. Autoantibodies in Autoimmune Diseases

Autoantibody	Associated Disease
Commonly Ordered Tests	
Rheumatoid factor	Rheumatoid arthritis, others
Antinuclear antibody	Systemic lupus erythematosus (SLE), others
Anticentromere	Limited scleroderma (CREST* variant)
Anti-ds-DNA	SLE
Anti-Sm	SLE
Anti-U1-RNP (anti-RNP)	SLE, mixed connective tissue disease (MCTD)
Anti-Ro/SSA	SLE, Sjögren's syndrome, others
Anti-La/SSB/Ha	SLE, Sjögren's syndrome, others
Less Commonly Ordered Tests	
Anti-Jo$_1$	Polymyositis
Anti-Mi	Dermatomyositis
Anti-PM-Scl (nucleolar)	Polymyositis–systemic sclerosis overlap
Anti-Scl-70	Systemic sclerosis (scleroderma)
Anti-neutrophil cytoplasmic (ANCA)	Systemic vasculitis

*The CREST syndrome (scleroderma with calcinosis, Raynaud's phenomenon, esophageal dysmotility, sclerodactyly, and telangiectasia) is a variant of systemic sclerosis and is sometimes classified as limited scleroderma.

heparinized or EDTA-coated tube. Routine examination of synovial fluid should include (1) notation of its gross appearance; (2) microscopic analysis, including cell count, leukocyte differential, and examination for crystals using polarized microscopy; (3) glucose concentration; and (4) microbiologic analysis, including Gram's stain and culture (see Tables 87–2 and 87–3). In cases of monarticular arthritis, a synovial biopsy may be necessary to exclude fungi, mycobacteria, and neoplasms.

Laboratory Tests

Rheumatoid factor is positive in at least 75% of patients with rheumatoid arthritis but may also be present in normal individuals and in other conditions. When the antinuclear antibody is positive at a significant titer ($\geq 1:80$), it may be helpful to obtain other serologies, including anti-ds-DNA antibody, anti-ENA (RNP/Sm) antibodies, SS-A and SS-B, and VDRL, among others (Table 87–4).

Other tests of potential value include the Westergren erythrocyte sedimentation rate (ESR), hepatic enzymes, creatine kinase, serum uric acid, creatinine, blood urea nitrogen, urinalysis, CBC, and white cell differential. Biopsy of the skin, lip, muscle, nerve, lung, or kidney may be necessary to exclude various disorders, including vasculitis, myositis, fasciitis, and amyloidosis. HLA-B27 or a radionuclide bone scan may be used to confirm the diagnosis of spondyloarthropathy, including reactive arthritis, Reiter's disease, or ankylosing spondylitis.

MANAGEMENT

During **acute flares** of arthritis, the joint should be rested or splinted.

In **chronic arthritis**, physical therapy and specific exercises are necessary to (1) maintain range of motion, (2) prevent joint contracture, (3) enhance muscle strength, (4) protect the joint, and (5) maximize func-

tion. Splints may also be useful in certain cases to protect and maintain joint structure and function. Surgery may be necessary to remove inflamed synovial tissues (synovectomy) or cartilaginous debris. Reconstructive surgery may be indicated to correct tendinous or bony deformities and to replace the destroyed arthritic joint with a prosthesis (total joint arthroplasty).

Septic arthritis should be treated with antibiotics and an appropriate drainage procedure (needle aspiration or open arthrotomy).

Osteoarthritis is treated with NSAIDs, but acetaminophen and other analgesics may also be useful and are generally less toxic.

Rheumatoid arthritis is treated with NSAIDs, analgesics, corticosteroids, and disease-modifying drugs, such as antimalarials (hydroxychloroquine), gold salts, methotrexate, sulfasalazine, and azathioprine.

SLE is treated with NSAIDs, corticosteroids, antimalarials, azathioprine, or cyclophosphamide.

Gout may be treated with some combination of NSAIDs, colchicine, allopurinol, or uricosuric agents. NSAIDs and colchicine are also useful in the treatment of **pseudogout**.

PATIENT AND FAMILY EDUCATION

Chronic arthritis may result in disability, financial hardship, and loss of spouse, family, and friends. Education is necessary so that both the patient and the family understand the prognosis and the reasons for therapy. The care giver should help the patient maintain the proper attitude and social relationships and should refer the patient for financial or social service assistance when necessary. Patients who are depressed or who are undergoing extreme stress because of their illness may require psychological counseling as well.

NATURAL HISTORY/PROGNOSIS

The prognosis depends on (1) the type of arthritis, (2) its severity, and (3) whether appropriate therapy was instituted before irreversible joint damage occurred.

Infectious arthritis carries a good prognosis if the diagnosis is made early and antimicrobial therapy initiated immediately. Patients with septic joints who are not treated within 3–7 days are at high risk for significant chronic morbidity including deformity, osteomyelitis, and death. The prognosis for rheumatoid arthritis and SLE is better when appropriate therapy is instituted early in the course of the disease. Osteoarthritis is usually a relatively mild disease compared to rheumatoid arthritis, but it can also result in significant disability. Gout can be effectively treated, especially in its early stages, but lifelong therapy may be required.

Research Questions

1. What causes the immune system to attack the joints in autoimmune diseases such as rheumatoid arthritis and SLE?

2. Why are corticosteroids and NSAIDs effective in reducing the inflammation of arthritis?

3. Why do certain viruses give rise to arthritis?

Case Resolution

Arthrocentesis of the right knee joint was performed, and the synovial fluid was consistent with inflammation rather than a bacterial infection. The CBC was normal, and the rheumatoid factor and antinuclear antibody tests were both negative. The patient was treated with ibuprofen for 4 weeks, which helped control her symptoms. At the end of that time, she felt much better, with significant decrease in joint pain and complete resolution of joint swelling. In retrospect, her physician believes that her arthritic symptoms were likely secondary to a viral syndrome.

Selected Readings

Gatter, R. A. *A Practical Handbook of Joint Fluid Analysis.* Philadelphia, Lea & Febiger, 1984.

Harris, E. D., Jr. Rheumatoid arthritis: Pathophysiology and implications for therapy. N Engl J Med 114:437–44, 1991.

McCarty, D. J. Differential diagnosis of arthritis: Analysis of signs and symptoms. *In* D. J. McCarty (ed.). *Arthritis and Allied Conditions.* Philadelphia, Lea & Febiger, 1993, pp. 49–62.

Polley, H. F., and G. G. Hunder. *Rheumatological Interviewing and Physical Examination of the Joints,* 2nd ed. Philadelphia, W.B. Saunders Company, 1978.

Schmid, F. R. Principles of diagnosis and treatment of bone and joint infections. *In* D. J. McCarty (ed.). *Arthritis and Allied Conditions.* Philadelphia, Lea & Febiger, 1993, pp. 1975–2002.

Wallace, S. L., J. Z. Singer. Therapy in gout. Rheum Dis Clin North Am 14(2):441–57, 1988.

CHAPTER 88

NECK PAIN

Ben Daitz, M.D.

H$_x$ A 27-year-old female receptionist was struck from behind last night while stopped in her car at a traffic light. This morning she is wearing a cervical collar given to her after a previous accident and complains of diffuse neck pain that radiates to the back of her head. She was wearing her seat belt, and her car was equipped with a head rest. She did not lose consciousness and did not go to the emergency room. In addition to what she describes as a "whiplash," she complains of general upper body muscle aching and stiffness and slight blurring of vision. Her health has been excellent except for a similar accident 3 years earlier. Cervical spine x-rays at that time were normal, and she was treated mainly with physical therapy with complete resolution of her symptoms. On the physical examination, motion of the head and neck is significantly restricted in all directions by discomfort. There is moderate tenderness to palpation over the spinous process of the seventh cervical vertebra and diffuse tenderness with taut muscle bands, and trigger points over the posterior cervical musculature and over both sternocleidomastoids and scalenes. A complete neurologic and general examination is otherwise unremarkable.

Questions

1. What is the differential diagnosis?
2. Are any other diagnostic tests or procedures indicated?
3. What is a trigger point in muscle, and what is its pathophysiology and treatment?
4. If imaging studies are normal, how would you treat the patient?

The term "pain in the neck," readily translatable across different cultures, aptly conveys the ubiquitous distribution of this nagging, disabling complaint. Epidemiologic studies indicate that more than one third of adults have experienced an episode of severe neck pain, often with a radicular component. Neck strain and whiplash injury are two of the most common traumatic musculoskeletal complaints in primary care practice. Acute and chronic neck pain frequently lead to a cascade of other musculoskeletal problems and significant long-term dysfunction.

PATHOPHYSIOLOGY

Diseases affecting the spinal cord, meninges, nerve roots, and nerves of the upper four cervical segments, or cervical plexuses, can produce a typical **neuropathic pain**. Neuropathic pain is described as sharp, burning, or aching and usually follows the course of the affected neural segment. Pain can be accentuated by movements that stretch the involved nerves or nerve roots. Neuropathic pain is frequently accompanied by sensory and motor disturbances such as hypesthesia, paresthesia, hypalgesia, and decrease in muscle strength, and in chronic conditions by a decrease in muscle mass. Disk herniation with radicular pain is a frequent and extremely disabling example of neuropathic disease.

Disease involving the first four cervical vertebrae and associated muscles, tendons, and joints constitutes a major source of pain and disability. Perhaps most common is **myofascial pain**, which is pain or autonomic phenomena referred from active myofascial trigger points. A myofascial trigger point is a hyperirritable spot, usually found in a taut band of skeletal muscle or in the muscle's fascia, that is painful on compression and can give rise to a characteristic pattern of referred pain, tenderness, and autonomic phenomena. Recent studies suggest that the trigger point may be associated with the muscle spindle and that sympathetic innervation of the spindle may be responsible for the autonomic symptoms such as tingling, dizziness, gooseflesh, and referred tenderness experienced by so many patients. All muscles may be involved in myofascial pain syndromes, either singly or in combination with other muscles in a functional unit. Each muscle with active trigger points produces its own characteristic, predictable, and reproducible pattern of referred pain and autonomic symptoms. Trigger points are activated by a number of direct and indirect stimuli (Fig. 88–1).

Nearly all individuals over the age of 50 years have **osteoarthritic changes** in the spine. Osteoarthritis is either primary (and genetically influenced) or secondary to traumatic, metabolic, or congenital problems. Joints are innervated by articular nerves, nerve branches serving adjacent muscles, and vasomotor sympathetic fibers. The periosteum is innervated, but there is no innervation of articular cartilage or subchondral bone.

Metastatic carcinoma is the most common tumor affecting the cervical spine. The odontoid process and the C7 and T1 vertebral bodies are most often involved, usually by hematogenous spread or extension along nerves to the contiguous vertebral body and epidural space.

DIFFERENTIAL DIAGNOSIS

Commonly, disease and injury of the neck involves nerve roots or nerves lying along the transverse processes or the paravertebral region of the spinal cord, thereby producing neuralgic pain felt in the occipital region, back, posterior ear and ear lobe, and anterior neck. If a deep cervical plexus is involved (i.e., distant from the vertebra) neuralgia can be experienced in the distribution of the cutaneous branches of the affected segments. A history of significant trauma, cervical arthritis, prior herniated disk, or herpes zoster infection, along with typical neuralgic pain and sensory disturbances, should alert the practitioner to consider a **neuropathic process**.

Myofascial pain is the most common cause of acute and chronic neck pain and other regional muscle pain syndromes. The location and intensity of the discomfort depend on the muscle or muscles involved. The upper trapezius and levator scapulae are perhaps the most frequent muscles involved in neck, head, and upper back pain, producing dull, aching, or burning pain and autonomic phenomena combined in characteristic patterns. Trigger points in taut muscle bands of the upper trapezius typically refer pain up along the posterolateral aspect of the neck, behind the ear, and into the temple, whereas levator scapulae trigger points refer pain to the angle of the neck and along the vertebral border of the scapula (Fig. 88–2). Trigger points in these and other muscles are readily palpated in their standard locations, using flat or pincer pal-

FIGURE 88–1. *The apparent relation of the trigger point (* ✱ *) to factors that can activate it and to its pain reference zone. The triple arrows (A) from the trigger point to the spinal cord represent the multiplicity of effects originating at the trigger point. The arrow returning to the trigger point (B) completes a feedback loop that is evidenced by the self-sustaining nature of many trigger points. The long arrow (C) to the pain reference zone represents the appearance of referred pain in neurologically distant sites that may be several segments removed from the trigger point. Arrow D indicates the influence on the trigger point of the vapocoolant-stretch procedure applied to the reference zone. Arrow E signifies the activating effect of indirect stimuli on the trigger point. Dashed arrow F denotes effects of trigger points on visceral function. (Reproduced, with permission, from J. Travell and D. Simons. Myofascial Pain and Dysfunction: The Trigger Point Manual. Vol. 1. Baltimore, Williams & Wilkins, 1983.)*

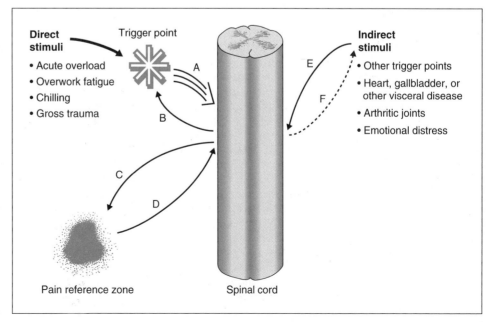

Direct stimuli
- Acute overload
- Overwork fatigue
- Chilling
- Gross trauma

Trigger point

Indirect stimuli
- Other trigger points
- Heart, gallbladder, or other visceral disease
- Arthritic joints
- Emotional distress

Pain reference zone

Spinal cord

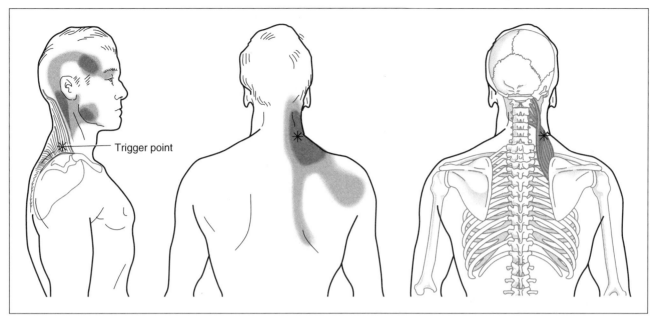

FIGURE 88–2. *Pain patterns for the right upper trapezius and right levator scapulae muscles. The essential pain pattern is solid colored, and the spillover pattern is stippled. (Reproduced, with permission, from J. Travell and D. Simons.* Myofascial Pain and Dysfunction: The Trigger Point Manual. *Vol. 1. Baltimore, Williams & Wilkins, 1983.)*

pation techniques. The diagnosis of myofascial pain is clinical, based on history and physical examination. Laboratory tests and imaging studies are helpful only in excluding other diseases, many of which, like arthritis and herniated disks, are accompanied by a significant myofascial pain component.

Neck sprain is the most common neck injury in which the four upper vertebrae and associated joints, muscles, ligaments, and tendons are involved. A sprain may produce minor tears of soft tissue and significant stretching of muscle. Deceleration and acceleration injuries (**whiplash**) sustained in motor vehicle accidents commonly cause neck sprain. Collision from the rear causes a deceleration injury in which the lower body comes to a sudden stop while the head is first thrown backward, hyperextending the neck, and then forward in extreme flexion, often meeting resistance from the steering wheel or windshield. Acceleration injuries cause the head to move forward in extreme flexion and then backward into hyperextension. Mild to moderate injury generally produces microhematomas and edema and elicits the stretch reflex, which is followed by strong muscular contraction. Mild to moderate whiplash injury often is not immediately painful, and neurologic symptoms are typically absent because major nerves are usually unaffected. Severe whiplash produces overstretching of muscles, particularly the sternocleidomastoids, scalenes, and other long muscles of the neck. Overstretching of connective tissue and articular capsules also occurs. Laceration of tissue and subluxation of joints are common, and in severe cases the intervertebral disk and supporting fibers may be disrupted, producing concomitant neurologic signs and symptoms. Pain may be delayed by 12–36 hours in mild injury but usually occurs within

minutes in more serious cases and is exacerbated by movement of the head. Cervical spine films should be ordered for patients with moderate to severe injury.

Dislocations, subluxations, and **fractures of the cervical spine** are common and are usually the result of significant trauma. Patients with a prior history of degenerative and congenital disease of the spine and patients who have undergone cervical laminectomy are at greater risk of injury. Dislocation or subluxation can occur years after surgery and the incidence is increased when multiple laminae have been removed. Plain x-rays should be ordered first, followed by other imaging studies as necessary.

Infectious arthritis and **osteomyelitis** produce dull, aching, or sharp pain of varying intensity, often radiating to the occipital region and the shoulder. There is usually exquisite tenderness over the vertebral bodies and the paravertebral muscles.

The pain of **osteoarthritis** can be moderate to severe in intensity, is often unilateral, and is aggravated by movement. Myofascial pain and stiffness are common, and with involvement of nerve roots, radicular patterns can be elicited. Rheumatoid arthritis may involve the dural structures, producing paresthesias, hyperesthesias, and weakness.

Primary or metastatic tumors can produce severe neck pain, often owing to pathologic fracture of the skeleton with concomitant sensory and motor dysfunction, depending on the site of involvement.

Acute thyroiditis causes a dull aching pain in the region of the gland, which is generally enlarged and indurated. **Tonsillitis** and **pharyngitis** should be suspected on the basis of the history and confirmed by examination.

EVALUATION

History

The characteristics of the pain should be elicited: type of onset (sudden or gradual), distribution (local, referral patterns), quality (sharp, dull, burning), intensity (mild, moderate, severe, excruciating), diurnal variations distribution (better or worse in morning or evening), and duration. Other important questions to ask include the following: What makes the pain better or worse? Are there other associated signs and symptoms? Has the patient received any treatment? What kind? Was it effective? What has been the impact of the pain on the patient's life (self, family, work)? Particular emphasis should be placed on eliciting pain patterns, and it is helpful to have the patient draw the pain pattern on a body form diagram. Pain diagrams can be used to monitor progress and for medicolegal documentation.

Physical Examination

The patient should be made comfortable and placed in a position that ensures optimal examiner comfort and ease in performing the examination. Good palpation skills can be learned by practice coordinated with review of the relevant anatomy. A comprehensive examination of the neck encompasses the following: assessment of posture and gait, head position, symmetry, swelling, and abnormalities of curvature; palpation of all spinous and transverse processes for pain, tenderness, and paresthesias; and palpation of muscles and soft tissues with particular attention to the upper trapezius, posterior cervicals, sternocleidomastoids, levator scapulae, and scalenes. The examiner should also palpate the thyroid gland and cartilage, hyoid bone, and supraclavicular fossa. Active and passive range of motion is assessed in all dimensions.

The Spurling test is helpful in determining the effect of compression on the cervical spine. It should be performed judiciously and carefully. The examiner applies gradually increasing pressure downward on the top of the skull. This maneuver narrows the intervertebral foramina, compresses the disk, and exerts shearing forces on joint surfaces and pressure on muscles and ligaments. Pathology in the upper cervical spine will produce pain localized to the vertebra involved, or pain and paresthesia in the distribution of the cervical plexus. Pain and paresthesia referred to the upper limb indicate a process involving the lower cervical and first thoracic vertebra. Pressure applied in a similar manner in both right and left lateral flexion closes the foramina even more and aids in determination of the lesion.

The traction test is performed with the patient sitting and the examiner gradually applying upward traction with one hand under the chin and the other under the occiput. This procedure distracts the disk and joints, diminishing or eliminating pain, paresthesia, and muscle spasm.

Additional Evaluation

Simple neck sprain can be assessed and managed without imaging studies. For more complex problems, plain x-rays of the cervical spine should be obtained first, followed by more specific imaging techniques as necessary.

CBC and differential, erythrocyte sedimentation rate (ESR), rheumatoid factor, and other appropriate studies should be ordered for infectious and inflammatory disorders as indicated.

MANAGEMENT

In general, patients presenting with neck pain, with or without neurologic involvement, will need to be seen on at least several occasions to adequately assess response to treatment and need for further workup. Patients suspected of having disease such as neoplasm, infection, or neurologic compression need more immediate and complete diagnostic evaluation and may require hospitalization for intensive therapy.

The herniated intervertebral disk, a common cause of cervical neuralgia, is generally treated conservatively. The control of pain is a paramount consideration. If NSAIDs or other nonnarcotic analgesics in combination with physical therapy modalities do not help, narcotic medications, epidural steroid injections, or even surgery may be needed.

Uncomplicated neck sprain can usually be treated with nonnarcotic analgesics, but codeine or stronger analgesics may be indicated for severe pain. The neck should be carefully palpated for evidence of myofascial trigger points. Because myofascial pain results from taut, contracted muscle fibers, treatment involves gentle stretching of the affected muscle groups. Stretching is facilitated by the use of a finely calibrated stream of vapocoolant spray directed over the skin and following the course of the affected muscle, including the muscle's specific referred pain pattern. Myofascial trigger points can also be injected with 0.5 mL (or less) of a local anesthetic agent without epinephrine by means of a 25-gauge or smaller needle. Corticosteroids are not injected in trigger points. Injection should always be followed by stretch and active movement of the involved muscle. The patient will benefit from a continuing program of active and passive stretching of affected muscles. If the injury is more than 24 hours old, moist, heat packs, ultrasound, and diathermy are useful. Cervical collars may provide some benefit but should only be used intermittently, since prolonged immobilization can produce more spasm. Systemic muscle relaxants are generally not helpful and may produce uncomfortable side effects.

Patients suspected of sustaining a cervical fracture or dislocation should be evaluated first with anteroposterior, lateral, and oblique radiographs. If the patient is neurologically intact and the fracture or dislocation is unstable, the patient is usually treated with traction to achieve stability. Traction is contraindicated in patients sustaining disruption of the occiput from C1, or of C1 from C2. Appropriate analgesia and physical therapy are initiated. Overall, treatment is generally conservative.

Appropriate antibiotics and analgesics are used to treat pain due to infection. Pain due to inflammation can usually be managed well with NSAIDs or other analgesics in combination with various physical therapy modalities. Trigger point injections in muscle, local anesthetic infiltration in other areas of soft tissue tenderness, facet blocks, and segmental epidural blocks are helpful adjuncts to consider.

PATIENT AND FAMILY EDUCATION

Pain is more effectively treated when patients have a reasonable understanding of why they hurt. Because neck pain can become a chronic condition, it is important to educate the patient and family about the cause of the pain and ways to relieve it. Patients should be provided with information about stretch and exercise programs, ergonomic considerations, and other home and workplace factors that may exacerbate or relieve symptoms. Support groups and pain management programs can be helpful in assessing individual needs, teaching new therapeutic and coping skills, and suggesting other mechanisms to manage chronic disability.

Research Questions

1. Are cervical collars helpful in treating neck sprains?
2. Are muscle relaxants effective?

Case Resolution

The patient had suffered a deceleration injury. Injection of trigger points in the sternocleidomastoids significantly relieved her pain. The patient was instructed to begin gentle stretching exercises for the anterior and posterior neck muscles. Use of moist heat packs, NSAIDs, and some time off from the patient's computer work station resulted in almost complete resolution of symptoms in 3 weeks' time.

Selected Readings

(Also see the Selected Readings list for Chapter 93.)
Shaw, N., and B. Daitz. *Regional Stretching Exercises.* Baltimore, Williams & Wilkins, 1992.

CHAPTER 89

SHOULDER PAIN

Christopher A. McGrew, M.D.

Hx A 19-year-old female nursing student complains of 2 months of right shoulder pain. The pain is worse when she swims and plays volleyball, and the shoulder is painful to sleep on. It hurts when she combs her hair or lifts her arm over her head. At times it feels as though the shoulder is "slipping." Her pain started after "spiking" the ball in a volleyball match. She felt a sudden slip and "catch" in her shoulder joint. She rested the shoulder for several weeks but did not seek medical treatment, occasionally treating the shoulder with ice packs and aspirin tablets, which improved the symptoms. The patient is otherwise in good health. She has no allergies and takes no other medication. Right shoulder examination reveals a limited active range of motion in forward flexion and abduction from the side, with pain from 70 to 120 degrees during abduction. Passive range of motion is normal. On palpation, there is tenderness over the greater tuberosity of the humerus as well as the lateral subacromial area. There is decreased strength (4/5) in the rotator cuff, including external rotation and supraspinatus testing. Impingement, apprehension, and relocation tests are positive. Neurovascular examination is normal. Anteroposterior and axillary x-rays are normal.

Questions

1. What diagnostic possibilities should be considered?
2. What other questions should you ask this patient?
3. What treatment would potentially alleviate her symptoms?

Primary care physicians often encounter patients with shoulder complaints. Epidemiologic reviews indicate that 8%–13% of athletic injuries and 1%–2% of all general office visits involve the shoulder. Shoulder pain can result from either intrinsic or extrinsic causes. This chapter primarily addresses nontraumatic intrinsic shoulder pain.

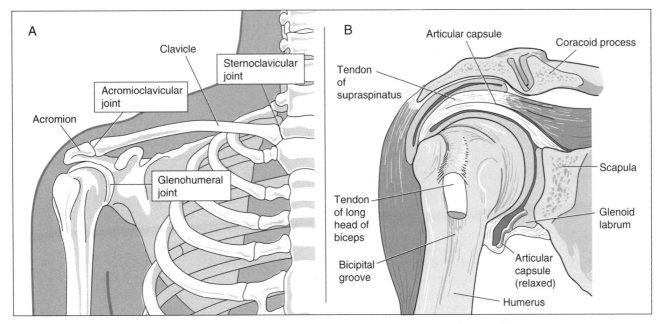

FIGURE 89-1. *A. Bony anatomy of the shoulder. B. Basic anatomy of the shoulder.*

PATHOPHYSIOLOGY

The shoulder bony anatomy consists of the scapula and humerus, which articulate at the glenohumeral joint, and the clavicle, which articulates with the acromion. The shoulder girdle is suspended on the thorax, primarily by the trapezius and serratus anterior muscle with only one skeletal attachment at the sternoclavicular joint. The glenohumeral joint is a ball-and-socket joint in which the head of the humerus articulates with the shallow glenoid cavity of the scapula. The cavity is deepened slightly by fibrous cartilage in its ridge, called the glenoid labrum. Stability around this joint is provided primarily by static restraints: ligaments and joint capsule (Fig. 89–1). Active restraint is provided by the muscles of the rotator cuff. The rotator cuff is made up of the supraspinatus, infraspinatus, subscapularis, and teres minor muscles. The supraspinatus and other cuff muscles stabilize the humeral head against the glenoid fossa during the process of abduction from the side. The primary mover for abduction is the deltoid. Other muscles that act in the shoulder include the pectoralis, latissimus dorsi, biceps, and teres major. The shoulder complex is innervated by the brachial plexus (C4–5), and the blood is supplied by the branches of the subclavian artery.

Between the acromion and the rotator cuff lies the subacromial space. This space is relatively narrow and contains musculotendinous structures as well as the subacromial bursa, which facilitates the glide motion of the rotator cuff. Under the cuff lies the joint capsule. Only if the cuff is torn is there a connection between the joint space and subacromial bursa. The long head of the biceps tendon lies in the bicipital groove located between the greater and lesser tuberosities. The biceps tendon enters the joint in this area by penetrating the

capsule and courses through the joint into its origin at the supraglenoid tubercle.

DIFFERENTIAL DIAGNOSIS

Extrinsic disorders that can refer pain to the shoulder include cervical spine disorders, brachial plexus neuropathy, postural/myofascial pain, neoplastic disease, thoracic outlet syndrome, diaphragmatic irritation, and myocardial ischemia. **Intrinsic** shoulder disorders include glenohumeral osteoarthritis, acromioclavicular arthritis, septic arthritis, rheumatoid arthritis, gout, osteonecrosis, rotator cuff impingement with or without glenohumeral instability, rotator cuff tears, biceps tendinitis, biceps tendon rupture, calcific tendinitis, and adhesive capsulitis.

Glenohumeral instability can be either traumatic or atraumatic. The classic traumatic cause of instability is shoulder dislocation. On the other hand, atraumatic instability can result from underlying connective tissue laxity or years of repetitive microtrauma, which gradually stretches the ligamentous glenohumeral capsule. Atraumatic instability is not the most common cause of shoulder pain but is probably the *most frequently underdiagnosed.* In some cases, glenohumeral instability can be unidirectional, such as the commonly occuring anterior instability. It may also be multidirectional and involve general laxity of the shoulder capsule and demonstrate anterior, posterior, and inferior laxity. One third of patients with instability will have had some significant trauma, such as shoulder dislocation. Some patients may have glenoid labrum tears, which may have resulted from a specific traumatic episode such as forced subluxation of the humeral head. Labral tears have also been reported in athletes without a significant history of a specific episode of trauma, especially in overhand throwing. This may result from weakness in the posterior stabilizing muscles of the glenohumeral area, which allows excessive forces to be placed on the anterior superior labrum during the acceleration phase of throwing. In some of these patients, there may be a voluntary component in which the patient can consciously and repetitively subluxate or dislocate the shoulder. In rare situations (e.g., Ehlers-Danlos syndrome), patients have an underlying connective tissue disorder.

Glenohumeral instability, no matter what the cause, results in excessive motion within the glenohumeral joint during activities involving abduction, elevation, external rotation, or overhand motion. This may result in "overstress" of the static restraint or of the active (muscular) restraint, causing pain and disability.

Impingement of the rotator cuff is defined as pinching or compression of the soft tissues within the subacromial space between the head of the humerus and the coracoacromial arch (most often during overhand motion). If impingement involves the bursa, bursitis occurs; if the long head of the biceps is involved, a bicipital tendinitis results; if the rotator cuff is involved, rotator cuff tendinitis occurs. Often, all three entities occur simultaneously.

Since impingement results from compression of structures within the subacromial space, any condition that further narrows this space (e.g., a calcium deposit, swelling of the soft tissues, excessive overhang of the anterior acromium) increases the chance for impingement. These possibilities are more likely to occur in the older patient. In the younger patient, underlying glenohumeral instability may result in excessive movement of the humerus on the glenoid. This may result in a secondary impingement of subacromial structures as the humeral head moves out of its normal relationship to the glenoid. This is probably the most common cause of impingement in the younger, athletic patient.

EVALUATION

History

The following should be elicited: the specific activity that causes pain, chronic versus acute onset, what makes the symptoms worse or better, instability or slipping sensation, dead arm symptoms, weakness, crepitation, and radicular symptoms. Family history, past medical history, and review of systems may uncover information suggesting a rheumatologic disorder.

Physical Examination

The physical examination begins with the neck, since cervical spine problems can result in referred pain to the shoulder. The shoulder should be inspected for atrophy or asymmetry. The examiner should observe the patient remove a coat or shirt to assess functional status. The shoulder girdle should be palpated gently and systematically, including the sternoclavicular joint, clavicle, acromioclavicular joint, acromion, scapula, and periscapular soft tissues. The arm should be extended passively and the rotator cuff palpated beneath the anterior acromial border. Tenderness palpated through the deltoid muscle suggests involvement of the subacromial bursa. Lymph nodes around the axilla may be enlarged. There may be myofascial trigger points, especially in the trapezius, rhomboids, and levator scapulae muscles. Active and passive range of motion should be assessed, including extension, flexion, abduction, adduction, external rotation, and internal rotation.

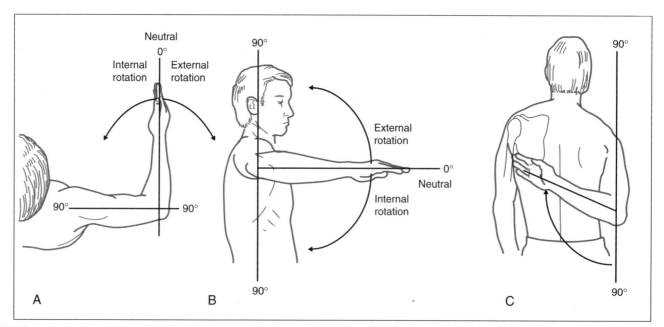

FIGURE 89–2. *Rotary shoulder motion.* **A.** *Rotation with arm at side.* **B.** *Rotation in abduction.* **C.** *Internal rotation posteriorly.* (Reproduced, with permission, from H. R. Brashear. Rotary shoulder motion. In H. R. Brashear (ed.). Manual of Orthopaedic Surgery, 6th ed. Park Ridge, Illinois, American Orthopedic Association, 1985, p. 137.)

TABLE 89–1. Special Tests Employed for Shoulder Examination

Name of Test	Position	Motion	Positive Result	Interpretation
		Stability Tests		
Apprehension test	Patient seated, shoulder abducted to 90 degrees and externally rotated with elbow at 90 degrees of flexion	Anterior directed force to humeral head	Apprehension or pain	Anterior instability
Inferior instability (sulcus sign)	Patient seated, arm abducted at side, elbow flexed 90 degrees	Arm pulled downward (inferior) with shoulder in neutral position at side	Inferior subluxation and presence of sulcus between humeral head and acromion associated with apprehension or pain	Inferior instability
Relocation (Jobe test)	Patient supine, shoulder abducted 90 degrees, shoulder at maximal external rotation	Anterior directed force on humeral head, then posterior motion	Apprehension or pain wth anterior force, decreased symptoms with posterior force	Anterior instability contributing to rotator cuff irritation. Relocation of humeral head reduces pain/anxiety
		Impingement Tests		
Neer test	Patient seated, extreme forward flexion of shoulder with forearm pronated	Maximal forced flexion	Pain	Inflammation or injury to the structures in the subacromial space suggested
Hawkins test	Patient seated, 90 degrees of forward shoulder flexion, elbow flexed 90 degrees	Forced internal rotation of shoulder	Pain	Same as for Neer test
		Biceps Test		
Speed test	Patient seated, shoulder forward-flexed 90 degrees, arm supinated	Resisted forward elevation	Pain at bicipital groove	Tendinitis of long head of biceps
		Thoracic Outlet Test		
Roos test	Arms abducted 90 degrees externally rotated, elbows flexed 90 degrees	Patient opens and closes hands for 3 minutes	Ischemic pain or paresthesias	Suggests thoracic outlet syndrome

Internal rotation can be measured by observing the highest spinal level that the patient can touch on his or her back with the thumb (Fig. 89–2).

The muscle groups should be tested for strength against manual resistance. Special tests for the shoulder are listed in Table 89–1. The primary care physician should be familiar with the impingement signs, apprehension test, relocation test, inferior instability (sulcus test), and Roos test.

Radiographic evaluation can vary but should include a true anteroposterior view, an axillary lateral view, and a scapular outlet view.

A subacromial injection of 8 to 10 mL of lidocaine 1% can be helpful in the diagnosis of impingement syndrome. If the impingement maneuvers can be performed painlessly following the injection, then impingement of subacromial structures is confirmed.

MANAGEMENT

Extrinsic disorders must be differentiated from intrinsic disorders before treatment can begin. Symptomatic treatment includes the use of NSAIDs, ice and heat (ice for more acute injuries, heat for more chronic injuries), and rest from the offending activity. Extrinsic disorders that cause shoulder pain are less likely to be relieved by these treatment modalities. For example, cervical spine disorders causing shoulder pain often improve with cervical traction. Myofascial pain in the neck and upper back with referred pain to the shoulder responds to special exercises, trigger point injections, and stretch and spray techniques. Extrinsic causes of shoulder pain often fail to respond to injections in the shoulder.

Maintaining and regaining range of motion, flexibility, and strength are critical in achieving successful functional results in any shoulder disorder. Physical therapy and rehabilitation are extremely important. Basic principles include maintaining range of motion, flexibility, and strength in all six directions (forward flexion, abduction, adduction, extension, internal rotation behind the back, and external rotation). Multiple, short exercise sessions are preferable to a few lengthy sessions and decrease the chances of irritating, damaging, or overtaxing periarticular soft tissues. Treatment progresses from passive range of motion exercises to active assisted exercises, isometrics, active strengthening exercises, and finally to late stretching and strengthening techniques. Local application of moist heat followed by ice precedes most exercise sessions. Any exercise causing lingering pain is temporarily omitted. As range of motion, flexibility, and strength improve, the functional capacity of the shoulder increases.

PATIENT EDUCATION

Patient education emphasizes maintaining range of motion and avoiding aggravating activities until appropriate healing and rehabilitation occur. Standard range of motion and strengthening exercises are illustrated in Figure 89–2.

NATURAL HISTORY/PROGNOSIS

Most nontraumatic shoulder disorders improve over time when treated with conservative measures. Patients without significant improvement in 3–6 months should be referred to an orthopedic surgeon.

Research Questions

1. What exercise could be used to prevent shoulder problems in overhand athletes?

2. Are "loose joints" (laxity) associated with increased injury rates?

Case Resolution

The diagnosis was anterior instability of the glenohumeral joint with secondary impingement. In this patient's case, a gradual increase in swimming frequency, intensity, and duration resulted in progressive improvement.

Selected Readings

Buschbacher, R. Shoulder girdle injuries. *In* W. Lillegard and K. Rucker. *Handbook of Sports Medicine: A Symptom Oriented Approach.* Boston, Andover Medical Publishers, 1993.

Goss, T. Shoulder and upper arm. *In* G. G. Steinberg et al. (eds.). *Ramamurti's Orthopaedics in Primary Care,* 2nd ed. Baltimore, Williams & Wilkins, 1992.

Julian, M. J., and M. Matthews. Shoulder injury. *In* M. Mellion et al. *The Team Physician's Handbook.* Philadelphia, Hanley & Belfus, 1990.

Travell, J., and D. Simons. *Myofascial Pain and Dysfunction: The Trigger Point Manual. Part 2. Upper Back, Shoulder and Arm.* Baltimore, Williams & Wilkins, 1983.

Zuckerman, J., S. Mirabello, D. Newman, et al. The painful shoulder. Part I. Extrinsic disorders. Am Fam Physician 119–28, January 1991.

Zuckerman, J., S. Mirabello, D. Newman, et al. The painful shoulder. Part II. Intrinsic disorders and impingement syndrome. Am Fam Physician 497–512, February 1991.

CHAPTER 90

WRIST AND ARM PAIN

Daniel C. Wascher, M.D.

H$_x$ A 34-year-old female office worker presents with a 3-month complaint of pain in her right arm occasionally associated with numbness in her right hand. Her symptoms occur while using a computer terminal but also awaken her at night. She denies any recent or past traumatic injuries. Her past medical history is unremarkable, but she does report a recent 4.5-kg (10-lb) weight gain. She previously took oral contraceptives but has not taken any medication for 3 months. She plays violin in a community orchestra. Physical examination demonstrates normal range of motion. There is no focal tenderness. Two-point sensation is intact in all digits. Her grip strength measures 15 kg (33 lb) on the right, 20 kg (44 lb) on the left.

Questions

1. What additional history should you obtain?
2. What primary diagnoses should be considered?
3. How can the patient's symptoms be localized to a specific anatomic structure?
4. What factors may contribute to her symptoms?
5. Which provocative tests should be performed?

Arm and hand pain is a common presenting complaint. Repetitive demands placed on the arm by

TABLE 90–1.   Common Locations of Tenosynovitis

Activity	Tendons Involved	Location	Eponym
Wrist/finger extension	Extensor carpi radialis brevis Extensor carpi radialis longus Extensor digitorum communis	Lateral epicondyle of elbow	Tennis elbow
Wrist flexion	Flexor carpi radialis Flexor carpi ulnaris Pronator teres	Medial epicondyle of elbow	Golfer's elbow
Thumb extension	Abductor pollicis longus Extensor pollicis brevis	First dorsal wrist compartment	de Quervain's disease
Grip	Flexor digitorum	Beneath A_1 pulley	Trigger finger
Wrist extension	Extensor carpi radialis brevis Extensor carpi radialis longus	Crossing over abductor pollicis longus and extensor pollicis brevis	Intersection syndrome

occupational and recreational activities frequently exceed the functional capacity of the tissue, resulting in injury and disability. The exact presentation depends on the offending activity and the structures involved.

PATHOPHYSIOLOGY

Nontraumatic arm and hand pain usually is caused by inflammation or compression. **Inflammation** generally occurs in muscle-tendon units or synovial joints. Musculotendinous inflammation is produced by an acute strain or a chronic repetitive stress. A variety of arthritides can affect the joints of the arm and hand. Continued use of the inflamed structures produces further inflammation and pain.

Compression generally affects the peripheral nerves as they pass through a narrowed anatomic compartment. Impaired blood flow from pressures as low as 30 mm Hg has been shown to affect axonal transport and cause focal demyelination, resulting in deterioration of nerve function. The extent of the damage is related to the severity and the duration of the compression. The cause of nerve compression is often unknown (idiopathic) but may be instigated by repetitive activities.

Ganglia are mucin-filled cysts that usually occur in young adults. The cysts may be multiloculated. Although their exact cause is unknown, they often occur following major or repetitive minor trauma.

DIFFERENTIAL DIAGNOSIS

Overuse injuries are common causes of arm and hand pain. The repetitive microtrauma that can occur with occupational or recreational activities can cause tenosynovitis or peripheral nerve compression. **Tenosynovitis** is an inflammatory condition due to repetitive overload of a muscle-tendon unit. The specific tendon involved depends on the offending activity (Table 90–1). Inflammation produces localized pain and weakness in the involved tendon. The resulting swelling may predispose the tendon to further injury. The inflammatory process may interfere with the normal gliding function of the tendon, producing a gritty sensation (crepitus) with tendon action. Chronic cases can result in tendon degeneration.

Although a variety of conditions may predispose patients to develop **peripheral nerve compression** syndromes (Table 90–2), symptoms in most patients are provoked by repetitive activities. Each nerve is subject to potential compression from multiple anatomic areas (Table 90–3); the most common disorders are compression of the median nerve as it passes under the transverse carpal ligament (**carpal tunnel syndrome**) and involvement of the ulnar nerve behind the medial epicondyle of the elbow (**cubital tunnel syndrome**). Peripheral nerve compression usually presents with numbness along the distribution of the nerve involved, often accompanied by pain. Weakness may occur in more advanced cases. Symptoms usually occur distal to the site of compression but may radiate proximally. Sometimes a nerve can have two separate sites of compression (**double-crush syndrome**).

A **ganglion** is diagnosed by the appearance of a cystic mass on the dorsal or volar aspect of the wrist joint; it can also occur along tendon sheaths or at interphalangeal joints. Ganglia can quickly be distinguished from neoplasms by their ability to transilluminate. Large ganglia may restrict joint motion, but generally pain and swelling are the predominant features. Ganglia tend to

---

TABLE 90–2.   Conditions Associated with Peripheral Nerve Compression

Anatomic
Old trauma
Neoplasm
Abnormal muscle bellies
Acromegaly

Neuropathic
Diabetes mellitus*
Alcoholism
Amyloidosis

Inflammatory
Rheumatoid arthritis*
Gout
Systemic lupus erythematosus

Altered Fluid Balance
Pregnancy*
Oral contraceptive use
Hypothyroidism
Hemodialysis

*A common association.

TABLE 90–3. Sites of Peripheral Nerve Compression

Median Nerve

Carpal tunnel
Flexor digitorum superficialis arch
Musculus pronator teres
Lacertus fibrosus
Arcade of Struthers

Ulnar Nerve

Guyon's canal
Musculus flexor carpi ulnaris
Cubital tunnel

Radial Nerve

Radial tunnel
Musculus supinator

---

fluctuate in size in proportion to the patient's activity level. Occasionally they spontaneously resolve.

Degenerative processes may be a cause of joint pain in older patients. **Osteoarthritis** is commonly seen in the wrist and first carpometacarpal joint. Proximal and distal interphalangeal joints also can be affected. The hallmark of degenerative joint disease is pain brought on by activity and relieved to some extent by rest. Crepitus and decreased range of motion are also noted. The triangular fibrocartilage complex is a dense fibrous structure interposed between the distal ulna and the carpal bones. Age- or activity-related degeneration can produce pain and clicking on the ulnar side of the wrist.

Systemic illnesses often begin with arm and hand pain. **Rheumatoid arthritis** commonly presents with symmetric pain and swelling of the wrist and metacarpophalangeal joints. **Psoriatic arthritis** often is manifested by proximal interphalangeal joint symptoms. Other inflammatory diseases can have arm and hand involvement (Table 90–4).

Nerve compression above the arm can mimic peripheral nerve compression. A disorder of the cervical spine, brachial plexus, or thoracic outlet can result in arm pain. Occasionally symptoms may be related to occult or distant trauma such as a stress fracture or fracture nonunion. A list of primary nerve disorders

TABLE 90–4. Differential Diagnosis of Arm and Wrist Pain

Common Causes

Tenosynovitis
Peripheral nerve compression
Ganglion
Osteoarthritis
Rheumatoid arthritis

Uncommon Causes

Cervical radiculopathy
Brachial plexus injury
Pancoast's tumor
Thoracic outlet syndrome
Occult trauma
Stress fracture
Other inflammatory arthropathies
Vasculitis
Neuropathy
Infection
Self-inflicted injury

---

and other causes of upper extremity pain are given in Table 90–4.

EVALUATION

History

The physician should ask about the nature and location of pain, paresthesias, and weakness. Symptoms can usually be localized to a specific anatomic structure. A detailed search must be made for occupational or recreational activities that may have precipitated or aggravated the symptoms. Identification of the dominant upper extremity will assist in the search for overuse injuries. A thorough review of systems should identify any associated systemic conditions. A family history of arthritis should be obtained.

Physical Examination

Range of motion, swelling, and crepitus of joints need to be assessed and compared to the uninvolved extremity. Areas of tenderness should be localized to specific anatomic structures by careful palpation. The examiner should transilluminate any soft tissue masses noted. The sensory examination should measure and compare vibratory, light-touch, and two-point sensation. Motor function is assessed by manual testing of individual muscles; pain associated with resisted muscle activity should be noted. Muscle atrophy needs to be noted. Quantitative functional testing can be performed using grip and pinch dynamometers. The brachial, radial, and ulnar pulses as well as the venous return should be assessed. A complete cervical spine examination must be performed in the presence of any radicular pain or numbness.

Provocative tests can be used to reproduce symptoms. Percussion of a nerve over the site of compression will produce an electric shock sensation along the course of the affected nerve (Tinel's sign, Fig. 90–1*A*). Occult symptoms may be provoked by placing the arm in a position that increases compression of a nerve; prolonged wrist flexion can compress the median nerve, reproducing carpal tunnel symptoms (Phalen's sign, Fig. 90–1*B*). Tension on an inflamed tendon can reproduce symptoms. For example, de Quervain's tenosynovitis is seen in patients who use their thumb in a repetitive manner. Forced ulnar deviation with the thumb grasped in the ipsilateral palm elicits symptoms in these patients (Finkelstein's test, Fig. 90–1*C*).

Additional Evaluation

Laboratory studies can confirm a specific diagnosis and help identify other associated conditions. Selected patients suspected of having systemic arthritic conditions may be tested for erythrocyte sedimentation rate, rheumatoid factor, ANA, or uric acid level. Blood glucose and thyroid hormone measurements can identify endocrine abnormalities. Radiographs will characterize inflammatory or degenerative joint disease. Occult fractures not readily apparent on radiographs can be

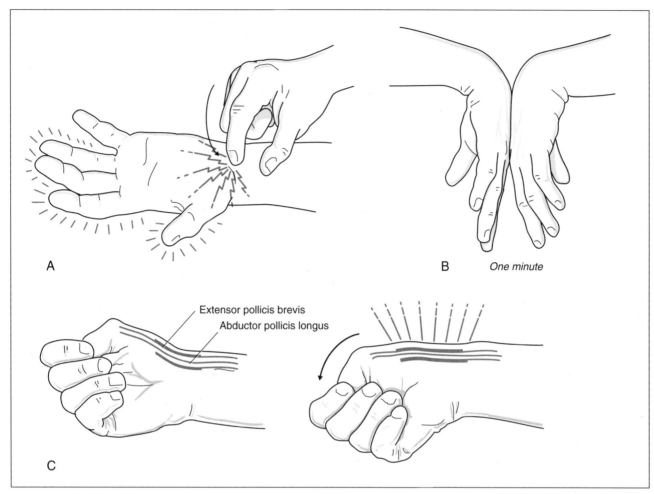

FIGURE 90–1. *A. Tinel's sign of median nerve at carpal tunnel. B. Phalen's test for carpal tunnel syndrome. C. Finkelstein's test for de Quervain's tenosynovitis. (Reproduced, with permission, from W. I. Newmeyer (ed.).* The Hand: Primary Care of Common Problems. *New York, American Society for Surgery of the Hand, Churchill Livingstone, 1985, pp. 76, 81, 82.)*

Extensor pollicis brevis
Abductor pollicis longus

visualized with a technetium bone scan. MRI or CT scans can identify cervical stenosis and protruding cervical disks. Abnormal nerve conduction studies will confirm and localize sites of nerve compression.

MANAGEMENT

Pain can be relieved by diminishing the inflammatory response. The injured structure should be rested by activity reduction or modification. Splints can provide rest and protection for injured tendons or can be used to position the arm to reduce nerve compression. Ice can diminish acute inflammation, while heat can help relieve symptoms in arthritic joints. Aspirin or other NSAIDs can provide analgesic as well as antiinflammatory effects. Corticosteroid injections can be used judiciously for inflammation unresponsive to other measures; however, repeated frequent injections may result in structural damage. When possible, underlying systemic disorders should be treated.

A rehabilitation program is important for restoring function to the injured extremity. A program of graduated stretching and strengthening exercises can speed recovery and prevent recurrence. Improper technique in the workplace or athletic arena should be corrected.

Surgery may be indicated when nonoperative measures have failed. Refractory lateral or medial epicondylitis responds well to release of the affected tissue from the epicondyle. Surgical release of anatomic structures compressing tendons or nerves can produce dramatic relief. Occasionally multiple sites need to be decompressed. Excision of a ganglion may be required for resolution of symptoms. Fusion of arthritic wrist or distal interphalangeal joints can provide great pain relief with little loss of function; joint replacement is preferred for degenerative metacarpophalangeal and occasionally proximal interphalangeal joints. Degenerative tears of the triangular fibrocartilage complex can be treated with arthroscopic excision.

PATIENT EDUCATION

The patient must be helped to identify and correct abnormal conditions or overuse patterns to prevent recurrence. Involvement of the employer, coach, or instructor sometimes is required in order to minimize any abnormal repetitive stress placed on the injured tissue.

NATURAL HISTORY/PROGNOSIS

Appropriate diagnosis and management of the offending activity or associated conditions can result in satisfactory treatment for many causes of arm and hand pain. Those cases unresponsive to nonoperative measures are usually managed successfully with surgical intervention.

Research Questions

1. What measures can employers or instructors take to minimize overuse injuries in the upper extremity?
2. What research models could be used for study of overuse injuries?

Case Resolution

The patient was found to have a positive Tinel sign of the median nerve at the wrist and a positive Phalen test.

Nerve conduction studies confirmed carpal tunnel syndrome; a urine pregnancy test was negative. She failed to improve with activity modification and use of a night splint; surgical release of the transverse carpal ligament gave complete relief.

Selected Readings

Freiberg, A., R. S. Mulholland, and R. Levine. Nonoperative treatment of trigger fingers and thumbs. J Hand Surg 14A:533–58, 1989.

Gelberman, R. H., R. Eaton, and J. R. Urbaniak. Peripheral nerve compression. J Bone Joint Surg 75A:1854–78, 1993.

Harvey, F. J., P. M. Harvey, M. W. Horsley. De Quervain's disease: Surgical or nonsurgical treatment? J Hand Surg 15A:83–7, 1990.

Newmeyer, W. I., R. J. Belsoe, A. S. Broudy, et al. Other commonly seen problems. *In* W. I. Newmeyer (ed.). *The Hand: Primary Care of Common Problems.* New York, American Society for Surgery of the Hand (Churchill Livingstone), 1985.

Osterman, A. L. The double crush syndrome. *In* G. K. Frykman (ed.). Peripheral Nerve Problems. Orthop Clin North Am 19:147–55, 1988.

Spinner, M. Management of nerve compression lesions. *In* J. A. Murray (ed.). Instructional Course Lectures. Am Acad Orthop Surg 33:498–512, 1984.

Stern, P. J. Tendinitis, overuse syndromes, and tendon injuries. Hand Clin 6:467–76, 1990.

Taleisnik, J. Rheumatoid arthritis of the wrist. Hand Clin 5:257–78, 1989.

Verhaar, J., G. Walenkamp, A. Kester, et al. Lateral extensor release for tennis elbow. J Bone Joint Surg 75A:1034–43, 1993.

CHAPTER 91

LOW BACK PAIN

Robert E. White, M.D., M.P.H

H$_x$ A 56-year-old female retail store buyer complains of dull low back pain that gradually began one morning 10 days ago and is accompanied by stiffness. The pain is present almost all day long, does not radiate from her lower back to any other location, and is most noticeable with bending or prolonged sitting. She is most comfortable lying supine and has found ibuprofen helpful. She cannot recall any special event that triggered or caused this pain. On another occasion 8 years ago she had similar pain. It resolved after 3 weeks without medical attention; however, this time her boss insisted she see a doctor before returning to work. Physical examination reveals no visible abnormalities of her back, but she does have some paraspinal tenderness to palpation in the L3–L5 region. Lumbar flexion is markedly diminished because of pain, but otherwise her range of motion is nearly normal.

Questions

1. Determining the precise pain location and sorting through a differential diagnosis is useful in evaluating most patients with pain. Is that true in this case?
2. What other history in addition to a description of the pain should you obtain?
3. In what other ways should this patient be examined?
4. Are x-rays or other imaging studies needed?
5. Can the patient return to work?

Acute low back pain (LBP) is one of the most commonly occurring human maladies. Almost everyone experiences it sometime in their lifetime, and as many as

20%–30% of North American adults report having had significant low back pain during the last year. Many will not need to see a physician, but enough do to make LBP the fourth most common symptom prompting visits to physicians. Contributing to this frequency, employers often require their employees to see a doctor, because LBP is the most common reason for employee disability up to the age of 45 years and the third most common for workers older than the age of 45 years.

PATHOPHYSIOLOGY

Back structures that can be a source of pain are ligaments, vertebral bone, facet joints, intervertebral disks, nerve roots, and muscles. Pain usually results from strain or degeneration of these structures, although serious inflammatory, infectious, or neoplastic conditions occur occasionally. Additionally, back pain can result from disorders of visceral structures immediately anterior to the spine: aorta, kidney, intestine, pancreas, stomach, gallbladder, prostate, uterus, and ovaries.

DIFFERENTIAL DIAGNOSIS

Table 91–1 provides a comprehensive list of conditions capable of causing LBP. However, 80% of the time a precise pathologic location or etiology will not be found. Furthermore, serious problems occur only 2 to 3

TABLE 91–1. Differential Diagnosis of Low Back Pain

Mechanical Low Back Pain	Nonmechanical Spine Disease	Visceral Disease
Lumbar strain	Neoplasia	Pelvic organs
Degenerative disease	Multiple myeloma	Prostatitis
Disks (spondylosis)	Metastatic carcinoma	Endometriosis
?Facet joints	cinoma	Chronic pelvic inflammatory disease
Spondylolisthesis	Lymphoma and leukemia	ease
Herniated disc	kemia	Renal disease
Spinal stenosis	Spinal cord tumors	Nephrolithiasis
Osteoporosis	Retroperitoneal	Pyelonephritis
Fractures	tumors	Perinephric abscess
Congenital disease	Infection	Aortic aneurysm
Severe kyphosis	Osteomyelitis	Gastrointestinal
Severe scoliosis	Septic discitis	disease
?Type II transitional	Paraspinous abscess	Pancreatitis
vertebra	Epidural abscess	Cholecystitis
?Spondylolysis	Bacterial endocarditis	Penetrating ulcer
?Facet joint asymmetry	ditis	Fat herniation of lumbar space
	Inflammatory arthritis (often HLA-B27 associated)	bar space
	Ankylosing spondylitis	
	Psoriatic spondylitis	
	Reiter's syndrome	
	Inflammatory bowel disease	
	Scheuermann's disease (osteochondrosis)	
	Paget's disease	

Reproduced, with permission, from R. A. Deyo. Early diagnostic evaluation of low back pain. J Gen Intern Med 1:328–38, 1986.

TABLE 91–2. Clinical Features of Low Back Pain (LBP)

History	Examination
Acute, Mechanical LBP	
Rest decreases pain.	There is palpable tenderness.
Posture affects pain.	Muscle spasm may be present.
Sitting increases and supine decreases.	Motion increases pain.
	Forward flexion is difficult.
Motion affects pain.	Sitting up and standing up are difficult.
Pain can be localized.	ficult.
Heat or cold may help.	Reversal of lumbar lordosis is impaired.
	paired.
Nonmechanical or Visceral LBP	
Pain at rest	Fever
Insidious onset	Abnormal abdominal examination
Pain less affected by motion or posture	Nonlumbar location of pain
or posture	Writhing pain
Evidence of systemic illness (fever, chills, weight change, morning stiffness, rash, or arthritis of other joints)	Visible inflammation
Visceral disease symptoms (gastrointestinal, urinary, or genital)	
Risk factors for underlying infection or tumor (age >50, recent surgery, immunosuppression, IV drug use, neoplasm history)	
LBP with Neurologic Deficit	
Dermatomal radiation of pain or numbness	Sensory, reflex, or motor confirmation of history
Accompanying weakness	Positive straight leg raising
Aggravation of symptoms by cough, forward flexion, or sitting	
Symptom improvement when supine	
Urinary or bowel incontinence	
Saddle anesthesia	

times in every 100 patients with LBP (even less commonly in patients below the age of 50 years).

EVALUATION

It is important to identify the occasional patient with significant nonmechanical, visceral, or neurologic disease (Table 91–2) and to address functional and occupational issues.

History

The physician should ask the patient to describe the pain and then listen for the features listed in Table 91–2. Symptom dimensions (quality, location and radiation, nature of onset, chronology, factors that relieve or enhance pain, and associated symptoms) should be clarified and smoking and inactivity (risk factors for mechanical LBP) asked about. Information related to antecedent injuries should be obtained; however, only 50% of mechanical LBP patients will be able to identify a specific incident. Asking direct questions about nonmechanical or visceral pain features (Table 91–2) helps exclude serious problems.

Physical Examination

The examiner should note whether the patient is obese (another LBP risk factor). If possible, the physician should watch the patient walk into the examination room and carefully observe movements during the visit (Table 91–2). The patient's back should be inspected while the patient stands. The examiner should palpate the back for paraspinal muscle spasm and areas of tenderness. Fist percussion or firm pressure over spinous processes may help localize pain. If the patient complains of pain in the buttock, thigh, or leg, the physician should palpate deeply into the sciatic notch for inducible sciatic pain radiation. Range of motion is tested next. Forward flexion is the most important movement to assess; extension and lateral flexion are tested if pain permits. A simple measure of forward flexion is the distance from floor to fingertips. Patients who are unable to stand should be asked to reach for their toes while sitting on the examining table. During flexion, the physician should note whether the normal lumbar lordosis is reversed into kyphosis; reversal indicates less severe impairment and spasm.

Neurologic function should be documented. Motor and coordination functions—gait, walking or standing on heels and toes, and quadriceps strength—should be observed. Ankle and knee reflexes should be elicited. Pinprick and touch sensation should be tested if there is a history of numbness or weakness. With the patient supine, the examiner should perform the straight leg raising (SLR) maneuver by lifting each leg separately, making sure the patient does not exert any effort. Patients will frequently experience LBP with this maneuver, but SLR is positive only when pain radiates down the leg in a dermatomal pattern after the leg is raised to 60 degrees, indicating nerve irritation as the sciatic nerve is stretched. The most commonly seen dermatomal patterns are L5 and S1 (Fig. 91–1).

Additional Evaluation

Functional and occupational evaluation is important in acute LBP, since many employers require physician orders for sick leave, permission to return to work, and workplace limitations. Patient expressions of pain and suffering do not always correlate with problem severity and functional capacity. In addition, the presence of persistent pain does not always indicate ongoing back injury, and x-rays define disease extent too poorly to reliably determine disability most of the time. Further complicating the assessment, patients' personal and social circumstances can affect suffering and disability. For example, patients who abuse alcohol, who describe pain patterns that do not make neuroanatomic sense, or who are dissatisfied with their jobs tend to recover poorly from either surgical or medical treatment.

Patients should be asked how LBP affects their activity, what type of work they do, and what was their past on-the-job experience with LBP. Jobs that require heavy lifting, repetitive lifting and twisting, chronic exposure to vibration, and prolonged sitting are more stressful on the back. The physician should try to gauge how patients cope with pain and how willing they are to "work" at recovery with exercises and habit change.

The physician also should listen for comments about job dissatisfaction and disputes, since these may suggest an eagerness to be declared disabled.

The examiner should look for inconsistencies. For example, ease in walking or changing positions when patients do not feel observed belies expressions of pain and immobility when they know they are under observation. Another mechanical LBP inconsistency is the patient's inability to forward flex yet have no paraspinal muscle spasm or pain on palpation. The physician should not conclude that every patient willfully exaggerates pain. However, many patients will regard pain as cause for alarm and disability, will be impatient with the pace of improvement, or will expect a cure without having to be actively responsible for their own back health.

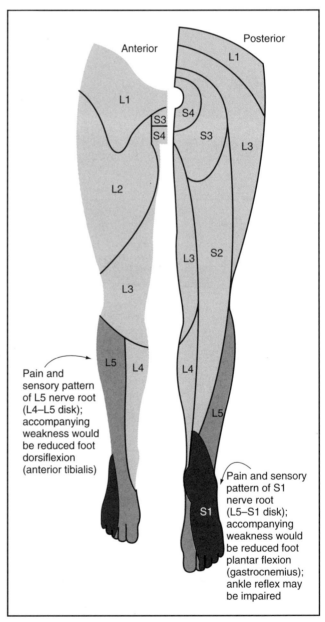

FIGURE 91–1. *Most common sciatica patterns.*

Laboratory evaluation is not necessary in patients who have ordinary mechanical pain. However, when visceral or nonmechanical disease is suspected, a urinalysis, CBC, and sedimentation rate should be obtained as well as additional testing, depending on the suspected cause.

Radiologic evaluation deserves special comment. Routine lumbosacral spine x-rays are inappropriate because they involve substantial radiation exposure, infrequently detect important abnormalities (only 1%–2% of patients with acute LBP have a serious disease as the cause, and only 1 in 2500 x-rays will reveal unsuspected disease), and frequently demonstrate "abnormalities" in normal individuals (e.g., 22% of symptom-free adults will have x-ray evidence of degenerative joint disease, compared to 26%–32% of adults with back pain). Therefore, x-rays should be ordered only when serious problems are more likely: age > 50 years, pain with no improvement after 4 weeks, neurologic deficit, a high suspicion of systemic or nonmechanical disease, or a history of trauma, cancer, immunosuppression, or intravenous substance abuse.

CT scanning and MRI are best reserved for patients needing clarification of neurologic impairment or for diagnosing malignant or inflammatory causes of acute LBP. If the history, examination, and clinical observation over 4 weeks do not suggest one of these circumstances, the usefulness of CT or MRI is limited. Like plain x-rays, they will reveal abnormalities in pain-free adults with surprising frequency and are costly.

MANAGEMENT

Approximately 75% of patients will have ordinary, acute mechanical LBP without evidence of serious or neurologic disease. About 2% will have a serious problem, and another 2% neurologic deficits. The remaining 21% will have more challenging presentations: recurrent pain, prolonged pain, or some feature suggesting a serious or neurologic problem. Older patients or patients in a referral clinic are more likely to be in the last three groups.

In **acute mechanical LBP**, management does not depend on identifying a specific painful structure or making a precise diagnosis. Time is the most important healing factor, and rest, pain control, reassurance, education, and appropriate activity promote recovery. Rest is useful, but strict bed rest is overprescribed and, if prolonged, may actually increase pain and disability. It should be reserved for patients whose pain and spasm preclude motion, and it should not exceed 3 days. Nonnarcotic and narcotic analgesia and muscle relaxants should be used freely and assertively in the first few weeks of acute pain and will be more effective if prescribed on a set schedule rather than "as needed." Traction, analgesic injections, and transcutaneous nerve stimulators are not beneficial in acute pain (although injections and stimulators can be beneficial in chronic pain). The usefulness of immediate exercises, physical therapy, and hot or cold compresses is unproven, but their use in later stages of recovery or in preventing recurrent LBP is more convincing.

Serious nonmechanical or visceral causes of LBP require treatment of the underlying inflammation, infection, fracture, or malignancy. If infection is suspected or if progressive neurologic deficits are present, hospital admission and prompt consultation with a neurologist or neurosurgeon is the usual course of action. Other conditions require less emergent referral or action.

The most common **neurologic** abnormality is sciatica due to a herniated disk (see Fig. 91–1). Because bed rest reduces intradiscal pressures, 3 to 7 days' bed rest is common practice. Narcotic analgesics are usually required, and follow-up within 2 to 4 weeks is essential. If weakness or reflex loss is present initially or develops later, neurologic or surgical consultation and MRI should usually be obtained. Patients with motor function abnormalities lasting longer than 12 weeks may incur permanent deficits. Though rare, cauda equina syndrome (with cord compression symptoms of saddle anesthesia, bilateral numbness or weakness, and incontinence) is an emergency necessitating neurosurgical consultation.

Patients with **complicated LBP** usually recover in the same way as those with ordinary, mechanical LBP, but uncertainty about the diagnosis requires additional testing and careful reevaluation in 2 to 4 weeks. The physician should pay greater attention to functional and occupational circumstances at each visit. Patients who show no improvement over 4 weeks or have multiple, recurrent LBP episodes need a thorough reevaluation and probably consultation. When pain lasts longer than 6 months, it is termed chronic and requires a different approach, if possible by rehabilitation and pain management specialists (see Chapter 103).

PATIENT AND FAMILY EDUCATION FOR ROUTINE, MECHANICAL LBP

Activity increases muscle tone and flexibility, increases endorphin production, and is associated with fewer LBP episodes. Specific exercises for the lumbar area should be encouraged (patient education pamphlets or physical therapists can assist). Walking or swimming are also valuable. Limiting activity to avoid pain can actually result in more pain and disability. Likewise, using pain as a guide to medication dosing and sick leave duration can be associated with a worse prognosis.

Most people will need either no sick leave or a period of only 3 to 5 days. Instead of prescribing prolonged sick leave, the physician should encourage the patient to return to work with a light-duty prescription (Table 91–3). Pain and stiffness do not preclude returning to work as long as limitations are practiced. A patient education pamphlet or physical therapy consultation may enhance patient motivation.

PROGNOSIS

Although one in four patients may experience worse pain and stiffness during the first week of LBP, 60% will improve. Seventy-five percent will recover within 4

TABLE 91–3. Light-duty Prescription for Use at Home or Work

Avoid	Encourage
Prolonged standing	Lumbar support
Prolonged sitting (especially in a car)	Frequent position changes
Lifting over 25 pounds	Maintain normal spine curvature
Listing and twisting motions	when standing or sitting
Slumping posture	Proper lifting technique

weeks and 90% by 8 weeks; 80% will be back to work within 4 weeks. Since only a minority of the remaining 20% will have clearly disabling injuries or diseases, many will need encouragement to cope, exercise, and return to work. Those not working after 6 months of LBP have a 50% chance of never being employed again.

Research Questions

1. What kind of activity best promotes healing of LBP?
2. Will back education or braces in the workplace reduce the incidence of LBP and resulting disability?
3. Using history and physical examination data, can a decision rule be developed to predict who has serious disease, who needs CT scanning or MRI, and who is prone to excessive disability?

Case Resolution

The patient's initial visit to the doctor had followed 2 days of sick leave and a request by her employer that a doctor specify her level of activity. The doctor prescribed ibuprofen and returning to light-duty work. One week later, the patient no longer needed ibuprofen and walking lessened the pain. Two weeks later, she was free of pain and stiffness.

Selected Readings

Bigos, S., O. Bowyer, G. Braen, et al. *Quick Reference Guide for Clinicians*, No. 14, *Acute Low Back Problems in Adults. Clinical Practical Guideline No. 14.* ACHDR Pub. No. 95–0643. Rockville, Md, Agency for Health Care Policy and Research, December 1994.

Deyo, R. A., J. Rainville, and D. L. Kent. What can the history and physical examination tell us about low back pain? JAMA 268:760–5, 1992.

Deyo, R. A. (ed.). Back pain in workers. Occupational Medicine: State of the Art Reviews 3(1):1–168, 1988.

Frymoyer, J. W. Back pain and sciatica. N Engl J Med 318:291–300, 1988.

Frymoyer, J. W. (ed.). *The Adult Spine: Principles and Practice.* New York, Raven Press, 1991.

Waddell, G. A new clinical model for the treatment of low back pain. Spine 12:632–43, 1987.

CHAPTER 92

KNEE PAIN

Edward N. Libby, M.D.

H$_x$ A 50-year-old male law enforcement officer presents with chronic right knee pain that has been present on and off for years. The patient thinks he may have injured the knee playing intramural sports in college, but he remembers no specific incident of trauma. Several years ago he stepped off a ladder too quickly, fell, and twisted his right knee. After the fall, the knee was mildly swollen. Since then the knee intermittently "swells up." His job performance had been unaffected by the knee pain until recently, when he was thrown to the ground and severely twisted the knee during a struggle with a suspect several weeks ago. He now experiences significant pain in the knee every day. He is concerned that his knee would never "be the same" should he require surgery and that the disability could cost him his job. Physical examination is remarkable for a small knee effusion, mild crepitus on knee flexion, a normal anterior drawer and Lachman maneuver, and a questionable positive McMurray test.

Questions

1. What structures of the knee may be damaged?
2. What was the mechanism of injury?
3. What additional tests should be performed?

Knee pain is a frequent complaint, and most knee pain can be managed by the primary care physician. The most common causes of knee pain seen in a primary care clinic are acute minor trauma, degenerative joint disease (osteoarthritis), rheumatoid arthritis, strains of the collateral and cruciate ligaments, and chronic meniscal damage. Rupture of the anterior cruciate ligament, septic arthritis, neoplasms, gout, and pseudogout are less commonly seen.

PATHOPHYSIOLOGY

The anatomy and function of the knee are deceivingly simple. The clinically significant bony structures include the femur, tibia, fibula, and patella, all of which interact as a ball-and-hinge joint. Menisci are the shock absorbers of the knee. They are generally of low vascularity with poor healing potential. Their presence is essential to normal knee mechanics.

The bony structures of the knee may be acutely injured by fracture or periosteal irritation. The menisci, collateral and cruciate ligaments, capsule of the knee, and patella are the major structural sites of knee pain. Knee injuries due to twisting may result in stretching or tearing of the ligaments. The menisci may also be torn or fragmented in twisting injuries. A severe twisting knee injury may result in damage to the medial collateral ligament, the medial meniscus, and the anterior cruciate ligament (O'Donoghue's triad).

Chronic knee pain may result from acute knee injuries. Meniscal damage results in abnormal distribution of forces in the knee joint and accelerates degenerative joint disease. Abnormal angulation of the knee, more commonly seen in women (genu valgum, "valgus knees"), also leads to more rapid joint degeneration. Severe valgus deformities can lead to dislocation of the patella.

DIFFERENTIAL DIAGNOSIS

In patients with acute knee pain, the differential includes infection, fracture, meniscal damage, gout or pseudogout, and ligament sprain or rupture. Chronic knee pain suggests osteoarthritis, meniscal problems, neoplasm, or autoimmune disorders (systemic lupus erythematosus or rheumatoid arthritis). A cyst of the semimembranous bursa (Baker's cyst) can cause pain posterior to the knee.

EVALUATION

History

Has there been any acute or previous trauma to the knee? If so, the physician should elicit the mechanism of injury. Was the leg flexed, extended, or rotated during the injury? Was there a direct blow to the knee and from what direction? Did the patient hear a pop or tear? Did the patient feel a ripping sensation in the knee?

The examiner should determine the degree of physical impairment in a patient with chronic knee pain. How active is the patient? How does the knee respond to stresses such as going up or down stairs, walking, kneeling, turning, or twisting? The sensation of an unstable knee ("it goes out from underneath me" or "I can't trust it") suggests serious ligamentous damage such as anterior cruciate rupture. Locking of the knee ("my knee gets stuck") with pain until manipulation and release, suggests a loose or torn meniscus or bone fragments that become trapped and subsequently interfere with joint movement. Early morning stiffness that improves after movement is consistent with osteoarthritis.

A search for systemic problems must be made. Fever may occur in lupus or rheumatoid arthritis. Is there a history of urethritis or conjunctivitis (as seen in Reiter's syndrome)? Does the patient have pain, swelling, or erythema in other joints (suggestive of inflammatory arthritis in multiple joints)?

Physical Examination

The physical examination of the knee begins by observing the patient during ambulation. Is the gait normal, or does the patient walk with a limp? This gives information about the degree of disability. Valgus or varus deformities of the knee can often be noted during ambulation. With the patient supine, the examiner should look for knee effusion or asymmetry. Quadriceps atrophy may occur after knee injury, and thus the musculature should be inspected. Adequate visualization of the patient's joints and muscles is ensured by having the patient change into shorts.

The physician should examine the normal knee first to gain the patient's trust and determine the normal range of motion. The anterior aspect of both joints should be observed for effusion. Palpation along the superior and inferior patella will "milk" the joint to demonstrate whether a significant effusion is present. Palpation of the joint line should be performed with the knee flexed at approximately 90 degrees. Pain during palpation of the joint line suggests meniscal damage. The knee should be moved through flexion and extension with the palm of the examiner's hand over the patella feeling for crepitus in the joint. Crepitus suggests degeneration in the knee or loose fragments of bone. Anterior cruciate strength may be tested using the Lachman maneuver (Fig. 92–1). The distal femur is held with one hand while the proximal tibia is grasped and pulled toward the examiner with the other hand. The examiner assesses the motion of the tibia anteriorly (in millimeters). An "end point" to the forward motion of the tibia suggests an intact anterior cruciate ligament, while the loss of this end point is often found in rupture of that ligament. End point determination may be difficult in large patients, especially those with powerful quadriceps. In these patients, MRI, examination under anesthesia, or arthroscopy may be necessary. The anterior drawer test is performed with the patient in the supine position with the knee flexed and the foot on the table. The examiner sits partially on the foot to stabilize it, then grasps the proximal tibia at the tubercles with the thumbs. The tibia is pulled toward the examiner (anteriorly) to test for an end point. This anterior drawer test reveals the integrity of the anterior cruciate ligament. Reversing the direction of tibial movement reveals the integrity of the posterior cruciate ligament.

The most commonly used maneuvers for meniscal damage are the McMurray and Apley tests. The McMurray test (Fig. 92–2) is an attempt to demonstrate a damaged meniscus trapped between the tibia and femur, which produces a clicking sound or feeling. The knee is palpated with the palm of the hand to feel for clicking while the joint is moved from flexion to extension with

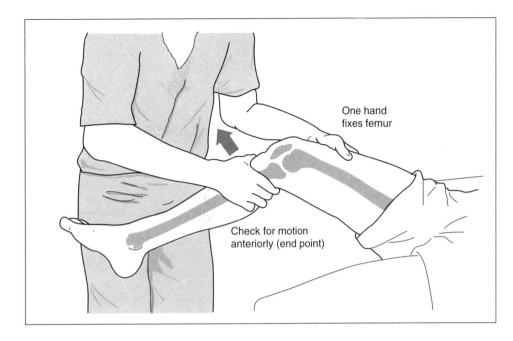

One hand
fixes femur

Check for motion
anteriorly (end point)

FIGURE 92–1. *Lachman maneuver.*

the foot rotated medially (to check the lateral menis-cus). The maneuver is repeated with the foot rotated laterally (to check the medial meniscus).

The Apley grinding maneuver is performed with the patient prone and the knee flexed and anchored by the examiner's knee or by an assistant. The foot (and therefore the tibia) is rotated while the examiner presses toward the knee in an attempt to "catch" a damaged meniscus between the tibia and femur. Pain during the compression suggests meniscal injury.

Collateral ligament testing is performed with the knee slightly flexed (15–30 degrees) (Fig. 92–3). The distal leg may be stabilized underneath the examiner's arm and force applied to the medial or lateral knee to test the amount of opening in the angle between the tibia and the

femur. Comparison between the normal and the abnor-mal knee is always made. A lack of end point to the motion suggests complete disruption of the medial or lateral collateral ligament.

In elderly patients, examination of the painful knee for osteoarthritis or rheumatoid arthritis should be per-formed. Although osteoarthritis does not cause any specific findings, crepitus of the joint is common. Rheumatoid arthritis may result in small effusions or warmth and thickening of the synovial tissues. Bacterial infections of the knee joint will cause an effusion, warmth, and pain on flexion and extension of the knee.

The physical examination of the knee requires prac-tice and experience. Only a few examination techniques are presented in this chapter. References listed at the

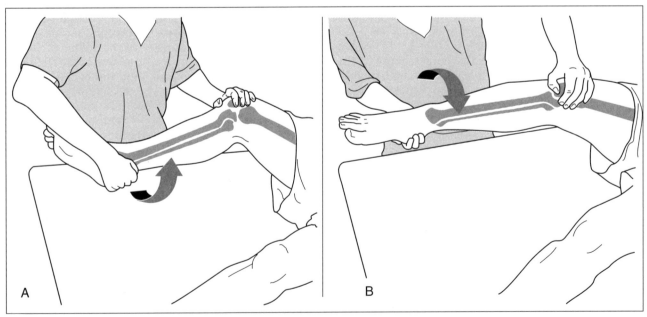

A

B

FIGURE 92–2. *McMurray's test.*

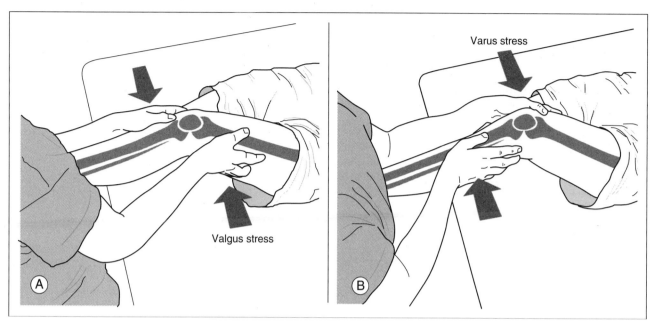

FIGURE 92-3. *Collateral ligament testing.*

end of the chapter provide more detailed information about knee examination.

Additional Evaluation

Laboratory testing is often unnecessary during the initial evaluation of knee pain. However, patients with chronic knee pain, knee effusion, fever, rash, or involvement of multiple joints may require laboratory investigation.

The erythrocyte sedimentation rate (ESR) is a nonspecific test that can be a clue to systemic inflammatory disorders. Marked elevation (i.e., > 100 mm/h) can be seen in patients with rheumatoid arthritis. Rheumatoid factor is commonly used to screen for rheumatoid arthritis. Antinuclear antibody testing for lupus erythematosus may be helpful. Elevated uric acid suggests gout. Suspected septic arthritis necessitates a peripheral white blood cell count and joint aspiration. An elevation of the white blood cell count in the synovial fluid greater than 50,000 cells/mL is strongly suggestive of septic arthritis. In an acutely injured knee with effusion, a grossly bloody aspirate is found in 90% of patients with anterior cruciate ligament rupture.

Radiography of the knee should be performed in cases of acute knee pain. Views should include anteroposterior, lateral, and a "sunrise" or "notch" view of the patella and patellar groove. Laxity of any supporting structure of the knee suggests severe injury and possible fracture. Severe knee pain also suggests fracture and requires radiographic assessment. In older patients, radiographs may help to measure the severity of osteoarthritis. Arthrography and computed tomography are not commonly used to evaluate the knee because MRI and arthroscopy offer superior information.

MRI offers a major advance in noninvasive imaging of the knee. MRI is especially useful in the evaluation of meniscal and cruciate injuries when the history or physical examination is inconclusive. If a patient's injury warrants an MRI study, it is usually serious enough to be evaluated by an orthopedist or primary care physician skilled in orthopedics.

Diagnostic arthroscopy may be indicated in patients with diagnostic dilemmas not resolved by the above assessment.

MANAGEMENT

In the majority of cases of knee pain assessed in a primary care practice, conservative management is effective. Rest, physical therapy (which may be carried out by the patient independently), over-the-counter medications (e.g., acetaminophen or ibuprofen), and education are the key components of conservative management. Osteoarthritis can be managed with rest, weight loss (if indicated), acetaminophen, or NSAIDs (e.g., ibuprofen). The severity of pain and disability are indicators of the degree of osteoarthritis. Radiographs can help define the extent of degeneration but are not always necessary. In severe osteoarthritis, pain and disability unresponsive to medical therapy may necessitate referral to an orthopedist for a surgical procedure (e.g., hip replacement).

Treatment of mild rheumatoid arthritis begins with NSAIDs or aspirin. Physical therapy can help increase flexibility and endurance. Intermittent heat therapy can improve joint function. Progressive or severe rheumatoid arthritis may necessitate consultation and comanagement with a rheumatologist. Corticosteroids (prednisone) and immunosuppressants (e.g., methotrexate) have significant adverse effects, and their use requires close monitoring and special expertise.

Contusions, ecchymoses, and minor strains can be treated symptomatically. The "RICE" regimen is frequently successful: rest, ice, (10–15 minutes per hour for 1–2 days), compression (wrap with an elastic bandage to decrease swelling), and elevation (to improve venous return and decrease swelling).

Ligament sprains are graded from first to third degree. A first-degree sprain is caused by stretching of the ligament with resultant pain and inflammation but no significant disruption of the fibers. A second-degree sprain results from partial disruption of the ligament fibers, but the ligament remains intact. In a third-degree sprain, the ligament is completely torn. The majority of collateral ligament sprains will heal with conservative treatment, including the use of crutches (to discourage weight bearing on the affected joint) until the time when ambulation causes only minor pain. NSAIDs or acetaminophen, elastic wraps or a knee brace for temporary support, and gentle reintroduction of activity approximately 2–4 weeks after the injury are recommended. Initial activities should be limited to walking and light lifting such as quadriceps extensions. Running straight ahead and then gradually testing the knee in zigzag patterns should follow. The total recovery time for ligament injury is approximately 4–8 weeks in young people and longer in the middle-aged and elderly.

Chronic meniscal problems can occasionally be treated with decreased activity and over-the-counter pain relievers. The recurrence of effusion, debilitating pain, or locking of the knee requires further evaluation and possible referral to an orthopedist. Arthroscopy with resection and repair of the damaged meniscus, removal of loose bodies, and smoothing of the articular surface may be necessary.

Knee effusions can also occur in osteoarthritis, rheumatoid arthritis, infection, and gout. Joint infection is a medical emergency. Rapid action is necessary to prevent permanent joint damage. If the knee is warm or erythematous, if the patient has systemic signs of infection, or if there is any suspicion of infection in the knee joint, the joint must be aspirated. The synovial fluid obtained should be sent for Gram's stain, culture, cell count, and crystal examination (to check for gout and pseudogout). The patient should be started on appropriate intravenous antibiotics and surgical consultation obtained.

PATIENT EDUCATION

Education can help patients understand and cope with their disease and empower them to participate in their rehabilitation. Simple exercises such as quadriceps extension, bicycling, and swimming can strengthen the supporting muscles of the knee and reduce pain. Over-the-counter medicines often give significant relief. Heated tubs and whirlpool baths may improve flexibility and decrease pain. Referral to physical therapy for range-of-motion exercises and quadriceps strengthening helps reinforce patient rehabilitation efforts. Weight loss can provide significant benefits by reducing joint stress and slowing the progression of osteoarthritis.

Patients should be aware of the warning signs that necessitate further evaluation, including sudden reduction in the ability of the knee to perform daily activities, locking of the knee, or increasing pain or disability.

NATURAL HISTORY/PROGNOSIS

Degenerative joint disease can become a serious, debilitating problem. Denuded joint surfaces can result in bone-to-bone contact. This accelerates knee joint destruction and may eventually necessitate joint replacement. Limitation in ambulation and significant pain unresponsive to medical management associated with radiographic findings of advanced joint disease (joint space narrowing, osteophytes, loss of normal joint contours) may require orthopedic referral and surgery. There are reasons, however, not to refer some patients (e.g., high surgical risk).

Most cases of knee pain seen in primary care will be due to benign causes such as mild degenerative joint disease or acute soft tissue and ligamentous injury. These problems will generally resolve within a matter of weeks to months with conservative medical management.

Research Questions

1. When is MRI indicated in the evaluation of knee pain?
2. What is the most cost-effective approach to the evaluation of knee pain?
3. At what point in degenerative joint disease is joint replacement indicated?
4. Should all anterior cruciate ruptures be repaired?

Case Resolution

The patient continued to have swelling of the knee despite conservative management. An x-ray demonstrated mild degenerative joint disease. The patient was referred to an orthopedic surgeon who suspected meniscal damage. Arthroscopy revealed a chronic tear of the medial meniscus and several fragments of bone ("joint mice"). Partial excision and repair were undertaken and the bony fragments evacuated. The patient has undergone successful physical therapy for knee strengthening and his symptoms have improved dramatically.

Selected Readings

Fries, J. F., and D. M. Mitchell. Joint pain or arthritis? JAMA 235:199–204, 1976.

Gaylis, N. B. Initial evaluation of the arthritic patient. Postgrad Med 80(5):65–72, 1988.

Hoppenfeld, S. *Physical Examination of the Spine and Extremities*. New York, Appleton-Century-Crofts, 1976.

LEG PAIN

Ben Daitz, M.D.

Hx A 65-year-old moderately obese male glazier complains of a crampy pain in his left calf, which he first noticed last month when walking up the stairs to his third floor apartment. Standing still for several minutes seems to relieve the discomfort. He says he is usually able to walk the block and a half to his bus stop without difficulty, but if he has to hurry, he might feel a "twinge." Three years ago, he had an uncomplicated myocardial infarction. He relates that 20 years ago a "ruptured disk" in his lumbar spine "made his calf hurt almost the same way."

Questions

1. What additional history would be important to obtain?
2. While examining the patient's legs, you notice that his feet are mildly hyperemic, his distal pulses are barely palpable, and he has a hair cutoff pattern above both ankles. His straight leg raising test is negative. What tests would you do next?

Pain in the lower extremity ranks just below backache and headache as a reason for visiting a primary care physician. According to the National Center for Health Statistics, hip and lower extremity impairments constitute about one third of all musculoskeletal complaints. To assess painful conditions affecting the lower extremity, the physician should first consider the intricate, individual, biomechanical mix that accounts for differences in the way people stand, walk, run, and experience discomfort. Leg pain usually is of musculoskeletal origin, the end result of transmitted forces from shoulders and backs, the effects of years of walking just a little out of kilter or standing up all day, or perhaps an episode of lifting the wrong way. This emphasis on biomechanics should also be paramount in the treatment of patients with leg pain. The primary care physician does not need to be an engineer or orthopedist but should observe how the patient stands and walks and correlate these observations to the anatomy.

PATHOPHYSIOLOGY

The major pathologic processes producing leg pain include trauma, arthritides, infections, myofascial syndromes and other muscle disorders, vascular syndromes, apophyseal disorders, extra-articular processes (e.g., tendinitis and bursitis), neoplasms, metabolic and endocrine problems, and neuropathic disease.

Leg pain is often referred from the low back, but conditions in the abdomen and pelvis also may be responsible. Lower extremity pain of neurologic origin more frequently emanates from the nerve roots and lumbosacral plexus and less commonly from the spinal cord and peripheral nerves. Perhaps the most frequent causes of referred pain to the leg are myofascial pain syndromes involving low back, pelvic, buttock, and hip muscles, which refer pain and autonomic symptoms distally in specific patterns. Vascular disease in the abdomen and pelvis may refer pain to the hip, thigh, and occasionally the knee.

DIFFERENTIAL DIAGNOSIS

Neurologic Causes

The herniated nucleus pulposus (HNP), or ruptured disk, is the prototypical example of a dorsal root lesion that may cause lower extremity pain and other neurologic symptoms. The distribution of pain depends on the level of the root involved and also on the degree of associated muscular spasm that invariably accompanies nerve root compression. The S1 root is most often compressed, followed in order by L5 and L4. The typical S1 dermatomal pattern may produce pain and paresthesia extending from the buttock down the posterior thigh to the lateral aspect of the leg, ankle, foot, and finally the fifth toe. L5 root compression produces pain in the low back, posterolateral thigh, dorsal foot, and medial toes. The L4 pattern includes the low back, anterolateral thigh, and medial leg and foot to the first toe. The paresthesia pattern is often more predictive of the lesion level than is the pain pattern. With acute disk rupture or more chronic degenerative disk disease, there is concomitant loss of disk space and consequent shortening and spasm of the paraspinal muscles on the involved side. This myofascial component may often produce a pain as severe as the nerve root lesion itself. HNP is a consequence of both trauma and the aging process.

Spinal stenosis is a syndrome characterized by bilateral and often severe leg pain, low back pain, weakness, and paresthesias—symptoms that are increased by exercise in the erect posture and relieved by flexing the lumbar spine by bending over or sitting. Spinal stenosis is produced by a gradual loss of space for the nerve roots or cauda equina, probably as a result of the aging process.

Diabetes mellitus is responsible for neuropathies and myelopathies that may cause lancinating pain and sensory deficits.

Nerve entrapment syndromes produce pain and neurologic symptoms most commonly as a consequence of ischemic compression of the nerve.

Meralgia paresthetica, entrapment of the lateral femoral cutaneous nerve, is a frequent cause of pain and paresthesia in the upper lateral thigh. Entrapment frequently occurs as the nerve exits the pelvis through the inguinal ligament rather than below it.

The sciatic nerve is the longest nerve in the body, gathering its constituent fibers from the L4 and L5 and S1, S2, and S3 roots. Although the nerve may become compressed at many points along its course, the most frequent lesion involves compression by the piriformis muscle as the nerve passes from the pelvis through the greater sciatic foramen. Pain is generally present in the buttock, along with tenderness over the sciatic notch. The pain may radiate along the course of the nerve to the foot. Motor symptoms and gait dysfunction are often present.

Vascular Causes

Arteriosclerosis obliterans is the cause of 95% of cases of chronic arterial occlusive disease. Intermittent claudication, the earliest symptom of the process, presents with extreme fatigue and cramping with exertion, with progression to sharp pain exacerbated by exercise and relieved by rest. The distribution of pain usually corresponds to the muscle group most affected by the arterial insufficiency. Aortoiliac disease produces claudication pain in the buttocks, hips, thighs, and calf (the Leriche syndrome), whereas occlusion in the femoral-popliteal system causes pain in the calf muscles. Rest pain occurs when the disease progresses to include multiple arterial segments and collaterals. The "five P's" signify the primary effects of acute occlusion in an extremity: pain, pallor, loss of pulse, paresthesia, and paralysis.

The venous side of the vascular system is frequently involved in painful conditions of the leg, and by far the most common affliction is varicose veins. Varicosities generally involve the greater and lesser saphenous networks and characteristically produce a mild, dull, aching discomfort.

Thrombophlebitis usually presents with moderately severe pain and marked tenderness extending along the course of the involved superficial or deep vein. Erythema and edema are often present. Multiple causes of thrombophlebitis have been postulated, including trauma, underlying venous stasis, and platelet aggregation disorders. Doppler studies provide a convenient and noninvasive method of diagnosis for vascular disorders.

Musculoskeletal Causes

Myofascial pain syndromes involving the quadratus lumborum muscle are one of the most common and distressing causes of low back, buttock, and thigh pain. The quadratus lumborum lies anterior to the long paraspinals and functions to extend the lumbar spine, laterally flex the spine, and hike the hip. Pain resulting from spasm in this muscle can be extremely severe and easily mistaken for lumbar radicular pain. Trigger points in the quadratus lumborum are often activated by the simultaneous motion of bending over and reaching to one side in order to pull or lift something. Recurrent quadratus lumborum spasm should alert the practitioner to look for skeletal asymmetries such as leg length and hemipelvic inequality. Simple lift devices can help correct inequalities and relieve symptoms.

Gluteus minimus trigger points, located over the anterior portion of the muscle, may refer pain down the lateral aspect of the thigh and lower leg to the ankle, simulating symptoms of L5 or S1 radiculopathies.

Trigger points in the iliopsoas refer pain to the anterior thigh as well as the low back.

Trauma

Hip fractures result in over 14 million hospital days a year and a prolonged outpatient recuperative process. Fractures involving the hip and femur frequently result from vehicular accidents or other high-force events. In the elderly, decreased bone mass contributes to fatigue fractures, which may then lead to falls. Dislocation of the hip is found in a younger population group, with posterior dislocation being the most common event. Emergency treatment of dislocations is imperative, as avascular necrosis may result from impaired vascular flow.

Infections

Infection of the hip joint occurs more often in infants and children than in adults, and should be treated as a medical emergency. Septic arthritis of the hip is usually seeded hematogenously, and organisms can quickly invade the richly vascular metaphyseal bone within the articular capsule. Gram-negative bacteria are the predominant organisms in infants, whereas gram-positive bacteria are more frequently found in older children and adults. Infants and children with septic arthritis present with decreased use of the extremity, while adults generally complain of acute groin pain and a limp.

Arthritides

Osteoarthritis involving the joints of the lower extremity is a major cause of pain and disability in patients over the age of 60 years. Over 100,000 hip replacements are performed each year in the United States because of degenerative arthritis. Factors predisposing to degenerative arthritis include congenital, developmental, traumatic, and other biomechanical abnormalities, which all contribute to tissue failure. Slipped capital femoral epiphysis and Legg-Calvé-Perthes disease are two such processes; they predominantly occur in children but no doubt contribute to the later development of osteoarthritis.

Epiphyseal Disorders

Legg-Calvé-Perthes disease, or osteochondritis of the epiphysis of the femoral head, is encountered more commonly in boys between the ages of 3 and 11 years. The process is often suggested by a limp or vague complaint of groin or medial thigh pain. Pathologic changes include an initial period of avascularity followed eventually by revascularization and bone healing. Slipped capital femoral epiphysis is suggested by the complaint of knee pain, limp, and leg weakness in a child undergoing a period of rapid growth. As a result of trauma, predisposing defects, or other shearing forces, the superior epiphyseal plate is forced posteriorly and inferiorly, producing a widening of the plate on x-ray.

Metabolic and Endocrine Disorders

Acute gouty arthritis most often presents first in the metatarsal-phalangeal joint of the big toe, producing pain, warmth, erythema, and exquisite tenderness of the involved joint. The pain is often so severe that patients cannot tolerate the pressure of a light sheet or minimal movement of the toe. Reduced renal excretion of uric acid is the responsible mechanism in about 90% of cases, while overproduction of uric acid is the cause in the remainder. Rapid fluctuation in serum urate levels, alcohol ingestion, fasting, and trauma are common precipitating events in gouty attacks.

Extra-articular Disorders

Plantar fasciitis is a frequent cause of heel pain, occurring often after extensive activity in an individual who has been relatively sedentary. Bony spurs, located at the attachment of the plantar fascia to the calcaneus, are thought to be a consequence of traction and pressure exerted by the fascia on the periosteum. The primary symptom is pain and point tenderness in the heel, radiating into the sole.

Metatarsalgia is a condition caused by excessive weight-bearing forces concentrating on the metatarsal heads. In people with pronated or splayed feet, or in women wearing high heels, the second, third, and fourth metatarsal heads bear greater weight and are typically tender to squeezing palpation. Patients may complain of the sensation of "walking on a pebble."

EVALUATION

The history is the critical factor in the diagnostic armamentarium. The pain diagram is an extremely important diagnostic tool; this anatomic contour drawing is given to the patient to help document the degree and distribution of pain and any associated autonomic and neurogenic symptoms. The pelvis and low back should always be considered as potential sources of referred pain. The patient's posture and gait should be carefully observed, and an appropriate neurologic examination performed. The musculoskeletal examination often yields the most findings. Joints should be assessed for active and passive range of motion and muscles palpated for trigger point pain and tenderness. All pulses should be examined. The appearance and texture of the skin and nails and changes in hair pattern may provide clues to underlying disease.

Occasionally, special testing is required for diagnosis or confirmation of diagnosis, e.g., x-rays, Doppler studies, MRI, or CT scanning.

MANAGEMENT

Trauma, including bruises, sprains, and nondisplaced fractures, is treated acutely with rest and appropriate immobilization, ice to reduce swelling, and pain medication. Moderate pain can generally be managed with NSAIDs or codeine. Early referral for physical therapy may significantly reduce rehabilitation time.

Myofascial pain responds most effectively to precise muscle stretching exercises, correction of underlying mechanical and systemic perpetuating factors, and when indicated, trigger point injections (Chapter 88).

Herniated disks, with or without radicular symptoms, should at first be managed conservatively. Timely referral for physical therapy and treatment of associated myofascial pain generally reduces the level of discomfort. The physician should explain that for most patients the prognosis for recovery is good given appropriate therapy, time, understanding of limitations, and commitment to preventive maintenance. However, many patients still do not respond well to conservative therapy, and chronic musculoskeletal back pain may become a frustrating management experience for both patient and practitioner. A full exploration of the patient's ergonomic environment and activities, life stresses and relationships, underlying disease factors, and coping mechanisms invariably yields helpful adjunctive management strategies. Narcotics should be avoided for all but intractable pain situations. Epidural corticosteroid injections are often helpful for HNP and other inflammatory conditions and should be considered early when medications and rehabilitation therapy are not effective. Surgery is considered only if neurologic involvement begins to produce progressive weakness, loss of function, or persistent and debilitating pain.

The pain of **osteoarthritis** of the lower extremity is best managed with a specific rehabilitation program and pain medications such as aspirin, acetaminophen, or other NSAIDs. Pain in weight-bearing joints is aggravated by obesity, faulty biomechanics, and over- or underusage.

Arterial vascular disease is managed by controlling the major cardiovascular risk factors. Good foot hygiene is important. Surgery is indicated for acute obstructive disease. Thrombophlebitis, if superficial, can generally be treated on an outpatient basis with rest, elevation, hot packs, and aspirin or other NSAIDs. Deep vein thrombophlebitis is best managed in the hospital with appropriate anticoagulation.

PATIENT AND FAMILY EDUCATION

After a diagnosis has been established, the patient should be given a full explanation of the pathologic process and a reasonable assessment of the prognosis and management options. In general, for conditions that have the potential of causing chronic pain, the earlier that rehabilitation modalities are instituted, the better the overall response. No discipline has a monopoly on the management of pain, and it is prudent for the practitioner to employ a multidisciplinary approach to care. It is important for the physician to become aware of professionals within the community who can assist in treating pain, including physiatrists, physical therapists, chiropractors, and massage therapists.

Research Questions

1. What are the mechanisms responsible for referred pain?
2. Why do disks degenerate?

Case Resolution

A Doppler study of the patient's lower extremities demonstrated 90% occlusion of the mid-femoral arteries bilaterally. The patient was started on aspirin therapy and ultimately underwent a bilateral femoral artery graft procedure with excellent resolution of symptoms.

Selected Readings

Bonica, J. *The Management of Pain.* Vols. 1 and 2. Philadelphia and London, Lea & Febiger, 1990.

Shaw, N., and B. Daitz. *The Travell Stretch Program.* Baltimore, Williams & Wilkins, 1992.

Tollison, C. D. *Handbook of Chronic Pain Management.* Baltimore, Williams & Wilkins, 1989.

Travell, J., and B. Daitz. *The Travell Tapes.* Baltimore, Williams & Wilkins, 1990.

Travell, J., and D. Simons. *Myofascial Pain and Dysfunction: The Trigger Point Manual.* Vols. 1 and 2. Baltimore, Williams & Wilkins, 1983, 1992.

COMMON NEUROLOGIC PROBLEMS

CHAPTER 94

HEADACHE

Glen H. Murata, M.D.

H_x   A 64-year-old male technical writer presents with a headache of 2 weeks' duration. The headache is described as a constant, "pressure-like" sensation over the left frontal region. It has been slowly increasing since its onset and has reached the point where the patient can no longer tolerate the pain. The patient's wife is worried that her husband seems to be somewhat forgetful and confused. A review of his past medical history shows that he was a heavy smoker but quit 3 years ago. He has consulted a physician for "tension headaches" several times in the past 20 years. Physical examination reveals a well-nourished patient who is bent over clutching his forehead in his hands. His temperature is 37.8° C (100.8° F), pulse 100/min, respiratory rate 20/min, and blood pressure 160/100 mm Hg. There is some tenderness over the left forehead but no conjunctival injection. Extraocular movements are intact. The pupils are 2 mm in diameter and minimally reactive to light. Visual fields are full. The fundi cannot be visualized because the patient is unable to cooperate. Neurologic examination reveals that the cranial nerves are intact, strength is 5/5 in all muscle groups tested, and sensation is intact with respect to touch, pain, and proprioception. The patient's gait and Romberg's sign are normal.

Questions

1. What is your differential diagnosis for this patient?
2. How are serious causes of headache distinguished from benign?
3. Should the patient undergo CT scan of the head?
4. If the CT scan is negative, should he undergo a lumbar puncture?

Headache is one of the most common causes of discomfort and disability in the United States. Up to 80% of normal adults report recurrent headaches, and a substantial proportion of sufferers describe their symptoms as severe enough to prevent them from attending school or going to work. Headache is the seventh most common symptom for which patients seek medical attention and accounts for 2% of visits to internists, general practitioners, and family physicians. Thus, it is important to have an orderly approach to this problem in order to identify the occasional patient who has a life-threatening disease.

PATHOPHYSIOLOGY

It is necessary to review the innervation of cranial structures, since the location and radiation of the headache often provide a clue to its cause. Much of our understanding of pain perception comes from observations made during neurosurgery. Pain-sensitive structures include the skin, muscle, and subcutaneous tissues of the head; the periosteum of the skull; the intracranial venous sinuses and their tributary veins; the dura at the base of the skull; the pial arteries; the trigeminal, glossopharyngeal, and vagus nerves; and the first three cervical nerves. The face and paranasal sinuses are innervated by the ophthalmic, maxillary, and mandibular divisions of the trigeminal nerve, while the pharynx is innervated by the glossopharyngeal nerve. The brain parenchyma and most of the dura are pain insensitive. Since structures in the anterior and middle fossae are innervated by the trigeminal nerve, pain from supratentorial lesions tends to be referred to the frontal area. The posterior fossa is innervated by the first three cervical nerves, and lesions in this area cause occipital headaches.

Detailed studies of the trigeminal nerve have established its role in the pathogenesis of vascular headaches. Innervation of intracranial arteries is most dense at the base of the brain. The trigeminal nerve has been shown to control vasomotor tone under a number of experimental conditions. Stimulation of this nerve also causes the release of vasoactive substances that lower pain threshold and cause edema of dural tissue. Thus, many features of vascular headaches can be explained by trigeminal nerve dysfunction.

DIFFERENTIAL DIAGNOSIS

The objectives for the outpatient evaluation of the headache patient are to (1) exclude life-threatening disorders that require prompt hospitalization and therapy, (2) identify headaches caused by diseases for which definitive outpatient treatment is available, and (3) provide symptomatic relief to those suffering from primary headaches, such as tension-type headaches and migraines. The success of this evaluation depends upon the ability of the physician to generate a complete differential diagnosis. Headaches can be caused by a wide variety of metabolic, infectious, traumatic, vascular, inflammatory and oncologic diseases (Table 94–1). Since the list is long, a systematic approach is needed. The most convenient way of generating such a differential is based on the anatomy of the head. As different structures are considered, different diseases come to mind. As the clinician considers each disease, he or she should decide whether the patient's history and physical examination are compatible with that possibility. Thus, the differential is continuously revised and shortened by repeated hypothesis testing during the history and physical examination.

It is most convenient to "start on the outside and work in;" i.e., consider extracranial diseases first, then secondary causes confined to the meninges, then secondary causes involving the cerebral parenchyma, and finally the primary causes of headache. This approach prompts the physician to consider the possibility of neuropathic pain syndromes, glaucoma, sinusitis, dental abscesses, and temporomandibular joint syndrome; then meningitis and subarachnoid bleeding; then tumors, abscesses, trauma, metabolic processes, and vascular events affecting the cerebrum; and finally primary headaches such as migraine.

EVALUATION

History

The patient's headache should be carefully described with respect to quality; location and radiation; severity; mode of onset; temporal changes; factors that precipitate, aggravate or alleviate symptoms; and functional debility. It is essential to determine whether there are associated neurologic symptoms, prodromes, and auras. Additional history should be elicited about diet and medications; menses; antecedent injuries and concomitant diseases; family history; and the results of any tests done by other physicians. One of the most important reasons for a careful description of the headache is to establish a baseline for patients who might develop recurrent symptoms. Changes in the frequency or severity of headaches may indicate a structural lesion that requires prompt evaluation.

Certain demographic and historical features are of diagnostic importance. Migraines tend to occur in young adults, while temporal arteritis occurs in the elderly. Most primary headaches are more frequent in women. Migraine headaches tend to be unilateral and "throbbing," while tension headaches are more often described as a "band-like" pressure. A headache with an explosive onset ("thunderclap" headache) suggests the possibility of a vascular catastrophe such as subarachnoid hemorrhage. Up to 10% of patients with headache worsened by exertion or changes in posture have an intracranial mass lesion. Patients with medulloblastomas or other midline tumors often find relief by sitting up and leaning forward. However, most of these findings are not very specific. In fact, the diagnostic criteria for primary headaches developed by the International Headache Society require the exclusion of an organic cause. Likewise, excruciating headaches causing marked disability are not always indicative of a life-threatening disease, since primary headaches often interfere with the patient's ability to work or attend school.

It is usually more productive to evaluate the patient for associated symptoms, prodromes, auras, and neurologic deficits; for exposure to dietary factors and medications; and for underlying disease processes. Migraines are often accompanied by scotomata, nausea, vomiting, photophobia, or phonophobia. They may be associated with menstruation or changes in sleep patterns or occur after exposure to certain dietary factors or drugs. Cluster headaches are characterized by lacrimation, rhinorrhea, and conjunctival injection. Certain medications such as nitrates and food additives such as monosodium glutamate routinely cause head-

---

TABLE 94–1. Differential Diagnosis of Headaches

Primary Headaches
Migraine*
Cluster headaches
Tension-type headaches*
Other headaches
  Cold stimulus ("ice cream") headaches
  Benign cough headache
  Benign exertional headache
  Headaches with sexual activity
  Posttraumatic headaches

Secondary Headaches
Disorders involving cerebral parenchyma
  Mass lesions
    Brain tumors*
    Brain abscesses*
    Parenchymal, subdural, or epidural hemorrhage*
    Hydrocephalus
    Benign intracranial hypertension
    Cerebral trauma*
  Metabolic causes
    Food additives and toxins (nitrites, monosodium glutamate, alcohol)
    Hypercapnia
    Medication side effects (nitrates, calcium channel blockers, minoxidil, oral contraceptives, indomethacin, trimethoprim-sulfamethoxazole)
    Febrile headaches*
  Vascular causes
    Embolic or thrombotic events
    Vasculitis
    Hypertension
Disorders involving the meninges
  Meningitis*
  Subarachnoid bleeding*
Disorders involving extracranial structures
  Neuropathic syndromes
    Trigeminal neuralgia
    Herpes zoster
    Retroorbital or parasellar disease processes
  Closed-angle glaucoma
  Paranasal sinusitis
  Dental abscesses
  Temporomandibular joint syndrome

*These are the most important causes of headache.

ache. Finally, it is important to determine whether the patient has had a malignancy that could metastasize to the brain; fevers, chills or sweats; or prior head injury.

Physical Examination

Physical findings should be interpreted within the same conceptual framework used for the history. Pain on percussion of a tooth or periorbital tenderness suggests the possibility of dental abscess or sinusitis. Facial pain induced by touching a trigger point is consistent with tic douloureux. Visual acuity should be examined to screen for an ocular or retroorbital process. Tenderness or redness over the temporal region is suggestive of temporal arteritis. The patient should be carefully examined for nuchal rigidity and changes in mentation. The type and duration of neurologic deficits should be described in detail, since the chronologic course helps distinguish migraine headaches from headaches due to vascular events or intracranial mass lesions. Headaches associated with alterations in mental status, nuchal rigidity, or protracted neurologic deficits should be attributed to a life-threatening intracranial process until proven otherwise. Edmeads has proposed a list of findings that are indicative of a serious process in patients with headache presenting to an emergency department (Table 94–2).

MANAGEMENT

Management depends on the severity of symptoms, presence or absence of neurologic deficits, and underlying medical conditions. Patients with severe headaches, neurologic deficits, or a history of trauma, malignancy, or fever should be referred to the emergency department for evaluation.

Emergency Management

In emergency departments, the most common types of headaches seen are those associated with extracranial systemic infections, tension headaches, and migraine. The proportion of headaches due to serious intracranial processes varies according to the community served and has been reported to be as low as 1%–2%. Thus, great care should be taken to select patients for radiologic evaluation of the head. Selection criteria have been shown to increase the yield of CT scanning for headache patients. These criteria include (1) suspicion of cerebellar hemorrhage or infarction, (2) stroke in evolution, (3) suspicion of intracerebral hemorrhage or mass lesion, (4) signs of increased intracranial pressure, (5) suspected cerebral abscess, (6) blunt head trauma with intracranial hypertension or neurologic deficits, (7) suspected depressed skull fracture, (8) open skull fracture, (9) penetrating head injury, and (10) head injury with depressed sensorium. Patients with a chief complaint of headache and one or more of these criteria had a 21% incidence of CT-detected abnormalities.

A lumbar puncture (LP) should be considered for any patient with high-risk clinical features if the CT scan is

---

TABLE 94–2. Findings Suggestive of Serious Underlying Causes of Headache

Advanced age
Worst headache ever
Onset with exertion
Decreased alertness or cognition
Radiation of the pain to between the shoulder blades (suggesting spinal arachnoid irritation)
Nuchal rigidity
Any historical or physical abnormality suggesting infection
Worsening under observation

---

negative. Ideally, a CT scan should be done before the LP because (1) it is noninvasive; (2) an LP increases the risk of cerebral herniation in patients with rapidly expanding mass lesions; (3) it is diagnostic for many lesions for which LP findings are nonspecific; and (4) certain conditions for which the LP is diagnostic, such as subarachnoid hemorrhage, also have characteristic features on CT scanning. The most appropriate candidates for LP are patients suspected of having meningitis or subarachnoid bleeding. These conditions can result in death or severe neurologic sequelae if left untreated but are not always suspected at the time of presentation.

Almost all patients with acute bacterial meningitis have fever, nuchal rigidity, altered mental status, and/or focal neurologic deficits. Since any febrile illness can cause a headache, the decision to do an LP is usually based on the results of a careful physical examination. Febrile reactions and nuchal rigidity are less common in chronic meningitis caused by mycobacterial or fungal organisms. Thus, an LP may be necessary to rule out infections in patients with chronic headache, even if there is no evidence of an inflammatory process.

One of the most perplexing problems for the emergency physician is to rule out subarachnoid hemorrhage in patients with severe headache. These patients can present with a premonitory headache in the absence of other findings. Although this group represents a small fraction of patients with headache seen in an emergency department, it is important to make an early diagnosis in this group. The outcome of subarachnoid hemorrhage depends on the extent of neurologic abnormalities at the time of diagnosis. CT scans show subarachnoid blood in 85%–90% of those who have bled. The remaining patients have to be diagnosed by lumbar puncture.

Migraine, cluster headaches, and tension headaches can be diagnosed in patients who have the appropriate clinical features and for whom serious abnormalities have been excluded. In most cases, a careful history and physical examination is all that is needed to screen for these secondary processes. A CT scan and/or LP may be necessary to establish the diagnosis with certainty in some patients.

The treatment of secondary headaches should be directed at the underlying cause. A large number of therapies are available for primary headaches as well. Recent studies have demonstrated the superiority of intravenous phenothiazines over ergotamine and narcotics for the treatment of acute migraines. Sumatriptan, which is a 5-hydroxytryptamine analog, has also been shown to be highly effective for migraine and cluster headaches. Its very low side-effect profile and rapid onset of action justify its use as a self-administered medication. Sumatriptan may become the treatment of choice for severe vascular headaches and may obviate the need for treatment in an emergency facility.

Edmeads suggested that those with primary headaches can be treated and released from the emergency department if all of the following are present: (1) previous identical headaches, (2) intact cognition, (3) supple neck, (4) normal neurologic examination, (5) normal vital signs, and (6) improvement under observation. Patients who do not fulfill these criteria should be admitted for further monitoring.

Outpatient Management

Patients with chronic or recurrent headaches pose some of the most difficult management problems for the primary care physician. Those with vascular, tension-type, or posttraumatic headaches can develop episodes so frequently that headaches become a daily occurrence. It is relatively uncommon for these patients to develop a serious intracranial abnormality months or years later. Nevertheless, it may become necessary to do a CT scan or LP if only to reassure the patient that there is no underlying disease process. Although headache patients may complain bitterly about the severity of their symptoms and the associated disability, the routine use of narcotics should be avoided. It is more appropriate to prevent headaches by using prophylactic and abortive medications. For vascular headaches, calcium channel blockers and β-blockers have been shown to reduce the frequency and severity of attacks. The effect of calcium channel blockers does not appear to be related to its vasodilatory properties, and not all types are efficacious. Verapamil is the agent most commonly used in the United States. Propranolol is also effective in preventing migraine attacks. The choice of calcium channel blocker or β-blocker should be based upon the patient's ability to tolerate potential side effects. Lithium is effective prophylaxis for cluster headaches. Abortive medications are those taken at the onset of an attack to decrease the severity and duration of symptoms. The most commonly used abortive drug for migraines is ergotamine, which is available as an oral or sublingual preparation, spray, or rectal suppository. There are too few studies to determine whether ergotamine or the more expensive sumatriptan is better for the self-treatment of vascular headaches. Oxygen aborts cluster headaches but is not available to most outpatients. Antidepressants should be considered for patients with incapacitating tension-type headaches, particularly if they are depressed.

It is important that patients with recurrent headaches not overuse ergotamine or NSAIDs, since excessive use of these preparations can result in "analgesic rebound" headaches that are indistinguishable from the primary disorder. A number of studies have shown that daily headache sufferers have a reduction in symptoms when analgesics and ergotamine are slowly withdrawn.

PATIENT AND FAMILY EDUCATION

Patient education is an important aspect of treatment for primary headaches, particularly if the patient's symptoms are severe and incapacitating. For those with migraines, a careful search should be undertaken for factors that precipitate attacks such as certain foods, dietary additives, and changes in sleep patterns or daily activities. Avoidance of these factors can result in a remarkable reduction in the frequency or severity of symptoms. In most cases, counseling can occur in the office or clinic. For severe symptoms, consultation with a psychologist may be necessary. Behavioral modification and biofeedback training can be highly effective in managing refractory cases.

Research Questions

1. How do dietary factors, menstruation, or changes in sleep patterns trigger migraine attacks?
2. What is the mechanism for migraine attacks in the absence of a provocative factor?
3. What is the pathogenesis of tension-type headaches, and how can they be prevented?

Case Resolution

The patient in question underwent a CT scan of the head, which revealed a mass in the left frontal lobe. A chest x-ray showed a right hilar tumor, a biopsy of which revealed small-cell carcinoma. The patient underwent palliative radiation therapy.

Selected Readings

Edmeads, J. Challenges in the diagnosis of acute headache. Headache Suppl. 2:537–40, 1990.

Edmeads, J. Emergency management of headache. Headache 28:675–9, 1988.

Fontanarosa, P. B. Recognition of subarachnoid hemorrhage. Ann Emerg Med 18:1199–1205, 1989.

Gordon, B., L. R. Barker, and M. L. Bleecker. Headaches and facial pain. *In* L. R. Barker, J. R. Burton, and P. D. Zieve (eds.). *Principles of Ambulatory Medicine,* 2nd ed. Baltimore, Williams & Wilkins, 1986.

Mills, M. L., L. S. Russo, F. S. Vines, and B. A. Ross. High-yield criteria for urgent cranial computed tomography scans. Ann Emerg Med 15:1167–72, 1986.

Olesen, J. The classification and diagnosis of headache disorders. Med Clin North Am 8:793–9, 1990.

DIZZINESS AND VERTIGO

Larry E. Davis, M.D.

Hx A 67-year-old female retired bank clerk complains of dizziness on bending over or looking up quickly. The patient describes the dizziness as a sense of imbalance and a feeling that the room is spinning for 5–10 seconds. She does not become nauseated and does not fall. She denies hearing loss or tinnitus. The episodes occur 1–3 times a day. Ten days earlier she was involved in a mild, rear-end automobile accident that resulted in a stiff neck for 3 days. Two days after the accident, the dizziness episodes began and have remained unchanged in severity. Her health has been excellent. The physical examination is normal. She has normal proprioception in her feet and normal vision, muscle strength, and coordination. Tandem gait is normal, and she does not have Romberg's sign. Cranial nerves appear normal on routine testing.

Questions

1. What systems are needed for normal balance?
2. What balance system is likely impaired in this case?
3. Would performing the Hallpike maneuver be useful?
4. What is the differential diagnosis and the most likely diagnosis?

Dizziness is a term used to describe a sense of light-headedness, imbalance, or disequilibrium. Patients often describe a feeling of "wooziness," a "swimming" sensation, or a feeling of impending faint. Dizziness is nonspecific and can be due to a variety of causes. Vertigo refers to the illusion of rotation or body movement through space. It is more specific for dysfunction of the vestibular system at the end organ, vestibular nerve, or brain stem level.

PATHOPHYSIOLOGY

Normal balance (Table 95–1) results from the proper brain stem and cerebellar integration of three sensory systems: vestibular, proprioceptive, and visual. Inappropriate integration of these sensory signals by the brain stem and cerebellum gives rise to dizziness or vertigo.

Vestibular System

The peripheral vestibular system is located in both temporal bones adjacent to the cochlea. The vestibulospinal system responds to changes in the body's spacial orientation to maintain body position and balance. Changes in spacial orientation are detected by movement of statoconia (tiny calcium carbonate crystals) that are embedded in a gelatinous matrix attached to hair cells in the macula of the utricle and saccule.

The vestibulo-ocular system maintains steady eye position in space during head movement. Moving the head increases or decreases the firing rate of hair cells in the cristae of one or more pairs of semicircular canals. If this system fails, a person who is walking has the illusion that the room is also moving. Abnormalities of either vestibular system give rise to several vestibular diseases (Table 95–2).

Proprioceptive System

The proprioceptive system sends afferent information from peripheral position receptors via peripheral nerves and spinal cord to the brain stem and cerebellum to determine the position of the legs in space and detect movement of the feet on the ground. Patients with diseases involving the proprioceptive system often complain of a feeling of imbalance while trying to walk on rough or uneven surfaces at night. These patients also may complain of numbness or paresthesias in their legs as well as frank weakness of foot muscles.

Visual System

The visual system serves to locate the horizon and detect head movement from the horizon. Inability to locate the horizon referable to head movement may result in dizziness.

Brain Stem/Cerebellum

The medulla, pons, and midline cerebellar structures integrate neural signals from the vestibular, visual, and proprioceptive systems. Either structural damage to the brain stem/cerebellum or metabolic dysfunction of

---

TABLE 95–1. Components of Normal Balance

Vestibular System
Detects changes in gravity
Causes eyes to remain steady during head movement
Proprioceptive System
Provides knowledge of position of feet
Detects leg and foot movement
Visual System
Detects head movement from horizon
Brain Stem and Cerebellum
Integrates signals from vestibular, visual, and proprioceptive systems

TABLE 95–2. Major Causes of Dizziness and Vertigo

Vestibular System
Benign positional vertigo
Meniere's disease
Vestibular neuritis
Chronic labyrinthine imbalance
Proprioceptive System
Spinal cord pathology
  Pernicious anemia
  Tabes dorsalis
  Spinocerebellar degeneration
  HIV myelopathy
Peripheral nerve pathology
  Sensory peripheral neuropathies (diabetic, alcoholic, carcinomatous)
Visual System
Recent diplopia
Cataract removal, with strong corrective lenses
Brain Stem and Cerebellum
Structural abnormalities
  Infarction (Wallenberg's syndrome, cerebellar infarct)
  Tumor (pontine glioma, cerebellar tumor)
  Degenerative (Shy-Drager syndrome, multiple sclerosis)
  Congenital (Arnold-Chiari syndrome, type 1)
Metabolic abnormalities
  Orthostatic hypotension
  Hypo- or hyperglycemia
  Severe anemia
  Hypothyroidism
  Heart failure
  Hyperventilation syndrome

these structures can give rise to vertigo or dizziness (see Table 95–2).

DIFFERENTIAL DIAGNOSIS

Occasional patients, especially teenagers and young adults, may become dizzy owing to **psychophysiologic causes**. The hyperventilation syndrome typically occurs in an anxious patient who hyperventilates to the point of significantly raising the arterial pH. These patients may complain of intermittent dizziness or a more chronic feeling of light-headedness.

Dizziness or vertigo can also be caused by many **drugs** (Table 95–3). The symptoms may be intermittent and occur only during times of peak blood drug levels.

TABLE 95–3. Commonly Used Drugs That Cause Dizziness

Vestibulotoxic Drugs
Aminoglycoside antibiotics (especially gentamicin, kanamycin)
Cancer chemotherapeutic drugs (especially cisplatin, chlorambucil)
Loop diuretics (especially furosemide, ethacrynic acid)
Quinine drugs (especially quinidine)
Central Nervous System Drugs
Sedatives (especially benzodiazepines, barbiturates)
Psychoactive drugs (especially phenothiazines, lithium carbonate)
Antidepressants (especially amitriptyline, imipramine)
Anticonvulsants (especially carbamazepine, phenytoin)
Salicylates (especially aspirin)
Circulatory Drugs
Antihypertensives (especially prazosin, ganglionic blockers)
Vasodilators (especially isosorbide, nitroglycerin)
β-Blockers (especially propranolol, labetalol)
Antiarrhythmics (especially mexiletine, flecainide, amiodarone)

Cessation of the offending drug will alleviate the patient's dizziness. While most offending medications affect the vestibular system, some drugs can produce dizziness via other actions including (1) a direct effect on the central nervous system (CNS), (2) changes in blood pressure, or (3) inducing a peripheral neuropathy. Permanent damage to the vestibular system can be caused by aminoglycoside antibiotics, furosemide, ethacrynic acid, and cisplatin. Generally, the ototoxic drugs damage both the left and right vestibular systems, thus giving rise to bilateral caloric abnormalities on electronystagmography (ENG) testing.

EVALUATION

History

A careful history will frequently suggest which of the systems contributing to balance is likely to be abnormal. If the complaint is vertigo, the impairment is usually in the vestibular system. However, a complaint of dizziness without vertigo does not rule out vestibular dysfunction. It is important to characterize the dizziness or vertigo with respect to (1) whether the symptoms are constant or intermittent, (2) the duration of symptoms, (3) whether the dizziness has a known trigger, and (4) what associated signs and symptoms accompany the main complaint. If the complaint is orthostasis, it is important to ask about symptoms that may be related to hypovolemia (e.g., vomiting, diarrhea, excessive sweating, melena, hematochezia). The physician should inquire about hyperventilation, including a sense of anxiety or apprehension, numbness or tingling of the hands, and periorbital numbness. It is also important to ask about syncope or falls.

Physical Examination

Vestibular System

Lying and standing blood pressures should be evaluated for the presence of orthostatic hypotension. A complete physical examination, including auscultation of the lungs and heart, should be performed. If the patient has a GI complaint, the abdomen should be examined. If excessive anxiety is suspected, it is important to hyperventilate the patient to see whether symptoms are reproduced. The external auditory canal should be inspected, and hearing acuity checked by the whisper test. The fistula test, performed by occluding the external auditory canal with the examiner's finger, will produce vertigo if a middle-inner ear fistula is present. The eyes should be examined for nystagmus.

There are several office tests to examine the vestibular system. The vestibulospinal system can best be examined by using the Romberg test and the tandem gait test. In the Romberg test, the patient is asked to stand with the feet together. In a normal test, the patient can stand without falling with the eyes open and closed. In an abnormal test, the patient can stand with the eyes open but not with the eyes closed. Closing the eyes removes sensory input from the visual system. Thus,

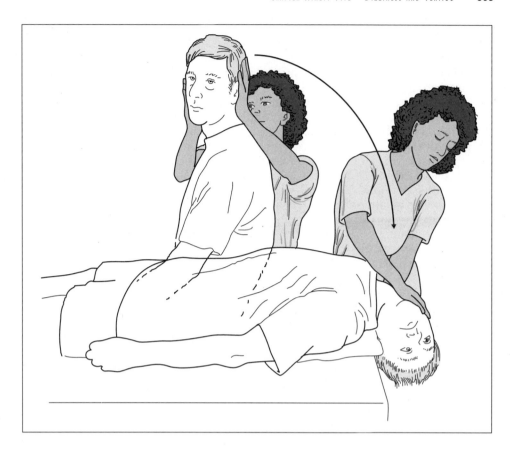

FIGURE 95–1. *Demonstration of the Hallpike maneuver to elicit vertigo.*

the patient must rely on the proprioceptive and vestibular systems for balance.

In the tandem gait test, the individual is asked to walk a straight line in heel-to-toe fashion. Vestibular or proprioceptive abnormalities will cause the patient to lose balance. If the patient can perform the Romberg and tandem gait tests, the vestibulospinal system is usually normal.

The vestibulo-ocular system is best examined in the office by testing the vestibulo-ocular reflex and performing a Hallpike maneuver. To test vestibulo-ocular reflex, the patient should be asked to read newsprint while walking about or while the head is moving. The Hallpike maneuver evaluates the effect of head position on the elicitation of vertigo (Fig. 95–1). The patient sits on an examining table with the head turned to one side. The examiner grasps the patient's head in his or her hands and briskly brings the patient to a supine position with the head hanging below the table top. The patient is asked to keep the eyes open. After 30 seconds, the patient is brought back to the original sitting position and the maneuver is repeated with the head turned to the opposite side. Normally, the patient does not experience vertigo and no nystagmus develops. Individuals with a peripheral cause of positional vertigo typically develop a moderate vertiginous sensation with lateral and rotary nystagmus after a short latency. The nystagmus disappears within 1 minute. Repeated Hallpike maneuvers usually fatigue the nystagmus and the sensation of vertigo in peripheral, but not central, causes of vertigo.

Proprioceptive System

Office testing of the proprioceptive system involves evaluation of position and vibratory sensation in the feet. Sensation can be measured using a 128 cycle-per-second tuning fork on the bony prominences of the toes or the ankle malleoli. Position sense is evaluated by determining whether the patient can detect passive movement of the toes. Patients with impaired proprioception usually have an abnormal Romberg test and cannot tandem walk.

Visual System

Office testing of the visual system includes an evaluation of the extraocular muscles for the presence of diplopia, an evaluation of visual acuity, and a funduscopic examination of the lens for the presence of cataracts.

Brain Stem/Cerebellum

Office examination of the brain stem and cerebellum involves evaluation of cranial nerves (particularly V, VI, VII, VIII, IX, and X) as well as assessment of coordination and gait (including tandem gait). The presence of Horner's sign may also suggest brain stem dysfunction.

Additional Evaluation

If abnormalities of the vestibular system are suspected, several laboratory tests may clarify the problem. Electronystagmography (ENG) is a series of tests that electrically record the velocity and direction of eye movements under a variety of test conditions. In the caloric examination, hot (44° C [111.2° F]) or cold (30° C [86° F]) water or air is irrigated into the external canal and against the tympanic membrane. The caloric test often indicates which side is involved.

CT scanning of the petrous bones allows excellent visualization of bony structures. CT is useful if a basal skull fracture or tumor causing damage to the bony labyrinth is suspected. However, in most situations, CT is of little help because it does not visualize the delicate membranous labyrinth. MRI poorly visualizes the bony and membranous labyrinth, but when gadolinium is administered as a contrast agent, it enhances the demonstration of inflammatory processes or tumors of the middle or inner ear. MRI is helpful in evaluating central causes of vertigo that involve the brain stem or cerebellum.

If structural damage to the brain stem or cerebellum is suspected, MRI of the head is indicated and possibly lumbar puncture. If anemia is being considered, a CBC should be ordered, while an ECG and Holter monitor are helpful in the evaluation of possible arrhythmias.

MANAGEMENT

The management of dizziness should be twofold. Primary treatment is directed at the underlying cause. In addition, if vertigo is present, symptomatic treatment should be prescribed. Anticholinergic drugs (e.g., scopolamine, atropine) are more potent than antihistamine drugs (e.g., dimenhydrate, diphenhydramine, meclizine, promethazine) in the management of vertigo. However, in the elderly, they may cause confusion or hallucinations and may precipitate urinary obstruction in men with prostatic hypertrophy.

In general, symptomatic treatment should be given only during the acute phase of vertigo. Chronic administration of these drugs actually may delay natural recovery. Patients with intermittent vertigo generally do not benefit from chronic administration of these drugs. Patients with dizziness due to visual, proprioceptive, or metabolic disturbances seldom benefit from antivertigo medications.

PATIENT AND FAMILY EDUCATION

Vertigo can be a frightening experience. Reassurance and simple explanations may help the patient cope with the problem until it spontaneously resolves. Individuals with partial damage to the vestibular system should attempt to avoid taking known vestibulotoxic drugs.

> **Research Question**
> 1. What is the pathophysiology of Meniere's disease?

Case Resolution

The diagnosis was benign paroxysmal positional vertigo secondary to the mild head trauma. The patient was treated with specific exercises for benign paroxysmal vertigo, and the symptoms resolved 3 days later.

Selected Readings

Baloh, R. W., V. Honrubia, and K. Jacobson. Benign positional vertigo: Clinical and oculographic features in 240 cases. Neurology 37:371–8, 1987.

Cohen, N. L. The dizzy patient: Update on vestibular disorders. Med Clin North Am 75:125–60, 1991.

Davis L. E. Dizziness in elderly men. J Am Geriatr Soc 42:1184–1188, 1994.

Herdman, S. J., R. J. Tusa, D. S. Zee, et al. Single treatment approaches to benign paroxysmal positional vertigo. Arch Otolaryngol Head Neck Surg 119:450–454, 1993.

Kroenke, K., C. A. Lucas, M. L. Rosenberg, et al. Causes of persistent dizziness: A prospective study of 100 patients in ambulatory care. Ann Intern Med 117:898–904, 1992.

Linstrom, C. J. Office management of the dizzy patient. Otolaryngol Clin North Am 25:745–80, 1992.

Paparella, M. M. Pathogenesis and pathophysiology of Meniere's disease. Methods of diagnosis and treatment of Meniere's disease. Acta Otolaryngol Suppl 485:26–35, 108–19, 1991.

Smith, D. B. Dizziness, a clinical perspective. Neurol Clin 9(2):199–207, 1990.

CHAPTER 96

SYNCOPE

Larry A. Osborn, M.D.

H$_x$ A 67-year-old male retired telephone company executive presents with a history of two episodes of "blacking out." He is known to have coronary artery disease, for which β-blocker and nitrate therapy have been prescribed. One episode occurred shortly after he arose from his living room chair, the other when he stood up after kneeling to find something in his refrigerator. Both episodes occurred yesterday, following a viral illness with associated vomiting and diarrhea. His physical examination reveals a supine blood pressure of 120/68 mm Hg and a standing blood pressure of 90/60 mm Hg. The supine pulse is 52/min, and the standing pulse is 56/min. The estimated central venous pressure is 3 cm H_2O, and the cardiac examination is remarkable only for paradoxical splitting of S_2. His electrocardiogram reveals a left bundle branch block.

Questions

1. What are the possible causes of the patient's syncopal episodes?
2. Are his faints likely to be unifactorial or multifactorial?
3. What further questions should he be asked?
4. What diagnostic studies would you recommend?

Syncope, or fainting, is a transient reversible loss of consciousness. It usually results from a temporary impairment of cerebral blood flow, but it may also result from metabolic derangements such as hypoglycemia. Syncope accounts for 3% of emergency room visits and 6% of medical hospital admissions. In approximately 50% of patients, an exact cause cannot be determined despite a comprehensive workup. Prognosis varies depending on the cause, with cardiac syncope having the worst outcome.

PATHOPHYSIOLOGY

Transient cessation or marked reduction of cerebral blood flow may result in loss of consciousness within 5 to 10 seconds. Factors that influence the susceptibility to fainting include body position, age, and the usual cerebral perfusion pressure. Syncope has an increased frequency in elderly persons, occurring at a rate of 6% to 7% per year.

DIFFERENTIAL DIAGNOSIS

In the evaluation of a patient who has had one or more episodes of loss of consciousness, syncope should be differentiated from a seizure disorder. Atypical seizures without the classic features of grand mal epilepsy may be difficult to distinguish from faints. Careful neurologic assessment, electroencephalography, and MRI or CT scanning of the brain may be required to establish the correct diagnosis.

One should attempt to determine whether proven syncope is cardiovascular or noncardiovascular in origin. The latter includes neurologic, metabolic, and psychiatric disorders. Cardiovascular causes include cardiac and reflex disorders. Cardiac faints may arise from mechanical causes, such as pulmonary hypertension or aortic stenosis, or from dysrhythmias, including tachyarrhythmias, bradyarrhythymias, or periods of asystole. Figure 96–1 outlines the differential diagnosis of syncope.

EVALUATION

History

Careful questioning of the patient and witnesses is important in order to determine the following: (1) the sequence of events; (2) provocative stimuli, such as cough, micturition, anxiety, head turning, or wearing of a tight collar; (3) positions in which the episodes occur; and (4) whether the syncope is exertional. The patient should be questioned about medications, present and past medical problems, and all symptoms associated with syncopal episodes, including any prodromal symptoms. Historical features favoring syncope over a major motor seizure include (1) patient oriented to place and circumstance upon awakening, (2) lack of tongue biting or incontinence, and (3) absence of preseizure aura.

Vasovagal syncope, in which various stimuli lead to vasodepressor (blood pooling) and cardioinhibitory

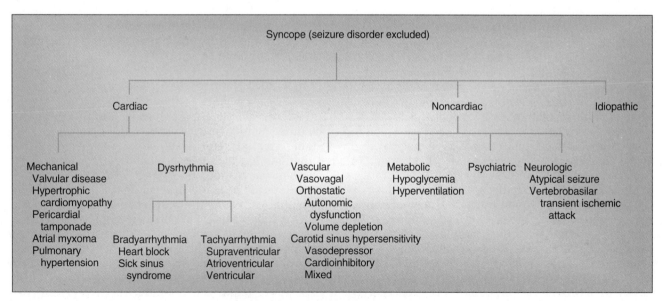

FIGURE 96–1. *Differential diagnosis of syncope.*

(heart rate slowing) responses, may be associated with micturition, defecation, coughing, the Valsalva maneuver, or straining. Vasovagal syncope is often heralded by premonitory symptoms, including nausea, sweating, and pallor. It usually occurs in younger patients. Syncope only in sitting or standing positions occurs with orthostatic or vasovagal syncope. Cardiac arrhythmias are often associated with abrupt-onset syncope without warning symptoms; fainting may occur while supine. Hypoglycemic syncope may be preceded by tremor, sweating, hunger, and headache. Cardiac syncope secondary to obstructive lesions is often exertional or postexertional. Fainting in elderly patients usually is not vasovagal but is due to other causes and is often multifactorial.

Physical Examination

A complete examination should be performed, including full neurologic assessment. Special emphasis should be placed on (1) measurement of the blood pressure and pulse rate in the supine, sitting, and standing positions; (2) careful cardiac examination for evidence of aortic stenosis, pulmonary hypertension, irregular rhythm, hypertrophic cardiomyopathy, or other conditions that could be related to fainting; and (3) examination of the carotid arteries. In patients without carotid pulse diminution or bruits, monitored carotid massage can be performed with an intravenous line established to determine whether carotid sinus hypersensitivity exists. The volume status should be assessed by estimating the central venous pressure from the jugular venous examination and by comparing the current to the usual weight. A careful mental status examination also should be performed.

Additional Evaluation

Laboratory Tests

Determination of the serum BUN and creatinine, along with the hematocrit, may assist in the diagnosis of significant plasma volume depletion, which would be manifested by an increased BUN to creatinine ratio and an elevated hematocrit. Blood glucose should be checked during near-syncope or syncope or as soon after an episode as possible, especially in diabetic patients taking insulin or oral hypoglycemic agents. An electrocardiogram should be obtained to screen for (1) prior myocardial infarction, (2) bifascicular or trifascicular disease, (3) prolonged QT interval, (4) delta waves indicative of pre-excitation, or (5) rate or rhythm abnormality. In patients with frequent symptoms, 24-hour Holter monitor testing may provide a diagnosis; ambulatory monitoring is less likely to be helpful in patients with infrequent symptoms. Echocardiography-Doppler study is valuable for the diagnosis of cardiac obstructive lesions and in assessing left ventricular global and regional function, looking for evidence of coronary artery disease or an arrhythmogenic substrate.

Special Studies

When the history, physical examination, and conventional testing fail to establish the cause of syncope, one or more of the following tests may be helpful.

1. **Cardiac event recorder**, which can be activated following an episode of syncope and which provides information about the heart rhythm during the preceding 4 minutes. It is especially helpful when symptoms are infrequent.
2. **Signal average electrocardiogram**, in which a computer analyzes several minutes of QRS complexes to determine whether or not low amplitude late potentials, indicative of ventricular scar tissue and potential susceptibility to malignant ventricular arrhythmias, are present. This examination is of greatest value in patients with coronary artery disease.
3. **Electrophysiologic testing** for evidence of sinus node dysfunction, conduction disease, or inducible tachyarrhythmias.
4. **Tilt table testing** to assess whether vagally mediated faints are present.

MANAGEMENT

The treatment of syncope involves both specific and nonspecific measures. Specific strategies are those tailored to the exact diagnosis. Examples include (1) pacemaker therapy for symptomatic bradyarrhythmias without an otherwise correctable cause (e.g., medications); (2) pharmacologic or nonpharmacologic (radiofrequency ablation, cryotherapy, or surgery) treatment of tachyarrhythmias; (3) withholding offensive medications when orthostatic hypotension is present (other measures for orthostatic dizziness or syncope in selected patients include support hose, mineralocorticoid therapy, and high-sodium diets); (4) surgery when mechanical cardiopulmonary causes are present, such as aortic valve replacement for aortic stenosis, heart-lung transplantation for primary pulmonary hypertension, and septal myectomy for hypertrophic cardiomyopathy with obstruction when medical therapy is ineffective; and (5) careful adjustment of insulin or oral hypoglycemic agents when hypoglycemia is deemed the cause of syncope.

PATIENT AND FAMILY EDUCATION

Patients should be taught syncope precautions, including avoidance of driving until determined to be stable (as per state law), and avoidance of other situations in which a faint could be hazardous, such as climbing on a roof or working with power tools. The house should be made as syncope-safe as possible, with potential exposure to sharp corners and other sharp objects minimized. Patients should be instructed to assume the supine-with-legs-elevated position when dizzy in an effort to abort frank syncope.

The family should be taught all these syncope precautions, and treatment measures should be fully explained. Family members, friends, and coworkers should learn cardiopulmonary resuscitation. In patients with as yet undiagnosed syncope, family members should learn to check the pulse and blood pressure, along with other observational information, during witnessed episodes.

NATURAL HISTORY/PROGNOSIS

Syncopal episodes may lead to considerable injury, particularly in elderly patients. Simple faints may be benign and self-limited, but cardiac syncope carries a 20%–30% yearly mortality. The mortality rate for unexplained syncope approaches 10%. Thus, an aggressive effort should be made to establish the exact cause of syncope, particularly in older patients.

Research Questions

1. Half of syncopal episodes currently remain unexplained despite comprehensive testing. What newer technologies can be developed to improve this diagnostic capability?
2. Can we improve the sensitivity and specificity of current tests for syncope and their ability to predict which treatment measures will be successful?

Case Resolution

The patient's diagnosis was orthostatic syncope related to volume depletion, resulting from vomiting and diarrhea secondary to a viral illness. Additionally, his nitrate and β-blocker therapy impaired the usual hemodynamic responses to volume depletion. He was admitted to the hospital for 1 day for intravenous volume repletion and was educated about slow position changes. His cardiac medications were resumed once he was stabilized. Because of his left bundle branch block, recurrence of syncope or near-syncope would warrant consideration of electrophysiologic testing, i.e., to determine whether intermittent infra-His heart block or ventricular arrhythmias were causative.

Selected Readings

Fitzpatrick, A. P., G. Theodorakis, P. Vardas, et al. Methodology of head-up tilt testing in patients with unexplained syncope. J Am Coll Cardiol 17:125–30, 1991.

Friedman, H. H. Syncope. In H. H. Friedman (ed.). *Problem-oriented Medical Diagnosis,* 5th ed. Boston, Little, Brown & Co., 1991.

Hanlon, J. T., M. Linzer, J. P. MacMillan, et al. Syncope and presyncope associated with probable adverse drug reactions. Arch Intern Med 150:2309–12, 1990.

Lipsitz, L. A. Syncope in the elderly. Ann Intern Med 99:92–105, 1983.

Manolis, A. S., M. Linzer, D. Salem, et al. Syncope: Current diagnostic evaluation and management. Ann Intern Med 112:850–63, 1990.

Winters, S. L., D. Stewart, and A. Gomes. Signal averaging of the surface QRS complex predicts inducibility of ventricular tachycardia in patients with syncope of unknown origin: A prospective study. J Am Coll Cardiol 10:775–81, 1987.

CHAPTER 97

SEIZURE DISORDERS

Douglas R. Jeffery, M.D., Ph.D.

Hₓ A 42-year-old right-handed male software engineer complains of spells in which he blacks out. These spells began about a month earlier and have occurred on four occasions. The patient states that he has some warning of their onset. He feels as though his stomach is "rising," and he has an intense sense of fear. His left arm tightens and starts to shake. Sometimes he smells an odor that he likens to burning plastic. This is usually the last thing he recalls. After a typical event, he feels confused and often is not sure where he is or even what day or month it is. He is fatigued and sleeps for several hours after the event. He reluctantly admits that urinary incontinence accompanies these episodes. Further questioning reveals that he was involved in an auto accident a year ago and was knocked unconscious for about 20 minutes. He suffered an injury to the right side of his head and for several weeks following the accident had persistent headaches. He has no other significant past medical history and no other complaints. He denies chest pain or palpitations with these episodes. The physical and neurologic examinations are entirely normal.

Questions

1. What do these episodes of loss of consciousness represent? What is the differential diagnosis of blackouts?
2. What factors in this case argue against a cardiac cause? Which aspects of the history suggest a seizure?

3. How would you proceed with more definitive diagnostic evaluation? How would you proceed with treatment?
4. Would you advise this patient to modify his life-style? If so, what activities would you advise against?

Epilepsy is one of the most common neurologic disorders encountered in the outpatient setting. Current estimates of prevalence range from 2 to 22 cases per thousand. This corresponds to about 2% of the population or about 4 million patients in the United States. Epilepsy may be described as an intermittent aberration of nervous system function due to the sudden and excessively disordered discharge of cerebral neurons. The resultant aberration of nervous system function is referred to as the seizure, or ictus, and may take on both convulsive and nonconvulsive forms. The convulsive forms, in which the patient experiences a generalized tonic-clonic convulsion (characterized by generalized tonic excitation of all muscles followed by relaxation and then again by tonic activity), are easily recognized. Nonconvulsive forms, characterized by alterations of consciousness and unusual stereotyped repetitive behaviors known as automatisms, often go unrecognized and hence undiagnosed.

Seizures will often occur as a single event, especially in patients who are currently controlled on antiseizure medication. Seizures may repeat themselves in the same setting. When seizures occur in succession such that the patient fails to completely regain consciousness between seizures or when seizures are so frequent or prolonged as to create a fixed and lasting epileptic condition, the patient is said to be in status epilepticus. This is a neurologic emergency that requires immediate intervention.

Seizures may either be idiopathic or occur as the result of acquired cerebral or systemic disease. Patients with idiopathic epilepsy tend to have generalized seizures in which there is a bilaterally symmetric onset without localizing signs. These patients will usually have their first seizure in adolescence. In contrast, patients with a secondary form of epilepsy tend to have their first seizure prior to the age of 10 years or after the age of 30 years.

PATHOPHYSIOLOGY

Seizures are generally considered to be a phenomenon of the cerebral cortex; therefore, lesions that give rise to seizure activity are generally located in the cortex. When a group of neurons initiates synchronous firing, there may be suppression of firing from neuronal inhibitory mechanisms. In the absence of adequate inhibition, there will be spread of abnormal electrical activity along fiber pathways. This spread may take place through efferent projections of the structure involved in ictal onset or through transsynaptic alterations in excitability; i.e., the activity may spread laterally from one axon to the next. Generalization of seizure activity depends on the ease of access from the site of initiation to other brain stem and forebrain structures and to the contralateral cortex. Once the abnormal electrical activity spreads to the opposite cortex, generalization has occurred.

DIFFERENTIAL DIAGNOSIS

Seizures represent a manifestation of underlying cerebral or systemic pathology, and a variety of possible causes exist (Table 97–1). In addition to structural lesions, a variety of metabolic abnormalities may give rise to seizures. The initial evaluation of a patient with new-onset seizures should include immediate measurement of glucose, calcium, magnesium, electrolytes, BUN, creatinine, liver function, and arterial ammonia (if indicated) and a toxicology screen. Because many of the conditions listed in Table 97–1 are potentially life-threatening neurologic disorders, any patient with new-onset seizure should undergo prompt diagnostic evaluation as an inpatient. A first seizure may serve as a forewarning that others will follow. The patient should be observed for 24 to 48 hours to ensure that there is no danger of status epilepticus.

While a comprehensive discussion of pseudoseizures is beyond the scope of this chapter, it should be noted that many patients with seizure-like symptoms actually have pseudoseizures. A pseudoseizure can be defined as a behavioral seizure not associated with electroencephalographic evidence of a seizure. Even well-trained observers may have difficulty distinguishing pseudoseizures from true seizures. If the treating clinician suspects that pseudoseizures are complicating the treatment or evaluation of a patient, it may be advantageous to refer the patient to a neurologist for ambulatory or video electroencephalogram (EEG) recordings.

Classification

The international classification of epileptic seizures is probably the most widely accepted classification sys-

---

TABLE 97–1. Differential Diagnosis of Cerebral Lesions Associated with Seizures

Infectious
Meningitis
Brain abscess
Viral encephalitis

Vascular
Arteriovenous malformation
Cerebral aneurysm
Stroke
Vasculitis
Cortical vein thrombosis

Neoplastic
Glioma
Meningioma
Metastasis

Metabolic
Hepatic encephalopathy
Uremic encephalopathy
Nonketotic hyperosmolar state
Hyponatremia
Hypoglycemia
Hypomagnesemia
Drug withdrawal (e.g., alcohol, benzodiazepines, barbiturates)

tem for seizure type (Table 97–2). It is not a classification system for epileptic syndromes; rather, it attempts to classify seizure types. This system categorizes seizures as either partial (seizures which begin focally) or generalized (seizures which are bilaterally symmetric without focal onset). It further divides partial seizures into those without alteration of consciousness (simple) and those associated with alteration of consciousness (complex). Seizures which begin focally are said to be partial in onset. At any time after the start of the seizure, abnormal electrical activity may spread to involve the contralateral hemisphere (secondary generalization). An example is the patient whose seizure begins with a jerking motion of the hand. With spread of the abnormal electrical activity along the motor strip, the forearm and arm may become involved ("Jacksonian march"). The activity may then spread to the face or leg before the seizure generalizes with onset of bilateral tonic-clonic convulsions and loss of consciousness. This type of seizure would be classified as one with partial onset (motor) with secondary generalization.

A postictal state characterized by confusion and fatigue is common after most types of seizures. It is not seen after classic absence seizures, which primarily occur in children. In that type of seizure, there is primary generalized onset of three-per-second spike-and-wave discharges on the EEG. It is a primarily generalized seizure with bilaterally symmetric onset. In its classic form, onset is sudden and there is no loss of motor tone. The patient seems to stare into space and may exhibit some lip smacking behavior or other automatism. The event lasts about 20–30 seconds, after which the patient returns to consciousness unaware that anything has occurred. Patients usually note that they have missed a few words in a conversation.

This type of seizure should be distinguished from a complex partial or psychomotor seizure seen in adults. Many adult patients tell their physicians they have petit mal epilepsy when in fact they have complex partial events. Patients with complex partial seizures have a focal onset (partial) and associated alteration of consciousness (complex). In true absence or petit mal epilepsy, the seizure is generalized at onset. This type of epilepsy is common in children and rare in adults. Complex partial seizures are common in both children and adults. A good clinical history and an EEG are helpful in making the distinction between the two types of seizures. The distinction is important because treatment of the two disorders is substantially different. In addition, absence epilepsy tends to have a strong familial genetic component, whereas complex partial seizures are more often associated with underlying central nervous system (CNS) pathology.

EVALUATION

History

The most important factor in the evaluation of any patient with new-onset seizures (or a previous history of epilepsy) is a careful and thorough clinical history. The patient should be questioned about the onset of the disorder and its relationship to antecedent events such

TABLE 97–2. International Classification of Epileptic Seizures

I. Partial (focal, local) seizures
  A. Simple partial seizures
    1. With motor signs
    2. With somatosensory or special sensory symptoms
    3. With autonomic symptoms or signs
    4. With psychic symptoms
  B. Complex partial seizures
    1. Simple partial onset followed by impairment of consciousness
    2. With impairment of consciousness at onset
  C. Partial seizures evolving to secondarily generalized seizures
    1. Simple partial seizures evolving to generalized seizures
    2. Complex partial seizures evolving to generalized seizures
    3. Simple partial seizures evolving to complex partial seizures evolving to generalized seizures
II. Generalized seizures (convulsive or nonconvulsive)
  A. Absence seizures
    1. Typical absences
    2. Atypical absences
  B. Myoclonic seizures
  C. Clonic seizures
  D. Tonic seizures
  E. Tonic-clonic seizures
  F. Atonic seizures (astatic seizures)
III. Unclassified epileptic seizures

as head injury, stroke, infection, or other illness. A carefully recorded description of seizure onset should be documented. Are there any warning signs such as nausea, odors, unusual sensations, motor signs, or feelings of fear or impending catastrophe? Many patients are able to tell when their seizures are forthcoming because of reliable warning signs. These warning signs are actually the beginning of the seizure and have electroencephalographic correlates. If the event has been witnessed by a family member or friend, the description can be helpful. The frequency of the seizures should be recorded as well as any triggering factors. Alcohol intoxication may lessen the likelihood of a seizure, but when blood alcohol levels fall, the likelihood of a seizure is greatly increased. Fatigue also will increase the likelihood of a seizure.

A history of a postictal state characterized by confusion and somnolence is important to obtain. In many patients with focal motor onset of seizures, the postictal state may be characterized by transient hemiparesis. This is known as Todd's paralysis and is thought to be mediated by postictal suppression of cortical neurons in the motor strip near the epileptogenic focus. The presence of Todd's paralysis in the postictal state may alert the physician to a seizure focus or other form of pathology along the motor strip. Except in patients with severe preexisting CNS disease, postictal paralysis should not last more than about 8 hours. A longer duration should prompt a search for more serious underlying pathology.

Neurologic Examination

The neurologic examination should include a careful search for focal deficits suggesting localized CNS pathology. Note should be made of the presence of bruits over the skull, a finding that suggests a possible arterio-

TABLE 97–3. Anticonvulsant Therapy for Seizure Disorders in Adults

Drug	Indication	Usual Adult Dose	Therapeutic Range	Major Adverse Effects
Phenytoin	Partial and generalized tonic-clonic seizures	300 mg/d	10–20 µg/mL	Fatigue, impaired concentration, blurred vision, postural imbalance, gingival hyperplasia, coarsening of features
Carbamazepine	Partial and generalized tonic-clonic seizures	200 mg twice daily to 1800 mg/d	4–12 µg/mL	Nausea, ataxia, postural imbalance, diplopia, impaired concentration
Valproic acid	Absence seizures, partial and generalized tonic-clonic seizures	250 mg twice daily to 1.5 g/d	50–100 µg/mL	Drowsiness, tremor, nausea, vomiting
Phenobarbital	Partial and generalized tonic-clonic seizures	90–120 mg/d in 2–3 divided doses	25–40 µg/mL	Sedation, vertigo, unsteadiness, impaired concentration
Primidone	Partial and generalized tonic-clonic seizures	250 mg twice daily	5–12 µg/mL	Sedation, impaired concentration, imbalance, unsteadiness

venous malformation (AVM). Other helpful signs include asterixis and tremulousness consistent with a metabolic encephalopathy.

Additional Evaluation

Neuroimaging is generally the next step. An MRI study is usually more sensitive than a CT scan for detecting lesions such as a brain tumor, brain abscess, stroke, AVM, or posttraumatic encephalomalacia (focal atrophy). Hemorrhage may be seen more easily on CT scan. If an MRI is not available, a CT scan may suffice. However, a noncontrast CT scan will frequently miss small tumors, brain abscesses, and other small structural lesions.

If the patient has a fever or other evidence of infection, a lumbar puncture is indicated if the initial imaging study suggests no evidence of a mass lesion and demonstrates free communication between ventricular spaces. If a mass lesion is identified, lumbar puncture may be contraindicated because of the risk of fatal herniation when significant pressure gradients exist. A lumbar puncture should not be attempted in the absence of an imaging study showing that all ventricular spaces are in free communication. If bacterial meningitis is suspected as a cause of new onset seizures, the patient should be treated immediately with antibiotics. Lumbar puncture can be delayed until the imaging study has been carried out. A brain abscess that has ruptured into the ventricle may mimic bacterial meningitis, and the risk of herniation following lumbar puncture can be quite high, especially if mass effect has occluded the flow of cerebrospinal fluid.

An EEG should always be obtained in patients with new-onset seizures. However, the absence of abnormalities on EEG should not be taken as evidence that a seizure disorder is not present. An initial abnormal EEG in patients suffering from known seizure disorders occurs about 65% of the time. With a second EEG, about 80% of such patients will show an abnormality. After

the third EEG, 85%–90% will show an abnormality. The most important piece of evidence suggesting a seizure disorder is the clinical history.

MANAGEMENT

Six main anticonvulsants are generally used in the treatment of adult seizure disorders: phenytoin, carbamazepine, valproic acid, phenobarbital and primidone (Table 97–3). The choice depends on the type of seizure. In general, the first rule of anticonvulsant therapy is to maximize control of seizures with one agent prior to the addition of a second compound. If adequate control cannot be achieved with one agent, then another compound can be added. Monotherapy greatly simplifies anticonvulsant therapy in addition to minimizing side effects associated with anticonvulsant use. With any anticonvulsant, the most common cause of breakthrough seizures is subtherapeutic drug levels. Side effects associated with most of these agents can be minimized by starting the drug at a low dose and slowly adjusting the dose upward to maintain it within the therapeutic range.

PATIENT AND FAMILY EDUCATION

Certain activities may need to be restricted, at least temporarily. For example, in most states there are laws stipulating that patients who have had a generalized seizure not drive until they have been seizure-free for 1 year. The physician must make the patient aware of such laws and carefully document that the patient has been informed and understands that there is a risk of breakthrough seizure activity while driving. The same consideration holds true for operating heavy or other potentially dangerous equipment. Otherwise, the presence of a seizure disorder need not prevent the patient from engaging in most normal activities. Patients should be cautioned against the use of alcohol and against excessive fatigue.

NATURAL HISTORY/PROGNOSIS

Approximately 40% of patients who suffer a first seizure and have no underlying CNS pathology will never have another seizure. For this reason, patients who suffer a first seizure and have no demonstrable CNS pathology are not routinely started on anticonvulsant medication.

Conversely, some patients will have recurrent seizures the frequency of which may vary from one or two per year to as many as several a week. For the latter group, referral to a neurologist is advisable. Those who have seizures only once or twice yearly can usually be managed by a primary care physician provided the proper therapeutic guidelines are followed.

Case Resolution

The patient had posttraumatic epilepsy most likely due to the presence of focal cortical glial scarring that formed as a result of his head injury. This served as an irritative focus giving rise to aberrant electrical activity at the site of injury.

Selected Readings

Engel, J. *Seizures and Epilepsy.* Philadelphia, F. A. Davis Company, 1989.
Forster, F. M., and H. E. Booker. The epilepsies and convulsive disorders. *In* R. J. Joynt (ed.). *Clinical Neurology.* Philadelphia, J. B. Lippincott Company, 1989.

CHAPTER 98

UNILATERAL WEAKNESS OR NUMBNESS

Askiel Bruno, M.D., and Molly K. King, M.D.

Hx A 69-year-old male retired tool-and-die maker presents with numbness and weakness of the right arm, which he noticed on awakening 10 hours ago. He denies any difficulty with vision or speech or symptoms involving the right leg. He also denies a prior history of right arm symptoms. He claims he drinks three to four "mixed drinks" most nights of the week but denies a history of recent or distant trauma, seizures, or delirium tremens. The rest of his medical history is noncontributory. The neurologic examination shows weak finger and wrist extensors on the right. The triceps, biceps, and deltoid muscles have normal strength bilaterally. The tendon reflexes are normal and symmetric in both upper extremities. Sensation to both light touch and pinprick is diminished over the dorsum of the right hand and forearm. The remainder of the physical examination is normal.

Questions

1. What is the most probable location of the lesion (or lesions) causing this patient's symptoms and signs?
2. What is the differential diagnosis?
3. What additional questions should the patient be asked?
4. What tests would be useful and why?

Unilateral weakness and numbness are common neurologic complaints. Any interruption of the motor or sensory pathways, from the cerebral cortex to the peripheral nerves and muscles, can result in one or both symptoms. Since the differential is so broad, a systematic approach to diagnosis is essential.

PATHOPHYSIOLOGY

The primary motor system originates in the motor cortex, located within the precentral gyrus of the frontal lobe. The fibers from these neurons travel through the subcortical white matter, the internal capsule, and the brain stem, crossing to the contralateral side at the level of the medullary pyramids. As they make their way down the ventrolateral columns of the spinal cord, these upper motor neurons synapse with lower motor neurons, which then carry the motor signals out through the ventral spinal roots—and the brachial and lumbar plexuses—to the individual peripheral nerves. Finally, these peripheral nerves synapse with their associated muscles, enabling muscle contraction and relaxation.

Pain, temperature, and touch are detected by sensory nerve endings throughout the skin. These sensory nerves then travel proximally along the peripheral nervous system until they enter the spinal cord. Near their point of entry, these sensory nerves cross to the contralateral side of the cord and ascend via the lateral columns through the brain stem to the ventral posterior nuclei of the thalami. The thalami are the main relay stations for sensory input. Within each thalamus, sensory nerves synapse with secondary neurons traveling to the primary somatosensory cortex, located within the postcentral gyrus of the parietal lobe. The primary somatosensory cortex is separated from the primary motor cortex (located in the adjacent frontal lobe) only by the fissure of Rolando.

DIFFERENTIAL DIAGNOSIS

Weakness and numbness can be unilateral or bilateral. Since a common problem in primary care practice is determining whether unilateral symptoms are due to a peripheral lesion (e.g., radiculopathy or compressive neuropathy) or to a more serious central lesion (e.g., stroke or brain tumor), this chapter deals exclusively with this issue. Suffice it to say that **bilateral extremity numbness or weakness** is usually caused by peripheral neuropathy (with diabetes and excessive alcohol use being the two most common etiologies) or myelopathy.

Unilateral weakness or numbness can be caused by disease affecting any of the sites along the motor or sensory pathways, including the brain, spinal cord, nerve roots, brachial or lumbar plexuses, peripheral nerves, or their associated muscles. For the sake of simplicity, the most common of these various disorders can be considered as being either central or peripheral.

Central Causes of Unilateral Numbness or Weakness

Central disorders that can cause unilateral weakness or numbness include stroke, transient ischemic attacks, subdural hematoma, brain tumor, brain abscess, multiple sclerosis, and migraine aura.

Stroke

Stroke is the most common central cause of unilateral weakness or numbness. Strokes can be either ischemic (80%) or hemorrhagic (20%). Ischemic strokes are caused by vascular occlusion due to (1) thrombosis without embolism; (2) embolism from the heart or from an atherosclerotic vessel; or less commonly, (3) vasoconstriction and focal cerebral hypoperfusion secondary to systemic hypotension. Cerebral vasoconstriction is the likely mechanism of the cerebral ischemia that can accompany migraine, subarachnoid hemorrhage, or abuse of sympathomimetic drugs (e.g., amphetamines, cocaine). Hemorrhagic strokes are caused by the rupture of a blood vessel with subsequent bleeding into the brain parenchyma or the subarachnoid space, the location of the hemorrhage depending on the location of the ruptured vessel.

Two key features of stroke are that (1) neurologic symptoms develop suddenly and (2) the symptoms can be explained by one lesion. Symptoms that develop slowly over days or weeks are very unlikely to represent a stroke. In that situation, an expanding cerebral lesion (e.g., tumor or abscess) is more likely.

Transient Ischemic Attacks (TIAs)

Transient ischemic attacks are defined as focal cerebral dysfunction due to focal cerebral ischemia, with symptoms that completely resolve within 24 hours. More than 90% of TIAs, in fact, last an hour or less. It is extremely important to distinguish TIAs from other transient "spells," since TIAs are often harbingers of subsequent cerebral infarction, and early initiation of treatment may prevent a stroke. In addition to unilateral weakness or numbness, the symptoms of carotid (anterior) circulation TIAs may include speech disturbance or amaurosis fugax (a perception of a veil or curtain descending over one eye); of note, however, numbness/weakness and eye symptoms almost never occur during the same episode. The symptoms of vertebrobasilar (posterior) circulation TIAs include combinations of vertigo, diplopia, dysarthria, dysphagia, and homonymous hemianopsia. TIA symptoms develop suddenly; when neurologic symptoms develop in a stepwise manner and progress from one area of the body to another in a noticeable sequence, a focal seizure or the aura of migraine is a more likely diagnosis.

Subdural Hematoma (SDH)

Subdural hematoma is an accumulation of blood between the dura and the arachnoid layers of the brain meninges. It compresses the brain and in severe cases can cause brain herniation. Early symptoms of SDH include focal numbness and weakness and a decreased level of consciousness. SDH should be suspected in the setting of head trauma, pharmacologic anticoagulation, or a bleeding disorder, especially in the elderly.

Brain Tumor

Brain tumors often present with focal weakness or numbness; unlike strokes, however, the symptoms usually progress relatively slowly, over days to weeks. Other associated (but not pathognomonic) symptoms include headaches and seizures. The exact symptoms and the rate of progression depend on tumor type and location. A history of extracranial malignancy (especially in the lung or breast) should lead to suspicion of a metastatic brain tumor. Meningiomas and gliomas account for approximately 60% of primary brain tumors in adults.

Brain Abscess

A brain abscess is another cause of weakness or numbness that progresses over days to weeks, and it thus resembles a rapidly growing brain tumor in its presentation. Brain abscesses are usually associated with headaches and signs of infection such as fever and leukocytosis. Causative organisms either reach the brain hematogenously (e.g., from the heart or lungs) or via contiguous spread from adjacent sites (e.g., the sinuses or middle ear).

Multiple Sclerosis (MS)

Multiple sclerosis often begins as focal numbness or weakness, with symptoms arising either relatively abruptly or over days to weeks. Although MS can occur at any age, its onset is most common in the 30 to 40-year-old age group. MS is distinguished from other neurologic disorders by its constellation of progressive or relapsing symptoms, which include (in addition to numbness and weakness) visual disturbances, bladder dysfunction, and incoordination.

Migraine

Migraine is common, affecting approximately 15% of the adult population. A migraine aura can consist of unilateral numbness or weakness in addition to visual symptoms such as bright lights or zigzag lines. These symptoms typically last 10–15 minutes and may or may not be followed by a headache. A key characteristic of the migraine aura is the relatively slow progression of symptoms, i.e., numbness that spreads from the face to the arm to the leg over several minutes. If such symptoms are associated with headache or nausea—or if the patient has a several year history of similar spells without serious sequelae—the diagnosis of migraine can be made with relative confidence.

Peripheral Causes of Unilateral Numbness or Weakness

Peripheral causes of unilateral numbness or weakness include neuropathies and radiculopathies; these should be suspected when symptoms are limited to only one extremity or to the face alone. In such situations, the distribution of numbness or weakness typically follows the known distribution of a particular peripheral nerve or nerve root. More extensive symptoms can result from dysfunction of multiple nerve roots (polyradiculopathy), the brachial or lumbar plexuses, or multiple peripheral nerves.

Most neuropathies or radiculopathies causing unilateral numbness or weakness are compressive in nature; i.e., they result from extrinsic pressure to the nerve or nerve root. However, it is important to keep in mind that other pathologic processes can lead to similar symptoms (e.g., radiculopathy due to herpes zoster or isolated neuropathy due to diabetes mellitus).

Radiculopathy

Radiculopathy typically causes pain or dysesthesia, an unpleasant "pins and needles" sensation. If the radiculopathy persists, focal numbness or weakness (as well as reflex loss) can also develop. Cervical and lumbar (or lumbosacral) radiculopathies are common causes of arm and leg pain, respectively (see Chapters 88, 90, 91, and 93).

Peripheral Neuropathy

These common causes of numbness or weakness in the upper extremity include (1) carpal tunnel syndrome, a pressure neuropathy of the median nerve that typically produces numbness and dysesthesias of the palmar surface of the thumb, index finger, middle finger, and the radial half of the ring finger; (2) ulnar neuropathy, causing numbness of the medial forearm, the fifth finger, and the ulnar half of the ring finger; and (3) radial nerve palsy, which results in weakness of finger and wrist extension.

BOX 98–1.   Key Questions to Ask Patients with Unilateral Weakness or Numbness

Where is the weakness or numbness located?
When did it begin?
Did the symptoms come on suddenly or gradually?
Have the symptoms improved, worsened, or remained the same since onset?
Is pain also present? If so, where is it located?
If the symptoms are intermittent:
    Are there provoking or alleviating factors?
    How long do the episodes last?
    How often do they occur?
    What are they like?
    Are all episodes similar?

The most common compressive neuropathy affecting the lower extremity is peroneal palsy, which causes weakness in foot dorsiflexion and eversion.

Bell's palsy, affecting the facial nerve (cranial nerve VII) is the most common peripheral neuropathy of the head and face. Its cause is often not apparent.

EVALUATION

History

Box 98–1 lists some of the key questions to ask a patient presenting with unilateral weakness or numbness.

The **location** of symptoms often helps pinpoint the cause, especially if it corresponds to the known distribution of a specific nerve or nerve root.

For central lesions, the rapidity of symptom onset is the key to differentiating vascular (e.g., stroke or TIA) from nonvascular (e.g., brain tumor) disorders. Did maximal symptoms develop suddenly, or over hours, days, weeks, or months? Stroke symptoms typically arise suddenly or over hours, whereas symptoms due to mass lesions tend to progressively worsen over days, weeks, or months. Sometimes a patient's family or friends can add further information, and an effort should be made to question them whenever possible.

Important clues may also be found in the patient's medical, occupational, and recreational history. A history of head trauma or anticoagulation raises the possibility of a subdural hematoma. Patients with a present or prior history of malignancy should be assessed for brain metastases or other neoplasm-related causes of their neurologic symptoms. Intravenous drug users are predisposed to developing brain abscesses (often secondary to septic emboli from an infected heart valve), cerebral lymphoma or toxoplasmosis (if they are HIV-positive), and strokes (if they are abusing amphetamines or cocaine).

Neurologic Examination

A thorough neurologic examination should be performed in all patients who present with a history of numbness or weakness. However, in patients with TIAs, the symptoms (by definition) are transitory, and a neurologic examination performed after the event will most likely be entirely normal. If TIAs are suspected, however, a systematic search should be made for possible sources of thromboemboli: the heart should be auscultated for murmurs and the carotid arteries carefully examined for bruits. However, recent evidence indicates that carotid bruits may be absent in up to 40% of patients with severe (> 70%) carotid stenosis.

Motor System Examination

In a patient complaining of weakness, the examination can determine whether the weakness is of the upper or lower motor neuron type (Table 98–1). Upper motor neuron dysfunction is caused by brain or spinal cord lesions, while lower motor neuron dysfunction is caused by lesions of the peripheral nervous system. The distribution of weakness should be meticulously assessed; e.g., is the entire hand weak or only muscles innervated by the radial nerve or the C7 nerve root?

Somatosensory System Examination

Examination of the somatosensory system is largely dependent on patient cooperation and, as a result, it is often more difficult to perform and interpret than is the motor examination. First, the patient should be asked to point out all areas of numbness, dysesthesia, and, if present, pain. When a patient's description of sensory symptoms corresponds to the distribution of a particular nerve or nerve root, then that is probably the affected structure. A careful sensory examination should then be performed, including assessment of both light touch sensation and pinprick sensation (e.g., using a discardable sharp object such as the pointed end of a split cotton swab).

Additional Evaluation

Once a diagnosis is made, blood tests can occasionally provide information about the underlying etiology. If, for example, carpal tunnel syndrome is diagnosed based on the history and physical examination,

then obtaining a blood glucose and thyroid-stimulating hormone (TSH) level will help determine whether diabetes mellitus or hypothyroidism is a contributing factor.

CT scanning and MRI are extremely valuable adjuncts in the diagnosis of cerebral lesions. CT helps distinguish ischemic from hemorrhagic stroke and should be performed as soon as possible after a patient presents with stroke symptoms. If CT done in the acute period is negative, the stroke is ischemic (i.e., nonhemorrhagic). If, after the initial CT scan, stroke location is uncertain or a brain stem or cerebellar stroke is suspected, MRI should be performed.

MRI is also the test of choice when brain tumor, brain abscess, or multiple sclerosis is suspected. In addition, MRI can be of benefit when a persistent radiculopathy is high on the differential, since it clearly delineates the vertebral bodies, the spinal canal, and the intervertebral foramina and disks.

If the patient presents with either a mild ischemic stroke or a TIA in the territory of the carotid artery—and the patient is a potential candidate for carotid endarterectomy—a carotid ultrasound should be performed to determine the degree of stenosis. If a stenotic lesion > 70% is identified (and a carotid endarterectomy is felt to be in the patient's best interests), a cerebral arteriogram should be performed to confirm the degree of stenosis and to evaluate the cerebral circulation for other possible anomalies such as aneurysms or arteriovenous malformations.

If a patient with an ischemic stroke or a TIA has evidence of heart disease (e.g., a murmur, significant left ventricular dysfunction, a recent myocardial infarction, or atrial fibrillation), an echocardiogram should be performed. Transesophageal echocardiography can be used to detect abnormalities not visible on the transthoracic approach.

Electromyography (EMG) is often helpful in further evaluating the patient with lower motor neuron weakness. By testing individual muscles, EMG can localize the lesion to a single nerve root, a single nerve, or multiple sites. In addition, EMG can provide information about the severity and chronicity of nerve injuries and can also indicate whether myopathy is present. Similarly, nerve conduction velocity (NCV) studies are useful in demonstrating sensory neuropathies and the slowing of conduction across compression points such as the

---

TABLE 98–1. Key Clinical Features of Upper vs. Lower Motor Neuron Weakness

Clinical Feature	Type of Motor Neuron Weakness	
	Upper	**Lower**
Facial weakness	Lower face only; sparing of muscles of forehead and eye closure	Lower and upper face, including muscles of eye closure (orbicularis oculi)
Hand weakness	Usually all hand muscles affected; painless	Only muscles innervated by a particular nerve or nerve root affected; often painful
Muscle tone	Increased several weeks after onset	Normal or decreased
Muscle bulk	Normal	Decreased several weeks after onset
Tendon reflexes	Increased several days after onset	Decreased from the beginning
Babinski reflex	Present from onset	Always absent

carpal tunnel (median nerve) and the medial epicondyle (ulnar nerve).

MANAGEMENT

An extended discussion of management is beyond the scope of this chapter, especially since management so clearly depends on the specific diagnosis. Very briefly,

- Stroke victims should be hospitalized promptly, with a CT scan performed on an emergency basis to distinguish between an ischemic and a hemorrhagic event. Several neuron-protective and antithrombotic drugs are currently being evaluated for use in the acute stroke setting.
- To prevent recurrent ischemic strokes, aspirin is usually recommended at a dose of 80–325 mg daily. For patients unable to tolerate aspirin, ticlopidine—another antiplatelet agent—should be considered, though its use requires periodic monitoring of the CBC because of the risk of neutropenia during the first 3 months of treatment. If the risk of recurrent stroke is high (e.g., in patients with atrial fibrillation or severe left ventricular dysfunction), anticoagulation therapy with warfarin is recommended in the absence of contraindications.
- Carotid endarterectomy should be considered in selected patients with carotid circulation TIAs (or mild strokes) provided they are good surgical candidates, have a > 70% stenosis of the corresponding carotid artery, and the anticipated morbidity and mortality from arteriography and surgery are < 5%.
- Lastly, patients with atherosclerotic cerebrovascular disease require scrupulous "risk factor" reduction, including smoking cessation and optimal control of hypertension, diabetes, and hypercholesterolemia.
- Selected compression neuropathies (e.g., carpal tunnel syndrome) will sometimes improve with nonsurgical management; i.e., using a splint or brace to immobilize the wrist. Similarly, compression of a nerve root by a herniated intervertebral disk often resolves if the patient remains at rest for several days. However, appropriate surgical consultation should be obtained if symptoms due to compressive neuropathy or radiculopathy persist or if weakness develops; in such situations, decompression procedures can often relieve symptoms as well as help patients regain lost function.
- Appropriate specialty consultation should be obtained for optimal management of brain abscess, brain tumor, or multiple sclerosis.

PATIENT AND FAMILY EDUCATION

Successful management often depends as much (if not more) on a well-educated and motivated patient as on a knowledgeable physician. Whether it be compliance with risk factor reduction measures or adherence to recommended treatment modalities, patient coopera-

tion is essential if an effective therapeutic alliance is to be realized.

PROGNOSIS

The prognosis after stroke largely depends on its size and location. Most of the recovery usually occurs during the first 30 days following the insult. Prognosis is also affected by stroke recurrence and cardiovascular co-morbidity.

Overall, the incidence of cerebral infarction in patients who have had a TIA is approximately 10% over the subsequent 3 years, and a large majority of these strokes occur during the first year. In two situations, the risk of stroke following TIA is higher than usual, thus warranting a more aggressive approach. First, patients with TIA or mild stroke due to severe (> 70%) carotid stenosis have a 13% annual stroke rate when treated medically (i.e., aspirin and risk factor reduction). This stroke rate can be decreased to 4% per year by carotid endarterectomy. Second, patients with TIA or mild stroke due to nonrheumatic atrial fibrillation have a 15% annual stroke rate when treated with aspirin. This stroke rate can be reduced to 8% per year with warfarin anticoagulation.

The prognosis of brain tumors depends on the tumor type. Meningiomas can usually be cured by excision. A solitary brain metastasis can sometimes be resected, thus enabling good-quality survival. Aggressive cerebral gliomas are typically fatal within several months after diagnosis.

The prognosis for brain abscess is good if (1) the diagnosis is established at an early stage; (2) effective antibiotic therapy is started promptly; (3) the patient is not immunocompromised; and (4) surgery, if required, is performed in a timely fashion.

The prognosis following nerve decompression is best when the compression is relieved relatively early in the course, i.e., before severe weakness or atrophy develops. After relief of a compressive mononeuropathy, approximately 90% of patients will have a > 90% improvement within 3 months.

Research Questions

1. Can anything be done to arrest or reverse acute cerebral infarction? If so, what is the time limit beyond which irreversible brain damage occurs?
2. Which patients with TIAs have the greatest risk of developing cerebral infarction? How can this risk be reduced most effectively?
3. How can the recovery of a decompressed nerve be enhanced?

Case Resolution

The neurologic examination established the diagnosis of a radial nerve palsy. On further questioning of his wife, it was determined that the patient's intake of alcohol was greater than he initially admitted and that he had been "binging" the night before the onset of his symptoms. In addition, the wife reported that after his drinking bout her husband had been "out cold" for over a dozen hours, resulting in prolonged compression of the right radial nerve against the humerus ("Saturday night palsy"). The patient was treated with a right wrist splint and physical therapy, with eventual resolution of his symptoms after several weeks. He was also referred to an alcohol rehabilitation program for further counseling and follow-up.

Selected Readings

Bruno, A. Ischemic stroke: 1. Early, accurate diagnosis. 2. Optimal treatment and prevention. Geriatrics 48:26–34, 37–54, 1993.

Dyck, P. J., P. K. Thomas, J. W. Griffin, et al. (eds.). *Peripheral Neuropathy.* Philadelphia, W.B. Saunders Company, 1993.

European Atrial Fibrillation Trial Study Group. Secondary prevention in non-rheumatic atrial fibrillation after transient ischaemic attack or minor stroke. Lancet 342:1255–62, 1993.

North American Symptomatic Carotid Endarterectomy Trial Collaborators. Beneficial effect of carotid endarterectomy in symptomatic patients with high-grade carotid stenosis. N Engl J Med 325:445–53, 1991.

Pulsinelli, W. Pathophysiology of acute ischaemic stroke. Lancet 339:533–6, 1992.

Suave, J. S., K. E. Thorpe, et al. Can bruits distinguish high-grade from moderate symptomatic carotid stenosis? Ann Intern Med 120:633–7, 1994.

CHAPTER 99

DEMENTIA

F. Claude Manning, M.D.

H$_x$ A 79-year-old widow was brought into the clinic by her granddaughter, with whom she now lives, for evaluation of confusion. The family reports that 2 years ago the patient was living alone in her own home and managing well. At that time, they became aware of her failure to pay several bills and her withdrawal from social activities. While normally meticulous in her personal appearance, she was recently noted to wear the same soiled dress for several days and not to have bathed. Two months ago, she had become lost while returning home from grocery shopping. Now the granddaughter reports that the patient cannot remember the names of her two great-grandchildren. The patient has a medical history of hypertension, adult-onset diabetes mellitus, hysterectomy, and cholecystectomy. Her medications are propranolol for blood pressure and diphenhydramine for sleep. She has no known history of head injury and denies any acute neurologic symptoms. In fact, the patient states that she feels perfectly well and that nothing is wrong with her. The physical examination is normal.

Questions

1. What syndrome or symptom complex does this patient exhibit, and what are its most common causes?
2. How can the severity of her problem be quantified?
3. What testing would be appropriate to establish the most likely cause of her condition?
4. Could her medications be contributing to her confusion? If so, what pharmacologic mechanisms might be involved?

Dementia is a common condition among the elderly. The prevalence increases dramatically with advancing age, affecting an estimated 10%–15% of persons over the age of 65 years and 40% or more of persons over the age of 85 years. Dementing illnesses often lead to substantial degrees of disability and dependence, resulting in enormous financial and emotional burdens for families.

Dementia represents a variable symptom complex of global cognitive impairment. By definition, the cognitive deficit of dementia involves significant memory loss plus an impairment in at least one other area of higher intellectual function: language, orientation, problem solving, calculations, insight, or judgment. Although minor changes in memory may occur with normal aging, the cognitive impairment of dementia is severe enough to interfere with the patient's customary affairs of life. Dementia is an acquired condition that usually appears over a period of months to years, and the cognitive deficits are present in the context of a normal level of consciousness. To avoid confusion, other terms implying dementia (e.g., senility, chronic brain syndrome) should not be used.

PATHOPHYSIOLOGY

Approximately 90% of dementia cases result from neurodegenerative processes or vascular injury (or both). The underlying mechanisms of the neurodegenerative disorders remain largely unknown. Current theories implicate abnormal deposition of neurotoxic substances, endogenous production of free radicals, and environmental toxins as potential causes. Gradual degenerative loss of neurons ultimately leads to the onset of dementia symptoms.

Vascular dementias may occur as a result of sudden thrombotic or embolic occlusion of intracerebral arteries (major stroke) but more often are a result of the gradual accumulation of multiple small strokes (multi-infarct dementia). Some cases are caused by chronic ischemic injury to subcortical white matter and nuclei (Binswanger's dementia). Nonvascular mechanisms of dementia include infections, toxins, and metabolic disturbances.

The causes of dementia are classified by their underlying pathophysiologic mechanism (Table 99–1). Degenerative dementias are the most common form and typically develop insidiously. They tend to occur sporadically in the aging population, although a few cases are inherited. Alzheimer's disease is the most common dementing illness, accounting for 50%–70% of cases. Vascular diseases are next in frequency, occurring in 10%–20% of cases. Mixed degenerative and vascular disease are responsible for another 10%–20% of cases.

A diverse spectrum of other conditions may also cause the symptom complex of dementia. A wide variety of prescribed and over-the-counter medications have been associated with cognitive changes in the elderly. Common offenders include anticholinergics, antihypertensives, antihistamines, and narcotic-analgesics. Chronic alcoholism can cause dementia through subcortical injury related to thiamine deficiency (Wernicke-Korsakoff syndrome) as well as through direct cortical toxicity. Hyperthyroidism and hypothyroidism are the most common metabolic disorders that may present with significant cognitive changes in the elderly. Intracranial causes of dementia include chronic subdural hematoma, brain tumor, and normal pressure hydrocephalus. The last disorder is characterized by the triad of dementia, urinary incontinence, and gait disturbance.

A distinction has been drawn between those conditions affecting primarily cortical regions and those involving primarily subcortical areas. Dementia due to cortical conditions is characterized by more severe memory loss with primary deficits in the cortical functions of language (aphasia), recognition (agnosia), and sequencing of actions (apraxia). Subcortical dementias are identified by a pattern of slowed mentation, apathy, and poor concentration, often in association with motor abnormalities and urinary incontinence. While these designations may be helpful in some cases, many patients will be found to have both cortical and subcortical features. Some authors have also advocated the classification of dementias based upon the potential for reversing or arresting the condition.

TABLE 99–1. Some Causes of Dementia

Degenerative

Cortical
  Alzheimer's disease
  Pick's disease
Subcortical
  Huntington's disease
  Progressive supranuclear palsy
  Parkinson's disease
  Olivopontocerebellar atrophy
  Multiple system atrophy

Vascular

Multi-infarct dementia
Major single-infarct dementia
Multiple lacunar infarcts
Binswanger's dementia
Cerebral amyloid angiopathy
Chronic subdural hematoma*

Toxic

Drug intoxication*
Alcohol-associated dementia*
Heavy metal poisoning*

Infectious

Neurosyphilis*
AIDS dementia complex*
Prion dementias (including Creutzfeldt-Jakob disease)
Postencephalitis dementia
Chronic meningitis*

Metabolic

Hypothyroidism*
Hyperthyroidism*
Vitamin B_{12} deficiency*
Wilson's disease

Other

Normal pressure hydrocephalus*
Brain tumor*
Anoxic encephalopathy
Demyelinating disease
Cerebral vasculitis*

*Potentially reversible or arrestable condition.

DIFFERENTIAL DIAGNOSIS

Dementia must be distinguished from other causes of mental confusion. The most important and most common of these are delirium and depression. Both conditions are prevalent in the elderly population. Clinical recognition is critical, since both delirium and depression carry significant risks of morbidity and mortality, and both can be effectively treated.

Delirium, also referred to as acute confusional state, is characterized by the onset, usually over a period of hours to days, of global disturbances in attention and thinking. The confusion often follows a fluctuating course and is typically associated with changes in the level of consciousness, either agitation or obtundation. Delirium may result from a multitude of underlying conditions (Table 99–2) and is considered to be a manifestation of widespread cerebral dysfunction. In severe cases, delirium constitutes a medical emergency that requires urgent diagnosis and treatment.

Major depression may also cause symptoms of mental confusion. Cognitive abilities may be impaired in depression as a result of poor concentration, uninterest, and psychomotor retardation. In addition, some patients with severe depression develop psychotic features, such as delusions or hallucinations. Such cognitive changes in depression have been referred to as "pseudodementia" because of their similarity to the deficits of true dementia. In contrast to demented patients, persons with depression are usually very aware

---

TABLE 99–2. Some Causes of Delirium

Systemic Illnesses

Acute infections
 Pneumonia
 Urinary tract infection
 Intraabdominal infection
Hypoxemic or hypotensive conditions
 Acute myocardial infarction
 Pulmonary embolus
 Shock from any cause
Metabolic disorders
 Fluid and electrolyte disturbances
 Hypoglycemia
 Hepatic encephalopathy
 Uremia

Adverse Drug Effects

Intoxications
 Anticholinergic medications (antihistamines, antidepressants, antispasmodics, others)
 Narcotic analgesics
 Sedative-hypnotics
 Corticosteroids
 H$_2$-receptor blockers
Drug withdrawal
 Alcohol
 Sedative-hypnotics

Primary Cerebral Conditions

Acute stroke
Subdural hematoma
Brain tumor
Meningitis
Encephalitis

Miscellaneous

Sensory deprivation ("sundowning")
Postoperative delirium

---

of their cognitive difficulties and tend to exaggerate their forgetfulness. Patients with depression also exhibit other symptoms such as depressed affect, loss of pleasure from previously enjoyed activities, feelings of guilt or worthlessness, and changes in sleep and appetite.

EVALUATION

The diagnostic evaluation of the patient with dementia has four purposes: (1) to verify the presence of dementia and exclude other look-alike conditions, (2) to determine the severity of the dementia, (3) to recognize potentially treatable causes, and (4) to identify treatable coexistent conditions that may result in excessive and unnecessary morbidity. The most common causes of dementia can be diagnosed on the basis of history and physical examination, while less common causes may require additional testing.

History

The **onset, duration,** and **course** of the dementia should be elicited. For example, Alzheimer's disease usually begins insidiously and progresses gradually over a period of years, while vascular dementias may have sudden onset and a stepwise pattern of deterioration. In addition, the **nature of the cognitive impairment and associated behavioral symptoms** should be described. Difficulties with word finding, recognizing

faces, and getting properly dressed are typical in Alzheimer's disease. Patients with vascular and subcortical causes of dementia are more likely to experience gait difficulties and urinary incontinence early in the course of their illness.

The **medication history** should include questions about prescription, over-the-counter, and illicit drug use. In frail elderly persons, almost any drug should be suspected as a potential cause of cognitive impairment. Careful inquiry should be made about alcohol use, and the daily/weekly intake should be quantified. The past medical history should ascertain whether the patient has at any time had a **significant head injury**. A history of **hypertension, stroke,** or **arteriosclerotic cardiovascular disease** increases the likelihood of a vascular cause. A **family history** of dementia in middle age suggests an inheritable form of dementia, such as Huntington's disease or familial Alzheimer's disease.

Physical Examination

In performing the physical examination, the physician should look for evidence of systemic disease. Findings of cardiopulmonary disease, infection, or metabolic disorders (e.g., hypo- or hyperthyroidism) may suggest an underlying cause or exacerbating component of the dementia. A thorough neurologic examination should be performed. Focal neurologic deficits can be associated with a vascular cause, such as multi-infarct dementia, or space-occupying lesions, such as subdural hematoma or tumor. Nonfocal neurologic signs, such as gait disturbances, tremor, or frontal release signs (snout or grasp reflexes), may be present in degenerative dementias.

An important addition to the usual physical examination is an appraisal of mental status. The assessment of orientation to person, place, and time, although important, is not sufficient. Mental status testing should also include evaluations of level of consciousness, affect, memory (short-and long-term), language abilities (e.g., naming, repeating, reading, and writing), attention and concentration (calculations and/or spelling), and the ability to copy geometric drawings or to draw a clock face. The use of a standardized mental status test, such as the Mini-Mental State Examination, offers three advantages: (1) it improves the reliability and validity of testing by different observers at different times, (2) it helps to quantify the severity of dementia, and (3) it provides a rough measure of disease progression on subsequent evaluations.

Additional Evaluation

Additional testing is usually warranted to exclude occult causes of dementia not detectable by the history and physical examination. A battery of laboratory studies has been recommended to detect potential metabolic or infectious conditions (Table 99–3). Controversy exists as to the necessity of a neuroimaging study in the evaluation of dementia. Some authorities recommend either a CT scan or MRI study of the head in all

---

TABLE 99–3. Recommended Studies in the Evaluation of Dementia

---

Complete blood count (CBC)
Sedimentation rate
Chemistry panel including glucose, electrolyte, calcium, creatinine, and liver function determinations
Urinalysis
Thyroid-stimulating hormone (TSH) level
Vitamin B_{12} level
Syphilis serology (RPR, VDRL)
HIV test, if indicated by risk factors

---

demented patients to look for subdural hematomas, brain tumors, normal pressure hydrocephalus, or undetected strokes. Others suggest that these studies may be reasonably limited to those patients with particular features (Table 99–4). When indicated by other findings, electroencephalography and lumbar puncture may be required.

MANAGEMENT

Management of the demented patient can be a difficult yet rewarding process. It requires a balanced approach that utilizes patient education, family counseling, drug therapy, and behavioral and environmental therapies. An important goal is to reduce excess morbidity by treating any associated medical diseases and depression. Equally important is to avoid and eliminate the use of unnecessary medications. Behavioral measures should be directed at providing a safe, familiar, and predictable living environment that reduces cognitive demands on the patient while allowing the opportunity to perform retained functional skills. Institutional care is often precipitated by the development of urinary incontinence or severe behavioral complications such as agitation or wandering.

Specific drug therapy for the cognitive deficit in Alzheimer's disease is now available. Tacrine is a centrally acting cholinesterase inhibitor that enhances cholinergic neurotransmission and may provide modest clinical improvement in some patients with mild to moderate Alzheimer's disease. Severe agitation or distressing psychotic symptoms may require cautious treatment with anxiolytic or antipsychotic medications, but all these drugs carry significant risks of adverse effects.

TABLE 99–4. Indications for CT Scan of the Head in Evaluation of Dementia

---

Recent onset of dementia
Rapid progression
Atypical presentation
Age less than 70 years
History of head trauma
Unexplained focal neurologic findings
Early urinary incontinence or gait disturbance

PATIENT AND FAMILY EDUCATION

Opinions differ over whether patients should be informed of the diagnosis of Alzheimer's disease or a related disorder. In most situations, the ethical principle of truthfulness would support the patient's right to participate in decision making, especially early in the disease course. The diagnosis should be explained in understandable terms, avoiding medical terminology and jargon. Patients and their families should be encouraged to establish advanced directives for medical care, including a living will and durable power of attorney.

Family members are often faced with increasing demands in response to the progressive dependency of demented patients. These demands place heavy emotional and financial burdens on care givers, who experience a confusing array of emotions, including anger, fear, and guilt. Medical providers should provide families with referral sources for educational materials, financial and legal advice, and support groups. All these services are usually available through local chapters of the Alzheimer's Association. Advice regarding respite services and residential or institutional care facilities should be offered before they become necessary.

NATURAL HISTORY/PROGNOSIS

Alzheimer's disease exhibits a gradual progression from mild memory problems in the early stages to an essentially vegetative state in the final stages. The time from clinical onset to death may vary from 2 to 15 years. Death usually results from malnutrition or pneumonia. Vascular forms of dementia typically have a more variable course of stepwise decline, and death often is due to other manifestations of vascular disease.

Research Questions

1. What is the role of amyloid protein in the pathophysiology of Alzheimer's disease?
2. Which areas of the brain are most crucial in the formation, retention, and recall of memory?

Case Resolution

The patient's mental status examination revealed a dementia of moderate severity. Recommended laboratory studies were all within normal limits. Both of her medications were discontinued successfully, and she subsequently showed significant improvement in her personal hygiene and capacity for self-care. However, the patient's memory and orientation did not improve appreciably, and she continues to reside with her granddaughter. The diagnosis was "probable" Alzheimer's disease; definitive diagnosis would require neuropathologic confirmation. The patient's granddaughter regularly attends support group meetings as recommended by the treating physician.

Selected Readings

Dilsaver, S. C. The mental status examination. Am Fam Physician 41(5):1489–96, 1990.

Foley, J. M., C. K. Cassel, P. Eastman, et al: Differential diagnosis of dementing diseases. JAMA 258:3411–6, 1987.

Katzman, R., and J. E. Jackson. Alzheimer disease: Basic and clinical advances. J Am Geriatr Soc 39:516–25, 1991.

Lipowski, J. Delirium (acute confusional states). JAMA 258:1789–92, 1987.

McKhann, G., D. Drachman, M. Folstein, et al: Clinical diagnosis of Alzheimer's disease: Report of the NINCDS-ADRDA Work Group under the auspices of Department of Health and Human Services Task Force on Alzheimer's Disease. Neurology 34:939–44, 1984.

Winograd, C. H., and L. F. Jarvik. Physician management of the demented patient. J Am Geriatr Soc 34:295–308, 1986.

SECTION XVII

COMMON PSYCHIATRIC PROBLEMS

CHAPTER 100

ANXIETY

Jonathan Lisansky, M.D.

H$_x$ A 47-year-old female complains of sudden attacks of shortness of breath, dizziness, heart palpitations, chest pain, and feeling like "the world is somehow unreal." She has had four attacks in the past month. Two occurred while she was driving to work and one occurred at work. One attack woke her up at night. During an attack, she feels like she is "ill and going to die." She also reports that she hates her job. She works at a children's hospital as a social worker and feels overwhelmed by the apparent expectation that she solve everyone's problems. There is a strong family history of alcoholism and anxiety in first-degree relatives. Her physical examination is normal.

Questions

1. What is the differential diagnosis? What is the most likely diagnosis?
2. What is the role of genetic predisposition in this disorder?
3. How common is this disorder?
4. What impact will the stress the patient experiences at work have on her recovery?

Symptoms of anxiety account for approximately 11% of all visits to primary care physicians; 18% of patients in primary care practices are prescribed minor tranquilizers, primarily to treat the symptoms associated with the anxiety disorders listed in Table 100–1. Approximately 2.9 million persons in the United States and approximately 6.5% of primary care patients suffer from panic disorder. One in five of these individuals receives treatment for this problem. Additionally, 15% of Vietnam veterans, 9% of Persian Gulf veterans, and one third of rape victims suffer from posttraumatic stress disorder (PTSD). Another 5% of the general population suffers from generalized anxiety disorder (GAD). Nearly half of all office visits to primary care clinicians are for one of 11 common symptoms associated with an underlying anxiety or depressive disorder. The primary care clinician is in an excellent position to diagnose and treat patients with these disorders.

Detailed diagnostic criteria for each anxiety disorder can be found in the American Psychiatric Association *Diagnostic and Statistical Manual of Mental Disorders: DSM-IV*. A defining feature of the patient with panic disorder is discrete episodes of anxiety with sudden onset and fairly abrupt termination. Episodes without the full array of symptoms are referred to as limited symptom attacks. For many individuals with panic disorder, anxiety provoked by the anticipation of (and desire to avoid) future attacks leads to agoraphobia. Agoraphobia literally means fear of the marketplace. Clinically it refers to the patient's fear of having another panic attack and to subsequent behavior designed to avoid circumstances that might provoke an attack or prevent escape in the event of an attack. The range of a patient's daily activity becomes severely restricted. The patient with panic attacks and agoraphobia may become housebound and unable to solicit professional help.

The core symptoms of PTSD include (1) reexperiencing the original stressor in the form of nightmares, intrusive daytime memories, and dissociative episodes (i.e., flashbacks); (2) hyperarousal; (3) intense distress in response to reminders of the traumatic event; (4) avoidance of stimuli associated with the traumatic event or "numbing" to stimuli in general; and (5) a foreshortened sense of the future. Frequently depression, difficulty with interpersonal relationships, and substance abuse are also present. In addition, a disturbance in the quality of sleep is often present in combat-related PTSD. These veterans may feel safer sleeping during the day when

---

TABLE 100–1. *DSM-IV* Classification of Anxiety Disorders

Panic disorder with and without agoraphobia
Posttraumatic stress disorder
Acute stress disorder
Generalized anxiety disorder
Social phobia
Specific phobia
Obsessive compulsive disorder
Anxiety disorder due to a general medical condition
Substance-induced anxiety disorder

they can quickly awaken and survey their perimeter. Many veterans have developed the habit of "sleeping with one eye open" and describe increased sensitivity to sounds while they sleep. Life is seen as unpredictable and dangerous. Panic attacks as well as generalized increased arousal and apprehension are common. In chronic cases, depression and suicidal ideation are a part of daily life. Worsening of symptoms at the time of year of the original trauma (i.e., anniversary reactions) are also common.

Generalized anxiety disorder has a prevalence of 1:20 in the general population. While the symptoms of anxiety in GAD are similar to those in panic disorder, the presentation differs in the distribution of symptoms over time, with panic disorder being paroxysmal and GAD more continuous in nature. In addition, the focus of concern is usually a variety of themes such as financial difficulty, health concerns, or interpersonal problems rather than specific symptoms such as dizziness or palpitations.

PATHOPHYSIOLOGY

Increased sensitivity of the presynaptic noradrenergic α_2-autoreceptor in panic patients and increased urinary epinephrine levels in patients with PTSD suggest the presence of increased noradrenergic activation in both disorders. This may be due to increased activity of the locus caeruleus. This cluster of neuronal cell bodies in the brain stem is the major CNS nucleus responsible for the distribution of norepinephrine throughout the brain. This nucleus also activates the sympathetic arm of the autonomic nervous system and partially regulates adrenomedullary epinephrine secretion.

Tricyclic and monoamine oxidase inhibitor antidepressants decrease the activity of the locus caeruleus, possibly explaining their efficacy in panic disorder. Alprazolam, the main benzodiazepine (γ-aminobutyric acid agonist) used in the treatment of panic, appears to decrease noradrenergic function by interfering with brain stem frontal cortex connections as well as by its gabaergic function. Paradoxically, antidepressants also induce a change in the number or sensitivity of the presynaptic noradrenergic α_2-autoreceptors in a direction that would increase noradrenergic tone and exacerbate symptoms of anxiety. This may explain the tendency of some patients with anxiety disorders to feel more symptomatic during the initial phases of treatment with tricyclic antidepressants.

Increased sensitivity to isoproterenol in some panic patients suggests that peripheral autonomic hyperactivity is present in this disorder. An abnormal pattern of regional cerebral blood flow in patients with panic disorder suggests that central mechanisms are responsible for, serve to perpetuate, or in some other way are associated with the pathophysiology of this disorder. Patients with PTSD have a unique pattern of disturbed pituitary adrenal function. This includes decreased excretion of urinary free cortisol, increased sensitivity to the feedback effect of dexamethasone, and an increased hypothalamic-pituitary ACTH response to naloxone. This is intriguing given the close relationship between central noradrenergic function and hypothalamic-pituitary-adrenal activity. The panic patient's negative or catastrophic interpretation of a wide range of normal physiologic stimuli may be central to the pathophysiology of this disorder. The fact that panic patients are more likely than matched controls to become symptomatic during exposure to diverse stimuli including CO_2, lactate infusion, yohimbine administration, and exercise, supports this theory.

DIFFERENTIAL DIAGNOSIS

Symptoms common in patients with anxiety disorders are also seen in patients with a wide variety of psychiatric and medical problems (Table 100–2). Shortness of breath, palpitations, sweating, numbness or tingling, and chest pain are all common symptoms in patients with angina pectoris and patients with primary anxiety disorders. To further complicate matters, there are times when a particular symptom may have both physical and psychological origins. For example, hypoxia may trigger dyspnea in patients with chronic obstructive pulmonary disease. However, dyspnea is, in and of itself, uncomfortable and anxiety provoking. The heightened state of anxiety may aggravate and worsen the subjective experience of dyspnea. In addition, a variety of medications can precipitate symptoms of anxiety. These include but are not limited to sympathomimetics (e.g., theophylline), antihistamines, bromocriptine, captopril, cimetidine, and quinacrine. Drug intoxication and withdrawal is an important consideration in the patient with anxiety. Stimulant abuse can precipitate irritability, agitation, anxiety, and psychosis. Cocaine, dextroamphetamine, and methamphetamine are commonly abused psychostimulants. Anxiety is a conspicuous feature of the withdrawal syndrome from alcohol, benzodiazepines, barbiturates, narcotics, caffeine, and nicotine. In addition, patients with other psychiatric conditions including personality disorders, somatoform disorders, adjustment disorder with anxious features, major depressive disorder, and alcoholism may also be troubled by anxiety.

EVALUATION

The evaluation consists of a careful history of the present illness and mental status examination followed by a physical examination and a standard battery of laboratory tests to help exclude the presence of one of the medical disorders listed in Table 100–2. Distinguish-

---

TABLE 100–2. Medical Conditions Mimicking Anxiety Disorders

Pheochromocytoma
Diabetes mellitus
Mitral valve prolapse
Temporal lobe epilepsy
Angina pectoris
Pulmonary emboli
Congestive heart failure
Hypoxia
Drug intoxication
Drug and alcohol withdrawal

ing between a primary anxiety disorder and a primary medical illness as the principal cause of symptoms such as dizziness, chest pain, or palpitations can be very difficult. It may be difficult for patients with anxiety disorders to discuss and describe the catastrophic stressors that first led to, or currently maintain, the intensity of their illness. In this case, it is helpful for the clinician to prepare the patient with an introductory comment designed to demonstrate empathy and establish rapport. For example, "I need to ask you some questions about your symptoms and your past experience that may be difficult or painful for you to answer. Please understand that I do not mean to deliberately cause you discomfort or pain. In order to arrive at an accurate diagnosis and a plan of treatment, I need to know something about what you have been through and the nature of your symptoms."

MANAGEMENT

Each anxiety disorder listed in Table 100–1 may be treated with either medications or cognitive-behavioral (CB) therapy.

Cognitive Behavioral Therapy

In the case of panic disorder, there is evidence that CB therapy is more efficacious than medication in achieving and maintaining a panic-free state. However, the need for rapid reduction in symptoms or the initial reluctance of some patients to accept a CB treatment approach makes medication an important treatment option. In practice, CB therapy and medication treatment are often complementary.

Cognitive-behavioral therapy involves the use of four techniques: interoceptive exposure, cognitive restructuring, in vivo exposure, and relaxation training.

Interoceptive exposure describes a process of deliberately provoking the somatic sensations the panic patient experiences during a panic attack. This may be accomplished by various maneuvers such as spinning the patient around or causing the patient to hyperventilate. Repeated exposure to these feelings allows the patient to become desensitized and less apprehensive about their return. Cognitive restructuring describes the process of identifying and correcting cognitive distortions and may be equally useful in panic disorder, GAD, and PTSD. A common example of a distortion is, "If my heart is beating fast, I must be having a heart attack." In vivo exposure is accomplished by identifying environmental cues that provoke the panic attack and desensitizing the patient using direct exposure to the feared object or circumstance. Relaxation training refers to diaphragmatic breathing and muscle relaxation techniques. These skills decrease the patient's tendency to hyperventilate and accumulate tension in various muscle groups. In the case of chronic PTSD, there are few data to help the clinician choose a primary treatment modality. However, for patients with acute PTSD, the initial intervention should be cognitive-behavioral and/or supportive psychotherapy with adjunctive use of medication if necessary. For many people, PTSD, like

generalized anxiety disorder and panic disorder, is a chronic illness with periodic remissions and exacerbations. No single course of CB treatment reliably provides significant reduction of the core PTSD symptoms beyond 6 months although further treatment may reestablish gains made during earlier treatment.

Pharmacotherapy

Since many anxiety disorders are intermittent or chronic, it is important to have specific goals in mind before initiating treatment with medications. For patients with PTSD, pharmacotherapy should be designed to decrease symptoms of hyperarousal, improve sleep, decrease avoidance, decrease impulsivity, improve mood, and if possible reduce intrusive symptoms. A positive and trusting relationship between patient and therapist is essential if pharmacologic or psychotherapeutic treatment is to be successful. For patients with panic disorder with agoraphobia, medication treatment is designed to provide a 6- to 12-month panic-free period. During this time, CB therapy should be used to decrease avoidance behavior. Helping the patient acquire CB skills to cope with symptoms of panic (should they return at a later date) is also advisable. If symptoms recur after a drug taper, some psychopharmacologists suggest an additional 12–24 months of treatment. For the patient with GAD, the treatment goal is reduction of symptoms to a point where vocational, social, and recreational functioning is minimally impaired and the patient is able to experience a subjective sense of well-being. For a significant number of individuals with panic disorder, PTSD, or GAD, the course of the illness is intermittent or chronic. During periods of increased psychosocial, interpersonal, occupational, or financial stress, or at the time of an anniversary reaction for patients with PTSD, symptoms may return or worsen. The risk of suicide is five times that of the general population. Accordingly, maintenance treatment with medication and psychotherapy may be a necessary and legitimate treatment option.

Specific Treatment
Anxiolytics

Benzodiazepines have the advantage of rapid symptom reduction, a low side effect profile, and few drug interactions. The common side effects are sedation, ataxia, and interference with short-term memory. In addition, use of the long-half-life benzodiazepines (e.g., chlordiazepoxide, diazepam, and flurazepam) in the geriatric population results in a fivefold increase in hip fracture compared with the rate in those with no drug use or use of short-half-life benzodiazepines. They should be used cautiously in patients with significant lung or liver disease because of the possibility that they may decrease respiratory drive or accumulate excessively, respectively. In addition, all benzodiazepines should also be used sparingly, if at all, in patients with a history of substance abuse.

The major disadvantage of benzodiazepines is the likelihood of withdrawal symptoms on discontinuation. Withdrawal symptoms from benzodiazepine discontinuation are impossible to distinguish from a clinical relapse (i.e., a return of the primary anxiety disorder). In the case of panic disorder, the patient must endure the symptoms for 1–2 weeks before it is clear whether or not a relapse will occur. The withdrawal protocol for alprazolam should be no greater than a 0.25 mg decrease in the total daily dose every 5 days.

Alprazolam is the most commonly used benzodiazepine for panic disorder. The total daily dose of alprazolam necessary to achieve a panic-free state may be as high as 6 mg/d or higher. The dose should be increased judiciously to minimize the sedative effect. Many people become tolerant to the sedative effect and to the ataxia seen in this dosage range. Insufficient drug dosage and inadequate duration of treatment are common causes of incomplete treatment response. Buspirone is an anxiolytic agent to which tolerance does not develop and from which there are no withdrawal symptoms. Although it has some efficacy in treating anxiety disorders, it takes 3–4 weeks before benefit is seen. While beta-blockers such as propranolol may be effective for treatment of mild generalized anxiety they are only marginally effective for social phobia and have little if any efficacy in the treatment of panic disorder.

Antidepressants

The anxiolytic effect of antidepressants makes them a first-line treatment option for patients with anxiety disorders. Antidepressants are also useful for treating the symptoms associated with a superimposed depression such as decreased energy, insomnia, anhedonia, irritability, and hopelessness. While they have the advantage of not being habituating, their major disadvantages include delayed onset of symptom reduction (3–4 weeks), a complex side effect profile, and potential for drug interactions. Tricyclic antidepressants are highly toxic when taken as an overdose. Some clinicians use a combination of benzodiazepines and antidepressants for the first few weeks to provide prompt symptom relief until the antidepressant can be expected to do so alone.

Antidepressants should be started in small doses (e.g., imipramine, 10–25 mg/d) to avoid the paradoxic exacerbations some patients with anxiety disorders feel at the beginning of treatment. Final dosages are comparable to the full dosage used to treat major depression. Tolerance is uncommon, and withdrawal symptoms are minor and can be avoided by a gradual taper. If abrupt discontinuation is necessary, withdrawal symptoms associated with cholinergic rebound can be avoided by the short-term use of anticholinergics such as diphenhydramine or benztropine. Common side effects include constipation, urinary retention, orthostatic hypotension, and dry mouth. Tricyclic antidepressants with the exception of nortriptyline and possibly protriptyline may be expected to increase the incidence of falls and subsequent hip fractures in the elderly.

The newer selective serotonin reuptake inhibitor (SSRI) antidepressants appear to be efficacious in panic disorder and possibly PTSD. They have few side effects compared with tricyclic antidepressants.

MAOIs, particularly phenelzine, may be useful and are relatively free of cardiovascular effects other than orthostatic hypotension. Combination with meperidine may be lethal. Patients must be able to adhere to a tyramine-free diet and understand the potential risks of a hypertensive episode.

PATIENT AND FAMILY EDUCATION

It is essential to inform both patient and family about the nature, course, and appropriate treatment of anxiety disorders. A variety of source materials are available for this purpose (see Selected Readings, below).

Research Questions

1. What role, if any, does GAD play in the development of coronary heart disease?
2. Would early counseling in patients with acute PTSD influence its course and help prevent the subsequent development of chronic PTSD?

Case Resolution

The diagnosis was panic disorder without agoraphobia. The patient was treated with imipramine and cognitive behavioral therapy. Her treatment also included instruction in relaxation techniques in the context of her workplace. With the therapist's help, she reexamined the extent of her responsibility for the children with whom she works. A year later, she was tapered off imipramine and was panic-free, but she remains vulnerable to exacerbations in times of extreme stress.

Selected Readings

Barlow, D. H., and M. G. Craske. *Mastery of Your Anxiety and Panic.* Albany, New York, Graywind Publications, 1989.

Charney, D. S., and G. R. Henninger. Noradrenergic function and the mechanism of action of antianxiety treatment. Arch Gen Psychiatry 42:473–81, 1985.

Integrated treatment of panic disorder and social phobia. Bull Menninger Clin 56(2 Suppl A), Spring 1992.

Kabat-Zinn, J. *Full Catastrophe Living.* Dell, 1990.

Nutt, D. J. Altered central α_2-adrenoceptor sensitivity in panic disorder. Arch Gen Psychiatry 46:165–9, 1989.

Roose, S. P., and A. H. Glassman. Cardiovascular effects of tricyclic antidepressants in depressed patients with and without heart disease. J Clin Psychiatry Monograph 7:2, May 1989.

Sheehan, D. V. *The Anxiety Disease.* New York, Bantam Books, 1983.

Symposium on Panic Disorder. Am J Med 92(Suppl 1A), January 24, 1992.

Wise, G. W., and S. O. Rieck. Diagnostic considerations and treatment approaches to underlying anxiety in the medically ill. J Clin Psychiatry 54:5(Suppl), May 1993.

DEPRESSION

Carol M.J. Larroque, M.D.

Hx A 35-year-old moderately obese female computer programmer who has been followed for mild hypertension for the past 3 years comes in for a routine medical follow-up. It is her first visit since the death of her husband 10 months ago. She has lost 17 pounds. She appears sad and reports that her appetite is poor, she has trouble staying asleep at night, and nothing is enjoyable to her anymore. She says she is always tired and has difficulty caring for her two small children. Tearfully, she reports that at times she wishes she too would just "pass away." The patient says she has been feeling this way "for months" but "things have become worse over the last 6 weeks." She speaks slowly and in a monotone. She tends to look down. Her grooming is adequate but not as stylish as in the past, and she lacks the vigor and sparkle that previously were characteristic of her personality.

Questions

1. What is causing this patient's change in mood, activity level, and outlook?
2. Can this change be explained by bereavement alone?
3. What criteria need to be met to diagnose a major depressive disorder, and if present how should it be treated?
4. What medical conditions often occur simultaneously with depression or can themselves cause symptoms of depression?
5. What must you consider when treating patients who have a history of hypertension as well as depression?

Feeling "depressed" or "down" is a universal experience with which all individuals must cope at one time or another. These feelings can be short-lived and often are a reaction to a disappointment, a loss, or the stressors of daily life. Indeed, "feeling depressed" may be an appropriate human response to a difficult event or circumstance. However, when the reaction is more extreme than might be expected, the individual is said to be experiencing an adjustment disorder with depressed mood. When the experience of depression becomes pervasive, interferes with functioning, and is a part of a specific constellation of symptoms, a major depressive disorder is likely to be present.

Major depression is a chronic, debilitating disorder that has a lifetime prevalence rate close to 6% in Americans 18 years of age and older. While the average age of onset is the late 20s, this disorder may begin at any age. Approximately 5% of children suffer from depression, often with symptoms of irritability and behavioral problems as key manifestations. Major depression occurs twice as often in adult females as in adult males, and there is an increased incidence in family members.

A cardinal symptom of major depression is the hopelessness experienced by those who are afflicted. Fifteen percent of those suffering from major depression will go on to commit suicide.

Interestingly, more patients with this disorder seek help in a primary care medical setting than in a psychiatrist's office. Major depression strongly correlates with chronic medical illness and substance abuse, especially alcohol and cocaine.

CLINICAL PRESENTATION

To diagnose a major depressive disorder, the criteria specified in the *Diagnostic and Statistical Manual of Mental Disorders: DSM-IV* must be met.

The essential feature of a major depressive disorder is a clinical course characterized by one or more major depressive episodes (Table 101–1). If a history of manic, mixed, or hypomanic episodes is present, or if criteria for a substance-induced mood disorder or a mood disorder due to a general medical condition are met, then the depressive episode does not count toward a major depressive disorder.

Symptoms must be present for at least 2 weeks. Symptoms that signal the probability of a major depression include (1) feelings of hopelessness, (2) changes in sleep or appetite, (3) the presence of anhedonia, and (4) suicidal ideation.

PATHOPHYSIOLOGY

Over the years there have been multiple theories to explain the etiology of depression: psychoanalytic, "learned helplessness," etc. Currently, the most widely held theories of depression emphasize its biological underpinnings. Depression is thought to be related to dysregulation of neurotransmitters in the brain, particularly the monoamine neurotransmitter system. The monoamine transmitters norepinephrine and serotonin are released by neurons originating in the locus caeruleus and the nuclei raphae, respectively. These neurotransmitters can activate both presynaptic and postsynaptic receptors. Their activity terminates when they are taken back up into the neuron, especially the presynaptic neuron.

The cyclic antidepressants interfere with the reuptake of both norepinephrine and serotonin. Other agents are highly selective for serotonin reuptake alone and thus are termed selective serotonin reuptake inhibitors (SSRIs). The monoamine oxidase inhibitor (MAOI) anti-

TABLE 101–1. *DSM-IV* Criteria for Major Depressive Episode

A. Five (or more) of the following symptoms have been present during the same 2-week period and represent a change from previous functioning; at least one of the symptoms is either (1) depressed mood or (2) loss of interest or pleasure.

   Note: Do not include symptoms that are clearly due to a general medical condition, or mood-incongruent delusions or hallucinations.

   (1) depressed mood most of the day, nearly every day, as indicated by either subjective report (e.g., feels sad or empty) or observation made by others (e.g., appears tearful). **Note:** In children and adolescents, can be irritable mood.

   (2) markedly diminished interest or pleasure in all, or almost all, activities most of the day, nearly every day (as indicated by either subjective account or observation made by others)

   (3) significant weight loss when not dieting or weight gain (e.g., a change of more than 5% of body weight in a month), or decrease or increase in appetite nearly every day. **Note:** In children, consider failure to make expected weight gains.

   (4) insomnia or hypersomnia nearly every day

   (5) psychomotor agitation or retardation nearly every day (observable by others, not merely subjective feelings of restlessness or being slowed down)

   (6) fatigue or loss of energy nearly every day

   (7) feelings of worthlessness or excessive or inappropriate guilt (which may be delusional) nearly every day (not merely self-reproach or guilt about being sick)

   (8) diminished ability to think or concentrate, or indecisiveness, nearly every day (either by subjective account or as observed by others)

   (9) recurrent thoughts of death (not just fear of dying), recurrent suicidal ideation without a specific plan, or a suicide attempt or a specific plan for committing suicide.

B. The symptoms do not meet criteria for a Mixed Episode.

C. The symptoms cause clinically significant distress or impairment in social, occupational, or other important areas of functioning.

D. The symptoms are not due to the direct physiological effects of a substance (e.g., a drug of abuse, a medication) or a general medical condition (e.g., hypothyroidism).

E. The symptoms are not better accounted for by Bereavement, i.e., after the loss of a loved one, the symptoms persist for longer than 2 months or are characterized by marked functional impairment, morbid preoccupation with worthlessness, suicidal ideation, psychotic symptoms, or psychomotor retardation.

Reproduced, with permission, from *Diagnostic and Statistical Manual of Mental Disorders: DSM-IV*, 4th ed. Washington, D.C., American Psychiatric Association, 1994.

depressants interfere with the breakdown of the biogenic amines intracellularly. Thus, theoretically it has been assumed that antidepressant medications enhance the activity of noradrenergic and serotoninergic neurotransmission, perhaps compensating for a deficiency of these neurotransmitters. However, the action of the cyclic antidepressants, SSRIs, and MAOIs occurs rapidly, within hours, but their full clinical effects do not appear for at least 4–6 weeks. This delayed action has led to a theory of down-regulation, a process by which antidepressants cause a reduction in the number of β_1-adrenergic receptors, α_2-adrenergic receptors, and serotonin 5-H_2 receptors.

DIFFERENTIAL DIAGNOSIS

Conditions other than a major depressive disorder may also cause a depressed mood. An **adjustment disorder with a depressed mood** occurs within 3 months of a specific stressor and does not persist for more than 6 months after the stressor has ceased. It generally causes marked distress (greater than normally

expected) or significant impairment in functioning. With a **dysthymic disorder**, a less intense depression is present for at least 2 years in adults. An individual with **bipolar disorder** will experience an episode of mania (a period of abnormally and persistently elevated, expansive or irritable mood) as well as an episode of major depression. **Bereavement** in some individuals may present with symptoms of major depression; however, such symptoms do not persist beyond 2 months following the death of the person missed.

Finally, certain medical illnesses as well as certain medications and illicit drugs can cause symptoms of depression. Such conditions are termed **mood disorder due to a general medical condition** and **substance-induced mood disorder**, respectively (Table 101–2).

EVALUATION

History

The history should include inquiry about (1) the presence or absence of criteria for the diagnosis of a major depressive episode (see Table 101–1), (2) precipitating and perpetuating factors, (3) medical illness, (4) medication use, and (5) patterns of alcohol and other substance use. In addition, the history should address possible homicidal urges as well as suicidal risk (including thoughts, plans, past attempts, and access to lethal means). The patient's system of social support should be assessed, since social isolation (including single or divorced marital status) increases suicide risk.

It is critical to ask the patient about delusional or hallucinatory experiences, symptoms that may be present in severe depressive episodes. Auditory hallucinations "commanding" the patient to harm himself or herself and "voices" making derogatory comments about the patient are especially worrisome in terms of suicide risk.

TABLE 101–2. Common Causes of Symptomatic Depressions

Type of Cause	Possible Cause
Pharmacologic	Steroidal contraceptives; reserpine, α-methyldopa, β-blockers; anticholinesterase insecticides; amphetamine withdrawal; cimetidine, indomethacin; phenothiazine neuroleptics; thallium
Infectious	General paresis (tertiary syphilis); influenza, viral pneumonia; viral hepatitis, infectious mononucleosis, AIDS; tuberculosis
Endocrinologic	Hypo- and hyperthyroidism, hyperparathyroidism, Cushing's disease, Addison's disease, hypopituitarism
Collagen-vascular	Systemic lupus erythematosus, rheumatoid arthritis
Neurologic	Multiple sclerosis, Parkinson's disease, head trauma, complex partial seizures (temporal lobe), cerebral tumors, stroke, sleep apnea
Nutritional	Pellagra, pernicious anemia
Neoplastic	Cancer of the head of the pancreas, disseminated carcinomatosis

Modified and reproduced, with permission, from R. Berkow (ed.). *The Merck Manual of Diagnosis and Therapy*, 16th ed. Rahway, New Jersey, Merck & Co., Inc., © 1992.

TABLE 101–3. Adverse Effects of Antidepressants*

Antidepressant	Usual Dosage	Adverse Effects			
	Dosage Range (mg/d)	Sedation	Anticholinergic Effect	Conduction Abnormalities	Lowering of Seizure Threshold
Tricyclics					
Amitriptyline	50–300	++++	++++	++++	+++
Nortriptyline	50–150	+++	+++	+++	++
Imipramine	50–150	+++	+++	++++	+++
Desipramine	50–300	++	++	+++	++
Doxepin	50–300	++++	+++	++	+++
Trimipramine	50–400	++++	++++	++++	+++
Clomipramine	50–300	++++	++++	++++	+++
Protriptyline	10–60	+	+++	++++	++
Newer Antidepressants					
Amoxapine	150–600	++	+++	++	+++
Maprotiline	50–300	+++	+++	+++	++++
Trazodone	150–600	+++	0	0†	+
Bupropion	200–450	±	±	±	+++++
Fluoxetine	20–80	±	0	±	+
Sertraline	50–200	±	0	±	?
Paroxetine	20–50	±	0	±	?

*High, 5 +; low, 1 +.
†May cause other cardiac difficulties.

Taking a complete psychiatric history (including past and present diagnoses, treatment, and treatment response) as well as a psychiatric history of family members helps in understanding the patient and in designing a treatment plan. A developmental and social history should also be obtained, including any instances of recent or past physical, sexual, or emotional abuse.

Mental Status Examination

The following characteristics are often identified in patients with significant depression.

Appearance-behavior: Poor grooming, decrease in eye contact, tearfulness, psychomotor retardation, agitation.

Mood: Sad, irritable.

Affect: Somber, constricted, anxious.

Speech: Slowed, soft, sparse; decreased spontaneity.

Thought content: Suicidal ideation, guilt, hopelessness, somatic concerns, ruminating obsessions, delusions of pervasive gloom and deserved persecution, nihilism.

Perceptual disorders: Auditory or visual hallucinations.

Cognition: Impaired memory, concentration, and insight.

Physical Examination and Additional Evaluation

A physical examination to screen for medical disorders is recommended. Patients being considered for treatment with a cyclic antidepressant should have a baseline electrocardiogram (ECG) performed, especially if they are over 40 years of age or have a history of cardiac disease. Thyroid function studies and a urine toxicology screen are frequently performed to assess for organic causes of depression. New-onset psychosis is an indication for careful neurologic evaluation and possibly neuroimaging and an electroencephalogram (EEG).

MANAGEMENT

Treatment for depression consists primarily of psychotherapy and pharmacotherapy. Electroconvulsive therapy or light therapy may be helpful for selected patients.

Psychotherapy during the acute phase of depression can provide support, guide treatment, and allow the therapist to be available during a crisis. Cognitive-behavior therapy to correct distorted thinking, psychodynamic therapy to help with past trauma, and family therapy to cope with current stressors are also important treatment modalities.

Pharmacotherapy is the cornerstone of treatment for major depression. For many years, the tricyclic antidepressants (TCAs) were the primary medication for major depression with MAOIs being used for atypical depression and dysthymia.

While effective, the TCAs have unpleasant and potentially dangerous side effects (Table 101–3). Their anticholinergic properties can cause serious problems in patients with acute narrow angle glaucoma or bladder outlet obstruction. Orthostatic hypotension can be dangerous in cardiac patients or the elderly. Daytime sedation and a decreased seizure threshold can also occur. However, the most serious side effects are related to prolonged cardiac conduction time and the induction of arrhythmias in certain individuals. TCAs appear to prolong both atrial and ventricular depolarization with a primary effect on the His-ventricular interval; at therapeutic levels, the PR, QRS, and QTc interval can each be prolonged. In individuals with preexisting (often unrecognized) cardiac conditions, TCAs can induce a significant atrioventricular (AV) block. Taken as an overdose, TCAs may cause deadly arrhythmias. Special precautions must be used when prescribing these potentially lethal drugs to suicidal patients. Consultation with a cardiologist is recommended before using TCAs in patients with a history of recent myocardial infarction or a history of arrhythmia, subclinical sinus node dysfunction, a prolonged QT interval, or other conduction defects.

Children and adolescents metabolize TCAs (and probably other antidepressants) differently from adults. Several episodes of sudden death have occurred in youngsters on TCAs. Therefore, consultation with a child psychiatrist is recommended to ensure proper administration of antidepressants to children. Special considerations should also be made in treating the elderly. MAOIs are less frequently used because of associated dietary restrictions: patients must adhere to a diet low in tyramine and other amines to avoid a sympathomimetic crisis.

Newer antidepressants have different side effect profiles (see Table 101–3). In particular, SSRIs (fluoxetine, sertraline, and paroxetine) are generally safer to use in patients with cardiac disorders or suicidal ideation. Common side effects of SSRIs are gastrointestinal disturbances, somnolence, headache, agitation, and insomnia. Sexual dysfunction, initial weight loss, and involuntary tremor may also be problematic. Fluoxetine and paroxetine should be used cautiously with other medications, since they can interfere with the hepatic metabolism of some drugs. Fluoxetine, MAOIs, and TCAs should not be used concurrently, since life-threatening reactions may occur. TCAs should be discontinued 1–2 weeks before starting an MAOI. Sertraline and paroxetine should be discontinued 2 weeks before starting an MAOI; fluoxetine should be stopped 5 weeks before starting a TCA or an MAOI.

NATURAL HISTORY/PROGNOSIS

A major depressive disorder usually develops over days to weeks although prodromal symptoms may be present for months. An episode may occur precipitously following a specific stressor such as the death of a loved one, childbirth, or an acute but debilitating virus. Unfortunately, many episodes of depression go unrecognized, and approximately 50% of depressed patients remain untreated.

Untreated, a major depressive episode generally lasts 6 months or longer. While many individuals have only one episode, over 50% of patients with this disorder experience subsequent episodes. These recurrences vary greatly. They may occur in frequent clusters or be separated by many years. In some people, recurrence is restricted to the later years of life. Most individuals return to premorbid functioning between episodes, but in 20%–30% of patients, residual symptoms remain. Most devastatingly, 15% of patients with major depression end their life by suicide.

PATIENT AND FAMILY EDUCATION

The following points should be stressed:

1. Depression can be devastating but is treatable. Hopelessness, irritability, and lack of motivation are symptoms of the disorder.

2. Medication may not be fully effective for 4–6 weeks, even with adequate doses.

3. After symptom resolution, at least 4–5 additional months of antidepressant treatment is necessary. Often patients require treatment for a year or so. Those with frequently recurring episodes of depression may require continuous maintenance medication.

4. Many patients stop taking antidepressant medications early in treatment because of their unpleasant side effects. If adverse effects occur, the treating physician should be notified promptly. Changing to an alternative medication usually proves helpful in such situations.

5. TCAs should be tapered, not stopped abruptly. Abrupt cessation of TCAs can cause a flu-like syndrome (i.e., anticholinergic withdrawal).

6. If the patient should become suicidal, psychotic, or severely depressed, emergency services should be sought. Hospitalization may be necessary.

Research Questions

1. How can major depressive episodes be prevented from recurring?
2. What biologic changes take place during depressive episodes that cause a patient to feel hopeless and suicidal?
3. How can the various forms of treatment available today be most effectively used to treat depression?

Case Resolution

This patient met the criteria for a major depressive disorder. In an uncomplicated bereavement, her severe symptoms would have diminished within 2 months following her husband's death. She was managed with psychotherapy and a tricyclic antidepressant (nortriptyline), with careful monitoring of her blood pressure. Within 1 month, she reported a more hopeful outlook and a significant decrease in her symptoms of depression.

Selected Readings

Arana, G. W., and S. E. Hyman. *Handbook of Psychiatric Drug Therapy,* 2nd ed. Boston, Little, Brown & Company, 1991.
Diagnostic and Statistical Manual of Mental Disorders: DSM-IV, 4th ed. Washington, D.C., American Psychiatric Association, 1994.
Practice Guidelines for Major Depressive Disorder in Adults. Washington, D.C., American Psychiatric Association, 1993.

THE SOMATIZING PATIENT

Michael Hollifield, M.D., and Albert V. Vogel, M.D.

Hx   A 34-year-old female temporary clerk presents with a chronic, intermittent history of dizziness and paresthesias. This condition has worsened over the past few weeks. The location of the tingling sensations varies. She also mentions "gas and stomach pains," which also are chronic and intermittent. Even though she has seen many doctors and has had many tests, she states that "no one can find out what's wrong" with her. She wants another opinion. She states she has been "sick a lot" since childhood and has been on various medications "on and off." Physical examination reveals a normotensive overweight woman. She has diffuse mild abdominal tenderness, without true guarding or rebound tenderness. Her neurologic examination is normal.

Questions

1. Does this patient have a diagnosable and treatable illness, or is her problem "functional" or untreatable?
2. How do you approach this visit, and how do you decide what workup to do?
3. What is a reasonable long-term plan for working with this patient?

The somatizing patient has one or more physical complaints for which appropriate medical evaluation finds no organic disease. When there is documented pathology, the symptoms or impairment grossly exceeds what would be expected from the physical findings. This phenomenon is referred to as somatization.

Stekel (1943) first used the term somatization to mean a bodily disorder that arises as the expression of a deep-seated neurosis. There is no general agreement on the definition of somatization. Somatization is not a discrete illness or pathophysiologic process but occurs in a variety of illnesses and diagnostic categories.

Somatization accounts for 10%–30% of all visits to primary care physicians. This percentage is higher in tertiary care settings. Ten to twenty percent of the American medical budget is spent on patients who somatize or have hypochondriacal concerns. Eighty percent of healthy persons have physical symptoms in any one week, and 4% of the public has multiple chronic functional symptoms. Somatic symptoms form a continuum—from mild to severe and from bothersome to incapacitating. Somatization may be primary or secondary to other illness. Up to 30% of these patients subsequently develop an illness that may be related to their symptoms. Many of these patients receive unhelpful or iatrogenically dangerous evaluations or treatment that fails to address the underlying problem.

In general, patients go to doctors to feel better, and doctors like to help patients feel better. Rapid and persistent symptom resolution is unlikely to happen with the somatizing patient. This leads to patient and physician frustration. Attention to the patient-physician relationship is crucial in caring for these patients. It may become curative or injurious, empowering or adversarial.

PATHOPHYSIOLOGY

There is evidence that people who somatize experience an amplification of normal bodily sensations. Minor symptoms may be caused by transient tissue pathology. Undetectable tissue pathology early in the course of physical illness can produce symptoms without an apparent physiologic explanation.

There are few good, and no compelling, studies demonstrating a genetic cause. Likewise, psychodynamic studies fail to establish a generally accepted cause. However, *DSM-IV* assumes the likelihood of a psychological cause or contribution in some somatoform disorders.

The pathophysiology, although not well understood, probably determines the symptoms of the patient. However, there is no unifying mechanism to explain somatization. In psychiatric syndromes with physical symptoms, the bodily sensations felt may be delusional, such as pain in major depression with psychosis. Symptoms may also result from a psychophysiologic process, such as the well-documented symptoms of panic attacks, or from stress-induced physiologic changes, which may lead to physical disease (e.g., the possible relationship between type A behavior and coronary heart disease). Also people with known physical disease may have psychophysiologic changes that cause their symptoms to worsen or to change in quality.

DIFFERENTIAL DIAGNOSIS

Adult patients presenting in primary care settings with somatization fall into four major overlapping categories (Table 102–1). There are pitfalls associated with both over-diagnosis and under-diagnosis of somatization. Over-diagnosis of somatization may result in failure to identify and treat other illnesses, thereby increasing morbidity and mortality. Failure to make the diagnosis of somatization may result in excessive diagnostic tests, unnecessary cost, and iatrogenic reinforcement of the patient's belief that an undetected

TABLE 102–1. Differential Diagnosis of the Somatizing Patient

Psychophysiologic Symptoms

Psychological factors affecting physical illness
Nonpathologic, transient psychogenic somatic symptoms (all are acute, but may become chronic)
  Grief/bereavement, with physical symptoms
  Fear, with physical symptoms
  Exaggeration or elaboration of physical symptoms (e.g., postaccident when litigation or compensation is involved)
  Sleep deprivation, with physical symptoms
  Sensory overload or deprivation, with physical symptoms

Psychiatric Syndromes (other than somatoform disorders)

Mood disorders (e.g., major depression and dysthymia)
Anxiety disorders (e.g., panic disorders)
Substance use, abuse, and withdrawal
Psychotic disorders (e.g., schizophrenia, psychotic depression, and monosymptomatic hypochondriasis)
Adjustment disorders with anxiety and/or depression
Personality disorders
Dementias

Somatoform Disorders

Somatization disorder
Hypochondriasis
Body dysmorphic disorder
Somatoform pain disorder
Conversion disorder
Somatoform disorder, not otherwise specified

Voluntary Psychogenic Symptoms or Syndromes

Factitious, with physical symptoms (e.g., Munchausen's syndrome)
Malingering, with physical symptoms

---

underlying physical illness remains. Some patients diagnosed with somatoform disorders do develop a physical illness that may explain the symptoms previously thought of as "somatoform." Whether this illness represents an existing condition that was not diagnosed or a new condition is sometimes difficult to determine.

Many somatizing complaints are ascribed by physicians to transient physical illness, such as acute viral illness ("It's the virus that's going around"), musculoskeletal injuries ("Maybe you slept on it wrong or hurt it and don't remember when"), soft tissue syndromes ("It is costochondritis"), or vague internal syndromes, and are treated successfully with reassurance and the passage of time. These unproven physical diagnoses are very common. When treatments for these diagnoses do not result in symptom relief, or when symptoms recur frequently, somatization may have been the problem all along. In fact, many somatizing disorders require the passage of a significant amount of time (chronicity) as an important diagnostic criterion. However, some somatoform and psychophysiologic syndromes do not require chronicity for diagnosis (e.g., conversion disorders, acute hypochondriacal symptoms, and physical symptoms of grief).

EVALUATION

The evaluation involves a thorough, relevant history and physical examination. Neither the presence of a physical examination abnormality nor a history suggestive of a physical illness eliminates the possibility of somatization. Somatization is commonly found in patients who have symptoms similar to those of a physical illness. An example is the presence of conversion seizures (pseudoseizures) in patients who have idiopathic epilepsy.

What clues can the physician search for, in addition to a thorough and reasonable search for physical illness? Here are several:

1. A screening questionnaire for new or established patients can be filled out by the patient in the waiting room or at home. Several standardized questionnaires are available that can be used as is or modified for the physician's patient population. This screen resembles a thorough review of systems with a symptom checklist. The questionnaire obtains information regarding patterns of visits to physicians and clinics, with the intent of understanding why a patient has chosen to seek help at this time, and asks how the presence of symptoms affects the patient's life and functioning. In addition, questions address the patient's medication use, alcohol and drug use, surgical history, and psychiatric and psychotropic medication history. Most new patients, whether somatizing or not, do not object to supplying this information. The same information can be obtained by physician interview, but the interview is more time consuming.

2. While the history is being taken, the patient should be given the opportunity to express what he or she thinks the underlying problem might be. Giving the patient a chance to tell the story will provide clues for more detailed inquiry in targeted areas. Certain interview styles improve the physician's ability to correctly diagnosis psychiatric disorders in primary care. In addition to specific questions about the medical history, general questions about recent or chronic stressful situations and commonly encountered human difficulties (such as deaths, troubles on the job or in a marriage, money worries, crises in faith) provide useful information. These questions also help establish a beneficial doctor-patient relationship. Specific questions aimed at suspected psychiatric disorders (e.g., delusions, paranoia, suicidal thoughts) are also helpful.

3. Attention to the manner in which the patient interacts with the physician is often revealing. Styles that are dramatic, anxious, depressed, angry, passive, bizarre, or paranoid give clues to underlying psychiatric syndromes. Do the physician's attempts to reassure the patient fall on deaf ears? Does it seem that the patient needs the relationship with the physician more than the relief of symptoms?

4. The subjective, emotional response of the physician to the patient hints at the presence of somatization, especially the chronic type found in somatization disorder and hypochondriasis. Patients who are disliked by physicians may be more likely to have organic brain disorders, somatoform disorders, personality disorders, and substance abuse than do those who are liked. Asking themselves a few questions (Box 102–1) may help physicians decide whether the patient has a somatoform disorder.

BOX 102–1. Questions Physicians Can Ask Themselves in Attempting to Determine Whether a Patient Has a Somatoform Disorder

Do you dread the phone call or the next appointment?
Are you angry, or do you feel that the patient is wasting your time and skills?
Does it seem that the patient is somehow working against you?

MANAGEMENT

Accurate diagnosis includes a biopsychosocial understanding of the patient. The most important part of the therapeutic process is to help the somatizing patient understand the disorder and its symptoms. It is only after this process begins that the patient will begin to attribute the symptoms to the correct cause. This process occurs slowly over many visits in the context of a supportive doctor-patient relationship. The indiscriminate use of multiple medications to treat symptoms usually has a paradoxical effect: it iatrogenically reinforces the notion of physical illness and may increase the risk of medication abuse.

These patients often develop a keen sense of not being treated correctly. If the somatizing patient does not feel understood, or is treated casually or randomly, the symptoms may be reinforced. If the patient senses that the physician is attempting to "get rid" of him or her, symptoms generally worsen. This increases the risk of iatrogenic harm through doctor shopping and repeated tests, which increases the chance of false-positive test results and unnecessary interventions. For the physician, emerging anger is usually a sign of frustration at not being able to effectively help or cure the patient. Professional impotence can occur in many medical settings but is very prevalent with the somatizing patient. Proper recognition, diagnosis, and management of these patients reduces the frustration. Peer support and Balint groups can help physicians cope with the emotions generated by these difficult medical situations.

Reassurance alone is often helpful in transient, self-limited conditions and acute somatization. The physician's task is to identify precipitating circumstances, allow the patient to ventilate, and provide supportive listening and education about symptoms. This may require a series of brief visits at short intervals. In the long run, this approach is time- and cost-effective because it may prevent chronic somatization. Attempts to talk the chronic somatizing patient out of symptoms usually fail and may result in an increase of complaints in order to "persuade" the doctor that he or she is "really" sick.

Psychopharmacologic treatment is effective in most psychiatric syndromes that present with somatic symptoms. For example, major depression and anxiety disorders are common primary care problems associated with somatic complaints. The somatic complaints disappear when the underlying depression or anxiety disorder is appropriately diagnosed and treated. Benzodiazepines are helpful for drug and alcohol withdrawal and may be of benefit adjunctively in the long-term treatment of selected substance abuse patients with somatization. Brief anxiolytic pharmacologic treatment may help in adjustment disorders, acute somatization, and transient, self-limited conditions, if coupled with supportive counseling. Medications are not the primary treatment indicated for personality disorders, voluntary psychogenic syndromes, or somatoform disorders.

Cognitive and behavioral treatment is indicated for certain mood, anxiety, and substance abuse disorders. A cognitive/educational approach is a major part of the treatment for somatoform disorders. Training is required for special treatment approaches (e.g., hypnosis, relaxation). Cognitive/educational approaches can be learned and effectively utilized by primary care physicians.

Individual psychotherapy is indicated for some psychiatric syndromes (especially dysthymia and personality disorders) that present with somatic complaints, and it may be helpful in patients with voluntary psychogenic syndromes and somatoform disorders. However, most patients seen in a primary care setting who experience psychiatric syndromes with somatic symptoms believe something is wrong with their bodies. Physicians must understand and explain to the patient the reason for the symptoms. Only when the patient reattributes from a strictly somatic to a psychosomatic explanation will a referral for psychotherapy be accepted.

Group psychotherapy is helpful for a variety of psychiatric and other medical disorders. However, it is not the primary treatment modality for patients with somatoform disorders or voluntary psychogenic syndromes.

PATIENT AND FAMILY EDUCATION

It is important to make an accurate diagnosis so that effective treatment can occur. However, effective treatment is also dependent on patient compliance, and compliance is dependent on whether or not the patient agrees with the physician regarding the diagnosis. When a patient is resistant to treatment, it may be essential to have one or a series of individual or family meetings for education and to come to an agreement on the explanatory model for the symptoms, so that treatment may proceed.

NATURAL HISTORY/PROGNOSIS

The outcome for the somatizing patient depends on the diagnosis. Most patients with acute somatization will not develop a chronic disorder if provided with brief supportive treatment and education. As mentioned above, somatic symptoms as part of nonsomatoform psychiatric disorders (e.g., major depression, panic disorder, and generalized anxiety disorder) will abate with accurate diagnosis and treatment. Some somatoform disorders become chronic and impair patients' functioning but can be alleviated by treatment.

SUMMARY

The somatizing patient in primary care is a challenge for the physician in many ways. Making an accurate diagnosis, understanding the patient, and helping the patient feel understood are essential to an effective treatment plan. Some treatments involve brief periods of medication, reassurance, and education. Others require long-term treatment of symptoms. The latter type is represented by patients with somatization disorder or chronic hypochondriasis. Iatrogenic harm and reinforcement of symptoms will be minimized by reducing excessive interventions. These patients should be given regular and predictable appointments—time-contingent rather than symptom-contingent. They benefit from prudent medical assessment coupled with cognitive and behavioral therapy in the context of a healing doctor-patient relationship. The physician is well advised to modulate the impulse to "do something" and to remember that offering honest, clear, sincere reassurance and education is doing something and has historically been a mainstay of medical care.

Research Questions

1. What are the physiologic mechanisms underlying centrally derived somatization?
2. In patients with somatoform disorders, can the treatments described above improve patients' lives and save money when compared to no treatment?

3. What is the prevalence of substance abuse and dependence in somatizing patients?

Case Resolution

Further history helped make the diagnosis of somatization disorder with a concurrent major depressive episode. The patient was treated with a tricyclic antidepressant and with regular, frequent follow-up visits to address her somatic complaints. After completion of medical treatment for 1 year, the patient was free of depressive symptoms and had less frequent somatic complaints. Long-term treatment will include follow-up visits at regular intervals in conjunction with behavioral therapy to manage her somatic complaints.

Selected Readings

American Psychiatric Association. *Diagnostic and Statistical Manual of Mental Disorders: DSM-IV,* 4th ed. Washington, D.C., American Psychiatric Association, 1994.
Balint, M. *The Doctor, His Patient, and the Illness.* New York, International University Press, 1957.
Barsky, A. J. Patients who amplify bodily symptoms. Ann Intern Med 91:63–70, 1979.
Escobar, J. I., A. Burnam, M. Kaino, et al. Somatization in the community. Arch Gen Psychiatry 44:713–20, 1987.
Ford, C. V. *The Somatizing Disorders: Illness as a Way of Life.* New York, Elsevier, 1983.
Goodwin, J. M., J. S. Goodwin, and R. Kellner. Psychiatric symptoms in disliked medical patients. JAMA 241:1117–20, 1979.
Kellner, R. *Psychosomatic Syndromes and Somatic Symptoms.* Washington, D.C., American Psychiatric Press, 1991.
Kellner, R. *Somatization and Hypochondriasis.* New York, Praeger-Greenwood, 1986.

CHAPTER 103

CHRONIC PAIN

Donald E. Stehr, M.D.

H$_x$ A 35-year-old male construction worker presents with the complaint of persistent low back pain. He is requesting an MRI and stronger pain pills. He also has some insurance forms to be filled out stating that he cannot return to work. He relates a history of a back injury at work 6 months previously. He has seen several physicians who have prescribed "muscle relaxers" and "antiinflammation medicine" but they are "not working." He states that he is unable to work and is applying for disability benefits. He is symptom-free other than the back pain. The physical and neurologic examinations are unremarkable.

Questions

1. Why might the patient want to change physicians?
2. Why is he still having the pain?
3. Does he require an MRI?
4. What is your role in determining his work status?
5. Could his problem have been handled better initially?

Few problems in medical practice are more difficult or frustrating than the problem of chronic, nonmalignant pain. The pain may involve any system of the body but musculoskeletal pain, headaches, chest pain, and abdominal pain are complained about most commonly. Pain is subjective and can be defined as an unpleasant sensory or emotional experience associated with actual or potential tissue damage, or described in terms of such damage. Chronic pain is usually defined as pain that has persisted longer than 6 months.

PATHOPHYSIOLOGY

Acute pain can usually be explained by a biomedical model in which the perception of pain is the result of tissue injury leading to the origination, conduction, and processing of pain signals by the central nervous system. This physiologic aspect of pain is referred to as nociception. However, in many cases of chronic pain, its persistence and severity is disproportionate to any apparent active tissue or organ pathology. To explain this phenomenon, it is necessary to consider a multi-factorial psychobiologic model that, in addition to tissues, organs and systems, includes psychosocial factors such as the individual's cognition, behavioral responses, and emotional responses as well as various societal factors.

DIFFERENTIAL DIAGNOSIS

Chronic pain can occur in many diseases. In conditions such as malignancy, rheumatologic diseases, and diabetic neuropathy, its cause usually is apparent. However, pain syndromes may be associated with conditions in which the pathology is less obvious, such as fibromyalgia, chronic headache, temporomandibular joint pain, low back pain, and irritable bowel syndrome. People with chronic pain frequently have symptoms of depression, but primarily depressed people may also have secondary headaches or other vague somatic symptoms. Patients with somatoform disorders may have pain complaints referable to multiple systems. Munchausen's syndrome, drug-seeking, malingering, and compensation-seeking patients may also present with chronic pain.

EVALUATION

History

The physician should allow the patient time to talk about the pain in an undirected manner in order to find out as much as possible about the pain. What is the nature of the pain? What is its location? What makes it worse or better? What does it feel like (e.g., "burning," "stabbing," etc.)? How severe is the pain, e.g., on a scale of 1 to 10? What is its pattern over 24 hours? When and where does it occur? What does the patient do when he or she has the pain, and what is the consequence? What is the patient's explanation of the pain and thoughts when experiencing it? Atypical pain patterns should alert the physician to look for psychosocial factors. The personal history will reveal the patient's activities of daily living and degree of dependency. If these are

disproportionate to the objective disease, the question of abnormal illness behavior is raised. Poor social functioning may suggest avoidance behavior. The family history may reveal exposure to chronic illness and caretaking as a child. Such exposure plays a role in the development of illness behavior in adulthood. The system review may reveal symptoms suggestive of depression such as emotional changes, sleep disturbances, or loss of libido.

Physical Examination

The physical examination provides important objective evidence of the patient's potential functional capacity as well as any organic pathology present. The neurologic examination is especially important. Sensory changes that do not conform to nerve distribution, pain reactions that can be distracted during the examination, gross guarding, grimacing, sighing, or distorted gait are all suggestive of a strong behavioral component.

Additional Evaluation

Patients with chronic pain have usually undergone a complete battery of tests at some point in the course of their symptoms. Simply repeating these tests will be unlikely to uncover anything new and will only shift attention away from the more important psychosocial factors.

MANAGEMENT

First, the provider must come to terms with the frustrating fact that once established, chronic pain does not usually go away and is essentially incurable. Treatment goals are thus supportive in nature and aimed at salvaging the patient from a pain-centered life-style. The physician needs to be direct in discussing with the patient that there usually is no "medical cure" for chronic pain. What you offer are options to help "control" and "overcome" the pain in order to improve the patient's functional status and quality of life and also to reduce his or her dependence on medical care.

The pain should be addressed in terms of its organic, emotional, cognitive, and behavioral components.

The organic (nociceptive) component will vary depending on the type of pain and its underlying pathology. For example, in severe rheumatoid arthritis, psychosocial factors may play only a minimal role and the treatment will be primarily biomedical (including the use of potent analgesics if needed). In contrast, there are patients with chronic abdominal pain in whom all studies are negative and psychosocial factors play the major role. In these latter cases, drug treatment should play only a minimal role and management efforts need to be directed at the psychosocial component. This distinction is important because "medical treatment" itself tends to reinforce pain behaviors.

Anxiety, depression, and sleep disturbances are common in chronic pain patients. There is a natural tendency to order antianxiety agents and sedatives.

However, patients quickly become dependent on these drugs and they do not relieve the pain. Low-dose tricyclic antidepressants are safer and may be of benefit in reducing depression symptoms, improving sleep patterns, and decreasing pain. If depression symptoms are severe, psychiatric consultation may be indicated, since chronic pain patients can be suicidal.

Chronic pain patients may have negative thoughts and self-talk while experiencing the pain. Cognitive therapy attempts to restructure these ideas by providing a variety of techniques to cope with the pain, such as relaxation training, biofeedback, altering pain appraisal, visualization of positive situations during the pain, changing self-talk, and learning to tolerate pain during activities.

Individuals can respond to illness in a variety of ways; some people may react "normally," whereas others may overreact (or underreact) in ways that are dysfunctional. The response to pain is simply one form of illness behavior. According to behavioral theory, these responses are learned and are shaped by their consequences. Behaviors that are followed by positive consequences tend to be maintained or to increase. Behaviors that are followed by neutral consequences tend to decrease. The behavioral modification approach, therefore, is to identify and reduce the reinforcing consequences of dysfunctional pain behaviors and at the same time reinforce "well" behaviors. Some typical pain behaviors and reinforcers are listed in Table 103–1. These behaviors involve the physician as well as the family. There are some basic behavioral techniques and principles that apply to everyday patient care. During visits, the conversation should be "shaped" along functional lines such as (1) increasing physical activities and exercise, (2) increasing social activities, and (3) decreasing dependence on medication. Ask the patient, "What have you been doing?" not "How do you feel?" Positive responses regarding function, no matter how minimal, should be reinforced by active listening (e.g., alert posture, eye contact, verbal support). Pain complaints and displays should be received passively (e.g., no eye contact or verbal responses).

It is appropriate to treat any organic component of the pain biomedically, including the use of analgesic drugs.

However, the physician must be aware of the behavioral consequences of medication taking, especially multiple drugs. Polypharmacy tends to gives patients the message that all the pain is secondary to tissue injury and therefore not under their control, thus reinforcing illness behavior. This can be minimized by limiting medication use and prescribing it on a fixed time schedule and not "as needed." Physiotherapy feels good but unless prescribed on a fixed schedule tends to reward the pain. Braces, splints, and transcutaneous electrical nerve stimulation (TENS) units may become symbolic badges of illness that induce sympathy and caretaking. Occupational therapy, therapeutic exercises, and general physical conditioning, on the other hand, focus on function rather than on symptom relief and reinforce "well behavior." Although the pain does not go away, pain perception tends to diminish as function improves.

We live in a society in which there is an accepted "sick role." The sick person is exempted from social responsibilities such as work or school as long as medical care is sought and an official (usually written) excuse obtained. This avoidance of responsibility can be a strong reinforcer of illness behavior. The physician's social role as validator of sickness is a powerful one and, in the case of chronic pain, a particularly thorny one, since disability benefits may also result.

Managing a chronic pain patient is difficult at best and unless the physician has special training, consideration should be given to obtaining consultation with a psychologist trained in behavioral medicine/health psychology or referring the patient to a comprehensive multidisciplinary pain clinic. Such clinics have the advantage of offering group therapy, including comprehensive cognitive/behavioral interventions and drug detoxification if needed. Participation in such programs does require motivation on the part of the patient, including a willingness to participate in group therapy and to make both the time and the necessary financial commitment.

Prevention

Some evidence suggests that chronic pain and disability from injuries may be at least partially preventable. The key seems to be the manner in which it is treated during the acute phase. Treatment should be based on objective clinical data rather than the patient's subjective complaints, with the goal of returning the patient to work as soon as possible to avoid disuse atrophy. Medication (including analgesic drugs) should be prescribed on a fixed schedule and not on the basis of symptoms. When the condition has had adequate time to heal, the patient needs to be sent back to work. A statement to consider using at this point is, "I know that you still do not feel one hundred percent, but we have allowed enough time for healing and if we baby the pain your muscles will get weak." This approach requires assertiveness on the part of the provider, but the alternative may, in some cases at least, lead to significant iatrogenic pain and disability.

TABLE 103–1. Common Pain Behaviors and Reinforcers

Behavior	Reinforcing Response	By Whom
Grimacing, posturing	Showing concern	Family
Complaining	Active listening	Family
Avoiding activity	Caretaking	Family
Avoiding social obligations	Providing excuses	Family
Missing work or school	Writing releases	Physician
Taking medication	Prescribing	Physician
Seeking medical care	Order more studies	Physician
Wearing braces, supports	Providing items	Physician
Not working	Authorizing compensation	Physician

PATIENT AND FAMILY EDUCATION

Since the family is usually the patient's primary support system, it is essential to get family members involved. Patients with chronic pain can be very demanding. Excessive caretaking or other reinforcing behavior needs to be identified and dealt with diplomatically. Patients with chronic pain have high divorce rates, and family therapy may thus be extremely helpful. Often there are associated sexual problems, and in such cases, sexual counseling may be indicated.

NATURAL HISTORY/PROGNOSIS

Once established, chronic pain is usually permanent. Disability payments, caretaking, and polypharmacy may reinforce and maintain it. With a comprehensive rehabilitation approach, however, both chronic illness behavior and functional status may be significantly improved. There is probably no greater test of a provider's behavioral skills and clinical sophistication than in the management of the patient with chronic pain.

Research Questions

1. How might a patient's cultural background influence chronic pain behavior?
2. How do age and sex influence the perception of chronic pain?

Case Resolution

The physician discussed the patient's situation at length with him, including exactly what he was and was not able to do, and referred him to a physical therapist, with the goal of gradually increasing his functional status.

Selected Readings

Caudill, M., R. Schnable, P. Zuttermeister, et al. Decreased clinic use by chronic pain patients: Response to behavioral medicine intervention. Clin J Pain 7:305–10, 1991.

Fordyce, W. Behavioral factors in pain. Neurosurg Clin North Am 2:749–59, 1991.

Fordyce, W., J. Brockway, et al. A control group comparison of behavioral vs. traditional management methods in acute back pain. J Behav Med 9:127–40, 1986.

Keefe, F. J., J. Dunsmore, and R. Burnett. Behavioral and cognitive-behavioral approaches to chronic pain: Recent advances and future directions. J Consult Clin Psychol 60:528–36, 1992.

Koch, H. The management of chronic pain in office-based ambulatory care: National Ambulatory Medical Care Survey. Advance Data From Vital and Health Statistics. National Center for Health Statistics. No. 123. DHHS Pub. No. (PHS) 86–1250. Hyattsville, Maryland, Public Health Service, Aug. 29, 1986.

Nicholas, M. K., P. H. Wilson, and J. Goyen. Comparison of cognitive-behavioral group treatment and an alternative non-psychological treatment for chronic low back pain. Pain 48:339–47, 1992.

Parsons, T. *The Social System.* New York, Free Press of Glencoe, 1951, pp. 433–9.

Pither, C. E., and M. K. Nicholas. Psychologic approaches in chronic pain management. Br Med Bull 47:743–61, 1991.

Sternbach, R. A. *Pain Patients: Traits and Treatment.* New York, Academic Press, 1974.

Waddell, G., J. McCulloch, E. Kummel, et al. Non-organic physical signs in low back pain. Spine 5:117–25, 1980.

CHAPTER 104

THE DIFFICULT PATIENT

Teresita McCarty, M.D., and Laura Weiss Roberts, M.D.

H$_x$ A college-educated, unemployed woman comes to the urgent care clinic in her sixth month of pregnancy requesting "a checkup and some help with a few things." For the past 3 weeks she has experienced intermittent abdominal cramps, spotting, and "maybe a fever." She has not received prenatal care, despite having "a few infections," because she felt "just fine." She denies the use of medications or illicit drugs, although her chart indicates that her urine was positive for marijuana and benzodiazepines 4 months ago when she came to the emergency room with a sprained wrist. She and her husband live in a rural area and do not have a telephone or access to a car.

According to the old chart, her husband is currently unemployed and "a little rough" with his wife when he is "stressed out." They ask to speak with a social worker about applying for "assistance." The patient develops a good relationship with a medical student in the clinic and declares that he is the "best doctor" she has ever met. She does not like the resident physician, however, and announces that she will talk only with the medical student or with the "boss around here." Despite some disagreement among members of the treatment team, it is decided that the patient will need at least 1 week of comprehensive outpatient evaluation. The social worker makes arrangements that would allow the patient and her husband to stay in a hotel room near the hospital. The patient, however, rejects this plan, stating adamantly that the room is a "dump" and that there is "a baby to consider!"

Questions

1. What is your personal reaction to the patient described above? Do you think others might share this reaction?
2. What makes this patient difficult? Is there a pattern to her seeming contradictions and inconsistencies?
3. What does the patient need medically? Which of the "difficult" symptoms require further evaluation? What aspects of her "difficult" style require intervention?
4. How can the medical student play a constructive role in this patient's care?

Caring for patients who are difficult to like or understand is a major challenge for clinicians. Even the most conscientious physician may find them inordinately taxing. Learning to care for troublesome patients nevertheless is an important task of clinical training. The approach presented in this chapter emphasizes four components: (1) recognizing what makes certain patients problematic; (2) assessing the clinical meaning of "difficult" symptoms and styles and how they influence the care patients receive; (3) learning to respond, not simply react, when caring for troublesome patients; and (4) understanding the pivotal role of the trainee in the medical team's management of difficult patients. By applying the strategies outlined, clinicians can ensure that all their patients, even the most difficult ones, receive optimal care.

A THERAPEUTIC APPROACH

The challenge in caring for difficult patients is to develop a well-defined but flexible approach that allows the physician to remain focused on the task of helping the patient. The practitioner must first determine what is clinically necessary for the care of the patient and then decide his or her responsibilities in achieving that objective. Though a simple idea, clarifying the medical problems posed by difficult patients is seldom straightforward, and the eventual problem list may have little correlation with the presenting complaints. Talking with the patient, reading the old chart, gathering collateral information, and comparing findings with other members of the multidisciplinary team are all key steps to take in determining which medical issues need to be addressed within what time period. The second task, deciding what responsibilities to assume in the care of a given patient, is often quite complex; some patients seem to clamor for the "moon," while others seem to resist all interventions. Despite these obstacles, the clinician has a duty to behave competently and compassionately, to communicate effectively with other members of the medical team, to help the patient as much as possible through clinically appropriate interventions, and to support the patient's ability to make informed choices.

IDENTIFICATION OF THE DIFFICULT PATIENT

There are seemingly endless ways in which patients can be difficult (Table 104–1). They can be unreasonable, dangerous, self-defeating, deceptive, repugnant, coercive, or recalcitrant. They can be so dissimilar to the care provider as to be enigmatic and unlikable. They can be so similar to the care provider—or the care provider's loved ones—as to be unnerving and upsetting. They can be so sick, physically traumatized, or intensely emotional that the professional burden of caring for them may feel overwhelming and, on some level, unfair. In short, they frequently require more than ordinary doctoring. Ironically, these issues may cause them to receive less than adequate care. Difficult patients are somehow not the patients they are "supposed" to be, and in their dealings with difficult patients, care providers may sometimes not feel or behave like the medical professionals they are supposed to be.

The medical literature focusing on the experiences of physicians provides some understanding of what makes patients "difficult." "Dependent clingers," "entitled demanders," "manipulative help-rejecters," and "self-destructive deniers" have been described as "hateful patients" dreaded by all physicians. Studies indicate that physicians are most troubled by patients who have a large number of ambiguous symptoms involving multiple organ systems, come in for treatment often, and are seen as treatment-resistant. These patients typically have significant psychosocial problems, are depressed, and believe they are powerless to change their life circumstances. Interestingly, there is some evidence that

---

TABLE 104–1. Identifying the Difficult Patient

Problematic First Impression	±	Problematic History	±	Problematic Behavior	=	Difficult Patient
Too "odd," too "talkative"		Thick chart		Agitated		
Too "sick," too "dumb"		Noncompliant		Demanding		
Too different (e.g., age, ethnicity, culture)		"Drug seeking"		Suicidal		
Too similar (e.g., young, professional, health care worker)		Diagnostic enigma		Angry		
Too threatening (e.g., attorney, criminal, violent person)		Past physician error		Tearful		
		Lawsuit		Independent		
		Nonresponsive		Nervous		
		Psychiatric problems		Controlling		
				Threatening		

the longer physicians have been in practice, the fewer difficult patient encounters they report. This may reflect a change in what is experienced as difficult and may correlate with an improved ability to respond to problem patients in a helpful and professional manner. Alternatively, it may indicate the experienced physician's ability to rid the clinic of these patients. One implication of this research is that the perception of "difficulty" may have more to do with the physician's attributes and expectations than those of the patient. This literature suggests that much of what is considered "difficult" about patients can be anticipated and minimized by the attentive physician.

ASSESSMENT AND DIFFERENTIAL DIAGNOSIS OF THE DIFFICULT PATIENT

Being "difficult" is a clinically important phenomenon with a distinctive differential diagnosis. Looking at the adaptive aspects of "difficult" characteristics, looking beyond the "difficult" for serious pathology, and looking for a mismatch between clinical resources and patient needs are all essential in the assessment of the difficult patient.

The "difficult" characteristics exhibited by a patient may have been adaptive in different circumstances. What works in certain families and ways of life may be perceived as problematic in the medical setting. The homeless person who is mistrustful of others is seen as uncooperative rather than as one who has adapted to a particularly harsh existence. The notoriously difficult physician-patient is an example of how a patient's need to know, to control, and to question may become intolerable to care givers. When a personality style has been useful to a patient since childhood or is vital to the patient's present adaptation to the world at large, it is presumptuous to insist that the patient be different to better fit into the clinic setting. In sum, a "difficult" presentation should be viewed as important clinical data, rich with information about the patient's past history and current coping mechanisms.

A patient's being "difficult" may obscure important pathology and should prompt thoroughness and curiosity in the treating physician. In an attempt to examine the connection between being difficult and having serious but unrecognized illness, a study was performed in which physicians were asked to identify their "most disliked" patients from the clinic roster. Interestingly, the most disliked patients included those with organic brain disease as well as those who were suicidal. The physicians perceived these patients as "immature" and "uncooperative" although they rarely associated their personal dislike with the patients' intellectual impairment or hopelessness due to depression. This work underscores the importance of remembering that a patient who seems unwilling to cooperate may actually be *unable* to cooperate because of undiagnosed organic or psychiatric illness. Encountering the "difficult" should serve as an important diagnostic indicator prompting a more detailed mental status examination, further evaluation, and appropriate consultation.

A mismatch between clinical resources, institutional style, and patient needs inevitably leads to difficult patient interactions. When patients' values and concerns differ from those of the institution, there is a tendency to question the patient's motivation and to pressure patients to conform. Seldom is there willingness (or are there sufficient resources) to alter the institutional routine to accommodate individual needs. An employed patient who seeks care during off-hours in an emergency room may be seen as an "inappropriate" user of medical services rather than as a conscientious employee who is reluctant to miss work. If the patient consults an alternative healer or requests a second opinion, the patient may be seen as recalcitrant rather than resourceful. Therefore, it is helpful to clarify the patient's values and needs and to define what resources are available to the patient through the medical system. By so doing, clinicians and patients may collaborate to obtain what is possible and beneficial within the institution and health care system and to minimize difficult encounters.

RESPONSE, NOT REACTION

Clinicians working with difficult patients need to pay particular attention to their own reactions (Fig. 104–1). Physicians may react with cynicism, disinterest, and detachment. Conversely, they may react by becoming overinvolved and by pursuing heroic efforts, with subsequent feelings of inadequacy. Because difficult patients tend to provoke a reaction, learning to think before reacting (i.e., to *respond*, not react) is a key skill to master.

There are several strategies clinicians can employ to improve their responses to difficult patients. It is essential first to remain calm and remember the duty to help and not harm. Arranging for the safety of the patient and members of the medical team, establishing communication, and developing a sense of connection with the patient as a person may require extra attention and time, but these measures are worth the effort. It is possible to create a therapeutic alliance—even with patients whose behavior seems incomprehensible or reprehensible—by exploring differences and seeking common ground. This alliance is essential as the clinician attempts to help the patient change detrimental behavior. One example is "teaching" the patient how to make a reasonable, clinically appropriate request in a way that allows the patient to be more successful in obtaining needed care. By supporting constructive choices made by the patient and encouraging appropriate self-advocacy, the clinician can help the patient act effectively in his or her own best interest. Whether newly struggling with difficult patients or approaching "burnout" for the umpteenth time, physicians may need to think about and reaffirm their own professional commitment to working with multiproblem patients. When a patient is confused, disrespectful, or diagnostically puzzling (or has another "difficult" attribute), this commitment may understandably require some bolstering. All these efforts will prevent unprofessional reactions by clinicians and will ultimately benefit the patient.

Identifying what has been learned from interactions with particularly difficult patients, preferably in discus-

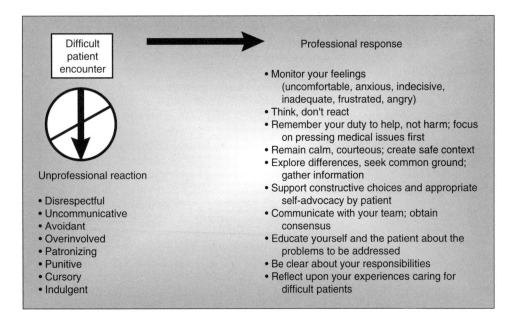

Difficult patient encounter

Unprofessional reaction

- Disrespectful
- Uncommunicative
- Avoidant
- Overinvolved
- Patronizing
- Punitive
- Cursory
- Indulgent

Professional response

- Monitor your feelings (uncomfortable, anxious, indecisive, inadequate, frustrated, angry)
- Think, don't react
- Remember your duty to help, not harm; focus on pressing medical issues first
- Remain calm, courteous; create safe context
- Explore differences, seek common ground; gather information
- Support constructive choices and appropriate self-advocacy by patient
- Communicate with your team; obtain consensus
- Educate yourself and the patient about the problems to be addressed
- Be clear about your responsibilities
- Reflect upon your experiences caring for difficult patients

FIGURE 104–1. *Professional responses versus unprofessional reactions*

sions with supervisors and consultants, is an important aspect of medical training. In this process, significant patterns may emerge: certain kinds of patients may be far more difficult than others for some physicians to work with, certain clinical sites may lead to predictable problem interactions, and certain team issues may arise consistently in dealings with difficult patients. Working with supervisors and consultants offers an opportunity to examine one's skill in providing competent, professional care to difficult patients. This approach will also improve the clinician's ability to give good medical care to all future patients.

THE PIVOTAL ROLE OF THE TRAINEE

Trainees—and medical students in particular—can play a crucial role in the management of difficult patients and help ensure that such patients receive good medical care (Box 104–1). Trainees are usually good listeners who empathize and advocate well for their patients. Patients recognize that trainees approach them as people and not as disembodied syndromes. Medical students usually talk to their patients and are generally available to answer their questions. Medical students also help their patients make informed choices. In addition, medical students often function as the conscience of a medical institution, since they are not yet bound by tradition or "standard procedure." Moreover, because trainees are not the ones on the medical team who enforce unwelcome treatment, they often can help facilitate a spirit of understanding and cooperation.

This capacity of medical students to form alliances with difficult patients is double edged; it can advance the patient's cause at the cost of alienating the trainee from other team members. The medical student's good relationship with the patient also can be exploited by a medical team eager for the patient's cooperation, placing the student in a potentially awkward position of conflicting loyalties. Miscommunication, accusations, disruption, and the taking of sides can occur—with the

trainee in the middle. To best utilize the constructive aspects of the patient-student alliance, all team members should be made aware of these potential problems and develop consistent ways of looking after the team as well as the patient. In this process, the team can better fulfill its ultimate aim: providing good care to all its patients.

LESSONS LEARNED FROM DIFFICULT PATIENTS

Working with difficult patients can yield many lessons of enduring value. Such experiences challenge clinicians to be rigorous and pragmatic in choosing a course of diagnosis and treatment. Dealing with difficult patients encourages resilience and good communication in the doctor-patient relationship. Difficult patients, with all

---

BOX 104–1. How to Help Difficult Patients Get Good Care

1. Make clear your commitment to the patient.
2. Maintain a respectful stance, and model compassionate behavior.
3. Carefully gather information about the patient's experience and illness.
4. Communicate all findings to the team, and discuss all findings with the team.
5. Educate yourself and your patient about the disease process.
6. Obtain consensus among team members about developing several acceptable treatment plans.
7. Clearly present tenable treatment options to the patient.
8. Be clear about the responsibilities of the physician and the patient in implementing a treatment plan.
9. To ensure consistency, discuss the treatment plan selected with all care providers.
10. Pay extra attention to communication and follow-up.
11. Find an acceptable professional setting to express any frustrations that are encountered.
12. Reward yourself for a task well done, and fortify yourself for the next difficult patient.

their associated challenges, blemishes, disguises, and aggravations, can remind us how hard illness and even survival can be. They infuse reality into the artificial context of the clinic or hospital and ensure that physicians recall the everyday world. Difficult patients also demonstrate how medical, psychiatric, and psychosocial factors may mask one another or impede care. Finally, working with difficult patients can have a beneficial effect on the functioning of medical care teams by improving joint decision making, communication, and trust.

Difficult patients offer physicians two remarkable gifts—an opportunity for greater self-knowledge and a chance to become better clinicians. Difficult patients allow capable clinicians to recognize both their strengths and their limitations. Though they are not immune to aggravation, such clinicians usually find acceptable professional settings in which to express the frustrations they have experienced. They pace themselves as best they can, take pride in their efforts, and fortify themselves in constructive ways for the next difficult encounter.

Research Questions

1. How does the initial impression of a patient influence the care he or she subsequently receives?

2. Which interviewing techniques can best assess patients who have subtle cognitive and psychiatric problems (and therefore seem "difficult")?

Case Resolution

The patient and her husband agreed to stay in the hotel room when the reasons for continued evaluation were carefully explained by members of the clinical team. The patient eventually revealed that she had intermittently used drugs to assuage overwhelming fears that began following an assault while she was in college. She immediately stopped her drug use when she realized she was pregnant; however, she worried that she may have harmed the baby and was terrified that physicians would question her "fitness" to be a mother. When the medical student asked her if these fears had anything to do with refusing the hotel room, the patient broke into tears.

Selected Readings

Drossman, D. A. The problem patient: Evaluation and care of medical patients with psychosocial disturbances. Ann Intern Med 88:366–72, 1978.

Goodwin, J. M., J. S. Goodwin, and R. Kellner. Psychiatric symptoms in disliked medical patients. JAMA 241:1117–20, 1979.

Groves, J. E. Taking care of the hateful patient. N Engl J Med 298:883–7, 1978.

Vaillant, G. E. The beginning of wisdom is never calling a patient a borderline; or, the clinical management of immature defenses in the treatment of individuals with personality disorders. J Psychother Pract Res 1:117–34, 1992.

Wright, A. L., and W. J. Morgan. On the creation of "problem" patients. Soc Sci Med 30:951–9, 1990.

CHAPTER 105

TOBACCO USE*

David B. Coultas, M.D.

H$_x$ A 50-year-old male plumber with a 35 pack-year smoking history complains of a persistent cough productive of clear sputum. The history, physical examination, and chest radiograph indicate that his cough is most likely due to chronic bronchitis secondary to smoking. Although he is reassured that he does not have lung cancer or "anything serious," he says that he does "not want to be told to quit smoking again" and is "not interested in quitting."

Questions

1. How would you respond to this patient?
2. What factors determine how successful patients will be in their attempts to quit smoking?

Cigarette smoking is the single most important cause of death in the United States, accounting for over 400,000 deaths per year. The estimate that 70% of cigarette smokers see a physician each year implies that physicians have direct contact every year with approximately 35 million smokers. No other group of health professionals has such wide contact with smokers and the potential to help so many smokers become nonsmokers. The role of the physician is further emphasized by the fact that 80%–90% of smokers use individual methods to quit, and only 10%–20% use formal cessation programs.

During the past 15 years a large body of information has accumulated providing strong evidence that physicians are effective in helping their patients stop smoking. Although interaction with individual patients is the most frequent context for helping smokers quit, other arenas may provide equally important opportunities for intervention (Box 105–1). Such opportunities include the prevention of cigarette smoking among children and adolescents, working closely with smoking cessation programs, and promoting private and public policies to create a nonsmoking environment. The focus of this chapter is on how to effectively intervene with individual patients.

PROCESS OF SMOKING AND SMOKING CESSATION

To maximize one's effectiveness and efficiency in helping patients quit smoking, it is important to understand why people smoke as well as the entire process of

---

BOX 105–1. Physicians' Roles in Smoking Cessation

INDIVIDUAL PATIENTS

ASK	Smoking habits, stage of change, perceptions about health consequences, past experiences, why smoke, why quit, concerns, resources, plans
ADVISE	To quit, personal benefits of quitting, other advice appropriate to information learned in ASK
ASSIST	Provide literature appropriate to information learned in ASK
ARRANGE	Negotiate plans for follow-up

COMMUNITY

SUPPORT	School-based programs for smoking prevention and cessation
	Workplace no-smoking policies and smoking cessation programs
	Legislative efforts to curb smoking

---

*Supported in part by a Preventive Pulmonary Academic Award, K07-HLO2474. National Heart, Lung and Blood Institute. National Institutes of Health.

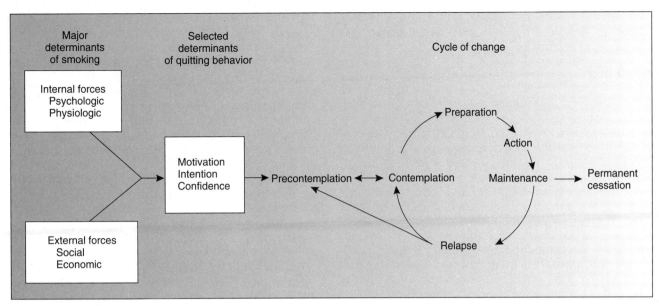

FIGURE 105–1. *Cigarette smoking and stages of change that can result in smoking cessation.*

smoking cessation. Initiation of cigarette smoking and smoking cessation are complex behaviors that are influenced by external and internal forces (Fig. 105–1). Major external forces include social factors (e.g., smoking by family members and peers) and economic factors (e.g., the cost of cigarettes). Internal factors that may influence an individual's smoking behavior include psychological (e.g., anxiety or depression, conditioning) and physiologic (e.g., nicotine addiction) characteristics. These external and internal factors also interact to affect the smoker's attitudes and beliefs about smoking and smoking cessation.

Initiation of smoking begins with experimentation in late childhood and adolescence. The incidence of starting smoking rises rapidly from the age of 11 years, peaks at the age of 17 to 19 years, and falls rapidly after the age of 23 years, with virtually no smokers starting after 35 years of age. Cigarette smoking by peers and family members are two of the most important determinants of smoking initiation. The rapid onset of powerful psychological and physiologic effects of cigarette smoke contribute to the maintenance of regular smoking and the great difficulty many smokers have with quitting.

Smoking cessation is a dynamic process, with changing levels of motivation to quit, intention to quit, and confidence in quitting (see Fig. 105–1). Investigations of smokers at various stages of change in the process of smoking cessation have contributed to our understanding of differences between successful and unsuccessful quitters. Predictors of outcome of smoking cessation efforts with the most clinical relevance for physicians include (1) motivation to quit, (2) intention to quit, (3) confidence in quitting, and (4) degree of nicotine addiction. Knowledge of these factors in individual patients enables the physician to target interventions for the smoker and to predict the likelihood of success.

A smoker's motivation to quit and intention to quit define his or her stage of change in smoking cessation. Prochaska and Goldstein suggest asking three questions

to assess a smoker's stage of change: (1) Do you intend to quit smoking in the next 6 months? (2) Do you intend to quit smoking in the next month? (3) Did you try to quit smoking in the past year? Smokers who answer "no" to the first question are considered **precontemplators** (about 35% of smokers). Smokers who intend to quit in the next 6 months but not in the next month are **contemplators** (about 50% of all smokers). Smokers who have tried to quit in the past year and intend to quit in the next month are in the stage of **preparation for action**.

For smokers who have quit, the stage of change is defined by the duration of cessation: if the duration of cessation is less than 6 months, the patient is in the **action** stage, while cessation for greater than 6 months is referred to as the **maintenance** stage. These stages of change are important to consider, as a high proportion of smokers in the action stage will resume smoking. Because relapse is common among smokers and may greatly affect their confidence about quitting, the physician's knowledge about a smoker's past experience with quitting is a necessary starting point for assisting smokers with future quit attempts. On average, smokers attempt to quit three or four times before they maintain abstinence. Because cigarette smoking and smoking cessation are complex processes that involve social, psychological, and physiologic influences, any intervention to help smokers quit that addresses only one of these areas (e.g., nicotine addiction) is unlikely to be successful. The approaches to helping smokers quit described in the next section combine determination of the smoker's motivation and intention to quit (i.e., stage of change) with a systematic assessment of factors that may influence the smoker's stage of change including his or her (1) understanding of the health effects of smoking, (2) past experience with quitting, (3) current concerns about quitting, (4) resources available to assist in quitting, and (5) specific plans for quitting. Careful questioning followed by discussion of these topics provides both physician and patient with the information needed to formulate realistic goals and plans for smoking cessation.

HOW TO HELP

As in all aspects of medicine, a structured approach to a patient's problem is necessary to maximize efficiency and effectiveness. The approach described here is adapted from available programs designed to improve physicians' skills in smoking cessation counseling. A program offered by the National Cancer Institute entitled "How to Help Your Patients Stop Smoking" includes four components, described as the "four A's": (1) **ask** about patients' smoking status at each visit; (2) **advise** them in a clear, direct manner to quit smoking; (3) **assist** the interested smoker in quitting by setting a quit date, providing self-help materials, and prescribing nicotine replacement therapy when appropriate; and (4) **arrange** follow-up visits (see Box 105–1).

Before any advice, assistance, or follow-up is arranged, the smoker's stage of change needs to be assessed as described previously. Frequently, this can be determined simply from the smoker's comments during the interview. For example, the patient profiled above is a precontemplator based on his statement that he "is not interested in quitting." The goal and thus the physician's approach to this smoker will be different than for smokers at other stages of change.

Although the ultimate goal is to help all smokers become nonsmokers, this is usually not realistic after only one visit; however, for many smokers it may become a realistic goal as the number of follow-up visits for smoking cessation increases. Thus, the foremost priority is to assist the smoker's progress through the various stages of change, as the patient learns the process of altering his or her smoking behavior and moves toward becoming a nonsmoker. Therefore, moving a precontemplator into the contemplator stage qualifies as a successful interaction.

Precontemplator

For smokers not interested in quitting, many of whom may become irritated or defensive when advised to quit, the first challenge is to put yourself and the patient at ease about openly discussing his or her cigarette use. Do not allow a patient's irritation or anger to dissuade you from attempting to move that patient from a precontemplative stage to a contemplative stage.

Your ability to engage the patient in further smoking-related discussion will depend upon your communication skills. To start, you need to (1) listen intently to understand your patient's perceptions, feelings, and attitudes, and (2) show your understanding by using empathic statements that reflect your interest, respect, and compassion (e.g., "You have obviously been told to quit smoking many times, and it really bothers you"). Next, you need to support the patient's autonomy (e.g., "I understand that smoking is your decision and it is no one else's business, but as your doctor . . ."), and then follow with a question to obtain permission to discuss the smoking issue further (e.g., "As your doctor, I am concerned about your health and would like to ask you some additional questions about your smoking. Is that okay?"). Attention to empathy, autonomy, and permission during the interview will frequently enable you to discuss the patient's smoking in considerable detail.

Having obtained the patient's permission to discuss smoking further, determine the patient's (1) understanding about the health effects of smoking, (2) past experience with quitting, (3) reasons for continuing smoking, and (4) reasons that would make him or her consider quitting. Although more than 80% of smokers are aware that smoking has adverse health effects, many underestimate the hazards. Therefore, you should assess the perceptions of current smokers about the health risks of smoking and provide accurate and understandable information, if needed, about those risks. Furthermore, you should attempt to *personalize* the information on the health consequences of smoking, emphasizing the benefits of cessation and avoiding "scare tactics," since they may interfere with efforts at cessation. Opportunities to personalize the message may arise when discussing symptoms, physical findings, laboratory values, and the presence of disease that may have been caused or worsened by smoking.

Learning about a smoker's past experience with quitting may provide valuable insights that will prove useful in formulating further advice and assistance. Smokers who are not interested in quitting have either never tried to quit in the past or relapsed after a previous quit attempt and, because of this prior experience, have decided not to try to quit again. For both types of precontemplators, an understanding of their reasons for smoking (e.g., relaxation) may help guide subsequent cessation advice (e.g., other methods for relaxation). A brief questionnaire published by the National Cancer Institute entitled "Why Do You Smoke?" will assist smokers in determining their reasons for smoking. Similarly, precontemplators who relapsed probably learned a great deal from this experience about obstacles to quitting (e.g., withdrawal symptoms, weight gain) and resources (e.g., family members, group programs, nicotine replacement) that may help during future quit attempts.

Although many precontemplators have numerous reasons for continuing to smoke, few have ever thought about what it would take to make them quit. Asking precontemplators to provide reasons that would make them consider quitting may help move them to the contemplator stage. These reasons may start them thinking about the balance between the risks and benefits of continued smoking.

To close the discussion, summarize what you have learned about their smoking history and offer (1) your concern about their continued smoking and (2) your willingness to provide assistance. Based on your interview, you may decide to provide them with appropriate literature that helps them understand why they smoke or that answers questions about the risks of smoking and the benefits of quitting (e.g., "The Most Often Asked Questions About Smoking, Tobacco, and Health and . . . The Answers"). Although your ability to provide ongoing assistance to the precontemplator may be limited, it is essential that the patient's smoking be addressed at all subsequent visits.

Contemplator

For smokers who intend to quit but have no plans for quitting and may be ambivalent about quitting, an approach similar to that described for the precontemplator may be the best initial step. However, the focus of your discussion should be on determining their reasons for hesitancy or ambivalence about quitting. Often, their reasons for not planning to quit are related to little self-motivation to quit, concerns they have about quitting, or problems they experienced during previous quit attempts. If smokers' only reason for thinking about quitting is because someone else wants them to quit, they are unlikely to be successful until they want to quit for themselves.

Numerous barriers to quitting have been described and include fear of "failing," disabling withdrawal symptoms, or concerns about weight gain. Fear of "failing" is a common obstacle and needs to be addressed by (1) informing the smoker of the common occurrence of relapse among those attempting to quit and (2) suggesting that relapse is not a failure but rather part of the process of learning to become a nonsmoker. During the first several weeks after cessation, withdrawal symptoms may be particularly acute. Pharmacologic interventions (i.e., nicotine patch or chewing gum) may be employed during this time to help relieve these symptoms and permit the smoker to concentrate on the task of behavior change. Weight gain of 2.5 to 4.5 kg (5–10 lb) is common after cessation and tends to be of particular concern to women. Limiting caloric intake and increasing exercise during smoking cessation are necessary to control weight gain. Only after you elicit and address the smokers' concerns about quitting will they move to the stage of preparing to quit.

Although specific advice and assistance for the contemplator will primarily focus on the issues identified during the interview, a few generic guidelines may also prove useful. Statements supporting their desire to quit and boosting their confidence in quitting may provide added impetus. Similarly, you can offer literature to help them choose the best way to quit (e.g., "Why Do You Smoke?") or self-help literature (e.g., "Clearing the Air") for specific advice about quitting. Finally, follow-up plans are necessary.

Preparation for Action

Although the methods outlined for contemplators also apply to smokers preparing to quit, the focus should be on helping them identify specific plans for dealing with anticipated obstacles to quitting. In general, obstacles can be classified as (1) behavioral factors (e.g., social/psychological situations or cues) that trigger smoking and (2) physiologic withdrawal symptoms. You may wish to focus their thinking by asking questions about how they plan to deal with certain "high-risk"

situations and by providing self-help literature (e.g., "Clearing the Air"). Common "high-risk" situations include (1) the time immediately after meals, (2) drinking coffee or alcoholic beverages, and (3) being around friends and coworkers who smoke.

Withdrawal is characterized by a wide array of symptoms that may develop as the nicotine level declines after cigarette smoking stops. The most common symptoms include anxiety, inadequate sleep, irritability, impatience, difficulty concentrating, restlessness, and craving tobacco. These symptoms are usually most intense during the first several weeks after cessation. In addition to a history of withdrawal symptoms during prior quit attempts, characteristics that suggest a high degree of nicotine dependence include smoking 21 or more cigarettes per day and smoking the first cigarette of the day within 30 minutes of awakening. However, the presence of withdrawal symptoms or evidence of high nicotine dependence should not be the sole guidelines for prescribing nicotine replacement, since smokers without these factors may also benefit from nicotine replacement. Furthermore, use of nicotine replacement without attention to the behavioral aspects of quitting (e.g., social and psychological cues to smoking) is not likely to be successful.

After developing specific plans for quitting, including a quit date, be sure the smoker receives self-help literature and makes plans for follow-up. Contact should be made with the patient on the quit date, either by telephone or mail, to reinforce your concern. In addition, the patient should be seen within the first several weeks after quitting to review any problems with slips or relapse.

Action/Maintenance

The major tasks during the action and maintenance stages are to continually review the patient's smoking status and to reinforce continued cessation. The action stage, the first 6 months after cessation, is the period of highest relapse. Therefore, reviewing reasons for slips and relapse and discussing new coping strategies should occur during the follow-up visits of all smokers in the action and maintenance stages of cessation.

SUMMARY

Physicians have many opportunities to effectively assist smokers in quitting. By means of a structured and empathic approach to obtaining a comprehensive smoking history, starting with determining the smoker's stage of change, realistic goals can be established—and advice and assistance targeted—to help patients during the smoking cessation process. Although this process takes time, it is the single most cost-effective intervention physicians can provide. By (1) dividing the approach described in this chapter over several visits, (2) utilizing self-help materials, and (3) obtaining assistance from trained nurses or health educators in the clinic, concern about lack of time does not have to be a major barrier to helping smokers quit.

Case Resolution

This patient was in the precontemplation stage and adamantly stated that he was not interested in stopping smoking. After acknowledging that smoking and quitting were the patient's decisions to make, the physician obtained the patient's permission to ask a few questions about his smoking. The patient reported feeling "sick" during a quit attempt several years ago, adding that he did not want "to go through that again." The physician advised him that he could effectively treat his withdrawal symptoms during future quit attempts, and the patient agreed to discuss this further at the time of subsequent visits.

Selected Readings

Clearing the Air: How To Quit Smoking...and Quit for Keeps. U.S. Department of Health and Human Services. NIH Publication No. 92-1647. Bethesda, Maryland, Public Health Service, National Cancer Institute, 1991.

Coultas, D. B. The physician's role in smoking cessation. Clin Chest Med 12:755–68, 1991.

Fiore, M. C., D. E. Jorenby, T. B. Baker, and S. L. Kenford. Tobacco dependence and the nicotine patch: Clinical guidelines for effective use. JAMA 268:2687–94, 1992.

The Most Often Asked Questions About Smoking, Tobacco, and Health and...The Answers. American Cancer Society (90-No. 2023-LE), 1982.

Ockene, J. K., J. Kristeller, R. Goldberg, et al. Increasing the efficacy of physician-delivered smoking interventions: A randomized clinical trial. J Gen Intern Med 6:1–8, 1991.

Prochaska, J. O., and C. C. DiClemente. Stages and processes of self-change of smoking: Toward an integrative model of change. J Consult Clin Psych 51:390–5, 1983.

Prochaska, J. O., and M. G. Goldstein. Process of smoking cessation: Implications for clinicians. Clin Chest Med 12:727–35, 1991.

Why Do You Smoke? U.S. Department of Health and Human Services. NIH Publication No. 92-1822. Rockville, Maryland: National Institutes of Health, 1992.

Williams, G. C., T. E. Quill, E. L. Deci, and R. M. Ryan. "The facts concerning the recent carnival of *smoking* in Connecticut" *and elsewhere.* Ann Intern Med 115:59–63, 1991.

C H A P T E R   1 0 6

ALCOHOL AND SUBSTANCE ABUSE

Celia A. Michael, Ph.D.

H$_x$ A 45-year-old male computer analyst comes for a "check-up" at his wife's urging. Although he reports good health in general, questioning reveals a 6-month history of gastrointestinal problems including nausea, cramping, and diarrhea. Although these symptoms occur only two or three times a week, he has lost 15 pounds and notes a general fatigue and lack of energy. He admits to "not taking good care of myself" because of a stressful job and financial concerns. On a daily basis, he smokes a pack of cigarettes, drinks several cups of coffee, and drinks a six-pack of beer. Other recent history includes a dislocated shoulder after a car accident several months ago. He is mildly hypertensive but takes no medication. He denies blood in his stools, vomiting, chills, and night sweats. Physical examination is unremarkable with the exception of mild abdominal tenderness, a coated tongue, a cigarette burn on the right hand, and a large bruise on the right knee.

Questions

1. What diagnostic hypotheses are you considering?
2. What psychosocial variables may be important?
3. How can you increase the accuracy of the patient's self-report?
4. Would you interview the concerned wife?
5. What tests would you order?

Primary care physicians have several unique advantages in the early diagnosis and treatment of substance abuse problems. First, people who drink excessively or abuse substances are seen more frequently in primary care settings. Second, intervention in this setting may be more effective because primary health care workers are viewed as helpful and credible. Third, the stigma attached to drug treatment centers is not present, and families can be more easily included in the process.

Substance abuse problems can be conceptualized as existing on a continuum of severity. The majority of the population either abstains from using addicting substances or uses them moderately. At the other end of the spectrum, approximately 5% of adults are heavy users. It is relatively easy for physicians to identify this group of individuals with severe abuse or dependence problems, but it is more difficult to diagnose the much larger number of excessive users who may be at increased health risk or who have accrued a negative health consequence related to excessive use (approximately 25%). This latter population, however, presents the best opportunity for intervention in a primary care setting.

PATHOPHYSIOLOGY

The *Diagnostic and Statistical Manual of Mental Disorders: DSM-IV* classifies nine substance groups associated with abuse and dependence: alcohol, cocaine, hallucinogens, inhalants, phencyclidine (PCP), opiates, amphetamines, cannabis, and hypnotics, sedatives, and anxiolytics. Although a discussion of the pathophysiology of each class of drug is beyond the scope of this chapter, these substances can produce acute effects that may present as intoxication, withdrawal, or delirium. In addition, the effects of chronic use are myriad, are substance specific, and include both psychological and physical consequences.

DIFFERENTIAL DIAGNOSIS

Many of the classic clinical and laboratory signs associated with substance abuse are not evident in the early stages despite heavy abuse. It is therefore unlikely that the diagnosis will be made on the basis of a single sign, but rather the problem may become apparent only if the clinician considers a constellation of medical, social, and psychological clues. It may be helpful to discriminate between screening and diagnosis. Screening is usually designed to cast a broad net that increases the chances for early detection. As such, it involves the use of only a few of the many procedures that are required for a more precise diagnosis. The second step, diagnosis, is a broader evaluation of signs, symptoms, and laboratory tests and leads to the establishment of treatment.

Contemporary approaches to the diagnosis of substance abuse avoid the use of such labels as "alcoholic" in favor of a more pragmatic, problem-based definition. Substance abuse may cause problems in many life areas including health, fitness, sex, legal, financial, interpersonal, and vocational domains. From this perspective, some individuals exhibit multiple life problems associated with substance abuse, while others exhibit milder or more intermittent problems. People vary considerably in the degree to which they are aware of their problems and in their readiness to change. By avoiding stigmatizing labels, the physician is able to focus on the negative consequences of the abuse and collaborate with the patient in making important decisions about the costs and benefits of change.

Substance abuse may be complicated by the presence of concomitant problems such as anxiety, depression, chronic pain, or marital distress and these problems may precede, accompany, or be the result of substance use. Young male substance abusers most frequently exhibit antisocial behaviors, whereas women are more likely to present with depression. Substance-abusing couples are more likely to be violent, and their children are more likely to be seen in primary care settings owing to abuse, neglect, or lack of supervision. Despite much research, attempts to identify a "substance abuse personality" have met with failure.

EVALUATION

Although it is rarely possible to conduct extensive interviews in a busy clinic, recent research shows that a brief checklist of clinical signs and medical history items yields a highly reliable diagnostic index. When combined with questions about consumption and problems related to substance use, this diagnostic process fits easily into a clinic framework. Corroborating data can be obtained from appropriate laboratory tests. Family members are a valuable source of information and can be routinely included in the interview if the appropriate groundwork is laid. In many clinics, the documentation of "vital signs" now routinely includes questions about alcohol and smoking.

The major categories of evaluation are described below. If medical history items exceed four, trauma history items exceed two, and clinical signs exceed four, there is a high likelihood of substance abuse. These positive responses should be followed by several additional questions and appropriate laboratory tests.

The checklists given in Tables 106–1 and 106–2 were derived from comprehensive analysis of a large number of clinical features and laboratory tests that were found to be predictive of substance abuse. Typically, greater diagnostic accuracy was obtained from clinical responses than from laboratory tests. In younger populations, slightly lower cutoff scores should be used across all categories. Conversely, in older populations, there is a greater chance for diagnostic inaccuracy owing to the increased frequency of other abnormal clinical findings.

Corroborating Information

If the initial evaluation is suspicious for substance abuse, further workup should include confirming laboratory tests and a brief, verbally administered questionnaire.

TABLE 106–1.   Medical and Trauma History

Medical History (Four or More Signs)	Trauma History (Two or More Signs After Age 18)
Frequent headache	Fractures or dislocations
"Shaky" hands	Traffic accident injuries
Sleep disturbance	Head injuries or falls
Poor memory	Violent injuries
Reduced concentration	Intoxication injuries
Gastrointestinal problems	Injuries from fights or assaults
Persistent cough	
Morning thirst	
Weight loss or gain	
Hallucinations	
Coated tongue	
Productive cough	

TABLE 106–2.   Clinical Signs of Substance Abuse (Four or More)

Alcohol	Cannabis	Opiates	Stimulants	Nicotine	Anxiolytics	Barbiturates
Hand tremors	Bloodshot eyes	Decreased pain	Increased heart rate	Increased heart rate	Sedation	Sedation
Facial redness	Drooping eyelids	sense	Nasal irritation	Increased blood	Dry mouth	Decreased respirations
Rhinophyma	Increased heart rate	Sedation	Dilated pupils	pressure		Decreased blood
Abnormal gait		Constipation		Cold toes and		pressure
Coated tongue		Constricted pupils		fingers		
Soft palate edema				Fine hand tremors		
Abdominal tenderness				Chronic cough		
Cigarette burns				Nicotine stains on		
Bruises, abrasions				fingers		
Trauma scars						
Spider nevi						
Flushed palm						

Laboratory Tests

Laboratory tests for alcohol abuse include γGT (γ-glutamyl transferase), MCV (mean corpuscular volume), and BAC (blood alcohol concentration). γGT is a hepatic enzyme that is sensitive but not specific for chronic excessive alcohol consumption (patients with nonalcoholic liver disease and those taking hepatic enzyme-inducing medications such as barbiturates will also have abnormal test results). Levels return to normal after short periods of abstinence. A test that is more reflective of chronic abuse is MCV, which indicates a toxic effect of alcohol on developing erythroblasts in the bone marrow. In the presence of a normal hemoglobin concentration and normal serum B_{12} and folate concentrations, this marker is moderately sensitive (it is also sensitive to cigarette smoking). The final marker, BAC, is the random measurement of blood alcohol concentration. Levels of more than 17 mmol/L (80 mg/dL) are suggestive of alcohol abuse, while a level of more than 33 mmol/L (150 mg/dL) indicates tolerance and dependence in a patient who is not obviously intoxicated. Blood and urine tests for the presence of various drugs can be obtained, but the physician must specify which classes of drugs are in question. The sensitivity of drug testing is limited by a number of factors, including when the drug was administered and its pattern of absorption and excretion.

Self-Report

While many instruments are too lengthy for clinic use, a widely used questionnaire, the CAGE (Box 106–1), is appropriate for screening purposes. Some research indicates a higher level of diagnostic accuracy for this one-minute instrument than for laboratory tests, which take longer and are more costly to obtain.

Two or more positive responses suggest that the patient has an alcohol abuse problem. Although an equally brief and valid drug use questionnaire has not been developed, the same questions can be modified to ask about abuse of other drugs. A final step is to ask questions about typical consumption patterns. A "standard drink" is defined as 360 mL (12 oz) of beer, 150 mL (5 oz) of wine, or a mixed drink containing 45 mL (1.5 oz) of liquor. Current evidence indicates that daily intake of more than 60 g of ethanol for men or 40 g for women is potentially hazardous to health. In addition to daily amounts, the frequency of heavy (greater than four drinks for women or five drinks for men) drinking days should be noted. For other drugs, little is known about the level of use that discriminates "safe" from "at risk."

The advantage of a problem-based definition of substance abuse is well illustrated here. The physician relies on a composite picture rather than a single isolated item of information. If a life problem related to substance abuse emerges from the inquiry, the physician can intervene without having to label or stigmatize the patient.

The diagnostic process relies heavily on self-report, and the accumulation of research indicates that substance abusers tend to underreport consumption patterns and minimize the negative consequences associated with abuse. Factors associated with accurate self-report are good rapport with the health care provider, the knowledge that laboratory test results are forthcoming, the assurance of confidentiality, and the use of careful questioning in a nonconfrontational manner.

MANAGEMENT

An impressive accumulation of research suggests that brief interventions in primary care settings can be effective in reducing substance abuse. In addition to being cost effective in the face of shrinking health care budgets, brief approaches are suitable for reducing the adverse health consequences seen in many patients who do not meet the traditional criteria for "alcoholism." Although severely impaired substance abusers are not the obvious target group for these strategies,

BOX 106–1.   CAGE is an acronym for four questions:

1. Have you ever felt you should **cut** down on drinking?
2. Have people **annoyed** you by criticizing your drinking?
3. Have you felt bad or **guilty** about your drinking?
4. Have you had a drink first thing in the morning to steady your nerves or to get rid of a hangover (**eye-opener**)?

application is justified when conventional services are unavailable. These strategies can be more or less elaborate depending on the setting, time constraints, availability of more intensive treatments, severity of the substance abuse, and ability of the practitioner to arrange for follow-up. The basic framework is adaptable for promoting a wide variety of health behavior changes. Two basic schemes are described here.

Basic Single-Session Intervention

This approach is suitable when severity is low to moderate, time is short, and the likelihood of follow-up is low. The intervention consists of assessment and one session of counseling. The physician engages the patient and a significant other in a discussion of concerns about the patient's health. This discussion should flow from the results of the assessment and should be seen by the patient as a logical extension of that process. In an atmosphere that emphasizes the patient's personal responsibility, the physician provides objective feedback and clear advice to change. If the patient chooses to change, a treatment option is selected and a referral is arranged. A return clinic appointment or some other system of follow-up should be established.

Ongoing Brief Interventions

When assessment indicates the presence of a more severe problem and the physician can follow the patient over time, the approach can include motivational strategies. These strategies can be matched to the patient's stage of readiness for change (see below) and are more suitable for those who may require greater therapeutic effort. The intervention consists of assessment and brief counseling during each clinic visit. The goal is to move the patient through the change process by means of a nonauthoritarian discussion of concerns. The procedure includes three steps:

1. The physician spends a few minutes establishing **rapport.** This can often be done while attending to the reason for the patient's clinic visit.

2. The examiner asks **open-ended questions** related to the substance abuse issue. Questions should be about life-style, stress, health concerns, a typical day, and details of substance use. Useful lead-ins are, "Tell me about...? How does this affect you? Are you concerned about...? What do you think? Where does this fit?" Questions that link substance abuse with the topic should follow, such as, "How does having a drink help with stress? Where does cocaine fit in with this? What effect does pot have on you? Would it be useful to look at how drinking fits in with your fatigue? Where should we go from here? What should the next step be?"

3. The physician ends the session by **summarizing** the patient's problems and concerns. The examiner should express support and a willingness to help, while emphasizing that the ultimate responsibility and decision to change belong to the patient. If the individual wants to change, he or she is ready to receive informa-

tion about treatment options. If the patient is not ready, the physician should not push or behave negatively but instead focus on maintaining the relationship and follow up at the next visit.

Equally important as the content of the intervention is the interactional style of the physician. Several elements enhance the likelihood for patient change:

1. The examiner should employ a **collaborative** instead of a confrontational approach. Authoritative confrontations tend to evoke resistance and arguments for the opposing viewpoint. Physicians who are perceived as warm, empathic, and optimistic are more likely to be successful in having their patients accept referral for treatment.

2. The physician should **elicit** the concerns and problems associated with substance abuse from the patient. Arguments for change are more powerful when given by the patient in response to the physician's questioning. Clear advice to the patient to make a change is important, but it should occur within a collaborative context.

3. Change should be thought of as a dynamic **process** that can best be conceptualized as a continuum of successive stages:

   a. **Precontemplation**—the patient is not interested in change.

   b. **Contemplation**—the patient weighs the pros and cons of change.

   c. **Preparation**—the patient exhibits some change behaviors or thoughts.

   d. **Action**—the patient is ready to select and implement a change plan.

   e. **Maintenance/relapse**—the patient learns to continue change.

4. The physician should provide a **menu** of options for change. These choices include self-help approaches, community groups, commercial programs, and more intensive programs. Individuals who select from a variety of options experience an increased sense of control and are more likely to follow through.

PROGNOSIS

Many patients cycle through the change process several times before achieving long-term success. Relapse rates for alcohol, heroin, and smoking are remarkably similar—approximately 70% within 3 months. Relapse is a normal part of the change process and should not be viewed as a failure. Instead, it should be regarded as an opportunity to learn what went wrong and to prepare for the next attempt.

Research Questions

1. What are the most effective components of brief office based interventions for substance abuse?

2. What brief techniques are most reliable for the early detection of substance abuse?

3. What are the most effective strategies that can be implemented in the clinic for assisting patients with relapse episodes?

twice. He has now been abstinent for a year. He and his physician discuss his progress and monitor potential problems at each visit.

Case Resolution

The comprehensive evaluation led the physician to suspect that alcohol abuse was responsible for many of the patient's complaints. Assessment of the patient's readiness for change indicated that he was not considering a change in drinking behavior. The physician expressed concerns for the patient's general health, which were addressed at follow-up visits during the next few months. Over the next 2 years, the patient progressed through the change cycle

Selected Readings

Hester, R. K., and W. R. Miller (eds.). *Handbook of Alcoholism Treatment Approaches.* New York, Pergamon Press, 1989.

Marlatt, G. A., and J. R. Gordon (eds.). *Relapse Prevention: Maintenance Strategies in the Treatment of Addictive Behavior.* New York, Guilford, 1985.

Miller, W. R., and S. Rollnick. *Motivational Interviewing.* New York, Guilford, 1991.

Skinner, H. A., and S. Holt. *The Alcohol Clinical Index.* Toronto, Addiction Research Foundation, 1987.

CHAPTER 107

OBESITY

Ann Gateley, M.D.

H$_x$ A 57-year-old woman presents with a chief complaint of bilateral heel pain. It is described as an ache in the morning that gradually eases up during the day. The patient does not engage in a regular exercise program. She has recently started working outside the home as a shelver in a discount merchandising mart. She is gravida 4, para 4. She has a 10-year history of hypertension and has been told that she has "sugar diabetes," which is diet controlled. She is 163 cm (5' 4") in height and weighs 90 kg (200 lb). Her blood pressure is 150/90 mm Hg, with her other vital signs being normal. The general examination is remarkable for obesity and an erythematous rash underneath both breasts and in the groin area. She has bilaterally tender heels at the insertion of the long arch.

Questions

1. Do you think the patient's heel pain, rash, hypertension, and diabetes mellitus are related to her weight?
2. How attainable is the goal of long-term weight loss in this individual?
3. How should you approach this patient and her problems?

over their ideal weight. Compared to similarly developed Western countries (e.g., Great Britain and Canada), our prevalence of obesity in adults is particularly high. In the Western world, weight often is inversely related to economic class, especially for women. This is most likely due to our high degree of industrialization combined with a sedentary life-style. The prevalence of obesity also varies with ethnic origin. In general, Native Americans are more overweight than African Americans who are more overweight than Hispanics who are more overweight than white Americans.

PATHOPHYSIOLOGY

Excluding weight gain secondary to organic disease or medications (Table 107–1), obesity is usually multifac-

---

TABLE 107–1. Biologic Causes of Obesity

Dysmorphic genetic obesities, e.g., Prader-Willi syndrome
Neuroendocrine obesities
   Hypothalamic obesity—secondary to trauma, malignancy, or inflammatory disorders
   Pituitary obesity—secondary to hypothyroidism or decreased growth hormone
   Ovarian obesity—secondary to Stein-Leventhal syndrome (polycystic ovary disease)
   Pancreatic obesity—secondary to insulinoma and hyperinsulinemia
   Adrenal obesity—secondary to Cushing's syndrome
   Exogenous obesity—secondary to medication use, e.g., glucocorticoids or tricyclic antidepressants

---

Approximately 40,000,000 individuals in the United States are at least 20% heavier than their ideal weight. Of these, more than 13,000,000 people are greater than 40%

torial in etiology. To put it simply, an individual becomes overweight when there is an imbalance between energy intake and energy expenditure. However, an individual's adult weight is the result of the complex interplay of several factors, including heredity. Unique differences in energy expenditure are seen at a very early age. If one compares infants of obese parents with infants of normal-weight parents, the resting metabolic rate of the former is discernibly less than that of the latter. Additional studies confirm that the rate of resting energy expenditure is inherited. Not only do resting metabolic rates differ among individuals, but there are also inherited differences in the level of spontaneous activity exhibited by individuals and the energy cost of light, submaximal exercise. The cultural milieu in which an individual is raised may be another factor contributing to obesity. In some societies, very heavy people are viewed as prosperous and healthy. Situational factors also can contribute to an imbalance between energy intake and energy expenditure. For example, if food intake remains the same, people will gain weight if they decrease their activity level. Examples of changes in activity level can be as subtle as a promotion from an ambulatory job to a desk job or as dramatic as incurring a disability that confines a person to a wheelchair. Lastly, animal studies suggest that an appropriate sense of satiety is at least partially based on inherited factors.

EVALUATION

The evaluation of obesity is best approached by performing a careful history and a thorough physical examination. The history should emphasize the patient's personal experience of weight gain and loss. A baseline exercise history should be obtained, including the nature of the patient's job and any exercise program that the patient follows. Of course, caloric intake can best be documented by having the patient maintain a careful food diary. The patient's sociocultural background should be ascertained as well as any family history of obesity. Finally, the clinician should assess (1) the patient's awareness of her or his overall health status and (2) the patient's motivation to effect a life-style change.

The physical examination should include the patient's height and weight and a determination of the body mass index (BMI). The BMI is a way to normalize weight for height in a manner analogous to the cardiac index and is obtained by dividing the patient's weight in kilograms by his or her height in meters squared (kg/m^2). The ideal BMI is between 20 and 25, and a value over 30 is indicative of severe obesity. If the appropriate equipment is available, a measurement of percentage of body fat also should be done. The easiest and least expensive way to estimate percentage of body fat is by using calipers. At least two determinations of skin-fold thickness should be made, and then a formula can be used to estimate the percentage of body fat. In addition, the waist-to-hip ratio (WHR) should be assessed using a tape measure. As this ratio approaches one (i.e., when the patient begins to resemble an apple), the risk of developing cardiovascular disease increases. The clinician should check for

TABLE 107–2. Medical Complications of Obesity

System	Complication
Cardiovascular	Hypertension
	Premature atherosclerotic disease
	Left ventricular hypertrophy associated with congestive heart failure
Pulmonary	Sleep apnea
	Alveolar hypoventilation
Metabolic	Gout
	Non–insulin-dependent diabetes mellitus
	Hyperlipidemia
Hepatobiliary	Cholelithiasis
	Hepatic steatosis
Musculoskeletal	Low back pain
	"Overuse" injuries
	Degenerative joint disease
	Aggravation of inflammatory arthritis
Reproductive/breast	Cancer
Renal	Proteinuria
	Renal vein thrombosis
Psychosocial	Impaired self-esteem
	Loss of mobility
	Subjection to discrimination
Miscellaneous	High operative risk
	Interference with diagnosis of other disorders

signs of obesity-influenced disease (Table 107–2) as well as mechanical problems induced by carrying extra weight. In addition, the clinician should consider requesting a small number of laboratory tests to confirm the presence or absence of associated disease (e.g., a blood glucose determination and a check for hyperlipidemia and hyperuricemia).

MANAGEMENT

The reasons to treat obesity are the same as the reasons to treat any other medical disorder. The clinician first must determine whether or not the condition has the potential to cause harm. Second, the clinician must be aware of whether effective treatment exits. Finally,

TABLE 107–3. Conventional Treatment of Obesity

Exercise
Unsupervised
Monitored
    Exercise prescription
    Personal trainer
    Class
    Community/hospital-based program

Diet
Unsupervised
    Individual
    Prescription
Monitored
    Weight loss program
    Inpatient unit
    Very low calorie diet (< 800 kcal/d)

Psychotherapy
Individual
Group
Lay

Medication
Surgery

TABLE 107–4. Pharmacologic and Surgical Options for Weight Loss

Mode of Action	Class of Drug	Surgical Therapy
Decreased appetite	Noradrenergic	
	Serotoninergic	
Decreased gastric emptying or reservoir	Cholecystokinin	Gastric stapling
Decreased energy stores by		
increasing adipose tissue lipolysis (currently in research and development)		
increasing fatty acid oxidation		
Increased energy expenditure	Thermogenic agents	
	β₂-Adrenergic agents	
	α₂-Adrenergic receptor antagonists	
Combination therapy	Serotoninergic plus noradrenergic agents	
Decreased energy absorption by		
blocking carbohydrate digestion	Glucosidase inhibitor	
blocking lipid digestion	Pancreatic lipase inhibitor	
decreasing absorptive surface		Intestinal bypass surgery

the clinician must be able to weigh the risks and benefits of treatment to determine whether treatment should be recommended.

Historically, the management of obesity has focused on interventions to achieve weight loss (Table 107–3). Most individuals in the United States who try to lose weight use a combination of exercise and diet. Pharmacologic and surgical options for weight loss are outlined in Table 107–4, and psychotherapeutic interventions are presented in Table 107–5. Diet, exercise, and various combinations of medication and behavioral modification techniques have been shown to produce modest weight loss (an average of 10% from the starting weight) in the majority of individuals who maintain these interventions for 6 months or longer. Medications are effective as long as they are continued. Surgery for obesity, such as gastric restriction procedures (e.g., stapling) or malabsorption procedures (e.g., intestinal bypass), is effective but should be reserved for patients with massive, refractory obesity. The cumulative cost of all these interventions is high—about 50 billion dollars annually in the United States.

PATIENT AND FAMILY EDUCATION

People in the United States are very successful at losing weight, but maintaining that weight loss is difficult, if not impossible, for most people. Furthermore, it has not been unequivocally demonstrated that weight loss *per se* reduces health risks. Therefore, primary care physicians should stress alternatives to the goal of weight loss. For overweight individuals, the overall goal should be to improve health (not appearance), and the specific goals should include improved fitness, increased mobility, greater flexibility, and increased self-esteem. The desired outcome should be improvement in complicating diseases (e.g., diabetes,

hypertension, hyperlipidemia) rather than loss of pounds. Specific suggestions for a healthier life-style include (1) increasing the level of exercise, (2) normalizing food intake (no fasting or binging), and (3) receiving less than 30% of the daily caloric intake from fat. Additionally, patients need to reset their negative body image and stop reproaching themselves for not being "movie-star thin."

NATURAL HISTORY/PROGNOSIS

Most people who initiate a weight loss program are able to achieve some weight loss. However, *maintenance* of weight loss has proved more difficult. Less than 5% of individuals who voluntarily lose weight are able to maintain their weight loss after 5 years. The majority of people gain back the weight within the first year. Additionally, the literature does not support the widely held view that achieving weight loss reduces morbidity and mortality risk. A meta-analysis of published studies analyzing the effects of long-term changes in body weight indicated that the highest mortality rates occur in adults who have either lost or gained excessive weight. The lowest mortality rates were associated with steady, modest weight gain throughout adulthood. Because of methodologic issues, however, the conclusions of this meta-analysis require additional investigation and validation.

Research Questions

1. Does voluntary weight loss, not associated with chronic disease or smoking, significantly lower morbidity or mortality in adults?
2. What factors are important in helping individuals achieve a long-term commitment to fitness and exercise?

TABLE 107–5. Psychotherapeutic Interventions

Individual psychotherapy
The addictive model (e.g., Overeaters Anonymous)
Behavioral modification—cognitive behavioral techniques
Hypnosis

Case Resolution

This patient had a body mass index of approximately 28. Her bilaterally tender heel pads were due to plantar fasciitis, an "overuse" injury often seen in overweight individuals. Both her hypertension and her diabetes mellitus were worsened by her weight. The rash was caused by candidiasis, which was promoted by diabetes mellitus as well as the warm, moist cutaneous environment provided by overlapping skin folds.

Heel cups and arch supports as well as a course of antiinflammatory medication helped the tender heels. She began a daily walking program and a low-fat diet. Over the next year, her hypertension and diabetes mellitus improved, and she currently feels better about her present state of physical fitness.

Selected Readings

Andres, R., D. Mueller, and J. Sorkin. Long-term effects of change in body weight on all cause mortality. Ann Intern Med 119(7 part 2): 737–43, 1993.

Bjorntorp, P., and B. N. Brodloff (eds.). *Obesity.* J. B. Lippincott Company, Philadelphia, 1992.

Gardner, D. M., and S. C. Wooley. Confronting the failure of behavioral and dietary treatments for obesity. Clin Psychol Rev 11:129–80, 1991.

CHAPTER 108

INSOMNIA

Amanda A. Beck, M.D., Ph.D.

Hx A 60-year-old female office manager complains of "insomnia." She states that her difficulty sleeping has been going on for years but seems to be getting worse lately. She gets sleepy at work, has had increasing trouble getting her work done, and drinks "lots of coffee" to help stay awake. She had a cholecystectomy about 5 years ago and takes a β-blocker for hypertension. She has tried various over-the-counter sleep aids. She considers her job stressful and drinks a "little wine" in the evening to relax. Most nights she enjoys watching television but often falls asleep while doing so. On weekends she likes to "catch up on her sleep" and go dancing with her husband.

Questions

1. What is this patient's major complaint?
2. What are the most likely causes of her problem?
3. What additional information (e.g., from the history, physical examination, or ancillary testing) should be obtained?
4. What options do you have in managing this problem?

Insomnia may be defined as trouble initiating or maintaining sleep. Trouble sleeping is a common problem. In a survey conducted in the United States, one third of respondents reported having trouble sleeping in the past year and one half of that subgroup considered their trouble serious. Insomnia is more common among those who are anxious, depressed, or ill. It is also more prevalent among women and the elderly. The vast majority of people who complain of this problem do not take either prescription or over-the-counter medications for it. Of those who do, however, such use is more common in women, the elderly, and those with symptoms of anxiety or depression.

PATHOPHYSIOLOGY

Sleep consists of two basic stages: REM (rapid eye movement) and NREM (non-rapid eye movement). Each is as distinctly different from the other as each is from waking. About one fifth of the night is spent in REM sleep and four fifths in NREM, which itself has four stages. Stage 1 of NREM is the transition from wakefulness to sleep. Stage 2 is light sleep. Stages 3 and 4 are often combined and called deep sleep or delta sleep. Each stage is distinguished by a characteristic electroencephalographic pattern. REM sleep is characterized by the presence of rapid eye movements, low or absent muscle tone in major muscle groups, and the occurrence of dreaming. NREM sleep may be thought of as an inactive mind in a moving body, while REM represents an active mind in a paralyzed body. The average length of the NREM/REM cycle is about 90 minutes. The purpose of NREM and REM sleep as distinct entities is unknown.

Almost all major functions of the body have cyclic activity, varying over a period of about 24 hours. Cardiac and respiratory function slows during NREM sleep, increases during wakefulness, and becomes variable during REM sleep. Endocrine function also varies, with this variability being quite complex. Thermoregulation is similarly altered during sleep. During NREM sleep, humans are less sensitive to heat or cold, and during REM sleep, inhibition of thermoregulatory mechanisms leads to a state approaching poikilothermy.

Most people are "entrained" to a 24-hour cycle; i.e., they adjust their behavior to operate within this time frame even though some intrinsic rhythms might differ. Light is the most important factor in synchronizing biologic cycles with the rotation of the planet. Other so-called zeitgebers (time-givers) like periodic eating, environmental temperature changes, arousal states, and social cues may influence the "clock." The main "clock" or oscillator for these cycles is the suprachiasmatic nucleus located just above the optic chiasm, and melatonin elaborated within the nearby pineal gland appears to be the hormone responsible for sleep onset and offset.

Two factors control the timing and duration of sleep: (1) sleep propensity, i.e., when a person sleeps in relationship to the underlying clock, and (2) sleep debt or pressure, i.e., how long a person has been awake. Sleep onset naturally occurs as body temperature begins to drop and melatonin secretion rises. This occurs normally in the late evening. The nadir of body temperature occurs in the early morning hours between 2 and 5 AM. Most REM sleep occurs near this nadir. Sleep offset occurs normally when body temperature rises and melatonin declines in the later morning hours, normally around 6–8 AM. This circadian rhythm adapts fairly easily to time changes of approximately 2 hours in either direction. Rapid changes larger than this exceed the "limits of entrainment."

Control of sleep within the brain is most likely facilitated by sleep-inducing areas in the brain stem as well as opposing wakefulness mechanisms such as the reticular activating system and the posterior hypothalamus. For sleep to occur, the wakefulness system must "shut off" so that the weaker sleep-inducing system can dominate. Insomnia may therefore have two neurochemical mechanisms—excessive arousal and insufficient strength of sleep induction. A variety of neurochemicals have been implicated in sleep and its various stages, such as acetylcholine and catecholamines in promoting wakefulness, and serotonin in sleep induction and slow-wave sleep enhancement.

Sleep deprivation has minor effects on many short-term tasks but significant deleterious effects on both creative and monotonous tasks. Deprivation of REM sleep has been reported to lead to excitability and anxiety, and the loss of slow wave sleep to intense fatigue, uneasiness, and withdrawal.

Normal sleep ranges from 5 to 10 hours. Having "enough sleep" enables a person to function competently during the day without struggling with sleepiness during prolonged quiet or monotonous situations. Age is the single most powerful determinant of sleep physiology. At about 3 years of age, a childhood pattern emerges with a sleep duration of about 10 hours. During adolescence, the total amount of sleep decreases to about 8 hours. Adolescents and young adults need as

much sleep as middle-aged adults but often have trouble falling asleep and arising, thus leading to chronic sleep deprivation. With advanced age, the total time in bed increases but the total amount of "true" sleep actually decreases. Deep sleep decreases, and REM sleep is maintained. Sleep efficiency (the ratio of time asleep to time in bed) falls from the level typical of middle-aged adults, i.e., from approximately 95% to 75%. Elders awaken more often and therefore report a greater degree of fragmented sleep. They also tend to go to sleep earlier in the night, thereby "phase advancing" their sleep in relation to the natural time of greatest circadian propensity.

DIFFERENTIAL DIAGNOSIS

Complaints of sleeping poorly can most simply be thought of either as difficulty with initiating and maintaining sleep (DIMS) or as difficulty with excessive daytime somnolence (DOES). However, people with severe DIMS sometimes feel quite fatigued during the day, and people whose major complaint is DOES often sleep very poorly at night but are unaware of it.

The differential diagnosis of insomnia may be categorized as follows: (1) transient situational factors outside the sleep process, (2) factors related to the sleep process itself, (3) circadian rhythm disturbances, and (4) psychiatric or medical illness. It is common for insomnia to be multifactorial. The following are some of the most common causes of insomnia as defined in the *International Classification of Sleep Disorders*.

Adjustment sleep disorder is a disturbance temporally related to acute stress or environmental change causing emotional arousal. Usually transient, this is the most common sleep disorder.

Psychophysiologic insomnia is a disorder of somatized tension and learned sleep-preventing behavior. It typically results in a complaint of poor-quality sleep and decreased daytime functioning. The true cause of the tension is often denied or repressed. There is often an overconcern with the inability to fall asleep so that a cycle develops in which the more the person tries to fall asleep the harder it is to accomplish. The association of sleeplessness with their particular bed or bedroom often results in patients sleeping better in places other than these. A hallmark is the near obsession of these patients with their sleep problem.

Inadequate sleep hygiene results from routinely performing activities that preclude good quality sleep and full daytime alertness. The complementarity and interdependence of sleep and waking practices must be recognized before successful sleep can occur. Proper sleep hygiene includes (1) adhering to regular times for going to sleep and arising, which are optimally related to the natural circadian rhythm, (2) limiting the amount of time in bed to little more than the time spent asleep, and (3) restricting naps if they result in reduced sleep the following night. Factors related to maintaining an optimal environment for sleep include (1) minimizing noise and light, (2) ensuring comfortable temperature and bedding, and (3) using the bedroom only for sleep-compatible behaviors, i.e., avoiding using the bedroom for paying bills, worrying, or watching television. Another component of proper sleep hygiene is avoiding stimulants such as caffeine and tobacco as well as other complex drugs such as alcohol. Stimulants may cause sleeplessness when initially used and withdrawal-related sleepiness when discontinued. The use of stimulants such as cocaine or other illicit drugs is often not reported and often not recognized. Alcohol initially induces sleepiness and is frequently used as a hypnotic. Since alcohol is metabolized later in the night, frequent awakenings occur, with increased REM activity and associated nightmares. Any drug that affects the central nervous system (CNS)—either as an intended effect or an unintended side effect—may disturb sleep.

Obstructive sleep apnea (OSA) typically presents as marked daytime sleepiness. It is characterized by repetitive episodes of upper airway obstruction that occur during sleep and are usually associated with snoring, multiple apneic episodes, hypoxemia, and repeated arousals. The hallmark snoring pattern consists of loud snores or brief gasps that alternate with periods of silence typically lasting 20–30 seconds. Snoring may be exacerbated by weight gain or by ingestion of alcohol before bedtime.

Central sleep apnea is characterized by decreased or temporary cessation of ventilatory effort during sleep, usually associated with hypoxemia. It usually presents with insomnia rather than daytime somnolence.

Periodic limb movements in sleep (PLMS) is a disorder manifested by repetitive episodes of highly stereotyped movements of the extremities, usually extension of the big toe in combination with partial flexion of the ankle, knee, and sometimes hip. These movements are often associated with partial or complete awakening, although in the morning the patient cannot recall either the movements or the frequent sleep disruption. Such patients typically complain of insomnia, unrefreshing sleep, or daytime fatigue. PLMS may be associated with a variety of medical conditions (e.g., renal failure) and can also be induced by drugs or drug withdrawal. It is especially common in the elderly, affecting one third of those over the age of 60 years.

Restless leg syndrome (RLS) is characterized by disagreeable leg sensations that usually occur prior to sleep onset and cause an almost irresistible urge to move the legs. Patients may describe an aching, creeping, tingling, or itching. It may be associated with pregnancy or anemia. Most patients with RLS also exhibit PLMS.

Sleep state misperception is a disorder in which insomnia with or without excessive daytime sleepiness occurs without objective evidence of sleep disturbance. "Insomnia" is often reported on the night a laboratory sleep study shows good sleep. Some patients may be grossly inaccurate in their estimation of time spent asleep. Inappropriate use of hypnotic drugs may result when this disorder goes unrecognized.

Circadian rhythm disturbances are characterized by a misalignment between the patient's sleep pattern and the pattern that is desired or regarded as the social norm. The time zone change syndrome (more commonly known as jet lag) follows rapid travel across multiple time zones and consists of varying degrees of difficulty initiating or maintaining sleep, excessive sleepiness during waking hours, a subjective decrease in alertness and performance, and somatic (primarily gastrointestinal) symptoms. Symptoms increase in proportion to the number of time zones crossed and when (1) a person travels from west to east, (2) takeoff or arrival is at variance with optimal sleep-wake times, and (3) the traveler is elderly.

Shift work sleep disorder consists of insomnia with or without excessive sleepiness that occurs in relation to work schedules. Typically work is scheduled during the "normal" sleep hours. Inability to maintain sleep characteristically shortens the sleep period by 1–4 hours, affecting mainly REM and light sleep. A marked increase in sleepiness can occur during the night shift. Despite many years of night shift work, adaptation rarely occurs, mainly because daytime activities are resumed on the days off work.

Psychiatric disorders can lead to sleep disturbances. Depression can cause difficulty in both falling asleep and maintaining sleep. This results in early awakening but usually not in objectively measurable sleepiness during the day. Insomnia associated with anxiety disorders is characterized by apprehension about one or more life circumstances. Panic episodes can be associated with sudden awakenings from sleep, and insomnia and excessive daytime sleepiness are common features of psychoses such as bipolar disorder.

A large number of **medical and neurologic disorders** also may cause insomnia, including Parkinson's disease, sleep-related epilepsy, chronic obstructive pulmonary disease, sleep-related asthma, fibromyalgia, peptic ulcer disease, and gastroesophageal reflux disease. As a rule, any cerebral degenerative disorder or any medical disorder that causes pain may lead to insomnia.

EVALUATION

History

Table 108–1 provides a checklist of questions that are helpful in assessing the complaint of insomnia.

Patients should be advised to keep a sleep log, completing a line each morning describing the previous night's sleep, including (1) the time they went to bed, (2) the time they last remember being awake, (3) the time of awakening in the morning, (4) the time out of bed, (5) the times of any awakenings and how long they lasted, (6) the use of any medications or other substances, and (7) any other conditions or circumstances that may have disturbed their sleep. From this data it can be determined whether a patient is attempting sleep at the optimal time of night (i.e., 12–6 AM) or is spending too much time in bed (i.e., > 110% of the total sleep time). "Efficiency" of sleep (the total time asleep/the total time in bed) is important to calculate, since it reflects success in sleeping during the attempted sleep period. Insomniacs are often frustrated because they spend a great deal of time in bed not sleeping. Latency (the time from lights-out to falling asleep) is also key, since it measures the ease with which someone falls asleep.

**TABLE 108–1.   Insomnia Checklist for
Assessment and Management**

Sleep Complaint

Duration
Factors associated with onset
Progression (Staying the same? Getting worse?)
Timing of complaint to the practitioner (Why now?)
Primarily poor sleep vs. daytime sleepiness
Reported sleep pattern
Beliefs about causes
Expectations of desired sleep

Environmental Factors

Absence of regular sleep place
Absence of bedtime routine
Use of bed and bedroom for other than sleep-enhancing activities (e.g., watching
    television, prolonged reading, paying bills, family disputes, eating)
Noise, light, or temperature not optimal
Bed partner movement, pet sleeping on bed
Bed uncomfortable for patient's needs

Diet and Drug Use

Stimulants such as caffeine or nicotine
Alcohol
Over-the-counter or prescription hypnotics
Other over-the-counter or prescription medications that may interfere with sleep

Sleep-wake Cycle

Irregular bedimes or arousal times
Sleep time does not coincide with natural sleep propensity time

Primary Sleep Disorders

Periodic leg movements during sleep (PLMS)
Nocturnal tingling, aching, or cramping (restless leg syndrome or nocturnal leg
    cramps)
Snoring and daytime sleepiness (obstructive or central sleep apnea)

Psychiatric Problems

Anxiety
Depression

Medical Problems

Any disorder causing physical discomfort before or during sleep

Neurologic Problems

Any degenerative disease of the central nervous system

Physical Examination

Examination focuses on the (1) body habitus (obesity
is common in patients with OSA), (2) neck (usually short
in OSA), (3) throat (often partially occluded in OSA), (4)
nasal passages (since occlusion may lead to mouth
breathing), and (5) lungs and heart (since OSA may
result in cardiopulmonary compromise).

Additional Evaluation

Polysomnography is the simultaneous recording during sleep of (1) an electroencephalogram (EEG), (2) eye
movement, (3) air movement through the nose, (4) an

electrocardiogram (ECG), (5) oxygen saturation, and
(6) limb and chest wall movement. Analysis of the resulting patterns can aid in the diagnosis of sleep apnea,
nocturnal seizures, PLMS, and other disorders.

MANAGEMENT

For the management of insomnia to be successful,
a large share of the work must be done by the patient.
The cornerstones of treatment are (1) realistic expectations of what can be accomplished, (2) appropriate
sleep hygiene practices, (3) behavioral therapy, and (4)
limited use of hypnotics.

Cognitive therapy focuses on correcting dysfunctional attitudes and beliefs regarding sleep. Individual
expectations about sleep vary, and it frequently is
necessary to dispel misconceptions. Improving sleep
hygiene is essential. Whatever the underlying diagnosis,
most sleep problems have an associated impairment in
sleep hygiene.

Some nonpharmacologic approaches can be helpful.
Chronotherapy is the use of bright light therapy to
entrain people to stay on a more appropriate sleep
schedule. Exposure in the morning helps people go to
sleep earlier at night, while exposure in the evening
helps people go to sleep later at night.

Stimulus control therapy focuses on maximizing the
association between the bedroom and sleep. As a
general rule, the patient should use the bedroom only
for sleep or sex and, if not engaged in either, should go
elsewhere.

Sleep restriction therapy attempts to improve the
efficiency of sleep. The patient restricts the time spent
in bed to little more than the nightly average actually
slept the week before.

Relaxation therapy focuses on ways to reduce anxiety symptoms that may be interfering with sleep.
Patients are taught how to physically and mentally relax,
thereby "allowing" themselves to fall asleep rather than
"making" themselves fall asleep.

Hypnotics are useful for patients who (1) are suffering
significant daytime consequences of their sleep disturbance, (2) have transient insomnia related to a personal
or environmental change, or (3) are entering into behavioral therapy for chronic insomnia and need occasional short-term assistance until a long-term nonpharmacologic regimen is established. The most effective
hypnotic is one with a rapid onset, relatively short
half-life, high therapeutic index, and specificity directed
toward sleep induction rather than relief of anxiety. For
these reasons, the benzodiazepines are the agents of
choice (Table 108–2) and medications such as antihistamines and barbiturates are not recommended. The
role of antidepressants in the treatment of insomnia not
caused by depression is unclear at this time. All
benzodiazepine hypnotics induce tolerance in approximately a month's time, thereby limiting their long-term
effectiveness. Long-acting hypnotics such as flurazepam
have been associated with daytime somnolence and an
increased risk of falls, while the short-acting agent
triazolam has been associated with amnesia. Lower
doses should be used in the elderly.

TABLE 108–2.   Benzodiazepine Hypnotics

Drug	Time to Reach Peak Levels (hours)	Elimination	Half-life (hours)	Dose Range (mg)
Triazolam	1.2 ± 0.5	Ultrarapid	2.6 ± 0.7	0.125–0.25
Temazepam	0.8 ± 0.3	Rapid	8.4 ± 0.6	15–30
Flurazepam	1.4 ± 0.7	Slow	40–103	15–30

Research Questions

1. What is the role of NREM and REM sleep?
2. Does light therapy have a role in the workplace or in institutions such as hospitals and nursing homes?
3. Can melatonin analogues be developed that will aid in the management of insomnia?

Case Resolution

The physician recommended that the patient (1) keep a sleep log, (2) enlist her husband's help in monitoring her sleep-related behavior, (3) maintain a consistent time for lights out and awakening, (4) watch television outside of the bedroom (and not nap in front of the set), (5) eliminate her evening wine, and (6) switch her blood pressure pill to a calcium channel blocker. At a follow-up visit 3 weeks later, she reported great improvement.

Selected Readings

American Sleep Disorders Association. *The International Classification of Sleep Disorders.* Rochester, New York, 1990.

Gillin, J., and W. Byerley. The diagnosis and management of insomnia. N Engl J Med 322:239–48, 1990.

Hauri, P. *Current Concepts: Sleep Disorders.* Kalamazoo, Michigan, Upjohn Company, 1992.

Kryger, M., T. Roth, and W. Dement. *Principles and Practices of Sleep Medicine*, 2nd ed. Philadelphia, W.B. Saunders Company, 1993.

Morin, C. *Insomnia: Psychological Assessment and Management.* New York, Guilford Press, 1993.

Printz, P., M. Vitiello, M. Raskind, and M. Thorpy. Sleep disorders and aging. N Engl J Med 323:520–5, 1990.

COMMON DERMATOLOGIC PROBLEMS

C H A P T E R   1 0 9

ACNE

Jerry Feldman, M.D.

H$_x$ A 19-year-old female sales clerk asks for help in treating her acne, which she has had for the past 3 years. A careful history reveals that she takes no systemic medications except birth control pills. She has no menstrual irregularities, abnormal hair growth, or history of occupational exposure to chemicals. Physical examination reveals a shy young woman with a large number of open comedones ("blackheads") and closed comedones ("whiteheads") and some inflamed papules on her face. Her back exhibits a moderate number of papules and pustules ("yellowheads").

Questions

1. What four factors are involved in the pathogenesis of acne?
2. Why does acne usually begin during puberty?
3. Why is it important to ask the patient about menstrual irregularities?
4. How does isotretinoin work, and what are the associated adverse effects?

Acne vulgaris is one of the most common skin diseases, accounting for approximately 25% of visits to dermatologists. Peak involvement occurs during adolescence, with nearly every teenager developing some degree of acne, ranging from extremely mild to severe. Although considered a benign disease, acne can result in permanent physical or emotional scarring. In women, acne may first develop in the late 20s or early 30s.

CLINICAL PRESENTATION

Acne vulgaris is a disease of a specialized type of pilosebaceous unit, the sebaceous follicle. Characteristic lesions include open comedones (blackheads), closed comedones (whiteheads), erythematous papules, pustules, and sometimes deep nodules or cysts (Fig. 109–1).

PATHOPHYSIOLOGY

The sebaceous follicle (Fig. 109–2) differs from the pilosebaceous follicle by having a much smaller hair and a larger sebaceous gland. These follicles are limited to the face, ear lobes, neck, shoulders, upper back, and V-shaped area of the chest.

Four major factors are involved in the pathogenesis of acne: (1) hyperkeratinization of the follicular duct, (2) increased sebum production, (3) increased local population of *Propionibacterium acnes,* and (4) development of inflammation.

The initial lesion in acne (the microcomedo) develops as a consequence of altered keratinization of the infrainfundibulum portion of the follicular duct. Normally, the corneocytes in this area are thin and separate easily. In acne vulgaris, they become thick and adherent, with a resultant failure to desquamate. The follicular duct becomes plugged, obstructing the follicular canal, causing cellular debris and sebum to collect behind the obstruction and form a solid mass known as a comedo.

Sebum is a complex mixture of lipids secreted by the sebaceous glands under endocrinologic control, primarily via androgens produced by the gonads and adrenal glands. The levels of these hormones (e.g., testosterone and dehydroepiandrosterone sulfate [DHEAS]) are usually normal in acne patients. Consequently, the defect is in end-organ hyperresponsiveness, leading to excess sebum production. Patients with acne produce more sebum on average, and sebum levels correlate directly with the severity of the disease.

P. acnes is a gram-positive diphtheroid that inhabits the lower part of the sebaceous follicle. The *P. acnes* population is dramatically increased in acne lesions, with the combination of increased sebum levels and altered follicular keratinization providing an ideal environment for its multiplication. As *P. acnes* multiplies, the microcomedo enlarges and forms a closed comedo or "whitehead." *P. acnes* manufactures lipases that degrade the sebum triglycerides into free fatty acids, breakdown products that are toxic to the follicular epithelium. *P. acnes* also produces a variety of other sub-

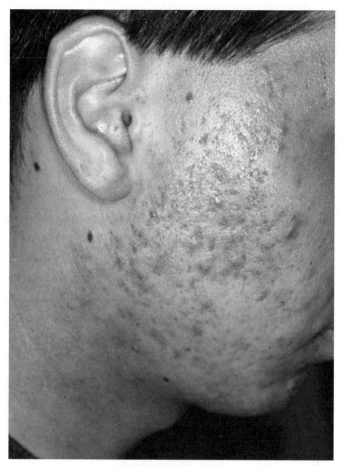

FIGURE 109–1. *Acne vulgaris.*

stances including proteolytic enzymes, hyaluronidase, and neutrophil chemotactic factors.

The inflammation that subsequently develops is multifactorial in origin. *P. acnes* secretes chemotactic factors that attract neutrophils to the follicular epithelium; these neutrophils then release toxic substances that breach the follicular wall. The sebum-derived free fatty acids also damage the follicular wall. As the weakened follicle expands and bursts, its contents (including keratin, hair, and *P. acnes*) are released into the dermis, eliciting an inflammatory response. In addition, the follicular epithelium secretes cytokines, attracting additional lymphocytes. Antibodies against *P. acnes* initiate the complement cascade, resulting in further escalation of the immune reaction.

The closed comedo ("whitehead") has two possible fates. It develops either into an open comedo ("blackhead") or into an inflammatory lesion, i.e, a papule, pustule, or nodule, depending on the depth and degree of inflammation.

DIFFERENTIAL DIAGNOSIS

The diagnosis of acne vulgaris is usually straightforward. At times, one must distinguish acne vulgaris from acne rosacea, perioral dermatitis, and folliculitis. Acne rosacea is characterized by papules, pustules, erythema, and telangiectasias in a central facial distribution. There are no comedones in acne rosacea. Acne rosacea usually develops later in life than does acne vulgaris. In perioral dermatitis, there are small erythematous papules in a perioral or perinasal distribution. The lesions are typically found in young women. Here, too, there are no comedonal lesions. Folliculitis is characterized by pustules in a follicular pattern, usually located on the chin, neck, and mandible in men.

EVALUATION

History

A thorough history should focus on possible etiologic factors. Is there evidence of a hyperandrogen state as manifested by irregular menstrual periods, hirsutism, or baldness? Is the patient taking any medications known to cause acne such as lithium, isoniazid (INH), androgens, corticosteroids, iodides, or bromides? Does the patient take oral contraceptives? Birth control pills containing certain progestational agents may provoke acne. Furthermore, acne may flare during the first two or three cycles of contraceptive usage. Does the patient have any habits that may induce acne? Mechanical trauma (e.g., friction, pressure, rubbing, squeezing) may aggravate acne lesions. Does the patient wear tight clothing, wear an occlusive chin strap, or continually wash? Is the patient exposed to comedogenic agents

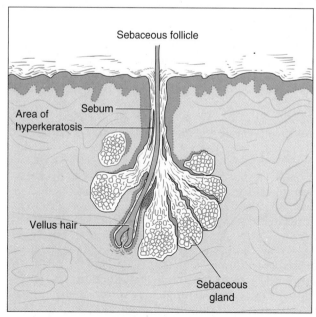

FIGURE 109–2. *Sebaceous follicle.*

such as heavy oils, greases, or tars? Most importantly, what treatments has the patient tried in the past?

Physical Examination

Careful examination of the skin is necessary to categorize the lesions as noninflamed or inflamed. Noninflamed lesions include closed comedones ("whiteheads") and open comedones ("blackheads"), each of which is typically 1–2 mm in diameter. Inflamed lesions include erythematous papules, pustules ("yellowheads"), and deep nodules or cysts. These lesions are graded on a subjective scale of 1+ to 4+. Inflamed lesions that are resolving appear as macules (flat red spots). In addition, patients may have scars of different types, including deep "ice pick" scars, soft scars, or hypertrophic or keloid scars.

Finally, the distribution of lesions should be documented. Do they involve the face, back, chest, arms, or buttocks? In patients with abnormal menstrual cycles or signs of hirsutism and in recalcitrant cases, an endocrinologic workup is indicated.

MANAGEMENT

The principles of treatment are based on correcting the pathophysiologic defects. These principles include (1) correcting the abnormal follicular hyperkeratinization, (2) decreasing the production of sebum, (3) decreasing the follicular population of *P. acnes,* and (4) decreasing the inflammatory response.

Agents that correct the abnormal follicular hyperkeratinization are called comedolytic agents. Topical tretinoin (Retin-A) is the most effective comedolytic agent. Since tretinoin causes irritation, it should be started at low concentrations on alternate days. Sulfur and benzoyl peroxide are less effective comedolytic agents. Currently available antiandrogenic agents are of limited use because of side effects. Estrogen decreases the production of androgen from the ovaries and is given most often in the form of birth control pills. However, it is important not to prescribe a birth control pill that contains a potent androgenic progesterone component.

The most effective sebostatic agent is isotretinoin (Accutane). Although it has revolutionized the treatment of acne, it should be reserved for recalcitrant cases of nodulocystic acne. The usual course is 16–20 weeks, with rare patients requiring repeat courses. The adverse effects of isotretinoin limit its usage. The most common side effects mimic the hypervitamin A syndrome, e.g., mucocutaneous effects such as dryness of the skin and lips, redness, scaling, and alopecia. Systemic side effects may include pseudotumor cerebri and decreased night vision. Even short courses of isotretinoin may cause skeletal hyperostoses. Moderate elevations of serum lipids are to be expected. Most significantly, isotretinoin is a teratogen and is absolutely contraindicated during pregnancy. Retinoic acid embryopathy occurs early in pregnancy and affects the central nervous system, craniofacial tissues, vascular system, and thymus. Contraception for the female patient is mandatory and should be extended for at least 1 month after stopping the drug.

Both topical and systemic medications are useful in suppressing *P. acnes.* Benzoyl peroxide is a topical and effective antibacterial agent that has been used in acne management for decades. This compound can produce irritation, dryness, and rarely allergic contact dermatitis. Currently, the two most effective topical antibiotics are erythromycin and clindamycin.

Tetracycline is the most commonly prescribed systemic antibiotic used in the treatment of acne. It often takes 4–6 weeks before improvement is seen. The absorption of tetracycline is inhibited by calcium, so it is recommended that the drug be taken on an empty stomach. Tetracycline also may cause irreversible yellowish-brown staining in developing teeth and consequently should not be used by pregnant women or children less than 12 years of age. Doxycycline and minocycline are related antibiotics that are also effective. Erythromycin and trimethoprim-sulfamethoxazole are alternative antibiotics that are often prescribed for patients who cannot tolerate (or do not respond to) the tetracyclines.

The tetracyclines, in addition to their antibacterial effect, exert potent antiinflammatory action by inhibiting neutrophil chemotaxis. Intralesional glucocorticoids are effective in decreasing the inflammation and size of moderately sized papules and nodules.

PATIENT AND FAMILY EDUCATION

Appropriate patient and family education is a vital component of acne treatment. Common myths must first be dispelled. No scientific studies indicate that diet plays a role in the pathogenesis of acne. Oily foods do not produce oily faces. Nor is acne a problem of dirt; in fact, overaggressive facial washing may aggravate the condition. Sunlight-induced erythema may mask active lesions, but sun exposure does not prevent acne.

Compliance with prescribed topical or systemic medication will be improved if the physician carefully explains both the disease and the adverse effects of the drugs. It is also important to stress the long-term nature of acne treatment. Many patients, for example, will need to remain on systemic antibiotics for 6 months or longer.

The physician must also be sensitive to the psychosocial consequences of acne, which can be significant. A sense of optimism should be conveyed, since acne—no matter how severe—can be improved by medical therapy. Self-esteem, self-image, and self-confidence can be destroyed during the especially vulnerable years of adolescence if acne is not kept in check with proper management.

NATURAL HISTORY/PROGNOSIS

Acne vulgaris usually starts in adolescence and resolves by the mid-20s. Acne develops earlier in females than in males and may persist in females into their late 30s. It is not unusual for women to develop acne for the first time in their late 20s or early 30s. The scarring of uncontrolled acne may persist forever.

Case Resolution

The patient's acne was treated with topical 0.025% tretinoin cream and oral tetracycline (500 mg twice daily). After 6 months of treatment, she had almost total resolution of her lesions.

Selected Readings

Cunliffe, W. J. *Acne.* Chicago, Year Book (Martin Dunitz), 1989.
Layton, A. M., and W. J. Cunliffe. Guidelines for optimal use of isotretinoin in acne. J Am Acad Dermatol 27, S2-S7, 1992.
Plewig, G., and A. M. Kligman. *Acne and Rosacea.* Berlin, Springer-Verlag, 1993.
Reingold, S. B., and R. L. Rosenfeld. The relationship of mild hirsutism or acne in women to androgens. Arch Dermatol 123:209–12, 1987.
Shalita, A. R., W. J. Cunningham, J. J. Leyden, et al. Isotretinoin treatment of acne and related disorders: An update. J Am Acad Dermatol 9:629–38, 1983.
Straus, J. S. Sebaceous glands. *In* T. B. Fitzpatrick, A. Z. Eizen, et al. (eds.). *Dermatology in General Medicine.* New York, McGraw-Hill Book Company, 1993.

CHAPTER 110

PSORIASIS

Irene Buño, M.D., and Jerry Feldman, M.D.

Hx A 27-year-old male forest ranger presents with a 1-year history of a red, nonpruritic, scaly rash on his trunk, extremities, and scalp. He feels well otherwise, has no history of medical problems, takes no medication, and denies any allergies. His family history is significant for an aunt with psoriasis. The physical examination reveals multiple well-demarcated red plaques with silvery thick scale on his scalp, elbows, knees, buttocks, and trunk. His fingernails have multiple small depressions.

Questions

1. What is the fundamental change in the epidermis of psoriatic patients? What factors can exacerbate psoriasis?
2. What are the social and psychological implications of a disfiguring disease?

Psoriasis is a chronic skin disease that is relapsing in nature. The worldwide prevalence of psoriasis varies from 1% to 3% depending upon race, geography, and environment. In the United States, psoriasis affects approximately 1% of the population. The prevalence among African Americans is very low, and psoriasis is almost nonexistent among Native Americans. Psoriasis affects males and females equally. The onset of disease is usually in the third decade of life. Earlier onset is predictive of greater extent of disease and less favorable response to therapy. One third of patients with psoriasis report having a relative with the disease. Other data suggesting a genetic predisposition include high rates of concordance among monozygotic twins and the association with the major histocompatibility antigens HLA B13, B17, Bw57, and Cw6. The relative risk of developing psoriasis among those who bear the Cw6 phenotype is 9–15 times normal.

CLINICAL PRESENTATION

The clinical presentation is highly variable in terms of the number, distribution, and type of lesions. The three important morphologic types of psoriasis include plaque-type, guttate, and pustular. The primary lesion in the first type is a sharply demarcated plaque with thick scale (Fig. 110–1). The lesion in guttate psoriasis is similar but smaller (Fig. 110–2). In contrast, pustular psoriasis is characterized by small, 2- to 3-mm sterile pustules. In all three forms, the lesions may be either localized or generalized.

PATHOPHYSIOLOGY

Abnormalities in epidermal cell kinetics, immune regulation, and genetics all play a role in the development of psoriasis. In psoriatic skin, there is evidence of excessive cellular proliferation and inflammation in the

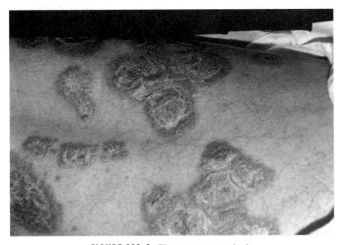

FIGURE 110–1. *Plaque-type psoriasis.*

epidermis, as well as decreased transit time of cells. Compared to normal skin, psoriatic skin lesions show a significantly shortened epidermal cell cycle (36 hours versus 311 hours for normal skin), a twofold increase in the proliferative cell population, and total involvement of the germinative cells of the epidermis (100% versus 70% in normal skin). Uninvolved skin in psoriatic patients may also display altered epidermal proliferation.

Involvement of the immune system is demonstrated by the (1) association between psoriasis and gene products of the major histocompatibility complex (i.e., HLA antigens); (2) presence of numerous activated T cells (CD4) within psoriatic lesions; (3) alterations in the number and distribution of Langerhans cells and dermal dendrocytes; (4) immune-dependent expression of adhesion molecules on psoriatic keratinocytes; and (5) antipsoriatic effects of treatments known to influence the immune system, such as cyclosporine and methotrexate.

Although the exact interaction between the immune system and epidermal proliferation is unclear, it is apparent that cytokines play a key role. Both immune cells and the epidermis secrete a wide variety of cytokines that initiate and maintain the psoriatic pro-

cess. Streptococcal proteins may act as superantigens triggering this self-amplifying cytokine loop.

Stress, physical trauma, and use of drugs (e.g., lithium, β-blockers, withdrawal from oral corticosteroids) also have been implicated as aggravating factors.

DIFFERENTIAL DIAGNOSIS

The diagnosis of classic untreated psoriasis usually is not difficult for the experienced clinicians. However, the early stages of psoriasis can pose a diagnostic dilemma.

Plaque-type psoriasis may be confused with nummular eczema, tinea corporis, lichen planus, Bowen's disease (squamous cell carcinoma-in-situ), pityriasis rubra pilaris, and cutaneous T-cell lymphoma (Table 110–1). Eczema has a diffuse, ill-defined border in contrast to the well-demarcated border of psoriasis. Tinea corporis will demonstrate fungal forms (hyphae) on a KOH preparation. Cutaneous T-cell lymphoma rarely has the distinct scale of psoriasis.

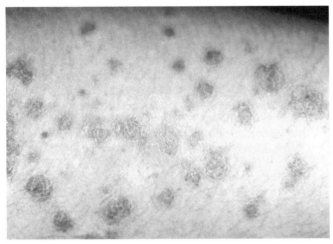

FIGURE 110–2. *Guttate psoriasis.*

TABLE 110–1. Differential Diagnosis of Psoriasis

Plaque Psoriasis
Nummular eczema
Lichen simplex chronicus
Tinea corporis
Discoid lupus erythematosus
Seborrheic dermatitis
Chronic dermatitis
Cutaneous T-cell lymphoma
Superficial basal cell carcinoma
Squamous cell carcinoma-in-situ (Bowen's disease)

Guttate Psoriasis
Pityriasis rosea
Secondary syphilis
Lichen planus
Drug eruption

Scalp Psoriasis
Seborrheic dermatitis
Tinea capitis
Pityriasis amantacea
Pityriasis rubra pilaris

Pustular Psoriasis
Subcorneal pustular dermatosis
Pustular drug eruption
Candidiasis

Palmar-Plantar Psoriasis
Eczema
Tinea manuum
Reiter's syndrome
Secondary syphilis

Guttate psoriasis may be confused with lichen planus, pityriasis rosea, and secondary syphilis. Lichen planus presents as violaceous, polygonal, flat-topped papules with fine white scaling. In contrast to the case for psoriasis, patients with lichen planus often have oral lesions. Secondary syphilis may be indistinguishable from psoriasis, but syphilitic disease tends to have more palmar lesions. A positive syphilis serology helps differentiate the two. Pityriasis rosea usually presents with a large herald patch and has a characteristic truncal "Christmas tree" distribution.

Scalp psoriasis may be confused with seborrheic dermatitis or tinea capitis. Patients with seborrheic dermatitis do not have lesions on the elbows, knees, and buttocks. In addition, the scale in psoriasis usually extends beyond the frontal hair line; this finding is rare in seborrheic dermatitis. Tinea capitis is unusual in adults.

EVALUATION

History

The history should seek to identify triggering factors (Table 110–2). Has there been a preceding infectious process? (Acute guttate psoriasis, for example, often follows a streptococcal infection by 1–2 weeks.) Since stress may stimulate psoriatic eruptions, inquiry should be made about recent stressful events. Has the patient taken any drugs (e.g., lithium or corticosteroids) that induce psoriasis? Does the patient have any joint pain or swelling (i.e., symptoms suggestive of psoriatic arthritis)?

Physical Examination

It is important to note the (1) distribution and extent of the lesions, (2) appearance of atypical lesions, and (3) presence or absence of diagnostic clues such as the Auspitz sign and Koebner's phenomenon. The Auspitz sign is very specific for psoriasis and refers to the appearance of small blood droplets on the erythematous surface a few seconds after removal of the hyperkeratotic scale. Koebner's phenomenon refers to the development of psoriatic lesions at sites of skin injury (e.g., scratch marks, surgical wounds, and areas of sunburn);

TABLE 110–2. Triggering Factors in Psoriasis

Drugs

Lithium
β-Adrenergic blocking agents
Systemic glucocorticosteroid withdrawal

Stress

Infection

(e.g., with *Streptococcus pyogenes*)

Trauma

Surgery
Chemical burn
Sunburn
Freezing
Pressure
Radiation
Laser burn
Scratching
Shaving

---

this phenomenon can be observed in up to 20% of patients with psoriasis.

Psoriasis may involve any area of the body, although the face is usually spared. Nail involvement occurs in 35%–50% of patients. Nail abnormalities range from pitting of the nail plate to the presence of yellowish macules subungually (so-called oil spots) to severe onychodystrophy. Nail changes are more frequent in patients with psoriatic arthritis.

The most common morphologic type is **plaque-type psoriasis**, also known as chronic stationary psoriasis or psoriasis vulgaris. Circular red, scaly plaques are typically present on the elbows, knees, lower back, and retroauricular areas of the scalp and may persist for months to years. Except in major skin folds, a large amount of scale is constantly produced.

Inverse psoriasis involves intertriginous areas such as axillary folds, inframammary creases, and intercrural regions.

Localized psoriasis is the presence of an isolated solitary lesion, e.g., on the glans penis. At the other end of the spectrum, psoriasis may be very diffuse, the most flagrant example being **psoriatic erythroderma**. In the latter condition, there is intense erythema (though with less severe scaling) involving all areas of the body, including the face and nails; psoriatic erythroderma may also evolve into a generalized exfoliative phase. This form of psoriasis may also occur as a response to topical therapy, representing a generalized Koebner phenomenon.

In **guttate** or **eruptive psoriasis**, lesions resemble small (0.5- to 1.5-cm) "raindrops" and are distributed over the upper trunk and proximal extremities. Guttate psoriasis is more common in young adults and is frequently preceded by a streptococcal throat infection 7–10 days before the cutaneous involvement.

Pustular psoriasis occurs in a variety of settings. Acute exacerbations of guttate psoriasis may be accompanied by 1- to 2-mm pustules surrounded by an intensive halo of erythema. Pustular psoriasis of the **von Zumbusch type** is a sudden generalized eruption of sterile pustules 2–3 mm in diameter associated with fever lasting several days; the lesions are typically distributed over the trunk, extremities, nail beds, palms, and soles. It can also occur in association with systemic infections.

Annular or **circinate pustular psoriasis** is a rare variant. Pustules appear on a ring-like erythematous base. Identical lesions are found in **impetigo herpetiformis**, a pustular and potentially fatal form of psoriasis associated with pregnancy.

MANAGEMENT

There is no cure for psoriasis, but many treatment modalities are available, including topical therapy, systemic medication, and phototherapy.

The most common form of treatment is corticosteroids applied topically. Topical corticosteroids are available in many different potencies as well as in a variety of vehicles (e.g., lotions, creams, and ointments). They are expensive and should be used sparingly, with application of a thin layer to the affected area once or twice daily, preferably to wet skin after a shower or bath. They become less effective over time, so the weakest possible preparation should be used for maintenance therapy, reserving the stronger preparations for more acute flares. Skin atrophy and systemic absorption is possible with overuse of the more potent steroids, and patients need to be warned of these potential adverse effects. Intralesional steroids can be of benefit in the management of selected plaques. Systemic steroids are generally contraindicated, since withdrawal of treatment may lead to a severe flare of disease and may even trigger acute pustular psoriasis or erythroderma.

Anthralin is a strong reducing agent with little systemic toxicity that has been used for many years in the treatment of psoriasis. It is available in different concentrations (0.05%–2%) in a petroleum jelly base or zinc paste. Treatment consists of daily application to affected areas, with a gradual increase in the concentration used and the length of time the paste is left on the skin prior to washing it off. Patients need to be warned that anthralin stains the surrounding skin, clothing, and hair. This treatment modality is especially effective for thick, scaly plaques.

Tar preparations (2%–5%) have been used for decades and are of great benefit in managing chronic plaque-type psoriasis. Tars contain a large variety of compounds, but little is known about their mechanism of action. There are few serious side effects even with prolonged treatment, although the pungent odor is sometimes commented on unfavorably by patients.

Calcipotriene, a topical vitamin D analog, is as efficacious as a potent topical steroid in clearing plaque psoriasis. If less than 100 g of calcipotriene ointment is used per week, there is little need to monitor serum or urine calcium levels.

Topical antiyeast agents are helpful to treat candidal superinfection in inverse psoriasis.

Systemic treatments are used in more severe cases of psoriasis. Methotrexate inhibits DNA synthesis and is thought to act primarily on the rapidly dividing epidermal cells within psoriatic lesions. It is indicated for generalized pustular psoriasis and psoriatic arthritis. It should not be used in patients with current infections or with significant renal, hepatic, or hematologic abnormalities. Pregnancy must be avoided by patients taking methotrexate. Liver biopsies need to be performed prior to initiation of therapy and after each cumulative 1-g dose to monitor for fibrosis and cirrhosis (which occur in 5%–10% of patients). The risk of hepatotoxicity depends on the (1) cumulative total dose, (2) length of treatment, (3) age of the patient, and (4) patient's daily alcohol intake.

Cyclosporine is an immunosuppressive drug often used in organ transplantation. It inhibits T-cell activation of IL-2 dependent pathways as well as proliferation of normal and transformed keratinocytes. Cyclosporine is indicated only for severe cases of psoriasis. Adverse effects include renal dysfunction, arterial hypertension, and increased levels of transaminases.

Etretinate, a derivative of vitamin A, is more popular in Europe than in the United States but can be effective in treating early forms of pustular and guttate psoriasis.

Etretinate causes rapid loss of scales. It has a long half-life in plasma and is a proven teratogen. Dose-related side effects include cheilitis, generalized pruritus, skin dryness, erythema, sore palms and soles secondary to loss of the stratum corneum, and thinning of scalp hair. Hypertriglyceridemia may also occur in the setting of liver disease, diabetes mellitus, obesity, or high alcohol intake. Thus, patients need to be counseled about avoidance of alcohol use as well as avoidance of pregnancy.

Phototherapy, from natural or artificial light, can be helpful in the treatment of psoriasis. Sunlight and ultraviolet B (UVB) therapy, for example, are frequently effective in the management of psoriasis.

Photochemotherapy combines the use of oral psoralen plus UVA light (PUVA). Psoralen is a photosensitizing agent that intercalates with DNA and irreversibly inhibits DNA synthesis and mitosis. Treatments are administered daily or several times per week, with the UVA dose gradually being increased. A course of 19–25 treatments is usually necessary to clear psoriatic lesions. Patients may complain of nausea, headache, and dizziness. In addition, patients should be warned about the need for eye protection and the possible increased risk of actinic sun damage and subsequent development of cutaneous cancers, especially squamous cell carcinoma.

Oral antibiotics effective against streptococcal organisms can improve guttate flares and acute exacerbations of psoriasis. Examples are dicloxacillin, cephalexin, and erythromycin.

For many patients, effective treatment entails a combination of the above-mentioned topical, systemic, and phototherapies. An especially popular combination is tar and ultraviolet light, known as the Goeckerman regimen.

PATIENT AND FAMILY EDUCATION

It should be emphasized to patients (and their families) that psoriasis is not infectious and thus not contagious. There is no scientific evidence that special diets are helpful. Aggravating factors should be identified and avoided insofar as possible.

Research Questions

1. Why are certain areas such as the knee and elbow especially prone to developing psoriasis?
2. How does a preceding streptococcal infection trigger psoriasis?
3. Are there any natural inhibitors of epidermal proliferation?
4. If the epidermis is more proliferative, wouldn't you expect a patient with psoriasis to be at greater risk of developing skin cancer?

NATURAL HISTORY/PROGNOSIS

Psoriasis is a chronic skin disease with an unpredictable course. It is treatable, although not curable. Spontaneous remission has been reported in 17%–55% of cases. Psoriatic arthritis occurs in 5% of patients.

Case Resolution

The patient's history and physical examination were consistent with moderate plaque psoriasis. Treatment included short-term high-potency topical corticosteroids initially, followed by mid-potency topical steroids as maintenance therapy. His psoriasis is currently under good control.

Selected Readings

Baker, B. S., and L. Fry. The immunology of psoriasis. Br J Dermatol 126:1–9, 1992.
Barker, J. N. W. N. The pathophysiology of psoriasis. Lancet 338:227–34, 1991.
Berth-Jones, J., and P. E. Hutchinson. Vitamin D analogues and psoriasis. Br J Dermatol 127:71–78, 1992.
Camisa, C. *Psoriasis*. Boston, Blackwell Scientific Publications, 1994.
Christophers, E., and W. Sterry. Psoriasis. *In* T. B. Fitzpatrick, A. Z. Eisen, et al. (eds.). *Dermatology in General Medicine*. New York, McGraw-Hill Book Company, 1993.
Fry, L. Psoriasis. Br J Dermatol 119:445–61, 1988.
Nickoloff, B. J. The cytokine network in psoriasis. Arch Dermatol 127:871–84, 1991.
Nikoloff, B. J., and L. A. Turka. Keratinocytes: Key immunocytes of the integument. Am J Pathol 143:325–31, 1993.

CHAPTER 111

CONTACT DERMATITIS

Jerry Feldman, M.D.

H$_x$ A 38-year-old female dietician recently had a punch biopsy performed for a skin lesion on her upper chest. After the procedure, she was instructed to wash the area and apply an over-the-counter topical antibiotic twice daily. Two days after beginning this wound care, she developed a pruritic, red, weeping rash at the site of her surgery. On physical examination, there were small blisters on an erythematous base in a rectangular shape at the surgery site. She takes no medication and is in good health. On further questioning, she stated that she had developed a similar rash on her ears many years ago after being given ear drops by her family doctor.

Questions

1. What is the immunologic mechanism underlying the rash?
2. What clues are provided by the configuration of the rash?

Dermatitis (eczema) is a common dermatologic reaction pattern seen in a variety of skin diseases including contact dermatitis, atopic dermatitis, lichen simplex chronicus, nummular dermatitis, and seborrheic dermatitis. The cutaneous morphology and histopathologic changes are similar in all these diseases.

Contact dermatitis can be classified as allergic or irritant (Fig. 111–1). Thousands of artificial and natural chemicals constantly challenge the skin barrier. Although many of these antigens have been described as contact allergens, only a relatively small number (e.g., metal objects, rubber articles, topical drugs, cosmetics, clothes, glues, and plants) are responsible for most cases of allergic contact dermatitis (ACD). In some studies, 25% of all women suspected of ACD reacted to nickel (Fig. 111–2). Ingredients in cosmetics account for about one third of positive patch test reactions. In addition, a significant number of lost work days each year are due to contact dermatitis, either allergic or irritant. Consequently, the diagnosis, prognosis, and treatment of contact dermatitis draws the physician into a complex network of medical, occupational, and social issues.

CLINICAL PRESENTATION

Clinically, three stages of ACD can be distinguished: acute, subacute, and chronic. The acute stage is characterized by a varied picture of erythema, edema, vesicles, and papules. Bursting of the vesicles leads to a weeping or crusted dermatitis. In the subacute phase, the vesicles disappear and the skin becomes scaly. In the chronic phase, the erythema fades and the skin becomes thickened (a process known as lichenification).

The actual clinical picture depends on factors related to the antigen (e.g., its concentration, localization, and duration of contact) as well as the immune reactivity of the patient. On the face, ACD often presents around the eyes with erythema, edema, and scaling. The thinness of the skin of the eyelids makes them especially susceptible to contact dermatitis. The offending antigen is

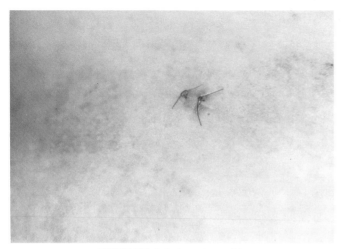

FIGURE 111–1. *Irritant dermatitis.*

often transferred to the face from the patient's normal-appearing hands.

Although usually localized, these dermatologic reactions can sometimes spread to distant sites. Autosensitization dermatitis, for example, is a poorly understood phenomenon in which eczematous lesions develop at distant sites without allergen contact at these sites.

PATHOPHYSIOLOGY

Allergic contact dermatitis is a model for type IV delayed-type hypersensitivity. The reaction has two phases: the afferent (or sensitization) phase and the efferent (or reaction) phase.

Most allergens are haptens, small molecules that require binding to a carrier to enhance their immunogenicity. Processing and presenting the antigen occur in the afferent phase of cell-mediated immunity. Within the epidermis, the bone marrow-derived Langerhans cells

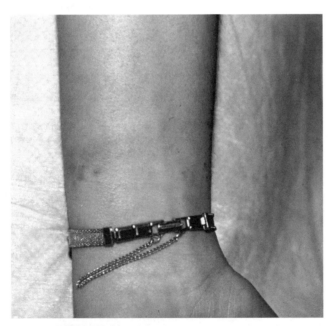

FIGURE 111–2. *Allergic contact dermatitis (nickel).*

ingest the antigen, process it, and present it on their cell surface bound to the HLA-DR molecules. This sequence of events enables the antigen to interact with naive T cells, either in the skin or in the regional lymph nodes.

The efferent phase is characterized by the proliferation of activated CD4 T cells, which contain receptors for the antigen–HLA-DR complex and which interact with the Langerhans cells to secrete interleukin-1 (IL-1). IL-1, in turn, activates CD4 T cells to synthesize and release interleukin-2 (IL-2). IL-2 acts nonspecifically to (1) activate antigen-specific memory and (2) cause antigen-nonspecific T cells to proliferate, expressing HLA-DR antigens and secreting interferon gamma (IFN-γ). Thus, the final response to the antigen includes both antigen-specific and nonspecific T cells.

IFN-γ plays a key role in localizing the reaction. IFN-γ causes expression of intracellular adhesion molecule-1 (ICAM-1), an adhesion molecule on keratinocytes and endothelial cells. ICAM-1 is a receptor for leukocyte function antigen (LFA-1), which is found on T cells. Thus, the interaction between ICAM-1 and LFA-1 appears to localize the inflammatory cells to the site of allergenic contact.

DIFFERENTIAL DIAGNOSIS

The differential diagnosis of contact dermatitis includes many other eczematous disorders. **Atopic dermatitis** appears as a symmetric, pruritic rash in infants, children, and adolescents with a personal or family history of atopy (e.g., asthma or allergic rhinoconjunctivitis). The lesions are commonly found on the antecubital and popliteal fossae, neck, and dorsal surface of the hands. **Asteatosis**, or "winter itch," commonly occurs in the elderly as dry, red, cracking patches. **Nummular eczema** appears as coin-shaped patches on the extremities. **Dyshidrotic eczema** manifests as small, extremely pruritic, deep-seated vesicles on the volar aspects of the hands, the lateral aspects of the fingers, and the soles. **Lichen simplex chronicus** appears as a localized thickened (lichenified) plaque, often on the nape of the neck or on the extremities. **Seborrheic dermatitis** appears as a greasy, red, scaly eruption centered around the nasolabial folds, eyebrows, scalp, and retroauricular areas. **Tinea corporis** at times may be confused with eczema, but a KOH preparation will show fungal hyphae. **Irritant dermatitis** may appear identical to contact dermatitis, but patch testing is negative.

D_x **Contact Dermatitis**

- Eczematous, pruritic plaques with sharp borders and thin scale.
- Lesions localized to areas of contact.
- Unnatural borders and asymmetry predominant.
- Acute weeping and oozing lesions.
- Chronic lesions lichenoid, scaly, and dry.

EVALUATION

History

The clinician should inquire about the duration of the rash, whether it is localized or generalized, and whether pruritus is a prominent feature. In addition, the patient should be questioned about exposure to potential irritants or allergens, occupational or household exposures, hobbies involving chemicals or plants, and use of topical medications or cosmetics. In difficult cases, the physician may want to observe the patient in the workplace.

Physical Examination

The physician should examine the entire skin surface. Is the rash localized or generalized? Symmetric or asymmetric? Are the borders "natural" or artificial appearing (i.e., unnaturally sharp borders)? Furthermore, are the physical findings more consistent with an acute dermatitis (e.g., erythema, vesiculation, weeping) or a more chronic process (e.g., scaling, lichenification)?

Additional Evaluation

The location of the rash sometimes points to the offending allergen (Table 111–1). In cases in which the allergen is not obvious, patch testing may be helpful. In patch testing, a small quantity of an allergen is applied in nonirritating concentration to clinically normal skin (e.g., the upper back). This application is left in place for 48 hours and then removed. The site is examined at 48, 72, and 96 hours for evidence of a positive reaction. When patch testing is negative but there is still a strong suspicion of allergic contact dermatitis, the repeat-upon-application test (ROAT) is used. In the ROAT, the patient applies the actual suspected product to the antecubital fossa once or twice a day for 1 week. The mechanics of patch testing are simple, yet the interpretation of the results may not be straightforward. False-positive and false-negative results can occur, and the final interpretation is more often an art than a science.

MANAGEMENT

The "cure" for allergic contact dermatitis lies in correctly identifying and avoiding the offending allergens. However, optimal management of symptoms can provide welcome relief for the patient.

Acute vesicular dermatitis should be treated with wet compresses and topical corticosteroid cream. If the dermatitis is widespread, a tapering dosage of systemic corticosteroids (e.g., prednisone) is the most efficacious therapy. Pruritus can be controlled with antihistamines. Subacute and chronic forms of allergic contact dermatitis are treated with topical corticosteroid ointments and emollients. The potency of the steroids required is determined by the location and duration of the dermatitis. Dermatitis involving the face, for example, should be treated with a weak (i.e., nonhalogenated) steroid preparation for a brief amount of time.

TABLE 111–1.   Localization of Allergic Contact Dermatitis

Scalp
    Hair dye
    Hair care products
Face
    Cosmetics, especially fragrances
    Preservatives
Upper eyelid
    Hair care products
    Nail polish
    Eyelid cosmetics
Lower eyelid
    Eye makeup
    Contact lens solution
    Ophthalmologic medicines
Ear
    Antibiotic drops, e.g., neomycin
    Hearing aid
    Earring (nickel)
Neck
    Jewelry
    Perfume
Trunk
    Clothing
    Soap
    Brassiere clasp (nickel)
Axilla
    Deodorant
Genitalia
    Deodorant
    Condom
    Spermicide
    Hemorrhoidal preparation
    Perfumed toilet paper
Wrist
    Watchband
Leg
    Stocking dye
Foot
    Shoe
Lower leg
    Medications for stasis dermatitis
Hand
    Latex glove
    Cleaning agents
    Dyes
    Food products
    Chromate

PATIENT AND FAMILY EDUCATION

Identification and avoidance of the allergen is the most important task for the patient; however, this seemingly simple request can be quite difficult to accomplish. For example, neomycin—a frequent cause of contact dermatitis—is found in a variety of over-the-counter preparations. It is a component of many creams and ointments designed for the skin as well as numerous otic and ophthalmologic preparations. In addition, patients sensitive to neomycin may also react to gentamicin and tobramycin. Cross-reactivity can occur among a wide variety of dissimilar compounds. For example, individuals who are sensitive to benzocaine may develop a reaction to procainamide, sulfonamides, p-aminobenzoic acid (PABA), hydrochlorothiazide diuretics, sulfonylurea oral hypoglycemic agents, and *p*-phenylenediamine hydrochloride (found in hair dyes).

For patients who cannot avoid exposure, the judicious use of barriers such as gloves may help prevent future episodes of contact dermatitis.

Research Questions

1. Why do some people and not others develop a contact dermatitis when exposed to nickel?
2. Why is contact dermatitis less common in the oral cavity than on the skin?

Case Resolution

This patient had developed an acute contact dermatitis in response to the neomycin in her topical antibiotic. She was given a potent corticosteroid cream and instructed to apply cool compresses three times a day. The pruritus decreased, and the rash slowly resolved over the next 10 days.

Selected Readings

Baadsgaad, O., and T. Wang. Immune regulation in allergic and irritant skin reactions. Int J Dermatol 30:161–72, 1991.

Fisher, A. A. *Fisher's Contact Dermatitis,* 4th ed. Baltimore, Williams & Wilkins, 1995.

Marks, J. G. Jr., and V. A. DeLeo. *Contact and Occupational Dermatology.* St. Louis, Mosby–Year Book, 1992.

Marks, R. (ed.). *Eczema.* London, Martin Dunitz, 1992.

Nethercott, J. R. Practical problems in the use of patch testing in the evaluation of patients with contact dermatitis. Curr Probl Dermatol 2(4):95–123, 1990.

CHAPTER 112

URTICARIA

Jerry Feldman, M.D.

Hₓ   A 37-year-old female postal clerk developed a pruritic rash on her trunk, arms, and face 6 days ago. She says the lesions come and go rapidly. On further questioning, she states that she was given penicillin for a sore throat 1 week before the eruption started. She denies any shortness of breath or arthralgias. The rash is so itchy that she cannot sleep.

Questions

1. What is the difference between urticaria and angioedema?
2. What factors can precipitate urticaria?
3. Which laboratory tests, if any, would you order for this patient?
4. What is the difference between acute and chronic urticaria?

Urticaria, frequently referred to as hives, is extremely common, with 15%–25% of the U. S. population experiencing at least one lifetime episode. These episodes are most often self-limited and not brought to the attention of medical personnel. Urticaria cases are artificially classified as acute or chronic. By definition, acute urticaria lasts less than 6 weeks, and these cases often have an easily identifiable cause. In contrast, chronic urticaria lasts longer than 6 weeks and the cause is rarely found. Acute and chronic urticaria have different pathophysiologic mechanisms.

CLINICAL PRESENTATION

Urticaria, or hives, is a cutaneous reaction pattern characterized by pruritic, transient, erythematous, edematous papules and plaques (often with central clearing) that may vary from a few millimeters to several centimeters in diameter (Fig. 112–1). These pleomorphic wheals are usually annular or circular, but occasionally bizarre serpiginous patterns may appear. Individual lesions are transient, often resolving in a few hours and rarely lasting longer than 24 hours. Angioedema, in contrast, is characterized by nonpitting edema, normal-appearing skin, and burning discomfort. Angioedema represents essentially the same histopathologic reaction as urticaria but occurs in the deeper subcutaneous tissues. Urticaria may occur anywhere on the body but usually spares the oral mucosa; angioedema, on the other hand, often affects the head and

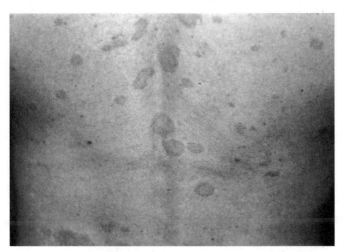

FIGURE 112–1. *Urticarial lesions.*

neck, especially the oral mucosa. Urticaria and angioedema may occur alone or together.

PATHOPHYSIOLOGY

Almost all forms of urticaria are due to mast cell degranulation with subsequent release of histamine and other chemical mediators (Table 112–1). Both immunologic and nonimmunologic mechanisms can cause mast cell degranulation (Table 112–2).

A type I hypersensitivity reaction (with cross-linking of IgE receptors on mast cells by multivalent antigen) is the most common pathophysiologic mechanism in acute urticaria. Type III immune complex activation of complement components (such as C5a and C3a) can also stimulate mast cell mediator release and is the underlying immunologic mechanism in collagen-vascular disease, serum sickness, and some drug-induced urticaria. Different immunologic mechanisms are involved in chronic urticaria. These patients often develop autoantibodies against IgE and the Fc portion of the IgE receptors. Even more important in chronic urticaria is the late-phase reaction, in which infiltrating lymphocytes release cytokines needed to maintain mast cell growth and stimulation.

Nonimmunologic mechanisms include direct degranulation of the mast cell. Factors capable of causing direct degranulation include opiates, radiocontrast

TABLE 112–1. Mast Cell Mediators

Histamine
Tryptase
Chymase
Carboxypeptidase A
Heparin
Eosinophil chemotactic factor
Neutrophil chemotactic factor
Prostaglandin D_2
Leukotrienes LTC_4, LTD_4, LTE, LTB_4
Platelet activating factor
Thromboxane A_2
Adenosine

TABLE 112–2. Mast Cell Stimuli

Immunologic Mechanisms

Allergens (IgE cross-linking)
Anti-IgE antibody
Anti-Fc receptor antibody
C3a
C5a
Cytokines

Nonimmunologic Mechanisms

Drugs
   Radiocontrast dyes
   Morphine sulfate
   Codeine
   Vancomycin
   Adriamycin
   Aspirin*
Physical factors
   Cold
   Heat
   Pressure
   Exercise
   Vibration
   Water
   Ultraviolet light

*Via arachidonic acid/leukotriene pathway.

dyes, and various physical stimuli such as heat, cold, pressure and ultraviolet light (see Table 112–2). Lastly, aspirin can cause urticaria by perturbing the arachidonic acid/leukotriene metabolic pathway.

DIFFERENTIAL DIAGNOSIS

Urticaria must be distinguished from erythema multiforme, early bullous pemphigoid, annular subacute cutaneous lupus erythematosus (SCLE), erythema annulare centrifugum (EAC), erythema chronicum migrans, acute febrile neutrophilic dermatoses, insect bites, cellulitis, and urticarial vasculitis (Table 112–3).

Erythema multiforme (see Chapter 113) is characterized by cutaneous target-like lesions and oral blisters. Early bullous pemphigoid will eventually transform into a bullous-vesicular pattern. Annular SCLE is usually found in sun-exposed areas and does not disappear within 24 hours. EAC is characterized by nonpruritic, slowly expanding, scaly plaques. Erythema chronicum migrans usually presents with a solitary annular lesion. Acute febrile neutrophilic dermatoses are thick, erythematous, edematous plaques that are not transient.

TABLE 112–3. Differential Diagnosis of Urticaria

Early bullous pemphigoid
Erythema multiforme
Acute febrile neutrophilic dermatosis (Sweet's syndrome)
Subacute cutaneous lupus erythematosus
Urticarial vasculitis
Erythema annulare centrifugum
Erythema chronicum migrans (Lyme disease)
Cellulitis
Arthropod bites

The lesions in insect bites contain a central punctum. Cellulitis is usually localized and accompanied by tenderness, fever, and leukocytosis. The lesions in urticarial vasculitis are often purpuric and usually last beyond 24–48 hours.

EVALUATION

History

Given the many possible causes of urticaria (Table 112–4), the history should be exhaustive. The following information should be sought: the location of lesions, their morphology (i.e., size, shape, and color), the pattern of attack (i.e., continuous or intermittent), and any associated symptoms (e.g., arthralgias or fever). The history should methodically review all possible causes of urticaria with special emphasis on the following factors: (1) prescribed drugs; (2) over-the-counter medications including vitamins, laxatives, and herbal remedies; and (3) aspirin-containing medications. Foods should be considered, including their associated preservatives, coloring dyes, and additives. The examiner

---

TABLE 112–4.   Causes of Urticaria

Food
Food additives
Drugs
Physical factors
   Dermatographism
   Cholinergic (elevated body temperature)
   Localized heat
   Cold
   Pressure
   Solar
   Vibration
   Aquagenic
Hepatitis B
Infectious mononucleosis
Streptococcal infections
Dermatophyte infections
Giardiasis
Endocrine
   Hypothyroidism
   Hyperthyroidism
Malignancy
   Lymphoma
   Solid tumors
   Myeloproliferative disorders
Contact urticaria
Blood products

---

should inquire about infections such as sinusitis, dental abscess, streptococcal disease, hepatitis B, infectious mononucleosis, and dermatophyte infection. A thorough review of systems should seek any symptoms of systemic lupus erythematosus, rheumatoid arthritis, vasculitis, malignancy, or thyroid dysfunction.

Certain forms of urticaria are precipitated by physical stimuli, including pressure, cold, heat, ultraviolet light, elevated body temperature, water, and vibration. These physical urticarias tend to be of short duration and mainly occur in young adults. Cutaneous involvement usually is limited to the areas subjected to the physical stimulation.

Additional Evaluation

Laboratory tests ordered without specific clues derived from the history are rarely useful. Skin prick tests or radioallergosorbent tests (RASTs) are also of little diagnostic value. Food diaries may occasionally be useful, but in general their yield is limited. Rarely, provocation testing may reveal the cause of urticaria. A physical challenge with the appropriate stimulus under the right conditions will confirm the diagnosis of physical urticaria.

MANAGEMENT

The best "treatment" for urticaria is avoidance of the offending agent. In most cases of acute urticaria, the offending antigen is identifiable, and exposure is self-limited. Symptomatic treatment with oral antihistamines (also known as H_1-receptor antagonists) is usually effective. When urticaria is chronic, the cause is rarely found and the need for prolonged symptomatic treatment becomes more important.

Nonspecific factors that aggravate cutaneous vasodilation (e.g., alcohol, aspirin, heat, exercise, and emotional stress) should be avoided. Topical agents are ineffective, and allergy hyposensitization is of little value. Dietary management may at times be helpful. Common foods that cause urticaria are shellfish, nuts, fish, eggs, chocolate, and cheese. The only definitive method to implicate a specific food as the cause is to perform a double-blind, placebo-controlled challenge test.

The drug management of chronic urticaria is based on a rational understanding of its pathophysiology. First, the effects of mast cell mediators, primarily histamine, can be blocked at the site of the cellular histamine receptors (H_1 and H_2) on blood vessels and nerves. Second, the release of mediators from the mast cell can be inhibited, primarily by agents that increase intracellular cyclic AMP or stabilize the cellular membrane.

It is important to remember that histamine functions as a chemical messenger, acting through the histamine receptors H_1, H_2, and H_3. The antihistamines are competitive antagonists that reversibly inhibit the interaction of histamine with its receptors. These agents can be classified as first-generation sedating agents, second-generation nonsedating agents, and tricyclic antidepressants.

The first-generation antihistamines are effective but frequently cause sedation as well as a variety of anticholinergic effects (e.g., blurred vision, urinary retention, and dry mouth). Before an older antihistamine is used, medical contraindications such as narrow angle glaucoma or severe prostatic hypertrophy should be ruled out. The newer nonsedating agents do not easily penetrate the blood-brain barrier and consequently have fewer side effects. These agents are metabolized by the cytochrome P-450 system, and coadministration of drugs that inhibit this enzyme may result in toxicity. Consequently, these agents are contraindicated in patients taking ketoconazole, itraconazole, erythromycin, or azithromycin. Finally, there is an art to prescribing antihistamines. Often, giving the antihistamine in the evening is sufficient to provide coverage during the day while minimizing the sedative side effects.

Because H_2 receptors are found on cutaneous blood vessels, the use of an H_2 blocker (e.g., cimetidine or ranitidine) in conjunction with an H_1 blocker may be useful in cases of recalcitrant chronic urticaria.

The antidepressant doxepin has been used successfully to treat chronic urticaria. Doxepin has both H_1 and H_2 blocking effects.

Mast cell mediator release inhibition has been attempted with β-adrenergic drugs such as epinephrine and terbutaline. Although cromolyn sodium can effectively inhibit mast cell release, it is of minimal value in treating urticaria because of poor gastrointestinal absorption.

Finally, glucocorticosteroids have a minimal role in treating urticaria. Adverse effects prohibit their long-term usage. However, in a difficult case, a brief trial may offer temporary relief.

PATIENT EDUCATION

The patient with chronic urticaria needs to know that these episodes of urticaria may persist for months or even years. Because the cause is rarely found, treatment is primarily symptomatic. Patients should be warned about side effects of antihistamines and questioned to determine whether they have conditions such as narrow angle glaucoma or benign prostatic hypertrophy. Although tolerance to the sedative effects of antihistamines often develops, these agents can cause severe drowsiness upon initiation of therapy. The patient also should be educated about the respiratory symptoms (e.g., wheezing, shortness of breath) that sometimes accompany urticaria and of the need to seek prompt medical attention if such symptoms arise.

NATURAL HISTORY/PROGNOSIS

Acute attacks of urticaria may last for hours or days. In contrast, chronic urticaria lasts for weeks, months, or even years. Some studies indicate that 50% of chronic urticaria cases remit within 6 months. Conversely, 15%–20% of patients with chronic urticaria may go on to have intermittent attacks over a span of 20 years or longer.

Research Questions

1. How would you go about isolating other mediators involved in the genesis of urticaria?
2. Why do some patients with chronic urticaria have only intermittent attacks?

Case Resolution

The patient's urticaria remitted after she stopped taking the antibiotic. She was informed that she was allergic to penicillin and was advised to avoid this class of medication in the future.

Selected Readings

Black, A. K., M. W. Greaves, R. H. Champion, and R. J. Pye. The urticarias 1990. Br J Dermatol 124:100–8, 1991.

Casale, T. B., H. A. Sampson, J. Hanifin, et al. Guide to physical urticarias. J Allergy Clin Immunol 82:758–62, 1988.

Champion, R. H., S. O. B. Roberts, R. G. Carpenter, and J. H. Rogers. Urticaria and angioedema. Br J Dermatol 81:588–97, 1969.

Hide, M., D. M. Francis, E. H. Clive, et al. Autoantibodies against the high-affinity IgE receptor as a cause of histamine release in chronic urticaria. N Engl J Med 328:1599–1604, 1993.

Huston, D. P., and R. B. Bressler. Urticaria and angioedema. Med Clin North Am 76:805–40, 1992.

Monroe, E. W. Urticaria. Curr Probl Dermatol 4:118–40, 1993.

Rothe, M. J., B. S. Nowak, and F. A. Kerdel. The mast cell in health and disease. J Am Acad Dermatol 23:615–24, 1990.

Soter, N. A. Urticaria: Current therapy. J Allergy Clin Immunol 86:1009–14, 1990.

DRUG RASHES

Carl Bigler, M.D.

H$_x$ A 72-year-old male retired barber presents with a generalized rash. The rash began on his trunk and abdomen and quickly spread to his proximal arms and legs. It is moderately itchy. He began treatment for prostatitis 5 days ago with trimethoprim-sulfamethoxazole. In addition, he takes enalapril for hypertension. There is no history of a drug allergy. Over-the-counter medications are limited to an occasional aspirin for headache. He denies fever, sore throat, or skin pain. The physical examination reveals a net-like pattern of erythema that blanches on compression with some fine scale on the back, abdomen, and proximal extremities. The rash is not tender to palpation, and there are no mucous membrane ulcers.

Questions

1. What are the diagnostic possibilities for a rash of this description?
2. Is this rash potentially dangerous?
3. What should be your course of action?

Drug rashes represent a common and difficult problem in primary care practice. A patient taking many drugs develops a rash. Is it a drug rash? If so, which drug is causing the rash? An effective drug may have to be stopped and never used again.

CLINICAL PRESENTATION

Drugs can cause almost any type of rash. Most drug eruptions, however, present as either (1) a morbilliform rash, (2) an urticarial rash, or (3) erythema multiforme.

Morbilliform, maculopapular, or **exanthematous** rashes are reticulated (net-like) rashes with red patches that blanch on compression. Some areas are smooth, while others show a fine, sandpaper-like scale (Fig. 113–1).

Urticarial drug rashes are characterized by hives, which appear as pink arches and rings that itch and subsequently move to other sites within hours (Fig. 113–2).

Erythema multiforme drug rashes are manifested by targetoid lesions that are often accompanied by mucous membrane ulcers. Targetoid lesions (so-called because they resemble a bull's eye target) are characterized by a central blister or area of brown-red discoloration surrounded by a pink, raised rim.

PATHOPHYSIOLOGY

The morbilliform pattern is the most frequently seen drug rash. Morbilliform drug rashes usually begin within 1 week after exposure to a drug. Occasionally, however, prolonged exposure may be required for sensitization, and a morbilliform rash is thus the most common skin pattern for "late" drug rashes. The pathophysiology is unknown.

Urticarial rashes are second in frequency. Drug-induced urticaria is caused most commonly by mast cell release of histamine and other chemical mediators. Histamine increases capillary permeability, resulting in edema and erythema. IgE-mediated urticaria is an immediate allergic reaction requiring prior sensitization. Such prior sensitization results in the production of IgE, which subsequently binds to mast cells. If this IgE–mast cell complex is later exposed to the same allergen (e.g., a particular drug or drug metabolite), within minutes the mast cell will release its granules of histamine and other mediators.

In addition to this IgE-mediated release of histamine, drugs can directly induce histamine release by nonimmunologic means. Narcotics, aspirin, and intravenous contrast dye can all directly stimulate mast cells to release histamine. In some patients with susceptible mast cells, the result is urticaria. No prior sensitization is required.

Drug-induced erythema multiforme is an unusual, but often severe, drug rash with significant morbidity and mortality. On biopsy, there is evidence of death of the top layer of skin (the epidermis). Dead epidermis cannot perform its barrier function, and the involved skin is susceptible to infection and loss of fluid. In addition, dead epidermis releases diffusible proteins called cytokines, which can cause fever and malaise but can also stimulate wound healing. Erythema multiforme reactions occur 3–10 days following drug exposure and are the result of a T-lymphocyte cell-mediated cytotoxic immune response against the epidermis. How drugs create this aberrant response is unknown.

DIFFERENTIAL DIAGNOSIS

Morbilliform drug rashes appear identical to viral exanthems. Diagnostic confusion can thus result when antibiotics are started during the early phase of a viral illness and a rash subsequently develops. These patients may be mistakenly thought to have a drug allergy. Morbilliform drug rashes must be differentiated from dermatitis; the former usually begin on the trunk and

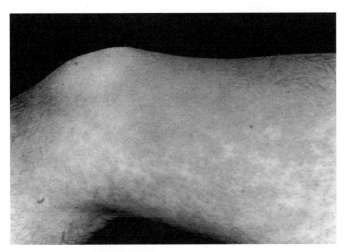

FIGURE 113-1. *A morbilliform rash.*

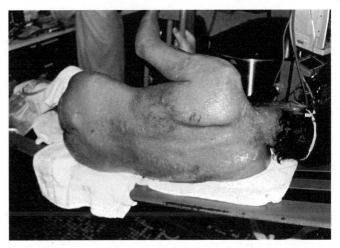

FIGURE 113-3. *Severe erythema multiforme–type drug reaction.*

spread, whereas dermatitis is more chronic, localized, and excoriated.

Urticaria may be confused with the target lesions of erythema multiforme. Urticarial lesions typically last only a few hours and new lesions are produced at a rapid rate, whereas erythema multiforme lesions are fixed for 1–3 weeks. Urticaria may be due to other causes such as infections or specific allergens. It is unusual for urticaria to be a reaction to medications used chronically.

Early, severe erythema multiforme reactions may be confused with morbilliform eruptions. In contrast, severe erythema multiforme reactions are characterized by mucous membrane (ocular, oral, or genital) involvement and skin tenderness rather than itching. In addition, targetoid lesions can often be found. Erythema multiforme can also be caused by herpes simplex. In these cases, targetoid lesions develop 7–10 days after a "cold sore" or genital lesion. As a rule, erythema multiforme drug reactions (Fig. 113–3) are more extensive and severe than erythema multiforme due to herpes simplex. The bullous lesions of erythema multiforme must be differentiated from other bullous lesions, including those associated with bullous impetigo, porphy-

ria cutanea tarda, and the autoimmune bullous diseases pemphigus and pemphigoid.

EVALUATION

In evaluating a patient on medication who develops a rash, a detailed drug history—including prescription drugs, over-the-counter drugs, illicit drugs, and herbal remedies—is essential. Any previous drug rashes should be classified as morbilliform, urticarial, erythema multiforme, or "questionable." This analysis of prior cutaneous reactions may provide a clue to the present drug culprit. Features that help distinguish among the different types of drug rashes are outlined in Table 113–1. Some drugs tend to cause a specific drug rash pattern (Table 113–2), whereas other drugs cause

TABLE 113–1.   Classification of Drug Rashes

	Morbilliform Rash	Urticaria	Erythema Multiforme
Onset	< 1 week	Minutes	3–14 days
Morphology	Maculopapular	Arches	Targets
Itchiness	+	++	+/–
Mucous membrane involvement	+/–	–	+
Fever	+/–	–	+
Tenderness	–	–	+
Duration	1–14 days	< 24 hours	7–21 days

TABLE 113–2.   Common Drug Reactions

Morbilliform Rash	Urticaria	Erythema Multiforme
Ampicillin	Penicillin	Sulfonamides
Sulfonamides	IV contrast dye	Phenytoin
Gold	Whole blood	Carbamazepine
Carbamazepine		Indomethacin
Phenytoin		
Naproxen		

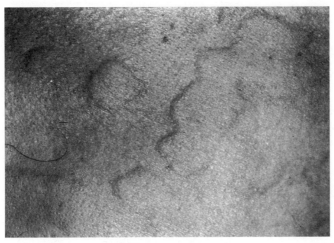

FIGURE 113-2. *An urticarial rash.*

TABLE 113–3. Drugs That Rarely Cause Rashes

Acetaminophen
Acyclovir
Antihistamines
Birth control pills
Digoxin
Gentamicin
Insulin
Prednisone
Tetracycline
Warfarin

rashes only rarely (Table 113–3). A skin biopsy is usually able to differentiate erythema multiforme from other bullous eruptions. This procedure is generally less helpful in urticarial and morbilliform rashes.

MANAGEMENT

The offending drug should be identified and discontinued. The drug allergy should be clearly noted on the patient's chart. The pruritus associated with morbilliform drug rashes may be lessened by applying topical corticosteroids (e.g., triamcinolone 0.1% ointment) or by taking oral antihistamines (e.g., diphenhydramine, hydroxyzine). Oral corticosteroids should be avoided, since their adverse effects may confuse the clinical picture. If a rash recurs following oral steroid therapy, the clinician is uncertain whether steroid therapy was stopped prematurely or the wrong drug was discontinued.

Urticarial drug reactions may progress to anaphylaxis, a medical emergency manifested by hypotension and laryngeal obstruction. Patients with the acute onset of drug-induced urticaria should therefore be monitored. Anaphylaxis should be treated with epinephrine and cardiorespiratory support as needed. Mild urticarial reactions often respond to antihistamines such as diphenhydramine.

Mild erythema multiforme reactions may be treated symptomatically. Drug-induced erythema multiforme should be followed closely, since blisters may progress for up to 10 days after the drug is stopped. Severe erythema multiforme reactions require hospitalization with expert wound care, nutritional and fluid support, ophthalmologic evaluation of eye lesions, and aggressive treatment of infection. Corticosteroids are contraindicated because of the risk of infection, impaired wound healing, and associated electrolyte abnormalities.

NATURAL HISTORY/PROGNOSIS

The clinical spectrum of drug rashes varies depending on the type of reaction. Morbilliform drug rashes may progress to erythroderma (redness of the entire skin surface). Urticarial reactions range from mild, transient urticaria to angioedema (swelling of the lips or genitals) to anaphylaxis. Erythema multiforme reactions range from a few lesions to involvement of the entire skin and mucous membrane surfaces.

Severe urticarial and erythema multiforme reactions are associated with significant morbidity and mortality. However, most drug reactions are self-limited and heal without sequelae. Drug rechallenge in patients who have experienced urticarial or erythema multiforme reactions is potentially life threatening. Rechallenge in patients who have experienced morbilliform reactions often results in a more severe rash and may cause erythroderma but is usually not life threatening.

Research Questions

1. What is the pathophysiology of morbilliform drug eruptions?
2. Why are certain drugs more likely to cause rashes than others?
3. What is unique about the rare patient who develops a rash among the thousands who take that drug?

Case Resolution

The patient had a morbilliform drug rash. Sulfa drugs frequently cause this type of rash, and the onset of the rash 5 days after trimethoprim-sulfamethoxazole was started also favors sulfamethoxazole over enalapril as the offending agent. Ciprofloxacin was substituted for trimethoprim-sulfamethoxazole, and the rash gradually improved over the next 7 days. The patient's chart was clearly labeled with a sticker indicating an allergy to sulfa drugs.

Selected Readings

Bigby, M., R. S. Stern, and K. A. Arndt. Allergic cutaneous reactions to drugs. Prim Care 16:713–27, 1989.

Blacker, K. L., R. S. Stern, and B. U. Wintroub. Cutaneous reactions to drugs. *In* T. B. Fitzpatrick et al. (eds.). *Dermatology in General Medicine,* 4th ed. New York, McGraw-Hill Book Company, 1993.

Bork, K. *Cutaneous Side Effects of Drugs.* Philadelphia, W.B. Saunders Company, 1988.

Bruinsma, W. (ed.). *A Guide to Drug Eruptions,* 5th ed. Amsterdam, American Overseas Book Company, 1990.

VIRAL INFECTIONS OF THE SKIN

Carl Bigler, M.D.

H_x A 4-year-old girl presents with a generalized rash that began 3 days ago. The rash appeared first on her face and scalp and spread rapidly to her trunk. The initial pink, flat (macular) lesions evolved into bumps (papules), then small blisters (vesicles), and finally crusts. She complains of itchiness and "not feeling well." She spends several days a week in daycare. Her temperature is 38.1° C (100.5° F), and numerous flat, pink patches, red papules, vesicles, and pustules are scattered over her face, scalp, and trunk. There are a few superficial ulcers on the hard palate.

Questions

1. What is the diagnosis?
2. Is this rash dangerous?
3. Is it contagious?

Viral infections may affect the skin in two distinct ways: as localized infections (e.g., warts) or as a manifestation of a systemic infection (e.g., measles). Systemic viral infections may produce a morbilliform rash or a vesiculobullous rash. A morbilliform rash is also called a maculopapular rash or an exanthem and is net-like with red patches that blanch upon compression. Some areas are smooth, while others have a fine, sandpaper-like scale (Fig. 114–1). The primary lesion in a vesiculobullous rash is a small, fluid-filled blister (Fig. 114–2). As the blister ages, it may evolve into a pustule or may rupture and create a superficial erosion (which may then develop a crust). Warts are discrete skin-colored papules with a rough or scaly surface (Fig. 114–3).

PATHOPHYSIOLOGY

Viruses are infective organisms composed of (1) a nucleotide core of DNA or RNA, (2) a protein coat, and sometimes (3) a carbohydrate and lipid envelope. Viruses are minimalistic in metabolic and reproductive function. Many structural and enzymatic proteins required by the virus are provided by the parasitized host cell. The nucleotide core contains little more information than is required for survival and replication of the virus. Viruses are highly specialized and often infect only certain cell types. An example is the papillomavirus, a double-stranded DNA virus that causes warts. It replicates only within stratified squamous epithelium such as skin or mucous membranes. Its environmental requirements are so strict that it does not grow in vitro,

in skin organ culture, or on the skin or mucous membranes of closely related species.

Systemic viral infections (e.g., measles, chickenpox) begin as respiratory infections due to droplet spread, with subsequent viremia and widespread tissue infection. Vesicular lesions are caused by viral infection of the epidermis, the top layer of skin. Morbilliform rashes are usually the result of a viral infection of endothelial cells within the superficial dermis of the skin, although they also require a host immune response. Localized infections such as warts often begin after direct inoculation of scratched or abraded skin. Table 114–1 lists the common viruses associated with morbilliform, vesicular, and papillomatous (wart-like) patterns.

Exposure to a virus does not always result in infection. The host must also be susceptible. For measles and

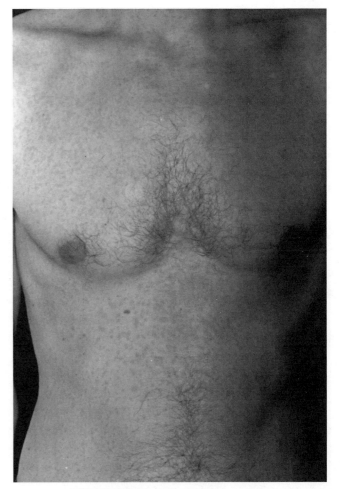

FIGURE 114–1. *Morbilliform viral exanthem.*

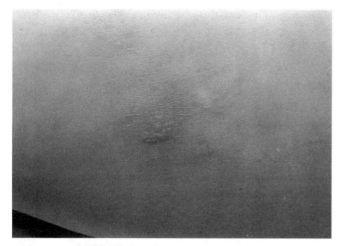

FIGURE 114–2. *Herpes simplex viral vesicles.*

rubella, previously uninfected children usually become infected after exposure to the virus, and infection conveys immunity from future infection. For wart viruses, most people are continuously exposed but not infected. A wart papule results when the immune system fails to recognize and contain a wart virus. Herpesviruses (responsible for chickenpox and "cold sores") are intermediate between these two examples. Primary infection is more severe clinically, and the subsequent immune response often protects against reinfection. However, the virus can remain latent within nerve ganglia, and its reactivation can result in localized disease. Examples include (1) herpes zoster ("shingles"), which typically occurs years after infection with chickenpox (varicella); and (2) recurrent herpes simplex infections (e.g., "cold sores," genital herpes), which often occur every few months after the primary infection. In all cases of viral infection, cell-mediated immunity is more effective than humoral immunity in clearing the virus, in providing immunity from future infection, and in maintaining latency (i.e., the symptom-free period following the primary infection).

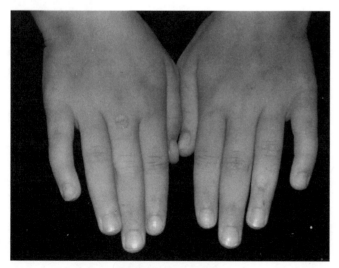

FIGURE 114–3. *Viral warts.*

TABLE 114–1. Patterns of Viral Rashes

Morbilliform/Viral Exanthems

Measles (paramyxovirus)
Rubella (togavirus)
Roseola (herpesvirus type 6)
Erythema infectiosum (parvovirus B19)
Many others

Viral Vesicles

Herpes zoster
   Chickenpox
   Shingles
Herpes simplex
   Oral (type 1)
   Genital (type 2)
Hand-foot-and-mouth disease (coxsackievirus type A16 most common)

Papillomas

Warts (papillomavirus)
Molluscum contagiosum (poxvirus)

DIFFERENTIAL DIAGNOSIS

Morbilliform rashes may be drug eruptions, scarlatiniform rashes due to streptococcal or staphylococcal bacterial infection, nonspecific viral exanthems, or rashes highly suggestive of a specific virus. In children, the appearance and progression of a rash associated with specific clinical features may point to a particular diagnosis.

Measles typically has a short but severe prodrome of fever and respiratory symptoms followed by mucositis (pinpoint white dots on an inflamed soft palate referred to as Koplik's spots) and then a generalized dark-red to brown morbilliform rash that lasts 3–5 days. Conjunctivitis, cough, fever, and preauricular nodes frequently accompany the rash. If measles occurs in partially immune patients who received the "killed" vaccine administered in the early 1960s, the prodrome is more severe and often includes abdominal pain and pneumonia. The rash frequently begins on the hands and may appear petechial (atypical measles).

Rubella has a mild clinical prodrome with mild respiratory symptoms and little or no fever. The rash is pink to light red in color and resolves in 1–2 days. Posterior auricular nodes are often easily palpable. Adults may have a persistent monarticular arthritis.

Roseola (exanthem subitum) occurs most frequently between 6 months and 2 years of age. The prodrome is characterized by a high fever lasting 3–5 days. Despite the high fever, the child is often active and appears well. The prodrome is followed by an exanthem that appears rapidly on the chest, back, and neck and lasts for 1–2 days. The individual erythematous lesions are often surrounded by a white halo.

Erythema infectiosum (fifth disease) has a 1- to 2-day prodrome manifested by a low-grade fever, usually followed by a facial rash that looks like "slapped" cheeks and a lacy, pink rash on the arms that may spread to the trunk and lasts 7–10 days. Adults and older children may develop a symmetrical arthritis.

Morbilliform eruptions in adults are often nonspecific. Viruses such as measles and rubella, which typically result in easily recognizable exanthems in children,

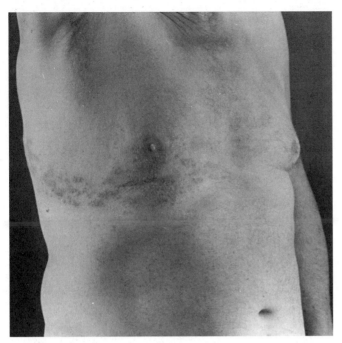

FIGURE 114–4. *Dermatomal vesicles of herpes zoster.*

often produce morbilliform rashes in adults that are indistinguishable from rashes seen with influenza, enteroviruses, or many other viruses.

Morbilliform drug eruptions may be difficult to distinguish from viral exanthems. Although symptoms such as fever, malaise, muscle aches, rhinorrhea, and cough may suggest a viral etiology, these symptoms are nonspecific and may occasionally occur with a drug reaction.

Scarlatiniform rashes due to streptococcal bacterial infections can appear similar to viral exanthems. Scarlatiniform rashes are often more prominent in skin creases, and the physical examination frequently reveals exudative pharyngitis.

The appearance of viral vesicles often implicates a particular virus. **Chickenpox**, for example, has a prodrome of mild fever and malaise followed by scattered showers of lesions that begin as pink macules and then progress to papules, vesicles, and finally crusts. Like all herpesvirus infections, the characteristic lesion consists of grouped vesicles on an erythematous base (the "dew drops on a rose petal" pattern). The diagnosis is difficult without these lesions and may be missed early in the infection. In adults, chickenpox is a more severe infection accompanied by malaise and cough.

Shingles (reactivation of chickenpox) characteristically follows a dermatomal nerve root distribution, thus making diagnosis easy (Fig. 114–4). Pain or paresthesias may precede the rash. Pain in the thoracic distribution may be misdiagnosed as a cardiac or pulmonary problem until the characteristic vesicles make their appearance. Shingles rarely recurs.

Herpes simplex infections (Fig. 114–2) appear as localized grouped vesicles or erosions on an erythematous base. Primary infections occur 3–10 days after exposure and are often more severe and painful

than recurrences. Recurrences are often preceded by paresthesias.

Herpesvirus may assume an unusual clinical appearance in the immunocompromised host. In patients with AIDS, herpesviruses may present with chronic perianal ulcers or widespread superficial ulcers (with or without secondary crusting). In patients with underlying dermatitis, herpesvirus may present with a worsening and crusted dermatitis, which may be rapidly progressive (a condition known as eczema herpeticum).

Hand-foot-and-mouth disease usually affects young children. A short, mild, viral prodrome is followed by scattered oral erosions. These findings are nonspecific unless the characteristic oblong vesiculopustules with surrounding erythema are found on the palms and soles. The lesions are also found rather frequently on the buttocks and typically resolve in 7–10 days.

Warts must be differentiated from **molluscum contagiosum** in children and young adults. Clinically, molluscum contagiosum appears in children as widespread, umbilicated, dome-shaped, skin-colored to yellowish papules. Common warts, in contrast, are usually more flat-topped and scaly. Molluscum contagiosum is caused by a poxvirus and is much more contagious (hence the term contagiosum) than are common warts. Molluscum in young adults appears in the genital region as a sexually transmitted disease (Fig. 114–5) and can be differentiated by clinical appearance from genital warts (condyloma acuminatum) (Fig. 114–6) and secondary syphilis (condyloma latum).

In older patients, warts may be difficult to differentiate from **seborrheic keratoses**. Seborrheic keratoses are benign epidermal tumors, usually pigmented; they are more common than warts in older patients.

EVALUATION

In evaluating a patient with a morbilliform rash, a detailed drug history will help exclude a drug eruption. Collaborating evidence for a viral etiology should be sought. In such cases, close acquaintances are often sick and the patient frequently complains of fever, sore throat, or malaise. There may be lymphadenopathy,

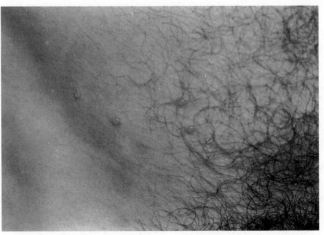

FIGURE 114–5. *Umbilicated papules of molluscum contagiosum.*

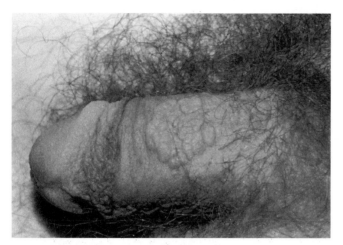

FIGURE 114–6. *Genital warts, or condyloma acuminatum.*

conjunctival injection, or pharyngeal erythema or exudate. The patient should be examined for the presence of specific viral exanthems as previously described. Exudative pharyngitis should be cultured for *Streptococcus*. A large number of viruses can cause exanthems, and viral cultures are usually not obtained for patients presenting with exanthems. Sometimes, however, the diagnosis is confirmed in retrospect by an increase in virus-specific antibody titers from acute to convalescent sera.

Most viral vesicles are caused by herpesviruses. Confirmation is readily obtained by performing a Tzanck test. The roof of the blister is removed with a sterile scalpel blade, and the base of the blister is scraped, applied to a glass slide, and processed with Wright's stain. The characteristic multinucleated giant cells are seen on microscopic examination. This technique does not discriminate between herpes simplex and herpes zoster. The virus may also be cultured, although false-negative results occur with some frequency in herpes zoster infections.

Wart virus cannot be cultured but may be specifically typed in research laboratories using DNA hybridization techniques. Molluscum contagiosum can usually be diagnosed by its clinical appearance. Confirmation may be obtained by skin biopsy.

MANAGEMENT

For morbilliform rashes, the possibility of a drug rash should be kept in mind and the patient's medications should be reviewed and evaluated (see Chapter 113). For viral exanthems, no therapy is required. Cool baths, moisturizing creams, and oral antihistamines such as diphenhydramine may provide symptomatic relief. The patient is often infectious for several days before and after the viral exanthem. Appropriate precautions should be taken to prevent spread of infection, particularly to immunocompromised people. For measles and rubella, local or state public health offices should be notified. The best "treatment" for measles and rubella is prevention through vaccination.

For cold sores or genital ulcers due to herpes simplex, short-term oral acyclovir therapy may decrease the number and duration of lesions but will not affect the recurrence rate. Topical acyclovir is not very effective. Both oral and genital herpes lesions are infectious with contact.

Chickenpox (systemic herpes zoster infection) is highly contagious and spreads via respiratory secretions and cough. Herpes zoster virus is present in the skin lesions but not the respiratory secretions of patients with shingles. Consequently, wound and hand-washing precautions should be followed to prevent transmission to others.

Shingles (localized, dermatomal reactivation of herpes zoster infection) often causes pain in the same nerve distribution as the rash. Occasionally, these painful paresthesias will persist after the rash has disappeared. Postherpetic neuralgia usually occurs in older patients and may be incapacitating. Treatment with acyclovir early in the course of shingles may decrease the incidence of postherpetic neuralgia in older patients. The benefit of corticosteroid therapy in these patients is less clear-cut. Acyclovir is also indicated in immunocompromised patients with herpes simplex or herpes zoster to prevent more severe localized disease and dissemination.

Hand-foot-and-mouth disease is self-limited, and no therapy is required.

There are many treatments for warts, all of which are destructive and not specific for the wart virus. For most diseases, satisfaction with therapy is inversely proportional to the number of treatments required, and warts are no exception to this rule. Even with adequate liquid nitrogen therapy, an average of three treatments are required to "cure" warts. Moreover, this "cure" is more apparent than real. Wart virus DNA can still be detected in normal-appearing skin. Treatment of warts often results in scarring, and no treatment is a reasonable option.

Genital warts should probably be treated with liquid nitrogen or podophyllin to prevent transmission to sexual partners. Because the wart virus may still be present even in the absence of visible lesions, condom use should be recommended. Female sexual contacts may be at an increased risk for cervical cancer and should have a Pap smear performed annually.

Because molluscum contagiosum can be transmitted to others, treatment is indicated. This condition can be treated effectively with destructive therapy, most commonly liquid nitrogen or simple curettage. Individual lesions resolve with treatment, but new lesions may appear for several weeks thereafter.

PATIENT AND FAMILY EDUCATION

The possibility of viral transmission among family members and appropriate preventive measures should be discussed.

NATURAL HISTORY/PROGNOSIS

Viral exanthems usually resolve spontaneously in 1–10 days depending on the type of viral exanthem and the individual's immune response. Pneumonia may complicate atypical measles or chickenpox in adults.

Erythema infectiosum may lead to transient red cell aplasia; this is typically more severe and prolonged in patients who are immunosuppressed or have a hemolytic anemia. In addition, erythema infectiosum may sometimes cause fetal demise in pregnancy. Rubella during the first trimester of pregnancy may cause the congenital rubella syndrome consisting of deafness, cataracts, and heart defects.

The vesicles of herpes simplex usually resolve without scarring. Recurrences can be as frequent as monthly, although many people have only a single episode. The number of recurrences tends to decrease with time. Herpes simplex recurrences on the lip (often referred to as "cold sores" or "fever blisters") may be precipitated by sunlight or fever.

The lesions of chickenpox and shingles may rarely result in scarring. Most people with a history of chickenpox do not experience reactivation of the herpes zoster virus as shingles. Herpes zoster, in contrast to herpes simplex, almost never recurs. Postherpetic neuralgia generally improves slowly with time, but this is little consolation to the minority of patients with excruciating pain or paresthesias. Disseminated herpes simplex or zoster in immunocompromised patients may be fatal if not treated aggressively.

Warts resolve spontaneously without scarring in most children, usually over months to years. In adults, spontaneous resolution occurs less frequently and it takes a longer time for warts to completely disappear.

Molluscum resolves spontaneously over months unless the patient is immunocompromised.

Research Questions

1. What causes herpes zoster to recur as shingles?
2. Why do only some people get warts?

Case Resolution

The patient has chickenpox. The disease is contagious, and she will have to miss school until her lesions crust over. Scarring will be minimal unless there is secondary bacterial infection or severe excoriations.

Selected Readings

Chang, T. (ed.). Viral exanthems. Clin Dermatol 7:1–128, 1989.
Hogan, P., J. Morelli, and W. Weston. Viral exanthems. Curr Probl Dermatol 4(2):35–94, 1992.
Maibach, H., and K. Beutner (eds.). Human infections with viral agents. Semin Dermatol 11(3):183–260, 1992.
Weston, W., and A. Lane. Viral infections. *In* W. Weston and A. Lane. *Color Textbook of Pediatric Dermatology.* St. Louis, Mosby–Year Book, 1991.

CHAPTER 115

BACTERIAL INFECTIONS OF THE SKIN

Mark D. Lehman, M.D., and Carl Bigler, M.D.

Hx An 8-year-old male child is brought to his primary care physician because of a facial rash that has been rapidly enlarging over the last 8–10 hours. The rash now encompasses the entire right cheek, eyelid, and forehead. He has not had fever or chills, although his mother mentions that he has had mild rhinorrhea for the last 3 days. He currently is taking no medications, and his mother reports that no friends or classmates are ill. The physical examination reveals a sharply demarcated brightly erythematous and edematous plaque involving the right cheek, eyelid, and forehead. The affected area is warm and tender to the touch. His temperature is 37.5° C (99.5° F).

Questions

1. What are some possible causes of this rash?
2. What potential risks should be considered?
3. What is the appropriate treatment?
4. Does this patient have a communicable disease?

Common bacterial infections of the skin present with a variety of clinical signs including superficial erosions with a golden crust, pustules, erythema, and fever. It is

**TABLE 115-1. Common Causes of
Bacterial Skin Infections**

Clinical Condition	Most Common Etiologic Organism
Superficial folliculitis	*Staphylococcus aureus*
Deep folliculitis	*Staphylococcus aureus*
Erysipelas	Group A *Streptococcus*
Cellulitis	*Staphylococcus aureus*, group A *Streptococcus*
Impetigo	Group A *Streptococcus*, *Staphylococcus aureus*
Ecthyma	Group A *Streptococcus*

important to determine whether the cause is infectious, since bacterial skin infections usually resolve completely with adequate antibiotic therapy. Failure to make this diagnosis will delay appropriate treatment and allow for local spread or rarely sepsis, as well as transmission to personal contacts.

PATHOPHYSIOLOGY

The skin serves many important functions, one of which is to provide a natural barrier to bacteria and thereby prevent cutaneous and systemic infections. The bacterial flora on the surface of normal skin provides additional protection. Any alteration of this cutaneous barrier may lead to skin infection. A primary infection usually arises within a small cut or hair follicle. A secondary infection occurs when a defect (e.g., eczema, a blister, or a burn) becomes colonized with bacteria. Most cutaneous bacterial infections are due to gram-positive cocci such as group A β-hemolytic *Streptococcus* or *Staphylococcus aureus* (Table 115-1).

DIFFERENTIAL DIAGNOSIS

There are three main types of cutaneous bacterial infections to consider: folliculitis, cellulitis, and impetigo. All three have distinctive characteristics that aid in identification.

The primary lesion in **folliculitis** is a pustule that originates in a hair follicle. Two types of folliculitis are commonly encountered: superficial and deep. **Superficial folliculitis** is identified clinically as a small pustule situated at the external opening of the hair follicle. This usually indicates a bacterial infection of the hair follicle, a process that may be facilitated by occlusion or chemical irritation although often there is no clear-cut precipitating event. The most common cause is *S. aureus*; other bacterial or fungal organisms are unusual unless the patient is immunocompromised. Several other conditions may look similar to superficial folliculitis (Table 115-2).

**TABLE 115-2. Differential Diagnosis
of Superficial Folliculitis**

Herpes zoster/varicella (chickenpox)
Acne
Milia
Pustular psoriasis (one type of psoriasis)

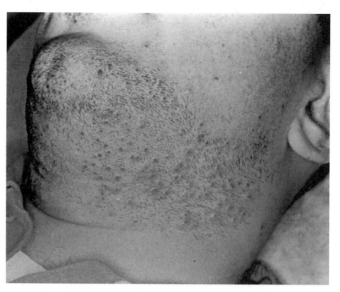

FIGURE 115-1. *Pseudofolliculitis barbae.*

If superficial folliculitis is not treated appropriately, it may progress to become a deep folliculitis. **Deep folliculitis** represents an infection deep within the follicle that creates an intense inflammatory response. When deep folliculitis presents in the beard area, it may become confluent to involve large portions of the face. This involvement of the surrounding tissue can create a cellulitis.

There are two main forms of deep folliculitis involving the head and neck. Both types are more common in men than in women, with blacks being more frequently affected than whites. **Acne keloidalis nuchae** is a chronic deep folliculitis occurring on the back of the neck that can eventually lead to scar formation. **Pseudofolliculitis barbae**, the other main form of deep folliculitis, is seen in the beard region of men (Fig. 115-1). In this condition, erythematous papules or pustules develop at the site of buried hair tips. The hairs appear to be growing in different directions in a disorganized pattern. The primary problem is that curved follicles tend to quickly reenter the skin and produce an ingrown hair. The inflammatory reaction is produced by the keratin in hair and by secondary infection. Both acne keloidalis nuchae and pseudofolliculitis barbae are usually initiated by close shaving.

"Hot tub" folliculitis occurs as a result of bathing in heavily used and inadequately chlorinated hot tubs and whirlpools. Characteristically, there is an eruption of pruritic follicular pustules or blisters concentrated on the trunk and buttocks. The folliculitis occurs 8-48 hours after soaking and clears spontaneously in 7-10 days. The causative organism is *Pseudomonas aeruginosa*.

Cellulitis is an acute, spreading, edematous, and inflammatory plaque. Warmth, erythema, and tenderness are the most helpful features in differentiating cellulitis from other clinically similar problems (Table 115-3). **Erysipelas** is a cellulitis that presents as an edematous, brawny, infiltrated, and sharply demarcated lesion that spreads peripherally. The skin is warm and

TABLE 115–3.   **Differential Diagnosis of Cellulitis**

Deep venous thrombosis
Stasis dermatitis
Contact dermatitis
Herpes zoster
Panniculitis (inflammation of subcutaneous fat)

bright red, although erysipelas caused by *Haemophilus influenzae* has a more violaceous hue and tends to occur around the eyes. The most common causative organism of erysipelas in adults is β-hemolytic *Streptococcus*. In children, the infection-producing bacteria is usually either β-hemolytic *Streptococcus* or *H. influenzae*. Recurrent erysipelas can occur.

In individuals with edematous extremities, an ulcer may develop with minimal trauma. The ulcer can be secondarily infected, with extension into surrounding tissue resulting in a cellulitis. In an acute or chronic dermatitis, *S. aureus* and β-hemolytic *Streptococcus* overgrow normal protective bacterial flora and predispose the dermis to cellulitis (see Table 115–1).

Impetigo (Fig. 115–2) is a contagious condition caused by direct inoculation of bacteria into superficial skin abrasions or hair follicles. The usual pathogens are group A streptococci and *S. aureus*. This condition is most commonly seen in children, occurring around the nose or mouth and less often on the hands. Impetigo is characterized by discrete, fragile vesicles surrounded by an erythematous border. These rupture easily to discharge an amber serous fluid that, when dried, forms a yellow crust that is the hallmark of the disease. New satellite lesions often appear in the vicinity of the original erosions and may coalesce to involve large areas of the skin.

Patients with eczema or psoriasis may become secondarily infected with the same organisms that cause primary impetigo. Secondary infection often causes a flare in symptoms of dermatitis. Clinically the dermatitis demonstrates exudate and crusts.

Untreated impetigo may worsen and extend deeper to become ecthyma. Ecthyma begins as an ulcerative pustule that becomes crusted and develops a raised border. It is usually caused by group A β-hemolytic *Streptococcus* entering a site of minor trauma. The disease occurs commonly on the shin or foot and frequently heals with scar formation. Ecthyma is more common in people who are immunocompromised or have poor nutrition.

EVALUATION

First, inquiry should be made about location, duration, previous trauma, preexisting cutaneous diseases, immunosuppressive diseases or therapy, and previous antibiotic therapy. A careful physical examination is also important, since most skin infections can be identified by their appearance. In addition, the appearance may point to a specific causative organism. The presence of erythema, warmth, and lymphadenopathy should be noted.

A Gram stain of vesicular/pustular fluid is a quick way to identify the causative organism in folliculitis and impetigo. In contrast, a Gram stain (or culture of a needle aspirate) identifies the causative organism only rarely in cellulitis. In addition, a skin biopsy for culture or blood cultures yield a causative organism less than 20% of the time in cellulitis. These procedures should be considered only if the cellulitis (1) appears atypical, (2) occurs in an immunocompromised patient, or (3) does not respond to empiric antibiotic therapy.

MANAGEMENT

Once the causative organism is identified, an appropriate antibiotic can be chosen. If no organism is initially identified, empiric therapy should be directed against the most common organisms causing the particular cutaneous infection. Oral dicloxacillin, cephalosporins, and erythromycin are usually effective in the outpatient management of staphylococcal and streptococcal infections. Coverage should be broadened in the immunocompromised patient and then made more specific after the final culture and sensitivity results are available.

Additional nonpharmacologic treatment of skin infections may help decrease spread and recurrence. For folliculitis, depending upon the location, wearing loose clothing and applying astringents may be useful in preventing occlusion of follicles. On the face and scalp, avoiding close shaving may prevent hairs from becoming ingrown. Povidone iodine washes or topical erythromycin may help prevent recurrent folliculitis. Some patients with recurrent folliculitis may be chronic carriers of *S. aureus*.

In the management of cellulitis, patients presenting with severe systemic symptoms, immunocompromised patients, and patients who are unreliable or unable to

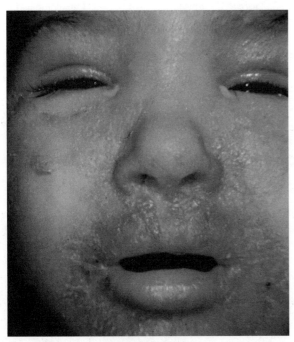

FIGURE 115–2. *Impetigo.*

care for themselves should be considered for hospitalization and treatment with intravenous antibiotics. Oral antibiotics are adequate for less severely ill patients. It is important to complete the full course of medication to prevent recurrences. Warm compresses and elevation of the affected area may aid in improving the symptoms.

The patient with impetigo should practice good hygiene (i.e., hand washing) to prevent further spread of the disease and to avoid transmission to personal contacts. Oral antibiotics should be used for severe or widespread impetigo. Less severe impetigo may be treated with the topical antibiotic mupirocin, which is effective against both streptococcal and staphylococcal infections. As the infection resolves, any underlying dermatosis should be treated to prevent recurrence of the impetigo.

PATIENT AND FAMILY EDUCATION

Patients with pseudofolliculitis barbae should be advised not to shave too closely. Patients placed on antibiotic therapy should be instructed to complete the full course of medication, barring intolerable side effects.

NATURAL HISTORY/PROGNOSIS

If left untreated, folliculitis becomes a chronic condition. While the patient rarely becomes seriously ill, the folliculitis continues to be painful and only infrequently resolves without treatment. An exception is "hot tub" folliculitis, which resolves spontaneously.

Cellulitis is potentially a life-threatening condition. If antibiotics are not initiated, the infection can spread systemically and lead to sepsis and even death. Intravenous antibiotics are indicated for severe infections or in an immunocompromised host. Uncomplicated cellulitis usually resolves in a few days with appropriate antibiotic therapy.

Impetigo infections will continue to spread (in size and from person to person) if untreated. Other complications include scarring (if the lesions are scratched or picked at) and the development of ecthyma. Rarely, the group A *Streptococcus* causing impetigo can lead to a poststreptococcal glomerulonephritis. Impetigo resolves quickly and without scarring when adequate treatment is started early in its course.

Research Questions

1. Why does "hot tub" folliculitis resolve without treatment while other forms of folliculitis require antibiotic therapy to resolve?

2. If a cellulitis involves a specific area of skin, why won't cultures from a biopsy grow the causative organism 100% of the time?

Case Resolution

The child's rash was diagnosed as erysipelas, and he was started on oral dicloxacillin. The infection resolved within 1 week with no complications.

Selected Readings

Berger, T. G., P. M. Elias, and B. V. Wintrub. *Manual of Therapy for Skin Diseases.* New York, Churchill Livingstone, 1990.

Maibach, H. I., R. Aly, and W. Noble. Bacterial infections of the skin. *In* S. L. Moschella and H. J. Hurley (eds.). *Dermatology,* 2nd ed. Philadelphia, W.B. Saunders Company, 1985.

Swartz, M. N., and A. N. Weinberg. Bacterial diseases with cutaneous involvement. *In* T. B. Fitzpatrick et al. (eds.). *Dermatology in General Medicine,* 4th ed. New York, McGraw-Hill Book Company, 1993.

Taylor, R. M. Bacterial infections. *In* T. T. Provost and E. R. Farmer (eds.). *Current Therapy in Dermatology—2.* Philadelphia, Decker, 1988.

Wortman, P. D. Bacterial infections of the skin. Curr Probl Dermatol V:193–228, November-December, 1993.

CHAPTER 116

FUNGAL INFECTIONS OF THE SKIN

Carl Bigler, M.D.

H$_x$ A 43-year-old right-handed male auto mechanic complains of dry scales on the palm of his right hand for the past 10 years. His right hand is often red and irritated, and painful fissures frequently develop after a difficult engine job. His left hand is unaffected. Moisturizers and hydrocortisone cream provide only temporary, mild improvement. On physical examination, his right hand has diffuse fine scale and mild erythema. His fingernails and left hand appear normal. His feet have thicker scale in a moccasin-shaped distribution, and many of his toenails are thickened and have yellow discoloration. When asked, he says that his feet do not bother him and he considers them normal, since his brother and father have similar-appearing feet.

Questions

1. Why is only one hand involved?
2. Can this rash be cured? If so, how?

Cutaneous fungal infections are a frequently encountered clinical problem. Who doesn't know someone who has had "athlete's foot" or "jock itch"? The physical disability is usually mild with some scaling, redness, and itch, but a fungal infection of the hands or fingernails may impair a person's ability to work or to interact with the public. The social disability is often heightened by concern about contagiousness.

PATHOPHYSIOLOGY

Cutaneous fungal infections are caused by fungi, or yeasts. Yeasts are usually round to oval in microscopic appearance but may have short, nonseptate hyphae. Dermatophytes have long, branching septate hyphae.

The yeast *Candida albicans* is not usually present on normal skin and requires an enriched cutaneous environment or a breakdown in host immunity to produce infections in skinfolds or mucous membranes. A moist, irritated cutaneous environment provides a nidus for *Candida* infection. Intertrigo is a candidal infection in skinfolds, often in the inguinal creases or under the breasts, and presents as beefy red, wet plaques with satellite pustules (Fig. 116–1). Diaper rash may be viewed as intertrigo in the gluteal clefts of babies or incontinent patients. Thrush and vaginal yeast infections are candidal infections of mucous membranes and often appear as adherent whitish material on an erythematous, slightly eroded base.

FIGURE 116–2. *Tinea versicolor on the back.*

Candidal infections are more common in (1) immunocompromised patients, (2) patients with diabetes, and (3) patients taking antibiotics.

The yeast *Malassezia furfur,* in contrast to *Candida albicans,* colonizes normal human skin. This organism has a nutritional requirement for fatty acids and thrives in the yeast form in sebaceous-rich areas of human skin. For unknown reasons, the yeast proliferates in certain individuals, developing pseudohyphae and producing an unusual rash (referred to as tinea versicolor) that has the appearance of scaly patches; these patches may be lighter or darker than normal skin color and often resemble candle wax dripping down the back (Fig. 116–2). Involvement of the face and distal extremities is unusual.

Dermatophytes have a predilection for the superficial, keratin-rich areas of skin and hair. The reason for this site specificity is not known, since keratin is not a nutritional requirement for these fungi. Dermatophytes extend into soft tissues only in severely immunocompromised patients.

Dermatophytes are classified by their living environment of choice. Geophilic fungi are most frequently isolated from soil, zoophilic fungi from animals, and anthropophilic fungi from humans. This classification system

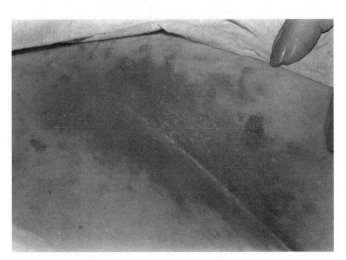

FIGURE 116–1. *Intertrigo due to* Candida albicans.

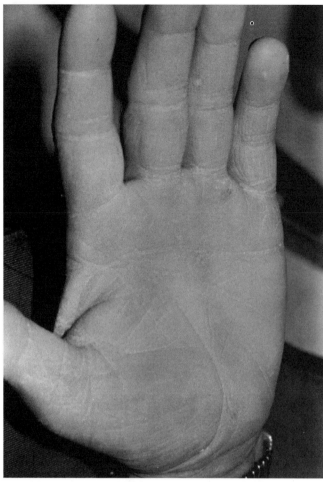

FIGURE 116–3. *Chronic tinea manuum.*

has important clinical correlates. Inflammatory tinea (with erythema, vesicles, and severe itching in addition to scale) is usually caused by "nonhuman" dermatophytes. Such infections are typically intense and self-limited. The host's immune reaction is responsible for the severe symptoms and also prevents these infections from becoming chronic. Nonhuman dermatophyte infections cannot be transferred from person to person.

Chronic tinea infections (e.g., chronic tinea pedis and chronic tinea unguium) are usually caused by "human" dermatophytes (Fig. 116–3). Affected individuals cannot mount an immune response to these fungi, and the rash is therefore difficult to eradicate even with optimal therapy. These rashes typically itch only mildly and intermittently. Fomites or personal contact may spread these fungi but only to susceptible individuals.

DIFFERENTIAL DIAGNOSIS

Dermatitis and psoriasis may appear similar to **tinea corporis**. Dermatitis caused by contact allergens (see Chapter 111), irritants, or dry skin presents as dry, scaly, erythematous patches. Psoriasis is most frequently manifested by multiple plaques with adherent white scale usually on the scalp, elbows, knees, and gluteal cleft. Tinea corporis is more likely to present as a solitary plaque with a peripheral rim of scale and central clearing (Fig. 116–4).

Tinea cruris is a dermatophyte infection of the groin that is often referred to as jock itch. For unknown reasons, this presentation of dermatophyte infection is unusual in women. The differential diagnosis includes dermatitis and intertrigo. A peripheral scaly rim favors tinea cruris. Scrotal or perianal involvement favors dermatitis. Red, macerated plaques within pendulous skin folds are characteristic of intertrigo (see Fig. 116–1).

The differential diagnosis for a scaly palm includes **tinea manuum** and chronic dermatitis. For unknown reasons, tinea manuum usually involves only one hand. Tinea infection of the nails (causing distal nail thickening and yellowish discoloration) also favors tinea manuum over chronic hand dermatitis.

Tinea pedis, or dermatophyte infection of the feet, may be difficult to differentiate from acute vesicular or more chronic scaly dermatitis. Nail involvement and maceration between the fourth and fifth toes favor a tinea infection.

Tinea capitis (ringworm of the scalp) has the appearance of (1) a scaly scalp (and nonscarring hair loss) when there is little host response or (2) an inflammatory mass with scarring alopecia if the immune response is brisk (Fig. 116–5). Tinea capitis is common in children and relatively uncommon in adults. The common causes of scarring alopecia in adults—including discoid lupus, dissecting folliculitis of the scalp, lichen planus, and morphea—are rare in children. The common causes of scaly scalp in adults—seborrheic dermatitis or psoriasis—may occur in children although alopecia and "black dots" (hairs broken at the follicular orifice) are features of tinea capitis and not of these diseases.

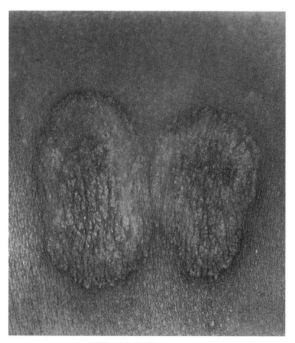

FIGURE 116–4. *Tinea corporis.*

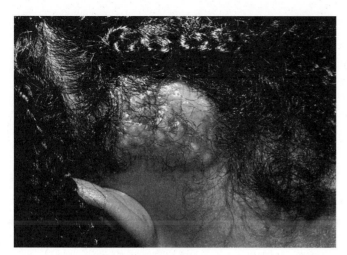

FIGURE 116-5. *Inflammatory tinea capitis.*

Tinea unguium (fungal infection of the nails; also called onychomycosis) shows thickening of the nail and crumbly material under the nail plate. Tinea unguium may occasionally be difficult to distinguish from traumatic nail dystrophy or psoriatic nails. Tinea of the nails does not cause the type of pitting seen in psoriatic nails and is usually accompanied by fine scale on the feet or hands.

Occasionally, a dermatophyte will extend down a hair follicle and present as folliculitis. This is especially likely to occur if a dermatophyte infection has been treated for a prolonged period with topical corticosteroids. The differential diagnosis includes bacterial folliculitis and acne.

The classical presentation of **tinea versicolor**—coalescing scaly, discolored patches dripping like candle wax down the back—is unique and diagnostic (see Fig. 116-2). The only other consideration is vitiligo, which shows complete absence of pigment, is not scaly, and rarely occurs on the back.

EVALUATION

The quickest and easiest method of diagnosing a cutaneous fungal infection is to scrape the scaly edge of a lesion or pull an involved hair and dissolve the keratin in 15% KOH. The long, branching, septate hyphae will appear among the keratin debris. Often 5 minutes or longer is required to dissolve the keratin, longer if the specimen is hair or nail. False-positive results can occur with clothing fibers. In tinea versicolor, the fungus appears as clumps of round yeast forms and short curved pseudohyphal forms (resulting in a characteristic "meatballs and hot dogs" appearance). *Candida* and dermatophytes—but not *M. furfur,* the cause of tinea versicolor—may be cultured on Sabouraud's dextrose agar. *Candida* grows relatively quickly, but dermatophytes may require up to 3 weeks for a positive culture. Saprophytic fungi cause cutaneous disease (with the exception of nail disease) only rarely, and cultured saprophytic fungi should be considered colonizers and not pathogens in most cases.

MANAGEMENT

Acute dermatophyte infections should be treated aggressively, including tinea capitis in a child or the first episode of inflammatory tinea pedis or cruris. Tinea capitis usually requires a 6-week course of oral griseofulvin. Giving griseofulvin with ice cream increases its gastrointestinal absorption and improves compliance. Topical antifungals are not effective in tinea capitis. Since a long course of systemic therapy is required, fungal culture is recommended to confirm the diagnosis. Because fungal cultures often take 3 weeks to grow, therapy should precede culture results, especially if there is scarring hair loss. Close contacts should be examined for infection. Selenium sulfide shampoo will decrease scale and may decrease contagiousness.

Acute tinea pedis, cruris, and corporis may be treated with topical antifungals. Even if the rash disappears in a week, treatment should continue for 3 weeks because recurrence rates are significant. Widespread tinea may be treated with oral griseofulvin for 4 weeks. Inflammatory tinea corporis may be transmitted to humans from cats, dogs, or cattle, and the patient should be questioned about the possibility of contact with these animals. If such is the case, the animals should be examined for tinea by a veterinarian.

Chronic dermatophyte infections such as chronic tinea pedis, tinea manuum, tinea cruris, or tinea unguium will not be cured by topical therapy. Systemic therapy with griseofulvin may be tried for tinea manuum, but if there is nail involvement recurrence is the rule. Long courses of griseofulvin are expensive and require monitoring of liver enzymes. For this reason, fungal culture is recommended before systemic therapy is started.

Although cure is not achieved, the symptoms of chronic dermatophyte infections can often be controlled by chronic topical antifungal therapy. Topical nystatin is effective against *Candida* but not against dermatophytes. Topical imidazoles (e.g., clotrimazole, ketoconazole, miconazole, oxiconazole, spectinazole, sulconazole) are effective against both yeasts and dermatophytes. There is no evidence that dermatophytes develop resistance to imidazoles with prolonged use. It is often helpful to add a keratolytic agent (containing salicylic acid, benzoic acid, or lactic acid) to remove scale, particularly in infections of the palms or soles.

Intertrigo requires initial therapy with nystatin or an imidazole cream or lotion as well as measures to correct the moist cutaneous environment. Washing with mild soap and drying with a hair dryer on low heat twice a day often help prevent recurrences. Chronic antibiotic therapy may contribute to yeast infections and should be discontinued if possible. Tight control of diabetes by diet or medication should also be achieved.

Tinea versicolor may be controlled with topical selenium sulfide solution applied overnight on a monthly basis. The yeast colonizes normal skin, so treatment does not eradicate the organism but decreases its density and prevents pseudohyphae formation. An effective alternative is occasional systemic therapy with keto-conazole, one dose with exercise, but this poses the hazard of systemic toxicity (including rare hepatotoxic-ity) for what is essentially a cosmetic problem.

NATURAL HISTORY/PROGNOSIS

Acute inflammatory tinea eventually resolves spon-taneously over a period of months although treatment will improve both itching and appearance within 3 weeks. Inflammatory tinea of the scalp may result in permanent hair loss and scarring if untreated. Chronic tinea infections of the hands, feet, and groin will persist indefinitely without treatment. Although treatment in these situations provides temporary relief, the rash eventually returns. Intertrigo may become chronic un-less the moist, macerated skinfold environment is im-proved. Tinea versicolor will persist indefinitely unless treated. None of these cutaneous fungal infections causes visceral involvement, even in immunocompro-mised patients. Acute, inflammatory tinea will not spread to close contacts, and chronic tinea will spread only to susceptible contacts. For such transmission to occur, the contact's immune system must "tolerate" the fungus and the appropriate cutaneous microenviron-ment must also be present. Moist, abraded skin without competitive nonpathogenic bacteria is preferred by pathogenic fungi.

Research Questions

1. Is the susceptibility to chronic fungal infections acquired or inherited?
2. Why do dermatophytes live only in the stratum cor-neum, the nonliving, keratin-rich scale on top of the skin?

Case Resolution

The patient's diagnosis was a chronic tinea infection of the feet and right hand. Treatment with clotrimazole cream and a moisturizer improved the appearance and decreased the painful cracking of his dominant hand.

Selected Readings

Borelli, D., P. Jacobs, and L. Nall. Tinea versicolor: Epidemiologic, clin-ical, and therapeutic aspects. J Am Acad Dermatol 25:300–5, 1991.
Elewski, B. *Topics in Clinical Dermatology: Cutaneous Fungal Infections.* New York, Igaku-Shoin, 1992.
Lesher, J., N. Levine, and P. Treadwell. Fungal skin infections: Common but stubborn. Patient Care 28(2):16–43, 1994.
Martin, A., and G. Kobayashi. Superficial fungal infections. *In* T. Fitzpatrick et al. (eds.). *Dermatology in General Medicine.* Vol. 2. New York, McGraw-Hill Book Company, 1993.
Martin, A., and G. Kobayashi. Yeast infections. *In* T. Fitzpatrick et al. (eds.). *Dermatology in General Medicine.* Vol. 2. New York, McGraw-Hill Book Company, 1993.

CHAPTER 117

MELANOMA

Carl Bigler, M.D.

H$_x$ A 25-year-old male law student comes in because he recently noted a changing mole on his upper back. The mole is asymptomatic. There is no family history of melanoma, but during childhood and adolescence, the patient used to sunburn severely. The nevus measures 5 mm in diameter and varies in color from brown to black with a small area of pink. The margins appear regular except for one small notch. Examination of the rest of the skin reveals multiple nevi and freckles. Some nevi appear similar to the changing mole. The patient's face and arms are suntanned.

Questions

1. Would you take a biopsy of this nevus?
2. Would you take a biopsy of the similar-appearing nevi?
3. What would you tell this patient?

More than 20,000 new cases of melanoma are diag-nosed each year in the United States. This number rep-resents approximately 2% of all cancer diagnoses. The incidence of melanoma does increase with age but un-like the case for lung, colon, and prostate cancer, mela-noma in a young person is not rare. The average light-pigmented person has approximately 30 nevi. Clearly, a biopsy cannot be performed on all nevi to rule out the possibility of melanoma. The clinician examining a pig-mented lesion must decide when to recommend a bi-opsy and when to reassure the patient that the lesion is benign. Early melanoma is curable by simple excision. Metastatic melanoma is almost uniformly fatal.

CLINICAL PRESENTATION

The clinical diagnosis of melanoma is based on four features, the so-called ABCD's of melanoma. If a line is

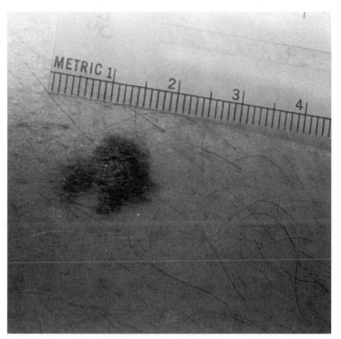

FIGURE 117–1. *Melanoma.*

drawn through the middle of the lesion and each side does not appear to be the mirror image of the other, then the lesion is *a*symmetrical (A). The *b*orders (B) of a melanoma are typically irregular or notched, and pigment may appear to leach into the surrounding skin. The *c*olor (C) of a melanoma may vary from shades of brown, black, or blue (deep pigment) to red (inflammation) or white (tumor regression). Melanomas are often greater than 6 mm in *d*iameter (D) at the time of discovery, though with increased public and physician awareness, many melanomas less than 6 mm in diameter are now being diagnosed and removed. Any lesion exhibiting these four features should be excised or a biopsy should be performed (Fig. 117–1). The likelihood of finding melanoma on biopsy depends on the prevalence of melanoma in the population studied. Melanoma is relatively rare in children less than 10 years of age, although it is during this time—and into the teens and early twenties—that common nevi are acquired and existing nevi may grow. Nevi may be acquired after age 30, but this situation is unusual enough to evoke suspicion and further evaluation, with a prejudice toward biopsy. Similarly, a biopsy should be done for a nevus that is changing out of proportion to other nevi.

PATHOPHYSIOLOGY

The development of melanoma appears to be related to periods of exposure to high-intensity sunlight. It occurs most frequently in areas of skin that sunburn frequently—the backs of men and the legs of women. In contrast, nonmelanoma skin cancer (see Chapter 118) is more closely related to *total* accumulated sun exposure and occurs more frequently on the face and arms. In melanoma, it is not clear whether the causative rays of

sunlight are the burning rays (ultraviolet B, UVB), which have been strongly linked to nonmelanoma skin cancer, or the longer wavelength (UVA) rays. The incidence of melanoma increases with proximity to the equator. Darker skin pigmentation is protective. People with a family history are at increased risk, as are people who tend to be mole formers.

Melanoma is a malignant tumor of melanocytes. Melanocytes provide melanin, which gives the skin color and protects it from the harmful effects of sunlight on cellular DNA. Melanomas begin superficially near the basement membrane zone of the epidermis where melanocytes are found in normal skin. Most melanomas undergo an initial period of radial growth and remain superficial for months to years before vertical growth and invasion—with a corresponding worsening prognosis—occur. The majority of melanomas arise de novo, i.e., as a "new mole," though as many as one third arise in a preexisting nevus, i.e., as a "changing mole."

DIFFERENTIAL DIAGNOSIS

For children and for adults through age 40, the differential diagnosis of melanoma includes nevus, dermatofibroma, lentigo, and vascular lesions. Nevi are generally symmetrical, with regular borders and uniform color. A nevus variant known as blue nevus has a uniform blue-black color and is symmetrical with sharp margins. Dermatofibromas are benign tumors of fibrous tissue and are often tan or brown, but, in contrast to melanomas and nevi, are firm like a scar. Lentigines are flat and small but may have irregular margins. Though the color variation among lentigines may range from tan to black, the color within each lentigo is uniform. Vascular lesions may have an alarming blue-black color, but with compression, these lesions blanch. In patients older than the age of 40 years, the differential diagnosis also includes seborrheic keratosis and pigmented basal cell carcinoma. These two epidermal tumors may be difficult to differentiate clinically from a melanoma. Seborrheic keratoses are benign tumors of the epidermis, the most superficial portion of skin (Fig. 117–2). These lesions may vary in color from tan to black. The most helpful clinical clues include scale (flaking), discrete margins, and the existence of multiple, similar-appearing lesions. Pigmented basal cell carcinoma may contain irregular pigment although the tumor often has a pearly, translucent quality not seen in most melanomas. In general, if an irregularly pigmented lesion cannot be positively identified as a benign lesion based on clinical examination, a biopsy should be performed.

Dx   MELANOMA

- Pigmented lesion that often is asymmetrical, has an irregular border, and varies in color
- May occur at any age but more frequent with increasing age

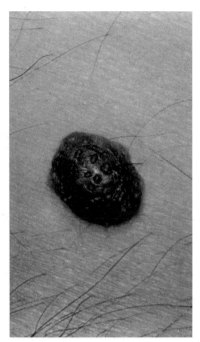

FIGURE 117–2. *Seborrheic keratosis.*

EVALUATION

Biopsy is the definitive test for melanoma. Excisional biopsy—complete removal including subcutaneous fat—is the procedure of choice. Prognosis in melanoma is directly related to the depth of tumor invasion in millimeters (Table 117–1). The depth of the melanoma also determines the margins of reexcision, the definitive mode of treatment (see below). Superficial biopsies (with tumor extending to the deep surgical margins) may provide only partial prognostic information. If a melanoma is so large that excisional biopsy is not possible, incisional or punch biopsy can confirm the diagnosis. Incisional or punch biopsies do not cause metastases. The clinical diagnosis of melanoma is never certain. Many lesions that meet the clinical criteria for melanoma will prove to be benign on biopsy. Prior to biopsy, the patient should be told that melanoma is one possible diagnosis of several. Patients often believe that the diagnosis of melanoma is a death sentence when, in fact, most melanomas are recognized early enough to achieve a complete cure. For this reason, it is preferable to communicate diagnosis and prognosis during a return clinic visit rather than on the telephone.

The histopathologic diagnosis of melanoma may occasionally be difficult, particularly in children or young adults. Multiple professional opinions may be requested before the final diagnosis is rendered. This may cause a delay in the diagnosis and be frustrating for both clinician and patient, but the diagnosis of melanoma typically has multiple effects on a patient's life. A patient who has a thin melanoma diagnosed and cured may still find it difficult and expensive to obtain life and health insurance. For this reason, a certain diagnosis is more important than a rapid one.

MANAGEMENT

Once the diagnosis is made, the definitive treatment is reexcision. As mentioned above, melanoma usually grows radially, often spreading as single cells along the basement membrane zone, before it becomes invasive. These cells are often present beyond the clinically apparent margin of the melanoma. An incompletely excised melanoma may recur, and recurrent melanoma has an ominous prognosis. For this reason, 1-cm surgical margins are recommended for melanomas less than 1 mm in depth and 2- to 3-cm surgical margins are advised for melanomas greater than 1 mm in depth. Prophylactic excision of lymph nodes is not recommended for most melanomas. The patient should have lymph node size assessed on physical examination as part of clinical staging. Once a melanoma is metastatic, radiation and chemotherapy offer palliation only.

The most effective "treatment" for melanoma is prevention and early diagnosis.

PATIENT AND FAMILY EDUCATION

Patients who have (1) a history of melanoma, (2) a family history of melanoma, or (3) multiple nevi are at higher risk of developing melanoma and should be educated in the technique of self-examination. These patients may also benefit from periodic examinations by physicians skilled in the diagnosis of melanoma.

Intense, burning exposure to sunlight should be avoided, especially in childhood and adolescence. The role of sunscreen is less clear for melanoma than for nonmelanoma skin cancers. Sunscreen blocks the burning UVB rays more effectively than it blocks the longer wavelength UVA rays. Most evidence links intermittent high-intensity UVB radiation to melanoma although some animal studies implicate UVA. UVA, in contrast to UVB, readily passes through window glass (which would thus be nonprotective). Of particular concern is the prevalence of tanning salons that utilize high-intensity UVA to tan their clients.

PROGNOSIS

Patients who have had complete excisions of thin melanomas can consider themselves cured, but they have about a tenfold increased risk of developing a second primary melanoma. Family members may also be at increased risk and should be so informed. The prognosis for thicker lesions is less certain. Melanoma, like breast and renal carcinoma, may occasionally present as metastatic disease many years after removal

TABLE 117–1. Relationship Between Melanoma Depth and 5-Year Survival

Risk	Melanoma Depth (mm)	5-Year Survival (%)
Low	< 0.76	99
Moderate	0.76–1.5	85
High	> 1.5	60

of the primary tumor. Metastatic melanoma has a predilection for brain and skin, and its prognosis is poor.

Research Questions

1. Why are melanomas more likely to metastasize than other types of skin cancer?
2. Why is the incidence of melanoma increasing in the United States?

Case Resolution

A biopsy was performed on the changing mole, and it was found to be melanoma-in-situ. It was treated by reexcision. Biopsies of several other nevi were benign. The patient's

outcome was excellent. He was pleased with the medical care he received but is suing the insurance company that denied him life insurance.

Selected Readings

Barnhill, R., M. Mihm, T. Fitzpatrick, and A. Sober. Malignant melanoma. *In* T. Fitzpatrick et al. (eds.). *Dermatology in General Medicine,* 4th ed. New York, McGraw-Hill Book Company, 1993.

Breslow, A. Prognostic factors in the treatment of cutaneous melanoma. J Cutan Pathol 6:208–12, 1979.

Diagnosis and treatment of early melanoma (NIH Consensus Conference). JAMA 268:1314–9, 1992.

Rigel, D. (ed.). Melanoma/skin cancer update. Dermatol Clin 9:617–702, 1991.

Wolf, P., C. Donawho, and M. Kripke. Effect of sunscreen on UV radiation-induced enhancement of melanoma growth in mice. J Natl Cancer Inst 86:99–105, 1994.

CHAPTER 118

NONMELANOMA SKIN CANCER

Jerry Feldman, M.D.

H$_x$ A 70-year-old farmer says he has a slowly growing "bump" on his nose that bleeds easily. Further history reveals that he has hypertension for which he takes an angiotension-converting enzyme (ACE) inhibitor. Physical examination of his nose reveals a 0.8-cm crusted, translucent, ulcerated nodule with a raised border. In addition, he has numerous scaly, red patches on his forehead and cheeks.

Questions

1. What are this patient's risk factors for nonmelanoma skin cancer?
2. What are the clinical subtypes of basal cell carcinoma?
3. What is the most important cause of nonmelanoma skin cancer?

One third of all cancers in the United States are nonmelanoma skin cancers, primarily basal cell carcinoma and squamous cell carcinoma. The incidence of nonmelanoma skin cancer has increased to an epidemic proportion in the past few decades. At least 500,000 basal cell carcinomas and 100,000 squamous cell carcinomas occur annually. Mortality due to these cancers is

infrequent, with most deaths arising from squamous cell carcinomas that have metastasized.

For whites, the incidence of nonmelanoma skin cancer correlates with increasing age and residency in areas of high ultraviolet B (UVB) exposure. The majority of cancers are located on the head and neck. Although nonmelanoma skin cancer is uncommon in African Americans, Asian Americans, and Hispanics, African Americans tend to develop squamous cell carcinoma more often than basal cell carcinoma.

CLINICAL PRESENTATION

Basal cell carcinoma (Fig. 118–1) has several different clinical and morphologic presentations. The most common subtype is the nodular basal cell carcinoma, which has the appearance of a translucent pearly white papule or nodule with a raised border. The nodule may be ulcerated, and the patient may complain that it bleeds easily. This complaint is often elicited in males in whom the bleeding is triggered by shaving. Superficial basal cell carcinoma presents as a well-demarcated, scaly red plaque, typically on the trunk and arms. It is commonly misdiagnosed as tinea corporis or dermatitis that has not responded to topical corticosteroid or antifungal therapy. Morpheaform basal cell carcinoma appears as

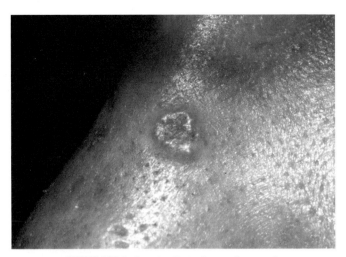

FIGURE 118–1. *Basal cell carcinoma (on nose).*

an indurated white or yellow plaque with indistinct margins that often resembles a scar. Morpheaform or sclerotic basal cell cancers are well known to extend far beyond their visible borders. Pigmented basal cell carcinoma is usually a nodular basal cell carcinoma containing a significant amount of melanin pigment.

Squamous cell carcinoma (Fig. 118–2) often presents as an ulcerated nodule, plaque, or erosion. A keratoacanthoma is a special type of squamous cell carcinoma that presents as a rapidly growing, berry-type nodule. Patients often state that this lesion has grown to a size of 1–2 cm within 4–5 weeks.

PATHOPHYSIOLOGY

Both squamous and basal cell carcinomas arise from keratinocytes. The most important etiologic factor in the development of nonmelanoma skin cancer is chronic cumulative sun exposure, primarily from the UVB (290–320 nm) spectrum. Several lines of evidence underscore the role of UVB in causing nonmelanoma skin cancer. First, the incidence is much greater among the following groups: (1) sun-sensitive phenotypes, i.e., fair-skinned whites; (2) whites living near the equator; and (3) albinos. In addition, the vast majority of skin cancers are located in anatomic areas with high UVB exposure, i.e., the head and neck. UVB has many detrimental effects on the skin including damage to DNA with probable mutations in tumor suppressor genes. In addition, UVB can induce localized and generalized immunosuppression.

Other known causes of nonmelanoma skin cancers include (1) ionizing radiation; (2) chemical carcinogens such as arsenic, nitrogen mustard, polycyclic hydrocarbons, and tobacco; (3) the combination of psoralen plus ultraviolet A radiation (PUVA therapy); (4) chronic ulcers and scarring dermatoses; and (5) viral carcinogens such as the human papillomavirus (HPV).

Immunosuppression is an increasingly recognized factor in the development of skin cancer. The risk of squamous cell carcinoma in immunosuppressed patients is 18 times that of the general population, while the risk of basal cell carcinoma is three times greater.

Certain genetic disorders, such as xeroderma pigmentosum, basal cell nevus syndrome, oculocutaneous albinism, and epidermolysis bullosa, may predispose a person to skin cancer.

The most important precursor lesion for squamous cell carcinoma is the actinic keratosis (Fig. 118–3). Histologically, these red, scaly patches represent early aberrant keratinocyte maturation. The probability of an individual actinic keratosis transforming into squamous cell carcinoma is less than 1%.

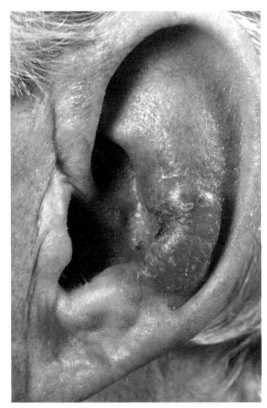

FIGURE 118–2. *Squamous cell carcinoma.*

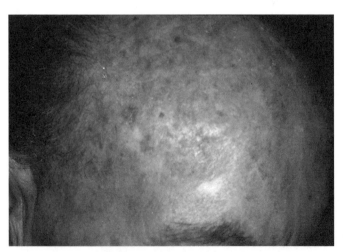

FIGURE 118–3. *Actinic keratosis.*

DIFFERENTIAL DIAGNOSIS

Nodular basal cell carcinomas may resemble melanocytic nevi, fibrous papules, sebaceous hyperplasia, hair follicle tumors, and squamous cell carcinoma. Morpheaform basal cell carcinoma must be differentiated from a scar, localized scleroderma, desmoplastic melanoma, and a desmoplastic trichoepithelioma. The pigmented basal cell carcinoma should be differentiated from a seborrheic keratosis, a nevus, and malignant melanoma. Finally, the superficial basal cell carcinoma may be indistinguishable from eczema, psoriasis, or cutaneous T-cell lymphoma.

Squamous cell carcinomas look similar to warts, irritated seborrheic keratoses, fungal infections, keratoacanthomas, or ulcerated basal cell carcinoma. Squamous cell carcinoma-in-situ (Bowen's disease) appears as a scaly, erythematous, well-demarcated plaque and resembles a superficial basal cell carcinoma or a plaque of dermatitis.

EVALUATION

History

The patient may complain of a new growth during a visit to a primary care physician, or these cancers may be incidental findings on physical examination. Patients with fair skin, a history of excessive sun exposure, or previous skin cancers are at extremely high risk for skin cancer. The physician should inquire about (1) previous skin cancers and treatment received, (2) whether the patient has ever had radiation therapy, (3) whether sun exposure has been prolonged or excessive, and (4) whether sun protection is currently being used.

Physical Examination

The physical examination should be carried out under the proper lighting. The physician should examine the entire integument and not only the sites mentioned by the patient. The nasolabial folds, nasal tip, and area behind the ears should be carefully examined. When a patient complains of a new growth, the physician should ask about its duration, its rate of growth, and whether it bleeds easily. With the above information, the physician should be able to characterize a nonmelanoma skin cancer as either a basal cell or a squamous cell carcinoma.

It is especially important that the primary care physician evaluate the lymph nodes in patients with squamous cell carcinoma. All lymph node chains of the head and neck, even the contralateral ones, should be examined. In addition, a careful bimanual examination of the submental lymph nodes is mandatory.

Additional Evaluation

A biopsy should be performed on all suspicious lesions for histologic confirmation of the diagnosis. Basal cell carcinoma should be classified as aggressive or nonaggressive based on the histopathologic growth pattern. Similarly, the histologic depth and the degree of differentiation of squamous cell carcinoma needs to be carefully assessed. Size, location, and duration also are important variables when planning the management of these lesions.

MANAGEMENT

The treatment of nonmelanoma skin cancer is primarily surgical. The specific therapeutic approach depends on the (1) histopathologic type, (2) anatomic location, (3) clinical size, (4) natural history of the tumor (primary versus recurrent), and (5) age and overall health of the patient.

Commonly used treatments include (1) excisional surgery, (2) Mohs' micrographic surgery, (3) cryosurgery, (4) electrodesiccation and curettage, and (5) radiotherapy. With small, histopathologically nonaggressive tumors, all these therapies have high cure rates. Mohs' micrographic surgery is the optimal choice for recurrent skin cancers and those tumors with an aggressive histology. Mohs' micrographic surgery is a special technique of processing tissue such that the entire surgical margin can be evaluated for the presence of tumor.

The most important precursor lesion of squamous cell carcinoma is the actinic keratosis. Consequently, eradication of these lesions may prevent future squamous cell carcinomas. Acceptable treatments include (1) cryosurgery, (2) topical 5-fluorouracil, (3) curettage, and in many cases, (4) close observation with the knowledge that up to 25% will spontaneously remit if sun exposure is minimized through avoidance or regular sunscreen usage.

PATIENT AND FAMILY EDUCATION

The key to preventing nonmelanoma skin cancer lies in educating the public about the hazards of sunlight. Rational avoidance of midday sun exposure, protective clothing, and proper usage of sunscreens will dramatically reduce the number of UV radiation-induced skin cancers. One theoretical analysis predicted an 80% reduction in the lifetime risk of nonmelanoma skin cancer in people who appropriately use sunscreens during the first 18 years of life. In addition, regular sunscreen usage will facilitate the remission of actinic keratoses.

NATURAL HISTORY/PROGNOSIS

All patients with basal cell and squamous cell carcinoma should have meticulous follow-up, monitoring for tumor recurrences, metastases, and the development of new primary skin cancers. Between 30% and 50% of patients will develop a new skin cancer within 5 years, with the majority occurring within the first year. Patients who present with multiple primary tumors have an even higher risk of developing a subsequent tumor. Consequently, patients should be examined every 3 months for the first year and every 6 months thereafter (and, if a tumor is discovered, the "clock" should be reset). Patients with squamous cell carcinoma, especially those with lesions in high-risk areas such as the lip and ear, should be thoroughly examined for regional lymphadenopathy.

Research Questions

1. Why do basal cell carcinomas rarely metastasize?
2. Why do squamous cell carcinomas develop in scars?
3. Given two patients with the same skin type and the same amount of sun exposure, why does one develop skin cancer while the other does not?
4. What is the role of the immune system in preventing skin cancer?
5. Why are organ transplant patients more likely to develop squamous cell carcinomas than basal cell carcinomas?

Case Resolution

A biopsy revealed a basal cell carcinoma with nonaggressive histologic features. The tumor was removed by Mohs' micrographic surgery and the defect closed with a skin graft. The patient was advised about skin cancer prevention techniques, and to date there has been no recurrence.

Selected Readings

Del Rosso, J. Q., and R. J. Siegle. Management of basal cell carcinomas. *In* R. G. Wheeland (ed.). *Cutaneous Surgery*. Philadelphia, W.B. Saunders Company, 1994.

Glass, A. G., and R. N. Hoover. The emerging epidemic of melanoma and squamous cell skin cancer. JAMA 262:2097–2100, 1989.

Hendee, W. R., and Council on Scientific Affairs: Harmful effects of ultraviolet radiation. JAMA 262:380–4, 1989.

Johnson, T. M., D. E. Rowe, B. R. Nelson, and N. A. Swanson. Squamous cell carcinoma of the skin (excluding lip and oral mucosa). J Am Acad Dermatol 26:467–84, 1992.

Karagas, M. R., et al. Risk of subsequent basal cell carcinoma and squamous cell carcinoma of the skin among patients with prior skin cancer. JAMA 267:3305–10, 1992.

Marks, R., G. Rennie, and T. S. Selwood. Malignant transformation of solar keratoses to squamous cell carcinoma. Lancet 1:795–7, 1988.

Preston, D. S., and R. S. Stern. Nonmelanoma cancers of the skin. N Engl J Med 327:1649–62, 1992.

Salasche, S. J., M. L. Cheney, M. A. Varvares. Recognition and management of the high-risk cutaneous squamous cell carcinoma. Curr Probl Dermatol V:141–92, 1993.

Schreiber, M. M., T. E. Moon, et al. The risk of developing subsequent nonmelanoma skin cancers. J Am Acad Dermatol 23:1114–8, 1990.

Thompson, S. C., D. Jolley, R. Marks. Reduction of solar keratoses by regular sunscreen use. N Engl J Med 329:1147–51, 1993.

CHAPTER 119

DEVELOPMENTAL-BEHAVIORAL ISSUES IN PEDIATRICS

Andrew C. Hsi, M.D., M.P.H.

H$_x$ A 23-day-old infant is brought for a well-child visit by his grandmother, who has assumed his care because of his mother's legal problems. She expresses concerns about his "shaking all of the time." She also wants information about his "crying so hard." She states that the baby "eats very often, but he vomits a lot." In response to questions about birth records, she initially seems reluctant to offer information. On first impression, the baby seems small and fussy. He appears to hold his hands close to his mouth and displays bursts of active rooting and sucking. When placed on the examination table, he prefers lying on his side in an arched position with his back hyperextended. With stimulation, he extends his arms and splays his fingers. Marked jitteriness occurs with his arms extended, but he does not have seizure activity. His head size seems small for his age. As the examination progresses, his grandmother offers, "I think his mom may have gotten into trouble for using drugs."

Questions

1. What additional medical information is needed?
2. Does this infant have developmental or behavioral problems?
3. Will this infant's clinical presentation worsen over time?
4. Was the mother's use of drugs responsible for the current clinical presentation?

The primary care provider needs to understand the normal pattern of growth, development, and behavior of infants and children to assess their well-being. To evaluate growth, the provider should use standardized growth charts to compare the child's weight, length, and head circumference to age-specific norms as well as the child's growth trends. Abnormally small or large stature is associated with a higher prevalence of developmental disabilities including intellectual deficits. In normal infants, new abilities appear in a predictable sequence with advancing age. The absence of appropriate emo-

tional and environmental stimuli can interfere with this expected sequence of development. The provider can assess development and behavior by using standardized screening instruments such as the Denver Developmental Screening Test (DDST). DDST in combination with observations by the parents or other caretakers can be used to screen for developmental problems. Infants exposed to alcohol or other drugs *in utero* have added risks for abnormal growth and development. The primary care provider should particularly be aware of the physical signs associated with maternal use of these substances during pregnancy.

PATHOPHYSIOLOGY

Findings of abnormalities in muscle tone, behavior, and feeding suggest brain injury. A history of difficult labor or marked respiratory depression at birth suggests possible hypoxic-ischemic encephalopathy. Infants at risk for developmental delays include those exposed to alcohol, tobacco, other drugs, and toxins during gestation. In the United States, 5–15% of infants may be at risk for developmental delays based on such exposure. The presence of tremors, jitteriness, feeding problems, and irritability accompany withdrawal from narcotic exposure during gestation. Early problems with glucose homeostasis or a maternal history of gestational diabetes can cause brain injury from hypoglycemia. Similarly, a history of severe infection, such as congenital viral infections or meningitis, might explain the presenting problems. The presence on physical examination of major or minor anomalies may lead to a diagnosis of a syndrome (e.g., Down syndrome), with a constellation of birth defects and developmental and behavioral problems. Genetic syndromes associated with short stature almost always include mental retardation or learning disability. Acquired injuries from head trauma occur frequently in motor vehicle accidents or child abuse. Findings associated with specific problems are summarized in Table 119–1.

TABLE 119–1. Signs and Symptoms Related to Disorders in Early Infancy

	Jitteriness, Tremors	Seizures	Feeding Problems	Increased Tone	High-pitched Cry
Exposure to alcohol or drugs	+	+	+	+	+
Hypoxic-ischemic encephalopathy	+	−	+	+	+
Infections	−	+	+	−	+
Seizure disorders	−	+	+	+	−
Hypoglycemia	+	+	+	−	−

Progressive diseases account for causes of developmental and behavioral problems. Seizures are associated with past infections and brain injury. Poor seizure control may result in developmental delays. Developmental delays may occur if control through medication is not achieved. Pediatric AIDS is an increasing problem. A manifestation of HIV infection of the central nervous system is the loss of developmental milestones. Inborn errors of metabolism involving abnormal metabolism of amino acids, carbohydrates, lipids, purines and pyrimidines, mucopolysaccharides, and heme pigments cause loss of nervous system control and associated mental retardation. The clinical manifestations of inborn errors of metabolism include developmental delay, motor system abnormalities, and seizures. Degenerative brain diseases are characterized by the progressive loss of intellectual, motor, and sensory functions.

DIFFERENTIAL DIAGNOSIS

The differential diagnosis of behavioral and developmental problems in infants is listed in Table 119–2. Prolonged irritability with feeding problems and neuromotor abnormalities imply brain injury. Symmetric abnormalities usually derive from generalized injuries or chemical exposures to the brain. Unilateral or asymmetric findings are more commonly associated with structural insults to the brain substance.

Birth defects increase the risk of associated problems in development and behavior. Five percent of newborns present with birth defects: 40% of the defects result from problems with developing tissues and 60% from deformations due to the distortion of fully developed structures by constraints in uterine size. Malformations occur during organogenesis in the first 13 weeks of gestation. Malformations occur in the brain, heart, and kidneys and are often subtle at birth. Deformations are not associated with developmental delay.

Not all infants exposed to alcohol or drugs will manifest severe or permanent developmental or behavioral problems. Problems associated with drug use are shown in Table 119–3. Fetal development, individual susceptibility of the fetus, and the amount and pattern of alcohol, tobacco, or other drug consumption by the mother are interrelated factors that may lead to malformations. Not all effects are dose related. A single dose of cocaine, for example, can cause ischemic injury to the brain from its vasospastic actions. Similarly, investigators have found no "safe" threshold quantity or duration of alcohol use that reliably predicts the development of the constellation of birth defects, developmental delays, and behavioral problems known as fetal alcohol syndrome (FAS). While some studies estimate the appearance of AS at 30%–40% among mothers who have consumed 3 oz of absolute alcohol daily, physical abnormalities have occurred at lower levels of exposure. Lesser amounts of alcohol exposure have been associated with various learning and behavioral disabilities termed alcohol-related birth defects (ARBD).

The actual mechanisms of behavioral and developmental problems associated with gestational exposure to alcohol and other drugs are not well understood. FAS produces malformation of the brain with loss of gray matter in the cerebral cortex and smaller than normal head size. Some infants exposed to cocaine and methamphetamine have gross changes in the structure of the brain. The specific interactions of alcohol and drugs on neuroreceptor systems and synaptic signaling in the fetal brain may be responsible for abnormalities seen in the behavior and development of the infant. Longitudinal studies of children exposed to alcohol and drugs show that these children, in the absence of physical abnormalities, may develop disabilities that would benefit from early diagnosis and intervention services.

EVALUATION

History

The history should review the prenatal course, labor, delivery, and postpartum events. The need for oxygen, prolonged hospitalization, intensive care, or readmission may indicate hypoxic injury, intraventricular hemorrhage, or central nervous system infections. The history should explore exposure to alcohol, tobacco, and other substances during gestation. Asking about the baby's feeding pattern, the quantity consumed at each feeding, and the expectations of the caregiver about the baby's feeding abilities are important components of the history. Review of developmental progress should specifically look for loss of abilities or delay in the expected pattern.

Physical Examination

Growth data should be plotted on growth charts and compared with previous information, with particular attention to the size of the head as measured by the occipitofrontal circumference (OFC). Malformations associated with FAS include smaller head size than expected for age, lower weight and length, small eye openings, nearly smooth philtrum (the groove between the nose and upper lip), thin upper lip, and abnormally positioned ears. A neurologic examination should include a search for tremors and testing of reflexes and muscle tone for symmetry and strength. General obser-

TABLE 119–2. Differential Diagnosis of Infant Presenting with Developmental/Behavioral Problems

Brain injury by history without progressive loss of milestones
    Hypoxic-ischemic encephalopathy
    Infection
    Hypoglycemia
    Gestational exposure to toxins including alcohol and other drugs
    Head injury
Brain injury with progressive loss of milestones
    Seizure disorders
    Pediatric AIDS
    Inborn errors of metabolism
    Degenerative brain disorders

vation should include the quality of the cry and how the infant feeds. The structure of palate, gums, and jaw during feeding, as well as the quality of sucking and bonding between the infant and mother, should be noted. Review of the infant's ability to self-comfort and be comforted by the caregiver should be recorded.

Additional Evaluation

The combination of major or minor malformations, growth parameter disturbances, and neuromotor findings may require referral to a dysmorphologist for diagnosis of alcohol-related birth defects or to a neurologist familiar with infants and children. When the head size is larger than the 90th percentile (and the percentile has progressively increased since birth), a head ultrasound may detect hydrocephalus. Imaging studies such as CT or MRI scans usually are not indicated as part of the initial evaluation of an infant with microcephaly unless the head is not growing.

Abnormalities associated with gestational use of alcohol or other drugs require repeated observations over time to determine whether the findings are static or progressive. If slowing of development or behavior occurs, early referral for intervention services will reduce future speech, language, and other problems.

MANAGEMENT

Specific Treatment

The visit should include a review of appropriate feeding schedules and amounts of feedings for infants. As the examination concludes, the examiner can emphasize recognition of cues produced by the baby. A baby that refuses to make eye contact and becomes

increasingly fussy needs less stimulus. Inappropriate feedings, noises, or handling may overload the baby's sensory system and result in increased irritability and feeding difficulties. Secure swaddling and a quiet place to sleep are often helpful.

General Treatment

The physician should develop a plan for periodic assessment of growth and development and refer to specialists if indicated.

Developmental milestones should be reviewed to identify delays that may require referral to specialized early intervention services.

The physician should determine the range of support available to the family such as nutrition support, social security supplemental income, and others.

Prevention

Primary prevention is the key intervention. The use of alcohol, tobacco, marijuana, and other substances begins in the preteen and early teenage years. Although some cultures promote the social use of drugs like alcohol, women of any age contemplating pregnancy (and their partners) need clearly presented information discouraging *any* use of alcohol during pregnancy. The health professional should discourage the use of alcohol, tobacco, and other drugs during pregnancy.

PATIENT AND FAMILY EDUCATION

The family should receive specialized instructions for managing feedings and irritable behavior. A discussion of the long-term prognosis relative to learning disabilities will assist the family in understanding the rationale for continued close observation of the baby and the possible need for referrals for early intervention services. Finally, owing to the accentuated demands created by an infant exposed to alcohol or other drugs, the examiner should reinforce the skills needed by family members who care for the baby.

NATURAL HISTORY/PROGNOSIS

The identification of a prenatal alcohol or drug history cannot of itself be implicated in future problems for a child. Although research is limited, children who have been exposed prenatally to drugs show a continuum

TABLE 119–3. Teratogenic Properties of Licit and Illicit Drugs

Specific Effects	Alcohol	Opiates	Cocaine/Methamphetamine	Marijuana	Nicotine
Growth retardation	+	+	+	+	+
Specific dysmorphism (a pattern of birth defects)	+	–	+ (Cocaine only)	–	–
Behavioral changes (newborn sleep/wake)	+	+	+	+	+
Abstinence syndrome	–	+	–	–	–
Increased mortality	+	+	+	–	+
Structural injuries to brain	+	–	+	–	–
Increased risk of sudden infant death syndrome	+	+	+	–	+

from minimal effects to severe impairment in all areas of their development.

Case Resolution

After the first year of life, this baby grew well, maintaining the 25th to 50th percentile for all growth parameters. He began to speak, using four words besides "Mama" and "Dada," his names for his grandmother and her husband. The mother was imprisoned, and the baby was permanently placed in his grandmother's home.

Selected Readings

Azuma, S., and I. Chasnoff. Outcome of children prenatally exposed to cocaine and other drugs: A path analysis of three-year data. Pediatrics 92:396–402, 1993.

Fergusson, D. M., J. Horwood, and M. T. Lynskey. Maternal smoking before and after pregnancy: Effects on behavioral outcomes in middle childhood. Pediatrics 92:815–22, 1993.

Green, M. *Pediatric Diagnosis,* 5th ed. Philadelphia, W.B. Saunders Company, 1992, pp. 117, 205, 345.

Levine, M. D., W. B. Carey, and A. C. Crocker. *Developmental-Behavioral Pediatrics,* 2nd ed. Philadelphia, W.B. Saunders Company, 1992, pp. 285–91.

Spohr, H., J. Willms, and H. Steinhausen. Prenatal alcohol exposures and long-term developmental consequences. Lancet 341:907–10, 1993.

CHAPTER 120

COMMON PEDIATRIC INFECTIONS

Barbara E. Small, M.D.

H$_x$ A 12-month-old boy presents with a 5-day history of clear rhinorrhea, nasal congestion, and occasional cough. He developed fever, irritability, and listlessness 3 days ago. He is refusing his bottle and did not sleep well overnight. He attends a daycare center 4 hours a day. He has had three episodes of otitis media in the past 6 months; the first was at age 4 months. There is no history of otorrhea (drainage from the ear).

Questions

1. How common are upper respiratory infections in children?
2. Why are children more susceptible to ear infections than adults are?
3. How should upper respiratory infections in children be treated?
4. How should otitis media in children be treated?

Upper respiratory tract infections (URIs), including acute otitis media (AOM), are by far the most common infections in children. The average incidence of viral respiratory infections is six to ten per year for infants and preschoolers, and three to five per year for school-age children and adolescents. The incidence is higher in children attending daycare centers. Upper respiratory infections last, on average, 6–9 days depending on the child's age and the setting in which the child is cared for (i.e., shorter duration in 1- to 2-year-olds cared for at home than in older children in daycare centers).

Acute otitis media is the most common illness encountered by physicians caring for children, accounting for 26% of all visits by children under the age of 2 years. Most children will have experienced at least one episode of otitis media by the age of 3 years, with estimates ranging from 66% to 77%. In fact, if tympanometry or acoustic reflectometry is used to diagnose middle ear effusion, virtually all children will experience an effusion by the age of 3 years, although 50% of infections are silent. The incidence of acute otitis media is greatest before the age of 2 years, peaking at 7–9 months of age. Approximately one third of affected children will have multiple episodes of otitis media. As many as 20% of infants will have three or more episodes by 1 year of age.

The average duration of otitis media is 5 days. Approximately 5%–10% of affected children will develop chronic middle ear disease, termed chronic otitis media with effusion (COME). In the United States, the estimated cost incurred by this common pediatric illness is 1–2 billion dollars per year, not including costs in time or family stress.

CLINICAL PRESENTATION

The patient presents with a history of rhinorrhea, fever, and irritability. The rhinorrhea usually precedes the other symptoms by a few days. In older children, otalgia (earache) is a frequent symptom. In some cases, otorrhea (discharge from the ear) may be the presenting complaint.

PATHOPHYSIOLOGY

In order to understand the pathophysiology of otitis media, some definitions are required. In broad terms, infections of the upper respiratory tract include the common cold, rhinitis, conjunctivitis, and pharyngitis. Upper respiratory infection can be defined as nasal discharge or nasal congestion with or without cough. A complicated upper respiratory infection is one accompanied by sinusitis or otitis media. Otitis media is an inflammation of the middle ear (sometimes involving the tympanic membrane), which can occur with or without fluid in the middle ear. Otitis media with middle ear effusion is often accompanied by fever, otalgia, irritability, lethargy, anorexia, vomiting, diarrhea, otorrhea, or erythema or opacification of one or both tympanic membranes.

The key to understanding otitis media is recognizing the central role played by the eustachian (auditory) tube (Fig. 120–1). The eustachian tube serves to (1) protect the middle ear from the secretions and flora of the nasopharynx, (2) drain fluid from the middle ear, and (3) equilibrate pressure between the middle ear and the atmosphere, thereby preventing a vacuum within the middle ear. Dysfunction of the eustachian tube leads to the accumulation of fluid, which then becomes infected in acute otitis media. Several factors contribute to this dysfunction. First, because the eustachian tube is more flaccid and more horizontal in younger children, they are anatomically predisposed to acute otitis media. Second, children with anatomic abnormalities of the eustachian tube are also more likely to develop otitis media. For example, 75% of children with Down syndrome have chronic otitis media with effusion. Children with cleft palate have problems with recurrent otitis media, which, if not routinely treated by tympanostomy tubes, results in decreased auditory and articulatory performance. Third, some upper respiratory infections lead to eustachian tube dysfunction, presumably through inflammation. Situations that increase exposure to upper respiratory infections (e.g., winter months, daycare, or siblings at home) also increase the incidence of otitis media. Passive smoking results in a 38% higher rate of acute otitis media and in a longer duration of effusion. Lastly, there is controversy about the role that allergies play in precipitating otitis media; some believe that allergies are a frequent cause of serous otitis media, while others say allergies play only a minor role in children.

The epidemiologic risk factors for recurrent acute otitis media are shown in Table 120–1.

A large number of episodes of acute otitis media (25%–42%) are preceded by a viral infection. Respiratory syncytial virus is the most commonly associated virus, although adenovirus, influenza, and parainfluenza may also be present. The chinchilla model illuminates the pathophysiology involved. In this model, intranasal influenza A inoculation causes metaplasia of the eustachian tube epithelium, resulting in increased secretions and subsequent blockage of the tubular lumen. Negative pressure then develops in the middle ear. If pneumo-

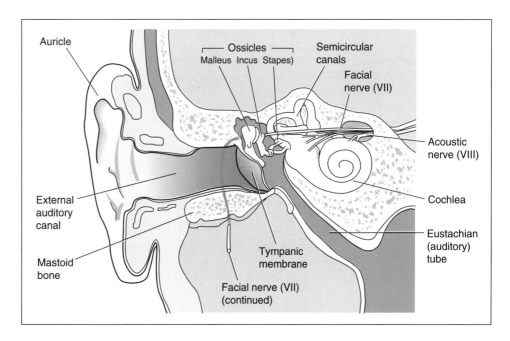

FIGURE 120–1. *Anatomy of the ear. (Reproduced, with permission, from B. J. Zitelli and H. W. Davis (eds.). Atlas of Pediatric Physical Diagnosis, 2nd ed. New York, Gower Medical Publishing, 1992, p. 22.2.)*

Auricle

Ossicles
Malleus Incus Stapes)

Semicircular canals

Facial nerve (VII)

Acoustic nerve (VIII)

Cochlea

Eustachian (auditory) tube

Tympanic membrane

External auditory canal

Mastoid bone

Facial nerve (VII) (continued)

TABLE 120–1. Epidemiologic Risk Factors for Recurrent Acute Otitis Media*

First episode occurs at less than 6 months of age
Male sex
Other siblings in the home (especially if they have a history of recurrent acute otitis media)†
Formula fed (especially if the bottle is propped for feedings)‡
Day-care attendance
Cigarette smoke in the home
Cold weather months of the year

*Adapted, with permission, D. W. Teele. *Pediatric Annals* 20:609–16, 1991.
†From C. J. Harrison and T. H. Belhorn. *Pediatric Annals* 20:600–8, 1991.
‡From V. M. Howie. *Pediatrics in Review* 14:320–3, 1993.

coccus is present, almost all animals develop acute otitis media, whereas few develop AOM if no bacteria are present.

Therefore, in addition to eustachian tube dysfunction, bacteria must be present in the nasopharynx for AOM to develop. There has been little change in the pathogens isolated from middle ear fluid over the last two decades. *Streptococcus pneumoniae* continues to be the most frequent isolate with *Haemophilus influenzae* a close second (Table 120–2). The etiologic agents in persistent or recurrent otitis media are the same as those seen in new cases, although the percentages vary. Antibiotic resistance is correlated with the presence of β-lactamase–producing bacteria.

The ultimate result of eustachian tube dysfunction and bacterial infection of the middle ear is inflammation. In acute suppurative otitis media, the tympanic membrane becomes thickened and erythematous, with purulent effusion of the middle ear occurring two thirds of the time as the middle ear tissues become edematous. In serous otitis media, edema is associated with a watery effusion of the middle ear. The tympanic membrane is often normal in appearance. Chronic mucoid otitis media is characterized by an uninflamed, chronically thickened tympanic membrane. The middle ear becomes filled with thick mucoid material owing to metaplasia of the epithelium lining the middle ear into mucus-secreting goblet cells. This is coupled with vasodilatation, subepithelial edema, and transudate of dense fluid. This inflammation is mediated by a variety of biochemical agents including arachidonic acid metabolites, antiprotease, and lysosomal enzymes.

TABLE 120–2. Bacterial Pathogens in Acute Otitis Media

Organism	Percentage of Cases Caused by	β-Lactamase Production
Streptococcus pneumoniae	30–40%	(−)
Haemophilus influenzae	25–45%	(+) ~20% of isolates
Moraxella catarrhalis	6–20%	(+)
Streptococcus pyogenes	2–3%	(−)
Staphylococcus aureus	2–3%	(+)

Dx Otitis Media

- Otalgia in older children
- Irritability in preverbal children
- Fever (23%–67% of the time)
- Presence of purulent fluid in the middle ear, usually associated with erythema or thickening of the tympanic membrane

DIFFERENTIAL DIAGNOSIS

The differential diagnosis of rhinitis and nasal obstruction includes viral or bacterial upper respiratory infection (including sinusitis), allergic rhinitis, vasomotor rhinitis, nonallergic rhinitis with eosinophilia, intranasal foreign body (presenting with unilateral symptoms), nasal polyps, tumors, rhinitis medicamentosa, adenoidal hypertrophy, choanal atresia, and an encephalocele draining cerebrospinal fluid.

Although suppurative and serous otitis media account for the vast majority of middle ear effusions, other conditions may also cause accumulation of fluid in the middle ear. These include allergy, environmental pollutants, pharyngeal obstruction due to tumors or adenoidal hypertrophy, hypothyroidism, amyloidosis, renal or heart failure, trauma to the nasopharynx, and barotrauma.

EVALUATION

History

It is best to begin with an open-ended question such as "What brings you to see me today?" This allows the parent or patient to tell his or her story while the physician integrates the information into a unifying diagnosis. Directed questions can then be used to confirm the diagnosis. The symptoms of acute otitis media are often nonspecific in infants, who are unable to communicate their experience. At the time of presentation with acute otitis media, 41% of children have rhinorrhea and 17% have cough. Irritability, lethargy, decreased appetite (especially for the bottle), disturbed sleeping patterns, vomiting, or diarrhea may be the predominant symptoms. Symptoms seem to worsen in the recumbent position. Fever is present in 23%–67% of patients. Otalgia is a reliable symptom in older children and is commonly related to acute otitis media. However, it may be caused by pain due to infection or a foreign body in the external auditory canal. Pain may also be referred to the ear from the mastoid, jaw, or pharynx. Pulling at the ears in a nonverbal child is not a reliable symptom of otitis media, because it may represent a habit unrelated to middle ear pathology. Otorrhea is seen most commonly in otitis externa but may occur in otitis media with rupture of the tympanic membrane or when tympanostomy tubes are in place. It may also be physiologic and due to liquefied cerumen. The history should include a thorough review of systems to determine whether more invasive disease (such as pneumonia or meningitis) is present.

Physical Examination

The physical examination should begin with an overall assessment of toxicity including level of responsiveness, temperature, and hydration status. The patient's weight is needed to calculate appropriate medication doses. Special attention should be paid to examination of the eyes, ears, nose, and throat. Conjunctivitis should alert the practitioner to the possibility of adenovirus or *Haemophilus influenzae* as a causative agent of infection. A pale, boggy nasal mucosa may indicate associated allergies. Tenderness over the frontal, ethmoid, or maxillary sinuses suggests sinusitis.

There are five general characteristics of the tympanic membrane to be observed: color, thickness (transparency), position, landmarks, and mobility. No single finding is diagnostic of acute otitis media. The healthy tympanic membrane is gray to pink in color. Erythema may result from crying alone. However, even in the absence of other pathologic findings, erythema may represent early myringitis (inflammation of the tympanic membrane). This is more likely to be the case if the redness is unilateral. Inflammation may change the thickness of the tympanic membrane and therefore its transparency. Normally one can see through the tympanic membrane into the middle ear cavity as through a thin sheet of cellophane. In some cases of acute otitis media without myringitis, pus can be observed in the middle ear cavity. This is the definitive finding in acute otitis media. However, chronic or acute otitis media may be associated with myringitis, resulting in a tympanic membrane that is slightly thickened (appearing like waxed paper) or very thickened and opaque-appearing.

The light reflex (in the anterior inferior quadrant) and the manubrium of the malleus are the most easily identified landmarks of the tympanic membrane. These landmarks are often lost in acute otitis media. The light reflex reflects the transparency or luster of the tympanic membrane and so can be lost in acute or chronic infection (or in resolving otitis media). The handle of the malleus may not be seen if the tympanic membrane is bulging into the external auditory canal as a result of middle ear effusion. In contrast, it may be seen in greater relief when the eardrum is retracted from negative ear pressure. The mobility of the tympanic membrane is a sensitive indicator of middle ear effusion and therefore otitis media. When fluid is present in the middle ear, there is decreased movement of the tympanic membrane on insufflation. This technique requires an airtight seal (not present with a tympanostomy tube) and some practice. It should be noted that infants (under approximately 4 months of age) tend to have a duller tympanic membrane with a diminished light reflex and decreased mobility. The tympanic membrane in infants is also more difficult to see because it is angled more steeply. A change in color or transparency in the presence of bulging of the tympanic membrane and decreased mobility is 95% predictive of acute purulent otitis media.

The pharynx should be examined for signs of concurrent infection. The neck should be checked for lymphadenopathy and nuchal rigidity, the latter being strongly suggestive of meningitis. The lungs should be auscultated for the presence of rales (crackles), which might indicate concomitant pneumonia.

Additional Evaluation

It is usually not necessary to order laboratory or radiographic tests to make the diagnosis of upper respiratory infection or otitis media. A nasal smear for eosinophils may be helpful in differentiating allergic rhinitis from a viral upper respiratory infection. However, a nasal smear containing eosinophils may also be seen in nonallergic rhinitis with eosinophilia. Sinus films in children older than 3 years of age may be useful in diagnosing sinusitis complicating upper respiratory infections. Tympanocentesis (extraction of fluid from the middle ear by means of a needle placed through the tympanic membrane) is the only reliable way to determine the etiologic agent of an episode of acute otitis media. However, it is not recommended for most cases and should be reserved for (1) patients less than 2 months of age, (2) immunocompromised or seriously ill patients, and (3) patients who have recurrent otitis media despite adequate treatment with antibiotics.

MANAGEMENT

Only a few medicines are useful in the treatment of upper respiratory infections and otitis media. Antihistamines and decongestants may offer symptomatic relief in cases of simple upper respiratory infections. However, they should be avoided in children less than 1 year of age. Topical decongestants should be used with caution and only briefly because they may cause chronic changes in the nasal mucosa that worsen nasal congestion. Neither antihistamines nor decongestants are indicated in the management of otitis media, since they are ineffective in preventing or altering the course of both acute and chronic cases.

Antibiotics are indicated in the treatment of bacterial rhinosinusitis manifested by fever, purulent nasal discharge, headache, and sinus tenderness. This condition may also present as a persistent cough with low-grade fever or halitosis. Bacterial sinusitis is characterized by the presence of nasal congestion and rhinorrhea for greater than 10 days (as well as abnormal sinus films) and should be treated with antibiotics. The antibiotic of choice is amoxicillin for 10–21 days depending on the response. Trimethoprim-sulfamethoxazole, cephalosporins, and amoxicillin-clavulanate should be reserved for nonresponders.

Antibiotics, specifically amoxicillin, have been shown to result in better outcomes than placebo in the treatment of acute otitis media, as measured by number of treatment failures and length of time of middle ear effusion (Table 120–3). Nearly half the patients with acute

TABLE 120–3. Antibiotics in the Treatment of Acute Otitis Media

Antibiotic	Advantages	Disadvantages
First Line		
Amoxicillin	Tastes good, inexpensive, fewest side effects	Limited spectrum, especially against β-lactamase producers
Trimethoprim-sulfamethoxazole	Two daily doses, inexpensive	Limited spectrum, displaces bilirubin in neonates, can cause aplastic anemia (rare)
Doxycycline (> 8 yrs old)	Two daily doses	GI upset, stains permanent teeth so cannot use under age 8
Second Line		
Amoxicillin-clavulanate	Broad spectrum, effective	Diarrhea (minimized if dosed at 30–35 mg/kg in three daily doses given with food), expensive
Cefaclor	—	Causes serum sickness
Cefixime	Two or four daily doses	Ineffective against *S. aureus*, expensive
Cefuroxime axetil	Two daily doses, broad spectrum	Tastes bad
Cephalexin	Broad spectrum, inexpensive	Ineffective owing to poor penetration into middle ear
Erythromycin-sulfisoxazole	Broad spectrum, moderately expensive	GI upset; three or four daily doses
Loracarbef, cefprozil, cefpodoxime	Very broad spectrum, two daily doses	Expensive, limited clinical experience

otitis media treated with a 10-day course of oral antibiotics have complete resolution of physical findings. However, many patients do not complete the full 10-day course. Noncompliance may result from medication spills, inability to give multiple doses during the day, or bad taste. A single dose of intramuscular ceftriaxone (50 mg/kg) is as effective as 10 days of oral amoxicillin (40 mg/kg/d in three divided doses) although it is more expensive. The presence of effusion after a case of acute otitis media does not signify treatment failure. Effusion normally takes 6–12 weeks to resolve. Treatment failure is defined by the persistence of symptoms 48–72 hours after starting antibiotics, or the recurrence of symptoms at the end of a 10-day course of antibiotics. Since physical findings cannot predict whether an effusion is sterile, the decision to treat empirically with antibiotics must be based on severity of symptoms. Antibiotics are successful in treating acute otitis media 83%–96% of the time, which correlates with the finding that 10%–15% of patients treated with antibiotics will have persistent acute otitis media, i.e., treatment failure.

In cases of recurrent otitis media, the next step is prophylactic antibiotics. A patient who has had three episodes within 6 months, or five to six in 1 year, should be given either amoxicillin, 20 mg/kg once a day, or sulfisoxazole, 50–75 mg/kg/d given in one or two doses, for 3 months. Recent recommendations are for this prophylaxis to be used only during symptoms of an upper respiratory infection. When prophylactic antibiotics have failed, or if there are signs of hearing loss, surgical intervention may be required.

The mainstay of surgical treatment for recurrent otitis media is tympanostomy or pressure equalization (PE) tubes. The tube overcomes the problem of eustachian tube dysfunction by providing a way to drain the middle ear and equalize pressure. It decreases the incidence of recurrent acute otitis media as well as the complications of cholesteatoma and chronic mastoiditis. Hearing is improved in most patients if there was hearing impairment before tube placement. However, there is little difference in long-term prognosis. Some studies report little advantage of pressure equalization tubes over the use of sulfa drugs alone for prophylaxis. The generally accepted indications for placement of tympanostomy tubes are (1) persistent or recurrent otitis media that has failed prophylactic antibiotics, (2) hearing loss of greater than 15 decibels, (3) language delay, (4) chronic adhesive otitis media, or (5) recurrent infections in children with an inherent predisposition to chronic otitis media. The latter includes children of Native American (Apache, Navajo) or Alaskan Eskimo heritage with an impaired ability to fight encapsulated organisms or children with craniofacial anomalies, such as cleft palate, Down syndrome, or other dysmorphic syndromes. The incidence of complications is low, and general anesthesia is not required. Tympanosclerosis and atrophy of the tympanic membrane are the most common problems associated with pressure equalization tubes. Persistent perforation is the most serious complication and is usually successfully repaired by further surgery. Adenoidectomy may be effective in older children in reducing the incidence of otitis media, but tonsillectomy offers no benefit.

PATIENT AND FAMILY EDUCATION

Parents need to be educated about the signs and symptoms that signal a new case of otitis media. They should be informed of the increased risk of recurrence if the first episode occurs in early infancy. They should know that tobacco smoke exposure, bottle propping, and daycare are predisposing factors that may be preventable. Instructions regarding the proper use and expected side effects of medications help maximize compliance. The need to seek prompt treatment and regular follow-up should be stressed.

NATURAL HISTORY/PROGNOSIS

Upper respiratory infections tend to be self-limited and last on average 1 week. Complications include sinusitis (5%–13% of the time) and otitis media (29% of the time), both of which should be easily treatable.

Acute otitis media usually responds well to antibiotics, with resolution of symptoms within 48–72 hours. Middle ear effusion commonly persists for up to 6 weeks in as many as 46% of cases. However, by 2–3 months after treatment for acute otitis media, 60%–90% of middle ear effusions have resolved. Recurrence of acute otitis media can be expected to occur in 30%–40% of children. The complications of otitis media include more serious systemic illness such as bacteremia, mastoiditis, meningitis, or damage to the ear resulting in hearing loss. The most common complication is hearing loss (usually conductive) due to (1) ossicular fixation or necrosis, (2) persistently perforated tympanic membrane, or (3) cholesteatoma. This hearing loss may be permanent. There can also be sensorineural hearing loss due to inner ear damage. Many of these complications can be avoided by prompt treatment and good follow-up.

Research Questions

1. What is the most cost-effective treatment of acute otitis media?
2. What measures could be used in daycare settings to decrease the incidence of upper respiratory infections?

Case Resolution

The patient was treated with amoxicillin (40 mg/kg/d in three divided doses). Symptoms persisted for 3 days, and the medication was changed to amoxicillin-clavulanate (at the same dose) with resolution of symptoms. At the end of 10 days, he was started on sulfisoxazole (50 mg/kg/d in two divided doses). At the 15-month well-child check, he had been free of recurrence for 3 months.

Selected Readings

Baker, R. C. Pitfalls in diagnosing acute otitis media. Pediatr Ann 20:591–8, 1991.

Cohan, R. T. The surgical management of chronic otitis media with effusion. Pediatr Ann 20:628–37, 1991.

Felder, H. The use of tympanotomy tubes. Pediatr Ann 17:616–9, 1988.

Giebink, G. S. Progress in understanding the pathology of otitis media. Pediatrics in Review 11:13–7, 1989.

Henderson, F. W. Viral respiratory infections. *In* A. M. Rudolph, J. I. E. Hoffman, and C. D. Rudolph (eds.). *Pediatrics*, 19th ed. Norwalk, Connecticut, Appleton & Lange, 1991.

Harrison, C. J., and T. H. Belhorn. Antibiotic treatment failures in acute otitis media. Pediatr Ann 20:600–8,1991.

Howie, V. M. Otitis media. Pediatrics in Review 14:320–3, 1993.

Le, C. Otitis revisited: Are ear tubes the answer? Contemp Pediatrics 5(9):24–45, 1988.

Potsic, W. P., and S. D. Handler. Ear, nose, throat, and mouth. *In* A. M. Rudolph, J. I. E. Hoffman, and C. D. Rudolph (eds.). *Pediatrics*, 19th ed. Norwalk, Connecticut, Appleton & Lange, 1991.

Wald, E. R., N. Guerra, and C. Byers. Upper respiratory infections in young children: Duration of and frequency of complications. Pediatrics 87:129–33, 1991.

C H A P T E R   1 2 1

SPECIAL PROBLEMS IN ADOLESCENTS

Victor C. Strasburger, M.D.

H$_x$ A 15-year-old female high school student complains of lower abdominal pain for the past 5 days. The onset of the pain was with her last menstrual period. The pains are dull, intermittent, and aching and are not associated with dysuria, frequency, urgency, or diarrhea. Her first menses (menarche) occurred at the age of 13 years. She had irregular menses for the first 18 months. Now her periods are regular, last 5 days, and require 2 to 4 pads a day. She has been having unprotected sexual intercourse with one sexual partner for the past month. She denies having breast tenderness, fatigue, nausea, vomiting, or vaginal discharge. Her parents do not know about her new sexual relationship. Physical examination reveals a fully sexually developed young woman (Tanner stage V breast and pubic hair development). She has papulopustular acne on her forehead and cheeks. Her abdominal examination shows no localized tenderness, guarding, or rebound. On pelvic examination (Box 121–1), she has a creamy white discharge (on saline and KOH wet mount preparations, this shows normal epithelial cells only). Her cervix is pink, firm, and not enlarged. An ectropion is present. The remainder of her pelvic examination is normal.

Questions

1. Why is this patient coming in now?
2. Could she be pregnant?
3. How can you best elicit her sexual history?

4. How should you deal with the issue of confidentiality?
5. Could she have a sexually transmitted disease? What other diagnostic possibilities should you consider?
6. How would you discuss the issue of contraception with her?

Adolescents represent a unique population of patients for several reasons: (1) they have a largely undeserved reputation as being difficult patients; (2) they engage in some risk-taking activities, such as early sexual activity, drug taking, or driving without seat belts, that frustrate their elders; (3) some physicians are uncomfortable with dealing with their early sexual activity; and (4) some physicians are not knowledgeable about the diseases that teenagers are likely to have and about adolescent psychology. From the adolescent's viewpoint, the "medical establishment" is either overly paternalistic or cold, impersonal, judgmental, expensive, and impossible to access easily. The issue that most concerns adolescents when seeing a physician is confidentiality ("Will this doctor tell my parents something that I don't want them to know?").

In the 1950s, the first Adolescent Medicine clinic was established, at Boston Children's Hospital. Since then, the field has grown into a board-certified subspecialty, with over 1000 members in the Society for Adolescent Medicine. The patient profiled above illustrates many of the subtleties involved in adolescent medicine: assuring confidentiality, taking a complete sexual history, and dealing with a teenager's stated—as well as unstated—concerns.

EVALUATION

The sexually active adolescent female puts herself at significant risk for pregnancy and sexually transmitted disease (STD). Although 55% of teenagers at menarche are anovulatory, 45% are not and are fully capable of becoming pregnant. In fact, 10% of all teenage pregnancies occur within the first month after initiation of intercourse, and half occur within the first 6 months

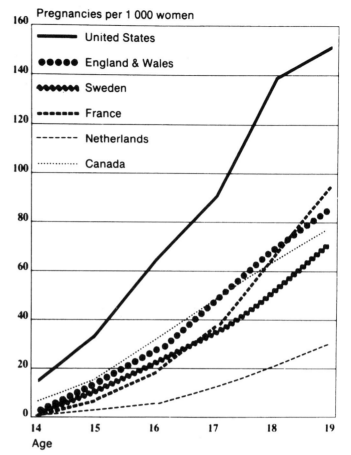

FIGURE 121–1. *Adolescent pregnancy rates, United States versus other Western nations. The United States has the highest teenage pregnancy rate in the Western world, despite the fact that American teenagers' rate of sexual activity does not differ from that of their European peers. Lack of comprehensive sex education in schools, inadequate access to birth control, and inappropriate portrayals of sexuality in the media are all important contributing factors. (Reprinted, with permission, from J. Trussel. Teenage pregnancy in the United States. Family Planning Perspectives 20:264, 1988. Copyright 1988, The Alan Guttmacher Institute.)*

(Fig. 121–1). A urine test will rule out pregnancy. Such tests are now sensitive to 25–50 mIU of human chorionic gonadotropin (hCG). In a normal pregnancy, the hCG level doubles every 2 days, reaching 50–250 mIU within 14 days after conception.

The risk of acquiring an STD in adolescence is also significant. One of eight adolescent females aged 15–19 years will develop pelvic inflammatory disease (PID). Sexually active teenagers have the highest rate of STDs of any sexually active age group. An estimated 2.5 million adolescents develop an STD annually. This risk is related to the number of teenagers having intercourse (Tables 121–1 and 121–2), their number of partners, and the unique biology of the adolescent cervix.

Cervical ectropion is common in adolescent females and represents the presence of columnar epithelial cells on the ectocervix. Such cells normally are confined to the endocervix, and with age, this transformation occurs, leaving the ectocervix lined with stratified squamous epithelial cells, which are relatively more resistant to infection.

BOX 121–1. When Does an Adolescent Female Need a Pelvic Examination?*

If she is sexually active
If she has unexplained lower abdominal pain
If she has a gynecologic complaint (e.g., vaginal discharge)
If she has severe dysmenorrhea or dysfunctional uterine bleeding (bimanual examination only if not sexually active)
If she requests one
If she is 17 years of age or older

*No formal written consent is required to do a pelvic examination; however, the patient's consent is mandatory.

TABLE 121–1. Premarital Sexual Activity Among Adolescent Women—United States, 1970–1988 (all races)*

Age	1970	1980	1988
15	5%	17%	26%
17	32%	36%	51%
19	48%	67%	75%
Overall	29%	42%	52%

*Source: Family Growth Survey, Centers for Disease Control, Morbidity and Mortality Weekly Report 39:930, 1991.

Confirmatory tests, using culture media to test for gonorrhea and a rapid fluorescent antibody test for *Chlamydia* (e.g., Microtrak, Chlamydiazyme), should be done. Sexual activity also places the adolescent female at risk for cervical dysplasia. Routine Pap test screening is essential. Increasing numbers of adolescents have abnormal Pap test results, probably related to acquisition of human papillomavirus (HPV). The Pap test is also useful as a backup method for diagnosing STDs, since it may show evidence of inflammation, organisms (e.g., trichomonads), or clue cells (i.e., bacterial vaginosis).

Dysmenorrhea often signals the onset of ovulatory periods and results from an excess of prostaglandins E_2 and $F_{2\alpha}$ in the endometrium, producing uterine ischemia and dysrhythmic uterine contractions. It is extremely common among adolescent females; it is the leading cause of short-term absence from school, and several surveys document that nearly 75% of all female teens experience it. However, in a sexually active teenager, it is a diagnosis of exclusion, since other, more serious conditions can cause lower abdominal pain.

MANAGEMENT

The typical teenager who begins sexual intercourse at a young age does not want to become pregnant. She will require sensitive counseling to determine the ideal contraceptive choice. In general, condoms are ideal for prevention of STDs, and oral contraceptives are preferred for pregnancy prevention. But other options should be explored as well: medroxyprogesterone acetate, levonorgestrel implants, foam, sponge, or perhaps even a diaphragm. Her choice will depend on her own comfort level, her knowledge about the various meth-

TABLE 121–2. Sexual Activity Among Adolescent High School Males—United States, 1990*

Race/Ethnicity	Percentage
White	56.4
Black	87.8
Hispanic	63.0
Grade in School	
9th	48.7
10th	52.5
11th	62.6
12th	76.3

*Source: Centers for Disease Control. Sexual behavior among high school students—United States, 1990. Morbidity and Mortality Weekly Report 40:885–88, 1992.

ods, the frequency of her sexual activity, how effectively she is counseled, and how closely she is followed. Compliance rates among adolescents taking oral contraceptives, for example, range from 30% to 50% after 6–12 months in certain populations. Compliance can be increased by scheduling regular follow-up appointments and by creating a feeling of trust and caring.

Papulopustular acne may cause irreversible scarring in teenagers, and they generally welcome help in treating their skin (although collectively they spend millions of dollars on over-the-counter products rather than seek medical help). Effective use of topical preparations such as retinoic acid and benzoyl peroxide, combined with the use of oral or topical antibiotics, can yield impressive results within a few weeks.

PATIENT EDUCATION

Identifying the sexually active adolescent is a crucial task for primary care practitioners. Every medical encounter with a teenager should be seen as an opportunity to update the history of risk-taking activities. But how does the physician ask "the sexual question"? First, teenagers must be assured that the physician is their physician, not their parents', and that health care will be confidential. In practical terms, this means telling the teenager at the outset that "what you tell me stays in this room, just between us, unless you're planning to hurt yourself or hurt someone else." At the present time, every state in the United States assures that teenagers can receive confidential treatment for STDs, and most guarantee, by statute, confidential treatment for pregnancy prevention as well. The doctrine of confidential health care for teenagers is also well established in common (i.e., judge-granted) law, at least for "mature minors"—those who are able to understand the risks and benefits of a particular treatment and who can therefore give an informed consent. Confidentiality also applies to taking a drug history from teenagers. Adolescents are unlikely to inform a doctor of their drug-taking behavior if they know that their parents will be told. In general, teenagers are reassured when practitioners explain about confidentiality and about the need to ask probing questions about sexual activity or drug-taking behavior simply to help them take care of themselves better. Such histories are far likelier to be reliable than when sensitive questions are asked with parents present in the examination room.

Treating sexually active teenagers may mean setting aside some personal feelings about human sexuality. Being understanding and nonjudgmental is critical. The teenager's medical well-being may depend entirely on the physician, who in turn may have to wrestle with some societal myths, such as (1) teenagers are promiscuous, (2) making birth control available to teenagers encourages them to become sexually active at a younger age, and (3) teaching young people about sex makes them more likely to have sex at younger ages. Different practitioners approach "the sexual question" differently. The direct approach is simply to ask, "Are you having sex with anyone?" If the answer is yes, the next

TABLE 121–3. Sources of Information About Sex for Teenagers*

Parents	53%
Media	48%
Friends	45%
Doctor or nurse	19%

*Data from L. Harris et al: American Teens Speak: Sex, Myths, TV and Birth Control. New York: Planned Parenthood Federation of America, 1986.

Research Questions

1. What is the extent of current teenage sexual activity, including intercourse and other sexual practices?
2. What determines the decision by both males and females to have first intercourse, and how can that decision be influenced?

question is, "With whom?" This method does not discriminate against those teenagers who may be gay or bisexual. But some teenagers and some practitioners may be reticent. For them, an indirect approach may work better: "Do you have any friends who are having sex?" If so, "What do you think about that?" There is a high likelihood that if their friends are having sex and they approve, then they, too, may be sexually active.

Finally, if the teenager is not sexually active, it gives the practitioner an opportunity to provide positive reinforcement for continued abstinence. In the United States, the average age at first intercourse is 15 years for males and 16 years for females. If a physician's practice includes high school students, many of them will be sexually active. Although much is still unknown about the sexual practices of American teenagers, there are currently severe constraints on studying any aspect of childhood or adolescent sexuality. For example, in 1991 U.S. Secretary of Health and Human Services Louis Sullivan canceled a planned 5-year, $18 million survey of 24,000 young people in grades 7 through 11 because he was worried about the "inadvertent message this survey could send." The survey would have provided invaluable information about teenagers' sexual habits and would have included several questions about their media habits as well. Although practitioners may not be able to change society's attitudes about such research, they do have a unique opportunity to engage in one-on-one interventions that may be extremely important in a young person's life. Providing confidential and thorough care for these teenagers can be both rewarding for the practitioner and lifesaving for the teenager. Physicians constitute an important potential source of information for teenagers about sex (Table 121–3).

Case Resolution

This 15-year-old young woman presented with dysmenorrhea and a "pregnancy scare"—she had been having unprotected sexual intercourse. Her pregnancy test was negative, and her Pap test was normal. Although she had not been using a barrier method of contraception (preferably condoms), she did not show evidence of an STD on laboratory testing. The most likely cause of her lower abdominal pain was dysmenorrhea. Treating this patient's dysmenorrhea with a prostaglandin inhibitor (e.g., ibuprofen, naproxen, mefenamic acid) helped forge an effective physician-patient bond, as did treating a condition that she came in with but did not seek help for—acne. After 6 weeks of treatment with oral tetracycline, topical retinoic acid, and topical erythromycin, her complexion improved greatly. The patient decided to take a low-dose oral contraceptive pill and use condoms for STD prevention.

Selected Readings

Braverman, P. K., and V. C. Strasburger. Adolescent sexuality. I. Adolescent sexuality. II. Contraception. III. STDs. IV. Office counseling. Clin Pediatr November 1993–February 1994.

Coupey, S. M., and L. V. Klerman (eds.). Adolescent sexuality: Preventing unhealthy consequences. Adolescent Medicine: State of the Art Reviews 3:2, June 1992.

Friedman, S. B., M. Fisher, and S. K. Schonberg (eds.). *Comprehensive Adolescent Health Care.* St. Louis, Quality Medical Publishing, 1992.

Greydanus, D. E., and R. B. Shearin. *Adolescent Sexuality and Gynecology.* Philadelphia, Lea & Febiger, 1990.

McAnarney, E., R. Kriepe, D. Orr, and G. Comerci (eds.). *Textbook of Adolescent Medicine.* Philadelphia, W.B. Saunders Company, 1992.

Strasburger, V. C. *Basic Adolescent Gynecology.* Baltimore, Urban & Schwarzenberg, 1990.

Strasburger, V. C., and R. T. Brown. *Adolescent Medicine: A Practical Guide.* Boston, Little, Brown & Co., 1991.

Strasburger, V. C., and G. Comstock (eds.). Adolescents and the media. Adolescent Medicine: State of the Art Reviews 4:3, October 1993.

CHAPTER 122

SPECIAL PROBLEMS IN THE ELDERLY

Richard J. Roche, M.D., and F. Claude Manning, M.D.

Hₓ An 83-year-old female who never married, has no children, and lives alone in a senior housing apartment complex, presents with a right wrist fracture after a fall in her apartment. She has had four other falls in the preceding 2 months and has been incontinent of urine for the past year. She previously complained of the urinary incontinence but stated, "It's just a normal thing you have to expect at my age." Her past medical history reveals prior diagnoses of atherosclerotic heart disease, chronic atrial fibrillation, congestive heart failure, diabetes mellitus, hypothyroidism, osteoarthritis, anxiety, and depression. She reports that she always follows her doctor's orders and has conscientiously been taking all 12 of her prescription medications. Her current medications are isosorbide dinitrate, sublingual nitroglycerin, digoxin, warfarin, furosemide, potassium chloride, chlorpropamide, levothyroxine, piroxicam, acetaminophen, chlordiazepoxide, and amitriptyline.

Questions

1. What factors might be contributing to the patient's incontinence?
2. What factors might be responsible for her falls?
3. What are the clinical implications of an altered or atypical presentation of disease in the elderly?

The elderly represent a unique group of patients. Currently, the over 65 years age group makes up 12% of the U. S. population. This proportion is expected to increase to 19% by the year 2025. The oldest old, those over age 85, represent the fastest growing segment of the population in this country.

Elderly persons are more susceptible than younger individuals to a variety of special problems, including incontinence, falls, and alterations in mental status (see Chapter 99). Evaluation of such problems often is complicated by the large number of potential causes. In addition, the geriatric population is also more likely to experience ill effects from the often multiple medications prescribed by health care professionals.

The combination of the physiologic changes of aging, chronic illness, adverse drug reactions, and declining social support systems render the elderly (especially those over the age of 85 years) vulnerable to progressive functional deterioration with the subsequent need for home care services or institutional care. The evaluation and management of older patients must encompass their social and functional status as well as their medical status. This is often best carried out by an interdisciplinary team.

Atypical Presentation of Disease

Elderly patients frequently do not manifest the "classic" symptoms of disease. Vague or nonspecific symptoms are often the first indication of a serious illness (Table 122–1). A number of physiologic changes of aging as well as several specific cultural beliefs and behavioral patterns may account for this phenomenon.

PATHOPHYSIOLOGY

Organ system function tends to decline with age and may not always be reflected by objective measures. For example, the serum creatinine level and liver function tests may be normal in the elderly even in the face of organ insufficiency. In addition, most individuals exhibit a *decrease in reserve capacity* as they age, and the ability to tolerate new diseases (e.g., infections)—or exacerbations of chronic disease—is diminished.

It has been estimated that 85% of older individuals are afflicted with one or more chronic diseases. Chronic illness may play a confounding role in disease presentation if symptoms due to an acute disorder are erroneously attributed to a preexisting condition.

Altered perception of pain in the elderly has also been postulated as a mechanism of atypical symptomatology. Higher pain thresholds have been ascribed to age-related neuronal degeneration, central mechanisms, peripheral neuropathies, and consistently elevated levels of pain from chronic diseases.

Behavior of the ill, aged patient is affected by a variety of social, ethnic, psychological, and clinical factors. These include (1) perception of illness severity, (2) perceived changes in functional status (ability to perform the activities of daily living), (3) denial, (4) access to health care, and (5) the attribution of symptoms to

---

TABLE 122–1. Symptoms of Atypical Presentation of Disease in the Elderly

Falls
Change in baseline mental or functional status
Decreased oral intake
Change in urinary continence
Failure to thrive
Delirium or confusion
Fatigue

---

the aging process rather than to disease. The elderly's perception of health is often influenced by their living environment. For example, the same symptom may be perceived as more severe and disabling by a person living independently in the community than by a person living in a nursing home, surrounded by infirmity and chronic disease. Generally, as people age their health expectations decrease regardless of health status. The elderly tend to overestimate their healthiness and underestimate their symptoms, contrary to the common stereotype of the hypochondriacal, complaining elder.

Both older adults and health care professionals often subscribe to the ageist view that certain symptoms "just happen when you get old." This may result in minimization of legitimate complaints, underreporting of symptoms, a pessimistic or helpless attitude, and delays in seeking care or prescribing treatment for reversible conditions. Health care professionals need to be aware that more than half the time elderly patients do not report significant symptoms when seen. Reasons include (1) patient beliefs that "nothing can be done about it, there is no need to bother anyone, and things will get better"; and (2) patient denial that the symptom might represent a serious condition. The health beliefs of the elderly thus play an integral role in the presentation of disease.

DIFFERENTIAL DIAGNOSIS

Table 122–2 summarizes the differential diagnosis to consider when an elderly patient presents with nonspecific symptoms or functional impairment. Myocardial infarction and bacterial infections are especially likely to have an altered presentation in the aged. Elderly patients with a myocardial infarction usually present with dyspnea and not chest pain; other presentations include syncope, fever, confusion, nausea, diaphoresis, weakness, falls, and stroke. Fifteen percent of patients may have no symptoms at all.

Elderly patients with bacterial infections usually manifest the classic signs of fever, inflammation, purulence, and leukocytosis. However, many present with vague, diffuse symptoms and few focal findings. Confusion, anorexia, lethargy, tachypnea and tachycardia may be the only manifestations of a serious infection. As is the case with fever, a normal white blood cell count (WBC) does not exclude an infection. However,

---

TABLE 122–2. Etiologies to Consider When an Elderly Patient Presents in a Nonspecific Manner

Depression
Polypharmacy
Myocardial infarction
Infections: urinary tract infection, pneumonia, cellulitis, decubitus ulcer, appendicitis
Vitamin B$_{12}$ deficiency
Thyroid disorders
Cerebrovascular accidents

---

the majority of elderly patients with a bacterial infection will demonstrate a bandemia or "left shift" (i.e., an increase in immature white blood cell forms) even if the WBC is normal.

EVALUATION

History

Eliciting an adequate history in an elderly patient can be an exasperating experience. Disease presentation is frequently less dramatic and specific than in younger patients (see Table 122–1). A deterioration in baseline functioning may be the only indication that an illness is present. Obstacles to obtaining an accurate history from an elderly patient include dementia, delirium, sensory deficits (e.g., deafness), and aphasia secondary to stroke. Consequently, it is essential that family, friends, and care givers be interviewed when obtaining a history. Taking a thorough social history is key, and the physician should inquire about the patient's living arrangements, support networks, and economic resources as well as family availability and the health status of the spouse or other care giver.

The medication profile may be the single most important aspect of the history to document. Patients over the age of 65 years take more prescription and over-the-counter medications than any other age group, and it is thus not surprising that they frequently suffer from side effects and drug–drug interactions. It is best to have an older person bring in all medications (i.e., the pill bottles themselves) for inspection, since drugs are commonly duplicated or their names are not recalled.

Physical Examination

A careful physical examination, though often more difficult to perform in elderly patients, is necessary to differentiate acute disease from chronic conditions or the aging process itself. The examination should focus on those organ systems most likely responsible for the patient's complaints. Emphasis should be placed on the cardiac, neurologic, pulmonary, and skin examinations. Vital signs sometimes provide valuable clues. Both a lying and a sitting blood pressure should be measured to assess for possible postural hypotension. It should be noted, however, that an orthostatic blood pressure drop normally occurs in 15%–30% of elderly patients. A weight measurement may assist in evaluating the patient's nutritional and fluid status. On examination of the skin, a careful search should be made for pressure sores. Decubitus ulcers may be an indicator of chronic disease, recent immobility, malnutrition, or neglect by a care giver.

The patient's temperature should be noted. Although the absence of a fever does not exclude an infection, the recent literature suggests that most elderly individuals with a proven bacterial infection *will* mount a temperature of at least 37.5° C (99.5° F). In addition, the higher the fever is, the greater the odds of the patient having a serious or life-threatening infection.

Additional Evaluation

A number of assessment tools are available to evaluate the elderly patient's functional, cognitive, and affective status. These include the Katz Activities of Daily Living (ADL) Scale, the Lawton-Brody Instrumental Activities of Daily Living (IADL) Scale, the Folstein Mini-Mental State Examination, and the Yesavage Geriatric Depression Scale. Utilization of these standardized assessments often reveals diagnostic and prognostic information that otherwise would be missed.

Certain disorders that are common in the elderly are especially likely to present in an atypical fashion (see Table 122–2), and thus several selected laboratory tests should be requested routinely when the diagnosis is not immediately apparent: urinalysis, CBC, electrolytes, thyroid-stimulating hormone, cobalamin (vitamin B_{12}), blood urea nitrogen, and creatinine. A chest x-ray to assess for pneumonia or congestive heart failure may be helpful, and an electrocardiogram to evaluate for ischemic changes should be considered.

PATIENT AND FAMILY EDUCATION

Patients and their families should be advised to regard changes in baseline functional status as a possible early sign of acute illness. They should also be informed that vague and nonspecific symptoms are not an expected consequence of normal aging and that such complaints should be promptly reported to a physician.

FALLS

Accidents are the fifth leading cause of death among the elderly, and falls are the leading cause of accidental death. About one third of community-dwelling elderly over the age of 75 years sustain a fall every year. Most falls occur at home during normal daily activities. While many falls do not lead to significant injury, about 5%–10% result in serious sequelae such as fractures. Even when an injury does not occur, the fear of future falls may lead to a self-imposed limitation on activity with subsequent adverse effects on mood and social functioning.

PATHOPHYSIOLOGY

Falls in the elderly may occur for many reasons (Table 122–3). True accidents can be viewed as falls resulting from unavoidable hazards in the absence of predisposing factors. However, nonsyncopal falls most often result from the interaction of (1) environmental hazards and (2) increased susceptibility resulting from disturbances of gait or balance. Falls due to syncopal episodes suggest a potentially life-threatening underlying condition and require urgent evaluation (see Chapter 96). A particularly common cause of falls among the elderly is the use of medications that may adversely affect gait, balance, or sensorium. Several factors acting in concert are often responsible for recurrent falls.

TABLE 122–3. Some Causes of Falls in the Elderly

True Accidents
Hazards in the home
Age-related decline in balance and gait

Disorders Affecting Gait
Stroke
Parkinson's disease
Normal pressure hydrocephalus
Myelopathy due to spinal stenosis
Arthritis
Foot disorders

Disorders Affecting Balance
Visual impairment
Vestibular disorders
Cerebellar disorders
Peripheral neuropathy
Parkinson's disease

Cerebral Hypoperfusion and Syncope
Orthostatic hypotension
Cardiac arrhythmias
Aortic stenosis
Vertebrobasilar insufficiency

Medications
Sedatives
Antidepressants
Antihypertensives
Diuretics

Multifactorial Etiology

EVALUATION

History

Patients who fall often do not present with this as their primary complaint. The history of falling may be elicited in the systems review, but more frequently patients present for treatment of the resulting injury. When managing the acute injury, it is important not to overlook the issue of *why* the fall occurred. The evaluation should include a history of the circumstances of the fall as well as a description of any environmental hazards that might have been involved. Any symptoms that preceded the fall should be elicited, with special reference to dizziness, syncope, palpitations, diaphoresis, and neurologic symptoms. Predisposing risk factors (Table 122–4) should also be identified.

Physical Examination

A general physical examination is necessary to identify possible predisposing conditions. Visual acuity should be assessed. The cardiovascular examination should include measurement of the blood pressure in

TABLE 122–4. Risk Factors for Recurrent Falls

Balance and mobility problems
Movement disorders (e.g., Parkinson's disease)
Cognitive impairment
Sedative medications
Arthritis
Foot problems
History of previous falls

both the sitting and the standing position. A drop in systolic blood pressure of > 20 mm Hg or in diastolic pressure of > 10 mm Hg is considered significant for orthostatic hypotension. The neurologic examination may reveal focal deficits (e.g., evidence of a prior stroke) or more generalized abnormalities (e.g., the tremor and cogwheeling rigidity of Parkinson's disease). However, the standard neuromuscular examination is relatively insensitive in uncovering important mobility problems. A performance-oriented assessment of balance and gait provides a more accurate picture of subtle impairments that may predispose to falls.

Additional Evaluation

Further investigation is often required, especially when the cause of the falling episode is not apparent based on the history and physical examination alone. An appraisal of hazards in the home may reveal environmental factors (e.g., poor lighting, loose throw rugs, or uneven stairs) that significantly contribute to the risk of falling. When falls occur as a result of syncope or suspected cardiovascular disease, ambulatory electrocardiographic monitoring or cardiac event recording to identify cardiac arrhythmias should be considered, as well as upright tilt testing to establish the presence of neurocardiogenic syncope (see Chapter 96).

MANAGEMENT

In addition to providing appropriate care for any resultant injuries, management of the elderly patient who falls includes (1) treating predisposing conditions and (2) eliminating or reducing risk factors for further falls (see Table 122–4). Medications that increase the risk of falling should be discontinued whenever feasible. Physical therapy aimed at improving gait and balance may (1) reduce the tendency to fall and (2) identify appropriate ambulation aids (e.g., canes or walkers) that may reduce the risk of recurrent falls. Finally, home safety devices (e.g., holdbars in the bathroom) that decrease falling risk may be suggested after a home visit by a nurse or physical therapist.

PATIENT AND FAMILY EDUCATION

Patients should be advised to report all medications they take, both prescription and over-the-counter. Fam-

ily support should be enlisted to install needed home safety modifications.

Research Questions

1. Is the process of aging primarily due to intrinsic or extrinsic factors?
2. Does an interdisciplinary approach and comprehensive geriatric assessment have advantages over traditional medical management in the care of the elderly?

Case Resolution

The physician concluded that polypharmacy (the use of multiple drugs) was a major problem for the patient, and a number of changes in her medication regimen were subsequently made: she was tapered off chlordiazepoxide and piroxicam, and amitriptyline was discontinued. The doses of furosemide and isosorbide dinitrate were lowered, and the long-acting chlorpropamide was switched to the shorter acting glipizide. When the patient returned for a follow-up visit 2 weeks later, she reported that she was feeling "more steady on her feet" and that her urinary incontinence was now occurring only intermittently.

Selected Readings

Nahemow, L., and L. Pousada. *Geriatric Diagnostics: A Case Study Approach.* New York, Springer Publishing Company, 1983, pp. 7–9.

Nevitt, M. C., S. R. Cummings, S. Kidd, and D. Black. Risk factors for recurrent nonsyncopal falls: A prospective study. JAMA 261:2663–68, 1989.

Rubenstein, L. Z., and L. V. Rubenstein. Multidimensional assessment of elderly patients. Adv Intern Med 36:81–108, 1991.

Tinetti, M. Performance-oriented assessment of mobility problems in elderly patients. J Am Geriatr Soc 34:119–26, 1986.

Tinetti, M., and M. Speechley. Prevention of falls among the elderly. N Engl J Med 320:1055–9, 1989.

Williams, M. E. Clinical management of the elderly patient. *In* W. R. Hazzard, E. L. Bierman, J. P. Blass, et al. (eds.). *Principles of Geriatric Medicine and Gerontology,* 3rd ed. San Francisco, McGraw-Hill Book Company, 1994.

SPECIAL ISSUES IN PRIMARY CARE

C H A P T E R   1 2 3

PATIENTS WITH CHRONIC DISABILITY

Kerrie R. Seeger, M.D., and Barbara Ludwig, Q.M.R.P., L.P.C.

H$_x$ A 22-year-old male college wrestler was returning to school from winter break when his car went out of control on an icy road and rolled over. Emergency medical technicians responding to the accident found him to be unconscious and hypotensive, with shallow respirations. After being extracted from the wrecked automobile, he was transported on a backboard to a hospital. A neurologic examination did not elicit reflexes or response to pain in his lower extremities. X-rays taken in the emergency room revealed a fractured left femur and left humerus and a fracture of the spinal column at T8. Urine showed gross blood. He required intubation for increasingly poor respiratory effort but remained otherwise stable. No skull fractures were identified, and CT scanning showed no bleeding. The patient's blood pressure was normalized with fluid administration, and his hematuria resolved over the next 48 hours. The patient's primary care doctor was called after his initial stabilization and subsequently coordinated his care. A neurosurgeon performed an operative intralaminar fusion on the second day after the accident to stabilize his spinal fracture. He was extubated following surgery and was able to maintain independent ventilation.

The postsurgery neurologic examination showed complete absence of all sensation, reflexes, and motor response below the level of the injury, indicating a complete disruption of the cord. There was also a loss of autonomic function (anhydrosis and paralytic ileus). Initially, the extremities were flaccid (because of spinal shock), but within a few weeks they became spastic. Normal bowel and bladder function were lost, as was normal sexual functioning.

Questions

1. If you were the physician on duty the night this patient came in, what else might you have done to minimize the development of chronic conditions?
2. Is this patient disabled? How would you assess this?
3. When and how would you talk to him about the prognosis for his current mobility, sexual, and elimination functions?

How extensive is disability? Data collected in 1992 showed that, of adults and children living in the United States, 19.4% had a disability, generally defined as a decreased ability to perform activities typically engaged in by people during any given stage in their lives. Among people 15 years of age and older, the prevalence of disabilities approaches 24%. This figure includes people with a wide range of types of disabilities and functional limitations. For example, 8.9% of American adults would have difficulty walking three city blocks, while 2% would have difficulty keeping track of money or bills, and 0.3% would need assistance with eating (Table 123–1).

WHAT IS DISABILITY?

Disability is a physical or mental impairment that substantially limits one or more major life activities of an individual. The World Health Organization (WHO) recognizes three components to disability: (1) impairment, (2) disability, and (3) handicap.

Impairment is what happens at the organ level; for example, a spinal cord injury, the brain injury in a person who has had a stroke, the limb of a person who becomes an amputee. WHO defines impairment as "any loss or abnormality of psychological, physiologic, or anatomic structure or function."

Disability is what happens at the person level, including "any restriction or lack (resulting from an impairment) of ability to perform an activity in the manner or within the range considered normal for a human being."

Handicap refers to effects upon a person at the community or societal level. Handicap is "a disadvantage for a given individual resulting from an impairment or a disability that limits or prevents the fulfillment of a

---

TABLE 123–1. Disability Facts

22 million Americans are hearing impaired; 2 million Americans are deaf.
2.5 million Americans are severely visually impaired (unable to read a newspaper).
120,000 Americans are totally blind and 600,000 are legally blind.
6 million American children and adults have mental retardation.
1 million Americans are wheelchair users.
2 million Americans with disabilities reside in institutions.

TABLE 123–2. Activities of Daily Living (ADLs)

Functional independence*/dependence of a person is measured in the following areas:
  Feeding
  Continence
  Transferring
  Going to toilet
  Dressing
  Bathing

*Independence means without supervision, direction, or active personal assistance.

role that is normal (depending on age, sex, and social and cultural factors) for that individual."

MEASURING DISABILITY

Disability can be assessed by a variety of indices that measure functional elements such as self-care activities, social interactions, physical abilities, and communication. One commonly used method of assessing disability is to gauge the patient's ability to perform six activities of daily living (ADLs): bathing, dressing, toileting, transferring, remaining continent, and eating (Table 123–2).

Handicap at the societal level is defined by scales such as the CHART (Craig Handicap Assessment and Reporting Technique), which objectively measures physical independence, mobility, activities, social integration, and economic self-sufficiency.

More comprehensive evaluation scales are now available. In addition to assessing the six basic ADLs, key functional activities such as having meaningful relationships, housekeeping, shopping, managing money, using a telephone, and using transportation are addressed.

DISABILITIES AND SOCIETY

Adults who are not institutionalized but are unable to work owing to disability face tremendous personal, financial, and emotional challenges and have an impact on society because of withdrawal from the work force. In 1992, an analysis was done of noninstitutionalized Americans' "days of disability" to determine the loss of work and school days and days of "bed-disability." Days of disability per person in the United States have increased since 1985 from 14.8 days to 16.3 days in 1992. If the average American loses 16 days of school or work annually to disability, the impact in terms of lost productivity is clearly significant.

Increasingly, people with disabilities are entering or reentering the American work force. Simple, inexpensive accommodations or adaptations often can help people with physical and mental disabilities increase productivity and decrease reliance on disability benefits. Workers with disabilities require an accessible workplace both physically (i.e., architecturally) and attitudinally (i.e., accepting of people using adaptive equipment such as wheelchairs or of those who speak or hear differently). The Americans With Disabilities Act of 1990 prohibits discrimination in the employment of people with disabilities and requires proactive steps to improve access in the workplace.

DEVELOPMENTAL DISABILITIES

Developmental disabilities (1) begin before adulthood, (2) most often include cognitive impairment (i.e., I.Q. < 70), (3) continue indefinitely, and (4) cause major functional impairments in key life functions. Up to 3% of the U. S. population has some type of developmental disability such as mental retardation, autism, or cerebral palsy. People with epilepsy, spina bifida, fetal alcohol exposure, and traumatic brain injury may be developmentally disabled. Down syndrome is genetically transmitted and associated with varying levels of mental retardation. People with developmental disabilities require lifelong support of varying types and intensities, designed to enhance quality of life and personal productivity. Areas of support may include financial security, personal safety, relationships with others, educational and vocational development, health care, and mental health concerns.

The most common cause of mental retardation is fetal exposure to alcohol (fetal alcohol syndrome, FAS). FAS is 100% preventable if the mother abstains from drinking during pregnancy. The significance of providing adequate "whole person" (biopsychosocial and environmental) supports and services increases as the life expectancy for people with lifelong disabilities improves. Today, over 80% of children with chronic conditions will survive into adulthood, and they have the right to lead productive, enjoyable lives.

THE DISABLED ELDERLY

The number of disabled elderly will continue to increase. Over the past few decades, elders with disabling conditions commonly were placed in nursing homes until death. The advent of home health care and government waiver programs (which allow the transfer of funds from institutional programs to home and community based programs) allows elders the choice of remaining in their homes in states in which appropriate resources exist. Community practitioners assume the primary care for elderly people with special and complex needs.

PSYCHIATRIC DISABILITIES

People who have disabilities such as schizophrenia, bipolar disorder, and personality disorders often require long-term, multidisciplinary treatment. Treatment typically includes counseling or psychotherapy, case management, ancillary support services for daily living needs, periodic inpatient services, and medication management. Some people with psychiatric disabilities may require care and support throughout their lifetime.

During the 1970s, large numbers of people with chronic mental illness were deinstitutionalized with little thought given to long-term community planning. Negative effects included decreased access to health care, increased substance abuse, homelessness, and exacerbation of disability. There were few organized and adequately funded community mental health programs to help these people make the transition into communities. The paucity of community-based mental health treatment and support programs for people with chronic mental illness continues to be a major societal problem.

PREVENTION OF DISABILITIES

Certain areas of disability warrant special mention because of the potential for prevention. Disabilities related to trauma such as amputations, spinal cord injuries, and traumatic brain injuries can be reduced through (1) aggressive public education campaigns (e.g., "buckle up for safety") and (2) legislative actions that impose severe penalties for high-risk activities such as driving while intoxicated. Educating women about alcohol use during pregnancy can help decrease fetal alcohol syndrome (FAS) and fetal alcohol effects (FAE).

DISABILITY AND THE FUTURE

Disabling physical conditions and mental illness have enormous impacts on individuals as well as on society as a whole. Economic and ethical issues challenge American society as quality-of-life expectations increase and new health care delivery systems evolve.

Research Questions

1. What drugs or techniques can be developed to promote nerve regeneration?
2. What effect will the ongoing deinstitutionalization of people with developmental disabilities have on the future of medical practice?

Case Resolution

This patient is now a person with paraplegia who joins one million other Americans who are wheelchair users. He spent 3 months in a rehabilitation program. Two year postrehabilitation, the patient regained partial bladder control and skillfully uses a lightweight sports wheelchair. He was graduated from college, has a steady girlfriend, and is a high school math teacher.

Selected Readings

Americans With Disabilities Act of 1990. Federal Register, Public Law (PL) 101–336.

Chirikos, T. N. Aggregate economic losses from disability in the United States: A preliminary assay. Milbank Q 67(Suppl. 2, Pt. 1):59–91, 1989.

Katz, S., et al. Study of illness in the aged. JAMA 185:94–9, 1963.

Lee, B. Y., L. E. Ostrander, G.V.B. Cochran, and W. W. Shaw. *The Spinal Cord Injured Patient.* Philadelphia, W.B. Saunders Company, 1991.

Menter, R. R., et al. Impairment, disability, handicap and medical expenses of aging persons with spinal cord injury. Paraplegia 29:613–9, 1991.

Rice, D. P., and M. P. La Plante. Medical expenditures for disability and disabling comorbidity. Am J Public Health 82(5):739–41, 1992.

U.S. Bureau of the Census Statistical Abstract of the United States, 114th ed. Washington, D.C., 1994, pp. 136–7.

World Health Organization. *International Classification of Impairments, Disabilities and Handicaps.* Geneva, WHO, 1980.

Zejdlik, C. P. *Management of the Spinal Cord Injury.* Boston, Jones and Bartlett, 1992.

Zwick, W., et al. Accessing health care in Delaware for people with disabilities: A comparison of consumer and physician perceptions. Del Med J 62(12):1443–50, 1990.

C H A P T E R   1 2 4

TEAM APPROACH TO CHRONIC CARE

Janette S. Carter, M.D., Kara L. Catton, R.D., C.D.E., and Esther P. Reinhardt, R.N., C.D.E.

H$_x$ The patient is the same patient who is profiled in Chapter 77: a 50-year-old, obese man with diabetes. He was put on insulin 10 years ago after an unsuccessful trial of oral medication. At present, he takes 14 units of NPH and 6 units of regular insulin in the morning and 12 units of NPH and 8 units of regular insulin in the evening. Even though he reports glucose levels between 120 and 180 mg/dL, his

HbA$_{1c}$ measurement is 14%. He complains of polydipsia, polyphagia, polyuria, and nocturia. He is on antihypertensive medication with poor control. He does not exercise but states that he follows a diabetic diet to assist with glucose control. He is accompanied to the clinic by his wife, with whom he was arguing when the physician entered the examination room.

Questions

1. What types of questions does a diabetes nurse educator ask patients in order to determine the cause of poor glucose control?
2. How does a visit with a registered dietitian help in determining medication adjustments for patients?
3. Is it helpful for a pharmacist to assess all medications to determine drug interactions and potential effects on the patient's glucose control?
4. How does a patient's psychosocial circumstances affect glucose control?

WHY A TEAM APPROACH?

With the increased longevity of patients, the management of chronic disease has become an increasingly important function of primary care physicians. Managing such conditions demands different skills of both physician and patient. The physician must not only diagnose and prescribe medications but also employ knowledge and skills not usually taught in traditional medical school curricula. The physician needs to know (1) health education skills; (2) nutrition education skills; (3) drug information such as interactions, adverse effects, and effective delivery methods; (4) psychosocial interviewing and intervention techniques for patient and family; (5) supervision skills with regard to "physician extenders"; and (6) team member and team leader skills including effective communication and the ability to negotiate common patient care goals and medical management styles.

The team approach can assist in this enormous undertaking. By working as a team member, the physician can expand his or her knowledge base about the patient and about possible therapeutic interventions with little increase in patient contact time. Conversely, inappropriate use of team members will lead to suboptimal and costly care for the patient. The appropriate use of nonphysician health care professionals with expertise in specific areas will ensure state-of-the-art patient care and improve outcomes. The innovative physician will learn to communicate well with other team members, whether they deliver care in a joint clinic or in separate offices or even separate buildings. In a competitive health care environment where patient satisfaction is paramount, those physicians who learn good team skills, both as members and as leaders, will gain an advantage.

ROLE OF TEAM MEMBERS

The multidisciplinary team consists of professionals with specialized training who provide coordinated patient care, at either a single clinic or various locations. In either setting, good communication ensures good patient care. Communication may be formal or informal. Examples of formal communication are patient conferences, team meetings, and written documentation. They provide the means to establish patient care goals and management plans, to provide information necessary for outcome evaluation and modification of management, to provide documentation for regulatory organizations, and to assist in the reimbursement for services rendered. When nonphysician health professionals' chart notes and consultations are overlooked by physicians, important input from these other team members regarding a patient's knowledge, attitudes, and motivation goes unused for patient care. Informal communication can bridge the gap between providers. Team member conversations, whether face-to-face or by telephone, provide information for clinical decision making and management strategies. Generally, a combination of formal and informal communications works best.

Team structure and function can also be formal or informal. Team roles may be well defined (multidisciplinary) or have significant overlap (interdisciplinary). Frequently, the former evolves into the latter as teams build cohesion and understanding and as members learn new skills that enable them to expand their core roles. For example, while medication adjustment recommendations are not a traditional part of a dietitian's role, some dietitians may be comfortable with taking on this advisory function because of experience gained while working with and learning from other team members. Physicians usually are the patient's first contact with a health care system, and they initiate team involvement. All team members, however, can be referral sources for consultations or for initiating the team approach for a patient's care.

Most teams include a primary care provider, a nurse educator, a registered dietitian, a social worker, and a pharmacist (Table 124-1). Primary care providers include physicians, physician assistants, and nurse practitioners. In addition to the traditional functions of examination and diagnosis, they also serve as team leaders and team initiators. Their comfort with and skill in the use of the team approach can facilitate patient readiness for change and their own willingness to use information and guidance from other team members. They ultimately are responsible for patient care goals and management based on input from all team members.

TABLE 124–1. Role of Team Members

Team Member	Role
Primary care provider	Team leader
Physicians	Establish patient care goals and management
Physician assistants	plans based on input from all team members
Nurse practitioners	
Nurse educator	Provide information and disease management skills, assist with disease complication surveillance and medication adjustment, assist with life-style changes
Dietitian	Evaluate usual dietary habits, provide diet education and guidance, assist with life-style changes
Social worker	Assist with issues related to employment, finances, marital/family relationships, and patient's health beliefs
Pharmacist	Review medications for correct administration, interactions, and adverse effects and reinforce healthful life-style changes
Psychiatrist/psychologist	Assist with disease adjustment reactions, facilitate healthful life-style changes

Nurse educators play a major role in helping patients understand disease processes and teaching self-care and life-style modifications. Optimally, they use patient-centered and patient-initiated goals (empowerment) to encourage adherence practices. Nurse educators can follow patients between their primary care provider visits and perform supervised medication adjustment and complication surveillance. By discussing patient adherence/nonadherence to recommended treatment regimens with other team members, treatment decisions can be modified.

While dietitians' background includes knowledge of the impact of good nutrition and therapeutic diets on disease, their most important role may be that of "change agent." The dietitian evaluates dietary habits, teaches patients the significance of dietary changes, helps establish priorities for dietary change, and translates nutritional science into eating habit skills. Dietitians possess the skills to tailor dietary educational strategies to meet the needs of patients from varied cultural and socioeconomic backgrounds. However, dietary changes are difficult to implement and cannot be "fixed" by one visit with the dietitian. Most patients require ongoing follow-up with a dietitian to educate and empower them to practice healthier life-styles. Dietary modifications for one diagnosis usually will have a positive effect on the patient's other problems.

Social workers evaluate factors that impair a patient's ability to comply with treatment plans. These include employment, financial stability, living conditions, marital/family relationships, and cultural beliefs about health care. For medical management goals to be patient-centered, the social worker may be needed to provide the team with insights to help develop practical goals. For example, marital problems may need to be addressed before the patient can address dietary changes successfully. Removing psychosocial barriers improves the likelihood of successful disease management.

Pharmacists evaluate and teach patients about their medications and assist with medication evaluation to decrease polypharmacy and drug interactions. Many patients have more than one chronic disease and often take multiple medications, thus increasing the likelihood of drug interactions and adverse effects. Information about drug administration (including timing and dosage) is discussed. The pharmacist also reinforces messages given to the patient from the other team members about life-style changes.

Additional health care professionals may be part of the team, depending on the specific patient. Podiatrists often are members of diabetes care teams. Psychiatrists and psychologists assist patients and families adjust to chronic diseases and necessary life-style changes. Occupational and physical therapists evaluate and educate patients on methods to improve the activities of daily living.

THE TEAM APPROACH IN ACTION

Team management for the patient profiled above begins with a visit to the **physician**. Concerns identified are poor diabetes and hypertension control and a strained marital relationship. The physician initiates referrals to the diabetes nurse educator, dietitian, and social worker before making any changes in the present treatment regimen.

The diabetes **nurse educator** evaluates the patient's educational needs, then focuses on blood glucose monitoring, insulin timing and administration, and the interaction of diet and exercise on insulin needs. The patient had been monitoring his glucose only on his days off. He agrees to monitor his blood sugar three times daily and begins walking for 10 minutes four times a week. The nurse educator discusses the use of alcohol and its relationship to the control of blood glucose. The plan is documented (formal communication) and discussed with the physician (informal communication). The **dietitian** reviews the patient's dietary habits and is concerned about the high-sugar, high-fat snacks the patient consumes while working at the convenience store and bar. The dietitian reinforces the benefits of exercise and the need for home blood glucose monitoring. The patient reports drinking a six-pack of beer plus several "shots" of whiskey daily when working. He expresses a desire to take an active role in managing his health care. The **social worker** discusses the newly identified problem of alcohol use. The marital relationship is strained owing to sexual dysfunction and financial problems created by the patient's alcohol consumption. The social worker refers the couple for marital counseling, directs the patient to an alcohol treatment program, and relays the patient's concern of impotence to the physician. The clinic **pharmacist** identifies the use of a thiazide diuretic as possibly contributing to poor glucose control as well as to impotence. The medication is changed to an angiotensin-converting enzyme (ACE) inhibitor, and the pharmacist assists with periodic blood pressure measurements.

The participation of the various team members allows a wider range of observations and information on which to base a management plan. The team approach reinforces patient care goals.

PROGNOSIS AND SUGGESTED USES OF THE TEAM APPROACH

The team approach can be useful in a broad range of situations (Table 124–2) and has several advantages from the patient's perspective (Table 124–3). The primary advantage is that the patient is given the knowledge and skills needed to perform self-care activities and to make life-style changes necessary for improved

---

TABLE 124–2. When to Use the Team Approach

Newly diagnosed chronic disease
Multiple chronic diseases
Diagnostic enigma
Recent disease exacerbation/complication
Poor medical outcome
Limited patient/family understanding of disease/self-care skills
Need for the increased support provided by a team
Behavioral or psychosocial problems
Patient who has high motivation for self-care

TABLE 124–3.   Team Approach from the Patient's Perspective

Advantages

Provides improved education about disease
Teaches problem-solving and self-care skills
Provides patient-centered choices for intervention
Supports all aspects of patient's health and well-being
Reduces acute and chronic complications
Provides easier access to consultants
May assist patient in obtaining health coverage for nonphysician services when part of a physician's "visit"

Disadvantages

May increase time spent in clinic(s)
May increase costs initially, which may not be reimbursed by insurance
May give mixed messages if members of team communicate poorly

health and well-being. Physicians often lack the time or expertise to deal with these activities. Problem-solving improves because of each team member's special knowledge and skills. If the patient can be actively involved in problem solving and selection of interventions over time (empowerment), the success of treatment will be enhanced, including improved disease control and complication prevention, decreased hospitalization, decreased overall costs, and improved quality of life. Table 124–3 also lists the disadvantages of the team approach from the patient's perspective, with the primary one being increased clinic time and appointments initially. If the patient is paying out-of-pocket for all or part of the medical care or has difficulty getting time off from work, this may have a negative impact.

Table 124–4 lists advantages and disadvantages from the physician's perspective. Major advantages are that (1) physicians need not be "experts" in fields in which they have no formal training and (2) their time can be used more effectively in areas of expertise such as physical examination and diagnosis. After working together for a while, the physician and coworkers may find an improved work environment, increased job satisfaction, and improved outcomes and productivity. Disadvantages for physicians include (1) the need to keep in close communication with a number of other professionals and (2) the potential that their vision of

TABLE 124–4.   Team Approach from the Physician's Perspective

Advantages

Allows more time for physical examination and diagnosis
Increases physician productivity through time/expertise of team members
Improves problem-solving for diagnostic enigmas
Improves patient care goals and management
Increases awareness of other team members' expertise
Expands services available
Decreases complications
Improves medical outcomes and patient satisfaction

Disadvantages

May increase short-term health care delivery costs
Requires communication and team skills
May give mixed messages if members of team communicate poorly
Creates frustration if team members used inappropriately

what is best for the patient will not coincide with the viewpoints of other team members. Without agreed-upon goals and plans, there is poor interaction, inappropriate use of team members, and job dissatisfaction. It is incumbent upon the physician to realize the expertise and limitations of team members. Either denying them the opportunity to contribute their specific skills or giving them responsibilities outside their area of expertise is bad for patient care and for the team members themselves.

SUMMARY

The team approach utilizes the skills of each team member and is guided by their special knowledge and skills. Optimally, both formal and informal communication is ongoing among team members. The team approach uses a treatment system that centers around patients and empowers them to do their best. Interactions with team members can reinforce messages, and the patient who has not responded to one individual may respond to another. Successful team interaction results in patients taking a more active role in their health care and in improved medical outcomes. In an era of chronic disease, increasing specialization, and closer monitoring of outcomes by various accrediting organizations, a physician who is comfortable using a team approach to health care will be more appreciated by his patients and better able to provide state-of-the-art medical care.

Research Question

1. How can management by a health care team be made more cost effective?

Case Resolution

At a 6-month follow-up appointment, the patient had a decrease in glycosylated hemoglobin level, exhibited an approximately 1-kg (2.2-lb) weight loss related to exercise and dietary changes, and reported successful completion of the alcohol treatment program. He also had improved sexual function owing to alcohol cessation and the change in antihypertensive medication. His relationship with his wife had improved. His wife asked the physician to thank all the members of the health care team.

Selected Readings

Ducanis, A. J., and A. K. Golin. *The Interdisciplinary Health Care Team: A Handbook.* Germantown, Maryland, Aspen Systems, 1979.
Langlois, J. P. Patient education. *In* P. D. Sloan, L. M. Slatt, and P. Curtis (eds.). *Essentials of Family Medicine,* 2nd ed. Baltimore, Maryland, Williams & Wilkins, 1993.
McCann, D. P., and J. H. Blossom. The physician as patient educator: From theory to practice. West J Med 53:44–9, 1990.
Robertson, D. The role of health care teams in care of the elderly. Family Medicine 24(2):136–41, 1992.

CHAPTER 125

OCCUPATIONAL AND ENVIRONMENTAL DISORDERS

Frank D. Gilliland, M.D., Ph.D.

H$_x$1 A 62-year-old male medical center employee was recently discovered to have an abnormal chest x-ray during an emergency department visit for bronchitis. The x-ray showed a new 3-cm opacity in the left perihilar region, and subsequent diagnostic evaluation revealed a primary lung cancer. The employee had smoked for 40 years but quit 5 years ago. He reports that he had also been employed as a miner and worked in several other jobs over the years that involved the use of "lots of chemicals." He and his wife strongly feel that his cancer is related to exposure to chemicals at work, and he requests your help in receiving compensation.

H$_x$2 A 29-year-old single mother of two preschool-age children is in danger of losing her factory job as a result of frequent early departures from work because of headaches. She is referred to you by her social worker for further evaluation. On further questioning, the patient describes a 2-month history of intermittent throbbing headaches. The headaches are bilateral, occur daily at work, and last all day until retiring at night. Analgesics do not relieve the pain. The social worker asks you to determine whether the headaches are work-related.

H$_x$3 A 47-year-old female bus driver resides in a home that uses a shallow well for domestic water. Recently, the local Health and Environment Department found chlorinated organic chemicals in the well water in her township. The patient is concerned that she is at serious risk for cancer as a result of drinking contaminated water for many years.

Questions

1. How would you go about determining whether these three conditions are work- or environment-related or whether significant exposure occurred?
2. What are the elements of an occupational history?
3. What are the elements of an exposure history?
4. How would you conduct an environmental evaluation of these patients?
5. Do you think further testing or data collection would add to the decision-making process? If so, how?
6. How would you communicate your findings to each patient?

The U.S. work force includes 110 million economically active adults who each spend at least 25% of their time at work. Because many occupations and environments involve exposure to uncontrolled hazards, occupational and environmental health disorders are common in the United States. It is estimated that 20 million work-related injuries, 390,000 new work-related illnesses, and 100,000 work-related deaths occur each year. Further breakdowns of occupational injuries and illnesses are shown in Tables 125–1 and 125–2.

The burden of illness and injury related to environmental exposures has not been well defined; however, the estimated 20,000 lung cancer deaths per year associated with radon exposure indicate that environmentally related health problems are common. Practitioners may find themselves inadequately prepared to diagnose and treat occupational/environmental disorders, or to answer their patients' questions and concerns about a seemingly endless number of occupational/environmental hazards. Because the vast majority of individuals with occupational/environmental disorders will present to primary care physicians, practitioners need to integrate occupational/environmental medicine into routine clinical practice.

EVALUATION

Patients with occupational or environmental concerns present to their physicians for three main reasons: (1) it is suspected that their symptoms, signs, or abnormal laboratory results are related to occupational/environmental exposures; (2) the cause of their symptoms is

TABLE 125–1. Occupational Injury Incidence Rates in the United States Private Sector (1985)

Industry	Injury/100 Full-time Workers/Year
Construction	15.0
Agriculture, fishing, forestry	11.0
Manufacturing	10.0
Transportation and utilities	8.5
Mining	8.3
Retail sale trade	7.5
Wholesale trade	7.5
Services	5.3
Finance, insurance, real estate	1.9

Data from Bureau of Labor Statistics, U. S. Department of Labor, 1987.

TABLE 125–2. Occupational Illness in the United States Private Sector (1987)

Injury	Estimated No. of Cases	Percentage of Cases
Skin disorders	41,800	33
Disorders associated with repeated trauma	37,000	30
Respiratory conditions due to toxic agents	11,600	9
Disorders due to physical agents	9,000	7
Poisoning	4,200	3
Dust diseases of the lungs	1,700	1
All others	20,100	16

unknown, and occupational/environmental exposures are part of the differential diagnosis; or (3) they have experienced exposure to a suspected harmful agent.

Effective diagnosis and treatment demands a clear understanding of the following principles of occupational/environmental medicine:

1. A detailed history is the key to evaluating occupational/environmental disorders. Physical examination findings and laboratory test results may raise suspicions about an occupational/environmental disorder and add to the data base obtained from the history. The decisive information about work- or environment-relatedness, however, almost always comes from the history.

2. Occupational and environmental disorders are neither rare nor exotic. Diseases resulting from occupational or environmental causes tend to have clinical and pathologic manifestations identical to diseases resulting from other causes. Only a very limited subset of occupational/environmental disorders is likely to be uncovered by routine clinical tests.

3. Many health problems are multifactorial in etiology, and occupational/environmental factors can both contribute to disease causation as well as exacerbate preexisting conditions. For diseases of multifactorial etiology, identification of one cause does not preclude other causes. In some situations, the presence of one etiologic factor may increase the risk of disease following an environmental exposure. For example, the risk of lung cancer among smokers is greatly increased after asbestos or radon exposure. Thus, the risk of a work- or environment-related disease is increased in the presence of another known etiologic agent.

4. Evaluating the relevance of exposures requires consideration of temporality (i.e., exposure must precede the onset of disease), latency (i.e., the time between exposure and disease onset), and dose-response and dose-effect relationships. For an exposure to be involved in the pathogenesis of a disease, it must precede the onset of the illness by a period of time greater than the latency period. Furthermore, the toxicokinetic and pharmacodynamic characteristics of the agent must be considered in order to assess whether the dose was sufficient to cause the observed response or effect.

5. Individuals vary in susceptibility. It is generally recognized that the concentrations at which humans respond to chemicals may vary by a factor of 1000.

Exposures of the same intensity can produce a marked response in one individual and little response in another. The fact that many workers were exposed to an agent without adverse responses does not preclude a sensitive individual from responding at equal or lower levels.

6. All occupational and environmental disorders are, in theory, preventable. In practice, clinicians can prevent these disorders by influencing the behavior of employers and employees. Physicians can educate employees, union health and safety personnel, and management about workplace hazards and use their authority to convince employers and employees to make needed changes. In some situations, it may be necessary to call in regulatory agencies such as the Occupational Health and Safety Administration (OSHA). Because occupational disorders are preventable, their occurrence has legal implications.

History

In his classic treatise *De Morbus Artificum Diatriba* published more than 300 years ago, Bernardino Ramazzini advised,

> *On visiting a poor home, a doctor should be satisfied to sit on a three-legged stool, in the absence of a gilt chair, and he should take time for his examination; and to questions recommended by Hippocrates he should add one more—What is your occupation?*

An occupational history is an essential part of the medical history. For some patients, it is necessary to ask about only the current job, the longest held job, and two major past occupations. In patients in whom an occupational or environmental disorder is suspected, a more detailed occupational and environmental history is required (Table 125–3). This history should include job title, place of employment, detailed job duties, second or part-time jobs, work at home, military service, and a listing of all exposures. Exposures can be categorized as chemical, biological, physical, or psychological. Inquiry should be made about specific exposures such as radiation, asbestos, silica, and other less common exposures such as beryllium and benzene. The assessment of temporal patterns of symptoms in relation to exposure is critical (Table 125–4). In addition, several different dimensions of the exposure history should be obtained to estimate exposure intensity (Table 125–5). A nonwork exposure history—which includes smoking, alcohol use, hobbies, residence location and type, water source, and medical procedures and testing—also is necessary.

TABLE 125–3. Outline of Occupational History

Description of all jobs
Work exposures
Temporal patterns of exposures and symptoms
Health problems or symptoms in other workers
Other pertinent exposures (hobbies, etc.)

TABLE 125–4.   **Temporal Patterns of Symptoms**

Onset
Disappearance
Weekend/vacation
Related to specific tasks or locations
Latency (time between exposure and onset of disease)

Environmental Evaluation

The physician should become knowledgeable about the workplace (or other pertinent environments) of the patient under evaluation. A visit to the work site or residence may be necessary and may require the cooperation of company managers. The company's health and safety professionals should be able to provide a description of the organization's activities, processes, products, and production materials. In addition, information about the illness and injury history of the work force may be available. A team approach to the environmental evaluation is often necessary. Industrial hygienists are trained to recognize, assess, and control workplace hazards. Since many companies do not employ industrial hygienists, consultative evaluations may have to be made through insurance companies.

Laboratory Evaluation

The principal role of the laboratory is to help elucidate the effects of exposure by means of commonly available blood or urine tests. For example, liver function tests will aid in determining whether or not there is hepatic inflammation or dysfunction. In a limited number of situations, a specialized test may be necessary to quantify the magnitude of exposure (e.g., blood lead levels); however, the presence of a xenobiotic (foreign chemical) in biologic samples does not mean that an adverse effect has occurred. Appropriate use of a specialized laboratory test to measure the amount of a xenobiotic in a given patient depends on the (1) specific xenobiotic, (2) exposure scenario, and (3) effect under consideration. Accurate interpretation of laboratory results requires knowledge of (1) the performance characteristics of the test and the clinical laboratory, (2) the manner in which the test was conducted, and (3) valid comparison groups.

Economic, Legal, and Social Issues

Economic, legal, ethical, and social considerations commonly intersect during occupational/environmental evaluations. Patients may be self-referred, referred by another physician, or referred by such diverse individuals and groups as lawyers, social workers, employ-

---

TABLE 125–5.   **Exposures**

Amount
Use of personal protective devices
Personal hygiene measures
Accidental exposure
Episodic exposure

TABLE 125–6.   **Evaluating the Toxic Effects of Chemicals**

1. Identify and prioritize the relevant chemicals
   Ask patient for names of chemicals and products used
   Obtain Material Safety Data Sheet (MSDS) from employer, distributor of product, or manufacturer of product
2. Obtain generic names of the chemicals
3. Select compounds to explore in detail
   Selection criteria:
      Intensity and duration of exposure
      Chemical class
      Toxicokinetics
      Toxicologic profile
   Information sources:
      Poison control centers
      National Institute of Occupational Safety and Health (NIOSH)
      General reference books (toxicology, epidemiology, occupational medicine)
4. Research
   Pharmacodynamics *in vitro,* in animal models, and in humans
   Epidemiology
   Consult
      Specialists such as occupational physicians, industrial hygienists
      Medical libraries
      RTEC (a microfiche database of chemical properties)
      Computerized databases
         MEDLARS TOXNET, CHEMLINE, CANCERLIT, TOXLINE HSDB, CCRIS
            TRI, ETIC, IRIS
4. Consult with governmental agencies
   Occupational Safety and Health Administration (OSHA)
   National Institute of Occupational Safety and Health (NIOSH)
   Environmental Protection Agency (EPA)
   State and local public health and environmental departments
   Food and Drug Administration (FDA)
   Agency for Toxic Substances and Disease Registry (ATSDR)

---

ers, unions, or insurance companies. The purpose and content of the evaluation may differ in each situation. Understanding the expectations of the patient and the referring individual or group should be accomplished early in the evaluation process. Third parties and patients may have different agendas. Care should be taken to respect the doctor-patient relationship, especially when another individual or group requests and pays for the evaluation.

MANAGEMENT

Formulating and implementing a therapeutic plan should be accomplished only after the firmest possible diagnosis has been made (Table 125–6). Most occupational and environmental disorders are not medical emergencies, and removal from exposure does not have to occur immediately. The far-reaching effects of certain courses of action (e.g., removal from a job, change of employment, or labeling a disorder as occupational) mandates that a practitioner proceed with caution to avoid unnecessary harm. Although subjecting the patient to further exposure may appear to add to the problem, it is important to weigh this additional risk in the context of the exposure that has already occurred and the possibility that premature or unjustified actions may be more harmful to all concerned in the long run.

For some patients, the nature of the disorder dictates a specific treatment plan. For example, a patient with heavy metal poisoning must be removed from exposure until levels decrease to the nontoxic range. For other patients, several alternative strategies may be possible; the eventual plan should satisfy the needs of the patient and, whenever possible, other interested parties such as employers and worker's compensation administrators.

The choice of treatment plan should be discussed with the patient and with other parties whose cooperation is needed for optimal implementation. Patients need to be fully informed of the risks and benefits of each option and should be actively involved in the decision-making process. Because some choices may have the potential of disrupting the individual's normal life activities, family relationships, employment, or income, involvement of social workers or union officials may be helpful. Patients should be asked whether the relevant findings and plans may be communicated to other physicians or to employers. Monitoring the medical and nonmedical effects of the treatment plan during subsequent visits may lead to revisions in the initial management strategy.

Research Questions

1. How can practitioners most effectively influence public policy about occupational and environmental health issues?
2. How can health professionals most effectively communicate with each other about the health risks associated with occupational and environmental exposures?

Case Resolutions

1. The first patient was not eligible to receive compensation under the worker's compensation regulations of his state. He sought legal counsel and filed suit against his former employers. Several years after his death, his wife agreed to a settlement with undisclosed terms.

2. The second patient and several coworkers had been exposed to high levels of toluene, a volatile organic solvent. As a result, they experienced headaches, a common symptom of solvent exposure. After proper ventilation of the work area was established, this cluster of headaches disappeared.

3. The third patient's health concerns were recognized as valid concerns by her physician. Her medical evaluation proved to be normal, and the physician subsequently discussed the risks of low-level solvent exposure with her. Reference literature concerning cancer prevention and the telephone numbers of appropriate community groups were also provided. This information empowered the patient to understand her cancer risks and to take action to reduce those risks.

Selected Readings

LaDou, J. (ed.). *Occupational Medicine.* Norwalk, Connecticut, Appleton & Lange, 1990.

Levy, B. S., and D. H. Wegman (eds.). *Occupational Health: Recognizing and Preventing Work-related Disease,* 3rd ed. Boston, Little, Brown & Co., 1994.

McCunney, R. (ed.). *A Practical Approach to Occupational and Environmental Medicine,* 2nd ed. Boston, Little, Brown & Co., 1994.

Ramazzini, B. *Diseases of Workers.* Chicago, University of Chicago Press, 1983 (originally 1713).

Rom, W. N. (ed.). *Environmental and Occupational Medicine,* 2nd ed. Boston, Little, Brown & Co., 1992.

Zenz, C., O. B. Dickerson, and E. P. Horvath (eds.). *Occupational Medicine,* 3rd ed. St. Louis, Mosby, 1994.

CHAPTER 126

LEGAL ISSUES IN OUTPATIENT MEDICINE

Carl Bettinger, M.D., J.D.

Hx A 25-year-old male newspaper reporter presents to an outpatient clinic to begin disulfiram (Antabuse) therapy for alcoholism. The clinic is a community-based facility with five doctors and two physician assistants. Although the clinic strives to provide each patient with continuity of care via a single physician, it is not uncommon for a patient to see different physicians on different visits.

At the initial visit, Dr. First performs and documents a routine history and physical examination. Baseline liver function tests (LFTs) are obtained, and the patient is instructed to return in 3 days to review the laboratory tests and to begin taking disulfiram.

Three days later the patient returns. The LFTs are normal. The patient is given a 60-day prescription for disulfiram and instructed to return in 30 days. Dr. First later testifies that he felt it was "absolutely necessary" for LFTs to be repeated upon the patient's return, but he neglected to document this in the patient's record.

The patient returns in 40 days, feeling somewhat fatigued. He sees Dr. Second. Dr. Second writes, "Here for R$_x$ refill" in the chart. He also writes a new prescription for disulfiram but does not order a repeat set of LFTs.

Two weeks later, the patient is admitted to a local hospital with fulminant hepatitis due to use of disulfiram. He rapidly develops hepatic encephalopathy and is transferred to a large tertiary care hospital, where he undergoes liver transplantation.

Questions

1. What are the essential elements of a medical malpractice claim?
2. If you act in such a way that the care you provide falls below the "standard of care," yet does not cause the patient harm, does the patient have grounds for a suit against you?
3. If you meet the standard, yet nonetheless cause the patient harm, does the patient have grounds for a suit against you?
4. What specific "danger areas" for malpractice exist in the outpatient setting?

Because an increasingly larger portion of health care is being provided in the outpatient setting, primary care physicians need to be aware of the specific malpractice "pitfalls" that lurk in outpatient care. Since many of these pitfalls are ultimately matters of good medical practice, attention paid to these areas will result in improved medical care overall as well as a decreased likelihood of litigation.

ESSENTIAL ELEMENTS OF A MEDICAL MALPRACTICE CLAIM

Medical malpractice is a type of negligence. Negligence has four basic elements: (1) a legal duty to act in a certain way toward another person; (2) breach of that duty; (3) harm to the other person; and (4) causation, i.e., the duty breached caused harm to the person to whom the duty was owed (Box 126–1).

More specifically, in a medical setting, a malpractice claim exists when there is (1) a doctor-patient relationship, which gives rise to a duty to act as a reasonably well qualified doctor *should* act under similar circumstances (also known as the "standard of care"); (2) a breach of that duty, or failure to act as a reasonably well qualified doctor should have acted under similar cir-

---

BOX 126-1. Elements of a Medical Malpractice Claim

1. Duty to meet the standard of care
2. Breach of duty
3. Harm to the patient
4. Causation (harm caused by breach of duty)

---

cumstances; (3) harm to the patient; and (4) causation, i.e., the harm at issue was caused by the breach of the standard of care.

Two examples will serve to illustrate these concepts:

Patient A is put under general anesthesia and dies as a result of an idiosyncratic and totally unexpected reaction to one of the anesthetic agents. Are there grounds for a malpractice case? In this situation, there is a doctor–patient relationship between patient A and the anesthesiologist. There is irrefutable harm, i.e., the patient's demise. There is certainly causation—no one is denying that the anesthesia caused the death. But since there is no evidence that the anesthesiologist did anything substandard, there is no breach of duty and therefore no grounds for a malpractice claim.

Patient B presents to an emergency room with the classic findings of acute appendicitis, including McBurney's point tenderness, rebound tenderness, fever, and an elevated white blood cell count. Patient B even tells the emergency room doctor that he believes he has appendicitis, yet the doctor, for some reason, concludes otherwise and instructs the patient to go home and take an over-the-counter antacid. Instead of going home, however, the patient proceeds directly to the hospital across the street and is subsequently taken to the operating room that night, where his acutely inflamed appendix is removed. Every doctor in town agrees that the first doctor fell below the standard of care in missing the diagnosis. But here, too, grounds for a malpractice case do not exist, since no harm befell the patient in the scenario presented. A case *would* have existed, however, if the patient had followed the first doctor's advice and subsequently died of peritonitis.

DANGER AREAS FOR MALPRACTICE CLAIMS IN THE OUTPATIENT SETTING

Many factors combine to give rise to a malpractice claim, but certain considerations are especially pertinent to the outpatient setting, particularly if—as is often the case—the outpatient setting is a busy one with many patients and many providers. Patients receiving care in such a setting often sense that there is no one they can call "their doctor" because they may see different physicians on different occasions. Furthermore, physicians working in busy clinics often lack the long-term "feel" that doctors develop for a given patient over time. Even where good continuity of care exists between a given patient and physician, the hustle and bustle of a hectic clinic schedule can result in less time being devoted to the visit than is desirable. This all-too-common situation can lead to a breakdown in communication between doctor and patient. When such communication goes awry, the stage is set for a malpractice claim.

Much has been written about communicating with patients, but the essentials can be summarized in a few short precepts:

The physician should sit down with patients, look at them when they speak, and listen carefully to what they say, without interrupting.

When patients are finished speaking, the doctor should ask whether there is anything else they would like to add. Only when the patient is finished should the physician start asking more focused questions.

Physicians should never ignore the last comments patients make as the visit is coming to a close. Many times these comments will reveal the true reason for the visit.

After the encounter with the patient is completed, the physician should document what just occurred, and do so while the memory of the visit is still fresh. The temptation to postpone dictation or note-writing until later in the day should be resisted. Five patients and four phone calls later, the recollection of what occurred during the visit will surely be worse, not better.

The documentation should include information about the chief complaint, a detailed history of the present illness, pertinent information from the review of systems, social and family history, the findings on physical examination, and conclusions and therapeutic plans, *including* what instructions were given to the patient and what instructions subsequent providers should follow. In most cases, all this can be done on a single outpatient encounter form.

In a clinic situation with multiple providers—and the strong possibility that a given patient will be seen by someone else on the next visit—notes must be written in such a way that the subsequent physician can understand the first physician's thought process and plans for the patient. (That, after all, is one of the basic reasons for note-writing.)

If, for example, a specific diagnostic pathway has been initiated to evaluate a patient with chest pain, the recommendations for the next step should be written down in case the ECG proves normal. Should an exercise stress test be done? A barium swallow? A trial of antiinflammatory medication? Similarly, if a patient has just started a new medication and follow-up laboratory tests will be needed in the future to check for possible adverse effects of the drug, the practitioner should let the next physician know—*in writing*. What laboratory tests should be obtained? Why are they necessary? When should they be performed?

Good documentation not only makes for good medical care, it makes for an almost impenetrable defense in the event a malpractice claim is subsequently filed. Argumentative "he said–she said" situations can be avoided if the physician can point to a contemporaneous writing (namely, the chart) as proof of his or her side of the story. Conversely, the absence of documentation will always lead to the accusation that if something wasn't documented, it wasn't done.

A subsequent physician seeing someone else's patient for the first time should make it a practice to obtain the old chart, read the last few notes, and ask the patient about the last few visits. The laboratory and x-ray sections of the chart should be checked, even if the previous provider did not indicate plans for such studies (such information may have been inadvertently omitted). The most recent physician is the one who will be held responsible for reviewing the results of studies done since the last visit, and he or she should thus try to get a sense of the flow of the patient's care. In short, the physician should not operate in a vacuum. Good medical practice abhors a vacuum, whereas a good plaintiff's attorney loves one.

Preserving what has been documented is as important as *documenting* what has occurred. Documentation serves little purpose if it is lost or, even worse, intentionally destroyed. One might think that the intentional destruction of medical records is a rare event, but it can occur under the most innocent of circumstances. For example, many physicians dictate their outpatient notes from longhand notes made at the time of the visit; these longhand notes are frequently destroyed after the dictation is completed. In the event of a subsequent lawsuit, the obvious question becomes, was there information in the missing longhand note contrary to the information presented in the dictated note? Since very few physicians can say they made a word-for-word comparison between the discarded handwritten note and the preserved dictated note, it is the jury that will be asked to decide this question.

SUMMARY

Good medical practice is the best way to avoid a malpractice suit. In the outpatient setting, good medical practice means optimizing communication, both between the physician and the patient and between the physician and other health care workers who may care for the same patient in the future. Taking the time to listen to the patient will accomplish the first goal. Taking the time to document all the pertinent information will accomplish the second.

Research Questions

1. Does documentation differ significantly between fee-for-service and managed care providers? Between mid-level providers (e.g., physician assistants or nurse practitioners) and physicians? Between a private practice setting and a university medical center?

2. Which setting, outpatient or inpatient, is more likely to give rise to a medical malpractice claim?

Case Resolution

Two years and several hundred thousand dollars' worth of medical care later, the patient filed a malpractice suit against Dr. First. At the subsequent trial, the patient was awarded nearly one million dollars in damages.

Selected Readings

Furrow, B., S. Johnson, T. Jost, and R. Schwartz. *Health Law: Cases, Materials and Problems,* 2nd ed. St. Paul, Minnesota, West Publishing, 1991.

Kennedy, I., and A. Grubb. *Medical Law: Text and Materials,* 2nd ed. Salem, New Hampshire, Butterworth Legal Pubs., 1993.

ETHICAL ISSUES IN OUTPATIENT MEDICINE

David A. Bennahum, M.D.

H_x1 A 15-year-old high school student comes to your office. She tells you that she is pregnant and asks for an abortion, but asks that you not tell her parents.

H_x2 A 45-year-old male restaurant manager has been informed that he has a positive HIV test. In the privacy of your office, he admits to you that he is bisexual and begs you not to tell his wife.

H_x3 An 81-year-old woman who lives with her son and daughter-in-law is brought to your office. She has mild dementia and severe aortic stenosis. The cardiologist recommends immediate surgery and the children agree, but the patient adamantly refuses surgical treatment.

H_x4 A 43-year-old corporate executive in your town is referred to you for evaluation of his chronic back pain. You discover that he has been abusing alcohol. He asks you not to reveal this to his firm.

Question

1. How would you respond in each of the above cases, and why?

As medical technology advances, patients, families, and physicians often face increasingly difficult dilemmas. Although it is in the intensive care units of hospitals that ethical questions are most often recognized and debated, the primary care physician is also frequently confronted with ethical questions in the ambulatory care setting. Physicians have a long-recognized duty to ease suffering, relieve pain, keep confidences, and avoid harm to their patients. The 20th century has seen new values such as patient autonomy, truth telling, informed consent, and the right to refuse care added to the traditional Hippocratic values of beneficence, nonmalfeasance, and justice (see the glossary in Box 127–1). In the following few pages, some of the principal ethical issues common to primary care medicine are discussed along with ways in which ethical conflicts can be identified and resolved.

THE BASIS OF ETHICAL DECISION MAKING

Clinical ethics is the discipline that prepares the physician to recognize and resolve moral problems in medicine. Ethical dilemmas arise when individuals, based on their personal value systems, disagree about the choice of actions such as abortion, termination of care, and allocation of scarce resources.

The Hippocratic tradition recognizes that physicians have an obligation to (1) help patients (beneficence), (2) not harm patients (nonmalfeasance), (3) guard what patients tell them in strict confidence, and (4) treat all patients justly. In the 20th century, however, the locus of responsibility has shifted from the physician to the patient. Today society recognizes the patient's right to make medical decisions, including the right to refuse care. Physicians are expected to tell the truth and to provide all the information necessary for rational de-cision making. While truth telling is at the core of contemporary ethical relationships, the physician

---

BOX 127-1. Glossary

Autonomy: The principle of respect for persons. Individuals are unconditionally worthy and deserving of the right to make their own decisions.

Beneficence: The principle of doing good. This may conflict with the principle of autonomy.

Competence: The presence of decisional capacity. This may be diminished for some issues (e.g., financial management) yet remain intact for others.

Confidentiality: A physician will not reveal information related by a patient or pertaining to a patient. There are legal exceptions such as homicide and the potential of harm to others.

Decisional capacity: The ability to make a rational and appropriate decision.

Distributive justice: The fair allocation of social benefits and burdens to all members of the society.

Fidelity: The relationship of patient and physician is one of fidelity in which there are mutual obligations to respect integrity and personhood.

Justice: Individuals should be treated equally and fairly. Individuals should receive what they are entitled to. Physicians should not harm or betray patients or fail to care for them.

Nonmalfeasance: The commitment not to do harm.

Utilitarianism: The theory that one should seek the greatest possible good for the greatest number of people.

must listen to the patient to understand what the patient wants to know and when the patient is prepared to hear critical information. The patient should expect the truth, yet the physician must communicate this in a manner that allows the patient time to assimilate (and adjust to) new and sometimes alarming information.

Modern medical philosophers such as Edmund Pellegrino have come to believe that notions of beneficence, autonomy, and justice are perhaps too limited and that an ethic of integrity and fidelity between a physician and patient is also necessary. While patients can and should expect competence, compassion, and honesty from their physicians, so too the patient has an obligation to tell the whole truth and to comply with agreed-upon therapy. Some would go further and suggest that prevention and the avoidance of harm are additional ethical obligations of the patient.

Physicians have obligations to society as well as to individual patients, and at times these duties may conflict. Should physicians enforce immunization requirements over the objections of parents? Must a physician maintain confidentiality even when the information in question could harm another person? How should limited medical resources be allocated?

In answering these questions, it is helpful to follow certain ethical guidelines. The rights of patients and their legal surrogates should be honored. When harm may be caused to another person, the obligation of confidentiality is overridden by the duty to inform and protect potential victims. Rationing is ethical when it is planned in advance and when all share equally in available resources, although those who plan such rationing should have the consent of the population for whom they are planning.

AN APPROACH TO ETHICAL DECISION MAKING

When a physician recognizes or is advised of a potential ethical dilemma, a systematic approach should be employed and the following questions asked:

1. Have all the necessary facts been gathered?
2. Is the diagnosis correct?
3. Is a consultation necessary?
4. Does the patient have the decisional capacity (i.e., competence) to make decisions about treatment?
5. If not, does the patient have an advanced directive and/or a legal guardian?
6. Does the patient have a spouse, parents, siblings, or children?
7. What ethical issues are raised by the clinical situation at hand?
8. Is there a conflict between the patient and his or her family, or between the patient and family and the health care professionals? Will airing the issues (and subsequent mediation) resolve the conflict?
9. Would a consultation with members of an ethics committee be of help?

Any relevant discussion with the patient, family, staff, or ethics committee should be documented as well as the rationale behind any action taken.

COMMON ETHICAL ISSUES IN OUTPATIENT MEDICINE

Obligations to Outside Agencies

A host of organizations may request documents, letters, laboratory results, expert opinions, bills, and records from physicians. The physician must always have the patient's permission before relaying information either communicated by the patient or ascertained by the physician in the course of an evaluation. The physician should never lie to the requesting agency but should always inform the patient of the request and ask the patient what information, if any, may be released. In most circumstances, the physician has no obligation to disclose what the patient does not want disclosed.

Physicians who work for managed care organizations may find themselves in a conflict between the needs of the patient and those of their organization. They may be asked to control costs by (1) ordering fewer laboratory tests, (2) shortening the time spent with each patient in order to see more patients, or (3) creating barriers to consultation, hospitalization, surgery, and expensive medication. It is important for the physician to explain these issues to patients and to work with colleagues to maintain high standards of care. If rationing is to take place, it must be done for all patients and not for selected patients; it should not compromise life expectancy or cause pain and suffering. In addition, patients should be kept fully informed of the policies of the organization, including any changes that occur over time.

Assessment of Children and Adults for Sports

Primary care physicians are often asked to evaluate children and adults for sports programs. In some communities, parents and coaches exert considerable pressure on children to participate in competitive athletics. Some may even request that a physician administer anabolic steroids or growth hormone to make an athlete more competitive. Team physicians may be asked to send an injured player back into a game prematurely. Unfortunately, the abuse of steroids and analgesics and the overuse and burnout of young athletes and dancers are common phenomena. Physicians must recognize that their duty is to the athlete and not to the parent, teacher, coach, or school.

Issues of Confidentiality

The outpatient arena is often the setting for agonizing conflicts of interest. Physicians may see minor children who are pregnant or have venereal disease. Rather than simply assume that the parents have their child's best interest at heart, the physician should try to understand the actual home conditions. If the child has abusive parents, the physician may have to refrain from informing the parents if, in the physician's judgment, that is in the child's best interest. In such cases, it is wise to seek consultation with colleagues and social agencies.

A unique situation occurs when the patient poses a risk to others. In the precedent-setting *Tarasoff v. the Regents of the University of California* case, a California court found that a psychiatrist should have informed a woman that she was at risk from a patient who was articulating homicidal fantasies and who subsequently did murder the woman. Confidentiality cannot be maintained when a person may come to harm from the actions of another. How then should the physician respond to a husband with a venereal disease or HIV infection who refuses to tell his wife? The physician is caught between two principles: the obligation of confidentiality versus the duty to inform. In many states, it is specifically forbidden to disclose the HIV status of a patient to another party. In these cases, the physician should try to persuade the patient to disclose such vital information to his or her sexual partners; if that approach fails, the physician may have to make a very difficult choice between the principle of confidentiality and the obligation to prevent harm.

Care of Patients Infected with HIV

As noted above, patients who are infected with HIV often present difficult ethical issues. There may be considerable prejudice in the community against HIV-positive individuals, especially if they are homosexuals or drug abusers. Patients may lose their insurance benefits or employment if their condition is disclosed. The converse of the problem is the risk that patients may actually create for others. A patient may tell you that he or she has had numerous sexual partners and that "safe sex" practices have not been followed. A patient with HIV may require surgery and thereby place other health care workers at risk. A few surgeons may even refuse to operate on a patient who is HIV positive. In such cases, a thoughtful review of the situation and consultation with other physicians, social workers, chaplains, and—at times—a hospital ethics committee may help point out the most appropriate course to follow.

Truth Telling and Informed Consent

It is crucial that physicians tell the truth, but it is important to understand what the patient wants to know and when and how to tell the patient about a disease. Empathy and compassion are important attributes of the skilled physician and are essential if the patient is not to carry the burden of illness alone. In order for the patient to make necessary decisions, the physician must educate the patient by providing a full and clear disclosure as to the nature of the illness, its probable course, and alternative treatment options (including possible consequences, both good and bad). Patients who have agreed to participate in clinical research trials need to be fully informed of the possible risks—and lack of proven benefit—of the drug, device, or technique under study. Similarly, physicians contributing to research or submitting articles for publication should adhere to rigorous standards of accuracy.

Advanced Directives and the Right to Refuse Care

Many primary care physicians see patients in nursing homes or hospices and care for terminally ill patients in their office practice. Physicians have an ethical respon-

sibility and a legal obligation to inform patients about advanced directives. The Danforth Amendment to the U.S. Federal Budget of 1991 mandated that persons being cared for in a facility receiving federal funds (such as hospitals, HMOs, nursing homes, and hospices) be advised at the time of admission of their right to refuse care and of the availability of advanced directives. The latter include the Living Will, Durable Power of Attorney, and other expressions of a patient's wishes. The Living Will allows patients to state their preferences as to treatment and requires two witnesses. The Durable Power of Attorney permits the patient to designate another person as a health-decision proxy who can ensure that the patient's wishes are carried out (or who can make decisions for the patient) if the patient ever becomes incompetent.

Discussing advanced directives affords the patient and the physician the opportunity to explore the patient's values and wishes. Many patients have never examined their own views on death and dying and greatly appreciate being able to talk about these issues. Whenever possible, the physician and patient should bring close family members into the discussion, so that there is agreement on what the patient has decided.

Assisted Suicide and Euthanasia

Among the most difficult problems facing patients and physicians are those of assisted suicide and euthanasia. While most patients can be relieved of physical pain, not all can be eased of their suffering. Society, the courts, and the medical profession remain wary of permitting physicians to assist or cause the death of even terminally ill patients, but the advancing medical technology guarantees that these issues will not go away. For some physicians it is simply not possible to take a human life, while for others the duty to ease suffering outweighs the prohibition against killing. Physicians must consider these questions with great care but should also remember that fidelity to patients should not impel them to break the law. If and when the law is changed, then each physician can decide what is ethical in the care of a particular patient. Until such time, physicians should listen, empathize, and do their best to relieve the suffering of their patients.

Genetic Counseling and Treatment

The rapid pace of discovery in human genetics will accelerate as the Human Genome Project advances. With the sequencing of the human genome and the advent of gene therapy, the ethical dilemmas of the future may well dwarf those of the present. Primary care physicians will undoubtedly have to guide couples through the knotty problems of fetal selection as the genes for a host of diseases are recognized. Decisions will probably be especially difficult for diseases that are expressed late in life, such as cancer and adult-onset diabetes mellitus. Is it ethical to terminate a pregnancy because the fetus is at risk for a disease later in life? How will society allocate resources for the treatment of diseases as their genes are discovered? In a crowded world with diminishing resources, the fidelity of physicians to their patients may be an important bulwark against unfettered utilitarianism.

Ethical Issues Faced by Medical Students

While medical students should familiarize themselves with medical ethics in general, they should be especially aware of those problems unique to physicians-in-training. For example, many students are concerned that they not mislead patients into thinking that they are "real" doctors. Students should always identify themselves to patients as students and ask the patient's permission to take a history, do a physical examination, or draw a tube of blood. An inexperienced student may feel guilty about causing a patient pain when drawing blood or performing a procedure. Patients are almost always supportive of students and pleased to help them but want to be told that the "doctor" is really a "student doctor" and that a supervisor is nearby.

At times students may find themselves being ordered to withhold information from a patient. An example is the student who knows the result of a test but is ordered to withhold this information from the patient until a specialist has been consulted. The student may feel that silence is a lie in this setting. Students can feel compromised by such experiences, and they may also learn an unfortunate future pattern of behavior. When in doubt, the student should ask the resident or attending physician for an explanation of the instructions. This, of course, is not always easy and may even be received with hostility, but more often the student's earnest doubts can help clarify the ethical dilemma in question and thus serve the patient's best interest.

Research Questions

1. Given the finite resources available for health care, what criteria should be used to establish allocation priorities?

2. What will be the ethical implications of the Human Genome Project as information becomes available?

Case Resolutions

1. A 15-year-old is a minor. In treating her, the physician must be aware of his or her own values, the patient's values and needs, the responsibilities and rights of the parents, and state law governing the care of minors. The U. S. Supreme Court has recognized the right of women to an abortion but has also permitted the states to regulate that right. Thus, some states may require a waiting period and parental notification. The latter may be bypassed if the child petitions a court. Thus, the physician must determine whether the parents will understand and help the child or whether the child, as in a case of incest or abuse, will be harmed by a parent.

2. Confidentiality will be breached if the physician informs the spouse, but the physician also has a duty to inform the spouse that she is at risk. Thus, two values are in conflict. The physician should try to persuade the patient to inform his wife, offering to be present if that would help. If the patient refuses, then the physician must decide which duty to follow—that of confidentiality, here protected by law, or that of protecting another person from harm.

3. While this 81-year-old woman has mild dementia, that does not make her incapable of making selected decisions, such as what food she eats or what clothes she wears. The physician needs to help the family look at the patient's lifelong values. Would she have risked surgery when she was younger? Is she currently depressed? Is it possible that anesthesia will worsen her dementia? The physician must gather all the relevant information, bring everyone together in a case conference with the patient, and mediate a decision that the patient can accept.

4. The alcoholic patient, like any other patient, expects absolute confidentiality in the doctor-patient relationship. If the physician were an employee of the corporation, then duty to the employer might outweigh the duty of confidentiality, but this should be made clear to the patient from the outset. Therefore, this patient should expect and should receive absolute confidentiality. An exception might be the case of an airline pilot or bus driver whom the physician knows is drinking at work, thus placing other lives in danger.

Selected Readings

Beauchamp, T. L., and L. Walters. *Contemporary Issues in Bioethics,* 2nd ed. Belmont, California, Wadsworth Publishing, 1982.

Brody, H., and T. Tomlinson. Ethics in primary care: Setting aside common misunderstandings. Prim Care 13(2):225–40, 1986.

Christakis, D. A., and M. A. Feudtner. Ethics in a short white coat: The ethical dilemmas that medical students confront. Acad Med 68(4): 249–254, 1993.

Fletcher, J. *Morals and Medicine.* Boston, Beacon Press, 1954.

Gorovitz, S. *Doctors' Dilemmas: Moral Conflict and Medical Care.* New York, Macmillan Publishing Company, 1982.

Jonson, A. R., M. Siegler, and W. J. Winslade. *Clinical Ethics: A Practical Approach to Ethical Decisions in Clinical Medicine,* 3rd ed. New York, McGraw-Hill Book Company, 1992.

Lynn, J. *By No Extraordinary Means.* Bloomington and Indianapolis, Indiana University Press, 1989.

Pellegrino, E. D. *Humanism and the Physician.* Knoxville, University of Tennessee Press, 1979.

Quill, T. E. Death and dignity. N Engl J Med 324:691–4, 1991.

Rachels, J. *The End of Life: Euthanasia and Morality.* New York, Oxford University Press, 1986.

INDEX

Note: Page numbers in *italics* refer to figures;
page numbers followed by t refer to tables,
and page numbers followed by b refer to comprehensive material in boxes.